WOMEN'S GYNECOLOGIC HEALTH

SECOND EDITION

KERRI DURNELL SCHUILING,
PhD, NP-BC, CNM, FACNM, FAAN

Professor and Dean
School of Nursing
Oakland University
Rochester, Michigan
Co-Editor-in-Chief
International Journal of Childbirth

FRANCES E. LIKIS,
DrPH, NP-BC, CNM, FACNM

Investigator, Vanderbilt Evidence-Based
Practice Center
Institute for Medicine and Public Health
Vanderbilt University Medical Center
Nashville, Tennessee
Editor-in-Chief
Journal of Midwifery & Women's Health

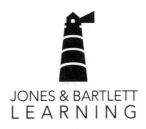

JONES & BARTLETT
LEARNING

World Headquarters
Jones & Bartlett Learning
5 Wall Street
Burlington, MA 01803
978-443-5000
info@jblearning.com
www.jblearning.com

Jones & Bartlett Learning books and products are available through most bookstores and online booksellers. To contact Jones & Bartlett Learning directly, call 800-832-0034, fax 978-443-8000, or visit our website, www.jblearning.com.

Substantial discounts on bulk quantities of Jones & Bartlett Learning publications are available to corporations, professional associations, and other qualified organizations. For details and specific discount information, contact the special sales department at Jones & Bartlett Learning via the above contact information or send an email to specialsales@jblearning.com.

The authors, editors, and publisher have made every effort to provide accurate information. However, they are not responsible for errors, omissions, or for any outcomes related to the use of the contents of this book and take no responsibility for the use of the products and procedures described. Treatments and side effects described in this book may not be applicable to all people; likewise, some people may require a dose or experience a side effect that is not described herein. Drugs and medical devices are discussed that may have limited availability controlled by the Food and Drug Administration (FDA) for use only in a research study or clinical trial. Research, clinical practice, and government regulations often change the accepted standard in this field. When consideration is being given to use of any drug in the clinical setting, the health care provider or reader is responsible for determining FDA status of the drug, reading the package insert, and reviewing prescribing information for the most up-to-date recommendations on dose, precautions, and contraindications, and determining the appropriate usage for the product. This is especially important in the case of drugs that are new or seldom used.

Production Credits

Publisher: Kevin Sullivan
Acquisitions Editor: Amanda Harvey
Editorial Assistant: Sara Bempkins
Production Manager: Carolyn F. Rogers
Associate Marketing Manager: Katie Hennessy
V.P., Manufacturing and Inventory Control: Therese Connell

Composition: Publishers' Design and Production Services, Inc.
Cover Design: Timothy Dziewit
Associate Photo Researcher: Lauren Miller
Printing and Binding: Malloy, Inc.
Cover Printing: Malloy, Inc.

Cover Image: The symbol on the cover is adapted from *The Changer* by K Robins and is used with the permission of K Robins Designs. The editors are very grateful to K Robins for allowing us to adapt her design for our cover, and we encourage readers to visit www.krobinsdesigns.com where *The Changer* and other symbols are available as pendants.

Some images in this book feature models. These models do not necessarily endorse, represent, or participate in the activities represented in the images.

Library of Congress Cataloging-in-Publication Data
Women's gynecologic health / [edited by] Kerri D. Schuiling, Frances E. Likis. — 2nd ed.
        p. ; cm.
    Includes bibliographical references and index.
    ISBN 978-0-7637-5637-6 (casebound)
    1. Generative organs, Female—Diseases. 2. Gynecology. 3. Reproductive health 4. Women—Health and hygiene.   I. Schuiling, Kerri Durnell.   II. Likis, Frances E.
    [DNLM: 1. Genital Diseases, Female. 2. Reproductive Physiological Processes. 3. Women's Health. WP 140 W872 2011]
    RG101.W773 2011
    618.1--dc22
                                                                                            2010018705

6048

Printed in the United States of America
15 14 13 12 11   10 9 8 7 6 5 4 3 2 1

Dedication

To our best teachers: our students and the women for whom we have provided care; and

To our colleagues, friends, and family members who have been encouraging and patient throughout the long labor of this second edition. There are too many to mention each of you by name, but you know that we know who you are. We truly appreciate the support you provided

—*Kerri and Francie*

To:

My longtime practice affiliates Earl Williams, MD, Jerry Irwin, MD, Kenneth Vanderkolk, MD, and the late Joseph Moore, MD, whose consistent advocacy helped pave the way for advanced practice registered nurses in Michigan to be credentialed and practice within their scope;

Virinder Moudgil, PhD, VPAA of Oakland University, who gave me the opportunity to work with the wonderful students, staff, and faculty at Oakland University;

My parents, Marie and Don Hall, whose belief that I can do anything makes me believe that I can;

Judd for his humor and companionship;

My children, Mary, Sean, and Sarah, who bring me life's greatest joys; and

Bode for his unconditional love.

—*Kerri*

To:

My husband Zan, your love is my haven, and your support makes anything possible;

My nieces Katherine and Elizabeth, my sister Mary, and my mother Katey, I have the best days with you; and

Robin, Amy, and Debi, your circle of friendship sustains me.

—*Francie*

Contents

Preface

Historically, women's health was framed within a biomedical model by clinicians. Textbooks typically used a biomedical framework to present women's health content. Although this approach can be useful on many levels, it also has limitations that can have significant negative effects on women's health, particularly gynecologic health. A biomedical model is disease-oriented and focuses on curing illness. This approach risks pathologizing normal aspects of female physiology. When a biomedical lens is used to assess women's health, there is risk of essentializing women and reducing them to biologic parts. An example of this proclivity is that for many years, women's health meant reproductive health, regardless of whether or not the woman planned to bear children. This reductionism transfers to practice where a woman's parts become the focus of diagnosis and treatment. The meaning of the diagnosis to the woman, as well as the impact that the diagnosis has on her, her significant others, and the work she does, is not addressed.

Feminist theories about women's growth and development provide a different perspective from earlier male-oriented models because they include women's lived experiences and the importance of relationships to women. Recognizing each woman as an expert knower supports women's agency. The focus is holistic, and health is assessed within the context of each woman's life.

It is important for our readers to know that we, as the editors of this book, are experienced women's health clinicians whose practice philosophy is grounded in caring for the whole woman within her lived experience. As teachers, we were repeatedly frustrated at the inability to locate a gynecologic textbook that we felt was suitable for our course. Many of the books that were available were written primarily from a biomedical perspective and, in our opinion, did not provide sufficient content about the normalcy of women's reproductive physiology. Books such as those authored by the Boston Women's Health Book Collective were extremely helpful with ideas about health and holism but lacked the necessary content to educate student clinicians. Other books did not provide the health-oriented perspective that is vital to the philosophy of care espoused by nursing and midwifery, in which we both strongly believe. Additional books provided elements of both biomedical and health-oriented views and had very useful decision trees or categorization of concerns or problems. We felt, however, that these books would not encourage students and practicing clinicians to think critically and to appreciate the importance of making decisions based on the most recent evidence.

For these myriad reasons, we embarked on producing a book that presents women's gynecologic health from a feminist and holistic viewpoint. Our goal was to create a book that emphasizes the importance of respecting the normalcy of female physiology, and provides medical content appropriate for assessment, diagnosis, and treatment of pathology. We believe this book embodies these perspectives and underlines the importance of collaboration among clinicians.

Some aspects of this feminist approach will be obvious to our readers, while others may be more subtle. For example, we used illustrations of whole women, rather than pictures of only breasts or genitalia, when possible. We refer to a woman who has a specific condition rather than referring to the woman by her condition. For example, we speak of the woman who is experiencing menopause, as opposed to the menopausal woman. We used the term *birth* as opposed to *delivery* because it situates the power to give birth within the woman versus transferring it to the clinician. We purposefully used *women's* rather than *gynecologic* as the first word of the book title. The goal is to help readers to keep first in their mind that they are treating a whole woman, not her body parts, and not just a condition. We hope this emphasizes the importance of treating women holistically within their lived experiences.

We were fortunate to have many excellent contributors to this book. Some are nationally known, and others might be new to many of you. The common thread among all of our contributors is their expertise in their respective areas and their recognition of the importance of evidence-based practice. Many of our contributors are expert clinicians and others are expert scientists. Frequently co-authored chapters represent a clinician and researcher team, whose collaboration provides readers with a real-world view that is grounded in evidence.

This book encompasses both health promotion and management of gynecologic conditions that women experience. All of the content is evidence-based. The first section of the book introduces the feminist framework of the book and provides readers with a context for evaluating evidence and determining best practice. The second section of the book provides a foundation for assessment and promotion of women's gynecologic health. The third and final section addresses the evaluation and management of clinical conditions frequently encountered in gynecologic health care.

We are gratified by how well the first edition of this book was received by clinicians, students, and faculty, and it was an honor to receive the 2006 Book of the Year Award from the American College of Nurse-Midwives. In this second edition of *Women's Gynecologic Health*, we have updated, and in many cases extensively revised, all of the chapters from the first edition. In response to requests from readers, we have added four new chapters that address diagnosis of pregnancy at the gynecologic visit, women's health after bariatric surgery, sexual assault, and urinary tract infections. In addition, we added critically needed content to existing chapters. For example, the chapter on lesbian health has been expanded to include gynecologic care for women who are bisexual and transgender individuals.

We believe this edition builds upon the precedents set in the first edition and hope it contributes to women receiving evidence-based, holistic, gynecologic care within their lived experiences. As before, we welcome feedback from our readers that will help us in future editions. Please contact us at womensgynhealth@comcast.net.

Kerri Durnell Schuiling, PhD, NP-BC, CNM, FACNM, FAAN
Frances E. Likis, DrPH, NP-BC, CNM, FACNM

Contributors

Ivy M. Alexander, PhD, APRN, ANP-BC, FAAN
Professor
Yale University School of Nursing
New Haven, Connecticut

Heather M. Aliotta, MSN, RNC
Nurse Practitioner
Women & Infants Hospital
Providence, Rhode Island

Christine L. Anderson, MSN, WHNP-BC, ANP-BC
Nurse Practitioner
Planned Parenthood League of Massachusetts
Boston, Massachusetts

Linda C. Andrist, PhD, WHNP-BC, RNC
Professor and Assistant Dean, Graduate Programs
School of Nursing
MGH Institute of Health Professions
Boston, Massachusetts

Alison Boehm Barlow, MSN, WHNP-BC
Instructor, Obstetrics and Gynecology
Vanderbilt University Medical Center
Nashville, Tennessee

Linda A. Bernhard, PhD, RN
Associate Professor, Nursing and Women's, Gender and Sexuality Studies
The Ohio State University
Columbus, Ohio

Jacquelyn C. Campbell, PhD, RN, FAAN
Professor and Anna D. Wolf Chair
Johns Hopkins University School of Nursing
Baltimore, Maryland

Katherine Camacho Carr, PhD, ARNP, CNM, FACNM
Professor and N. Jean Bushman Endowed Chair
Seattle University College of Nursing
Seattle, Washington

Susan Chasson, MSN, JD, CNM, FNP-BC, SANE-A
Sexual Assault Nurse Examiner
Coordinator, Utah Coalition Against Sexual Violence
Lecturer
Brigham Young University
Provo, Utah

Mary Ann Faucher, CNM, PhD, FACNM
Associate Professor
Louise Herrington School of Nursing
Baylor University
Dallas, Texas

Linda A. Fernandes, RN, MSN
Graduate, CNS Forensic Focus
Johns Hopkins University School of Nursing
Baltimore, Maryland

Catherine Ingram Fogel, PhD, WHCNP-BC, FAAN
Professor
School of Nursing
University of North Carolina at Chapel Hill
Chapel Hill, North Carolina

Nancy Gasiewicz, DNP, MSN, RN
Assistant Professor
Northern Michigan University
Marquette, Michigan

Mickey Gillmor-Kahn, MN, CNM
Course Faculty
Frontier Nursing University
Hyden, Kentucky

Janet Graham, DNP, MSN, FNP-BC
OB-GYN Associates of Marquette
Marquette, Michigan

Sandra H. Hines, PhD, RN, WHNP-BC
Assistant Professor
Eastern Michigan University
School of Nursing
Ypsilanti, Michigan

COL Nancy J. Hughes, LTC, AN, CNM
Commander
Moncreif Army Community Hospital
Jackson, South Carolina

Robin G. Jordan, PhD, CNM
Course Coordinator
Frontier Nursing University
Hyden, Kentucky

Holly Powell Kennedy, PhD, CNM, FNP, FACNM, FAAN
Professor and Helen Varney Professor of Midwifery
Yale University School of Nursing
New Haven, Connecticut

Suzanne M. Leclaire, MSN, MHS, RN
Landstuhl, Germany

Linda Ledray, PhD, RN, SANE-A, FAAN
Director, SANE-SART Resource Service MMRF
Minneapolis, Minnesota

Lisa Kane Low, PhD, CNM, FACNM
Assistant Professor
Coordinator, Nurse–Midwifery Program
School of Nursing
Program in Women's Studies
University of Michigan
Ann Arbor, Michigan

Janis M. Miller, PhD, APRN
Associate Professor and Research Associate Professor
School of Nursing
School of Medicine, Department of Obstetrics and Gynecology
University of Michigan
Ann Arbor, Michigan

Katherine Morgan, MS, WHNP, ANP
Assistant Professor (Clinical)
University of Utah, College of Nursing
Salt Lake City, Utah

Patricia Aikins Murphy, CNM, DrPH, FACNM
Professor and Annette Poulson Cumming Presidential Endowed Chair in Women's and Reproductive Health
University of Utah
Salt Lake City, Utah

Deborah Narrigan, CNM, MSN
Project Coordinator, Tennessee Connections for Better Birth Outcomes Study
Vanderbilt University School of Nursing
Nashville, Tennessee

Ellen Olshansky, DNSc, RN, WHNP-BC, FAAN
Professor and Director
Program in Nursing Science
University of California, Irvine
Irvine, California

Kathryn Osborne, PhD, CNM
Course Coordinator
Frontier Nursing University
Hyden, Kentucky

Nancy J. Schaeffer, MSN, NP
Nurse Practitioner
Massachusetts General Hospital
Gillette Center for Women's Cancers
Boston, Massachusetts

Beth A. Collins Sharp, PhD, RN
Senior Advisor, Women's Health and Gender
    Research
Agency for Healthcare Research and Quality
Rockville, Maryland

Daniel J. Sheridan, PhD, RN, FNE-A, FAAN
Associate Professor
Johns Hopkins University School of Nursing
Baltimore, Maryland

Katherine Simmonds, MSN, MPH, WHNP-BC
Clinical Assistant Professor
MGH Institute of Health Professions
Boston, Massachusetts

LTC Nancy M. Steele, PhD, RNC, CNS, WHNP
European Regional Medical Command
Landstuhl Regional Medical Center, Germany

Diana Taylor, RN, MS, PhD, FAAN
Professor Emerita, UCSF School of Nursing
Director, Research & Evaluation, UCSF Primary
    Care Initiative
Advancing New Standards in Reproductive Health
    Program (ANSIRH)
Bixby Center for Global Reproductive Health
University of California, San Francisco
San Francisco, California

Dawn M. Van Pelt, RN, MSN
Graduate, CNS Forensic Focus
Johns Hopkins University School of Nursing
Baltimore, Maryland

Carol A. Verga, CNM, ARNP
Center for Women's Health at Evergreen
Kirkland, Washington
Clinical Instructor
University of Washington
Seattle, Washington

Alida D. Wagner, RN, MSN, CEN
Central DuPage Hospital
Winfield, Illinois

Mary Wallace, RN, MSN, CFNP
Professor Emerita
School of Nursing
Northern Michigan University
Marquette, Michigan

Reviewers

Kristi M. Burdick, DNP, RN, FNP-BC
Assistant Professor
School of Nursing
Northern Michigan University
Marquette, Michigan

Nanci Gasiewicz, DNP, RN
Assistant Professor
School of Nursing
Northern Michigan University
Marquette, Michigan

Joyce King, PhD, CNM, FACNM
Clinical Assistant Professor
Nell Hodgson Woodruff School of Nursing
Emory University
Atlanta, Georgia

Lucy Koroma, MSN, WHNP-BC
Instructor
Department of Obstetrics and Gynecology
Vanderbilt University Medical Center
Nashville, Tennessee

Laurie Arnold Tompkins, ARNP, MSN, BC
Assistant Professor
Department of Obstetrics and Gynecology
Vanderbilt University Medical Center
Nashville, Tennessee

Introduction to Women's Gynecologic Health

Women's Health from a Feminist Perspective

Lisa Kane Low
Kerri Durnell Schuiling

What does gender have to do with women's health? The most obvious answer is that women's health is about women and their health; therefore, gender is an issue. However, gender is an issue only because the focus is women. The true challenge to answering this question accurately lies in gaining the understanding that its answer depends on the definitions used. For example, if we were speaking about gender only as if it was synonymous with sex, then the stated answer "Women's health is about women; therefore, gender is an issue" would be correct. Gender, however, is *not* synonymous with sex. *Gender* is defined as a person's self-representation as man or woman or the way in which social institutions respond to that person based on the individual's gender presentation. The term *gender* is used when referring to social and cultural influences based on sex (Pinn, 2003a). It is rooted in biology and shaped by the environment and experience (Pinn, 2003b). This broader definition of gender makes the answer to the question "What does gender have to do with women's health?" much more complex.

There are three aspects to consider when answering this question. The first is an aspect of comparison: exploring women's health as compared to men's health. The second aspect is context: exploring the context of gender, including how it affects the process of providing healthcare services. The third aspect to consider is the social construction of gender, including how it affects women's health. The significance of answering the question from each of these perspectives is that each viewpoint has implications for the manner in which women access, receive, and respond to health care. These three aspects provide opportunities for us to better understand women's healthcare experiences. They also assist in the identification of some of the underlying factors that influence the healthcare disparities that women experience. The purpose of this chapter is to provide an overview of women's health using gender considerations as a lens for exploring women's health in general and gynecologic health in particular.

Women's Health Care and Gynecologic Health

The state of women's health care today is a direct reflection of women's status and position in society. To date, many healthcare advances have been made under the rubric of women's health; however, there is still a long way to go before all women receive comprehensive, compassionate healthcare services that address the complexity and diversity of how women live their lives and experience health and disease.

This textbook is based on a feminist framework in an effort to advance the health care provided to women in today's society. The authors attempt to acknowledge the complexity of women's health by paying particular attention to women's status in society and their unequal access to opportunity, while focusing on women's gynecologic health and well-being.

Feminism

What is feminism? Feminism is not a singular "what." Indeed, there are multiple definitions of feminism. One definition that is well suited for addressing the context in which women experience health and wellness is that offered by bell hooks (2000): Feminism is a perspective that acknowledges the oppression of women within a patriarchal society, and struggles toward the elimination of sexist oppression and domination for all human beings. Acknowledging the oppression of women is increasingly more difficult within many Western societies. Affluence and increased opportunities within some sectors of employment or education are often construed as equal access or equity in opportunity for all women. However, oppression is defined as "not having a choice." When this definition is used, many more individuals are able to recognize constraints in their personal experiences, and acknowledgment of oppression in its various forms becomes possible. Examples include a range of extremes from forced marriage, forced sterilization, unfair labor practices, denial of access to pharmaceutical methods of contraception, to not being able to access desired healthcare providers. These ranges of extremes represent the vast breadth of experiences women may have within the context of a patriarchal society that denies equal access to power, resources, and opportunities for women.

Characteristics of a feminist perspective include the use of critical analysis to question assumptions about societal expectations and the value of various roles on both political and individual levels. The process of critical analysis is accomplished by rejecting conceptualizations of women as homogeneous. It acknowledges power imbalances, and uses the influence of gender as the foremost consideration in the analysis. Using a gender lens that is informed by feminism permits areas of disparity to be identified both between groups, based on gender, and within groups, based on the recognition of heterogeneity among women.

Feminism requires exploration of women's health within the context of how women live their lives both collectively and individually within a patriarchal society. The various

TABLE 1-1 Components of a Feminist Perspective in Women's Health

Works with women as opposed to for women
Uses heterogeneity as an assumption, not homogeneity
Minimizes or exposes power imbalances
Rejects androcentric models as normative
Challenges the medicalization and pathologizing of normal physiologic processes
Seeks social and political change to address women's health issues

social, environmental, and economic aspects become integral to understanding the context in which women are able to achieve health and well-being. Furthermore, feminism requires consideration of health, as influenced by the intersection of sexism, racism, class, nation, and gender, within a framework that acknowledges the role of oppression as it affects women and their health as individuals and as a group. **Table 1-1** offers components of a feminist perspective when considering women's health issues or models of care, which can help to reframe one's view of women's health in a feminist perspective.

A Model of Care Based on a Feminist Perspective

A model of care that is based on a feminist perspective contrasts sharply with a biomedical model, particularly in areas of power and control. A feminist model supports egalitarian relationships and identifies the woman as the expert knower. The woman is the center of the healthcare model. The following key points provide further insights into a feminist-based model of care:

1. The model of care must focus on being *with* women, not *doing for* women. This frames the model of care as a partnership with women as opposed to a model of care that is directed by others and then assigned to women through a process of authoritative knowledge being handed down on the assumption that it is correct.
2. Heterogeneity, rather than homogeneity must be used as an assumption. Considerations of "all women," or offering grand theories regarding women, or using broad gender-based assumptions all serve to essentialize women rather than acknowledge the diversity within the larger group that comprises women. An assumption of heterogeneity considers women on an individual basis, tailoring health care and services to each woman's unique needs rather than treating all women as a group with the assumption of similarity across all considerations of health.
3. The feminist model of care must seek to minimize or expose power imbalances that are inherent in most current healthcare models, especially those based on a biomedical model. Power should be distributed equally within the healthcare interaction, and the interaction should be based on a belief in a woman's right to self-determination. There-

fore, the role of the clinician is providing support, information, and skillful knowledge, as opposed to asserting authority over the decision-making ability of the individual.

4. A feminist framework rejects androcentric models of health and disease as normative. The pervasiveness of male-based models being extrapolated and applied to women on the assumption that a woman is merely a biologic variant of man serves to constrain a full consideration of women's health issues. This misapplication of androcentric models to women's health also serves to medicalize or pathologize normal physiologic processes of women such as menstruation, childbirth, and menopause (Lorber, 1997).

5. A feminist perspective challenges the process of medicalization and pathologizing by identifying and exploring women's unique health experiences and normalizing them. Medicalizing is the process of labeling conditions as "diseases" or "disorders" as a basis for providing medical treatment. The medicalization of women's biologic functions, such as menstruation and pregnancy, frequently has been cited as an illustration of both the social construction of the disease and the general expansion of medical control into everyday life (Conrad, 1992; Zola, 1972).

6. A feminist framework acknowledges the broader context in which women live their lives and the subsequent challenges to their health as a result of living within a patriarchal society. It argues for a process of social and political change that would eliminate gender bias and sexism and result in the betterment of all human beings.

The Social Construction of Gender and Health

A discussion of the social construction of gender is provided here as a basis for exploring the value of a feminist framework in understanding women's health. This discussion is followed by strategies to analyze women's health issues from a feminist perspective. As Lorber (1997) notes:

> [A]s a social phenomenon, illness has to be gendered because gender is one of the most important statuses in any society. Gender is also socially constructed. Girls and boys are taught their society's expectations of appropriate behavior; they grow up to enact their society's gendered social roles. Gender is a social institution that patterns interaction in everyday life and in major social organizations. (p. 5)

Gender influences which health services are offered, which health risks are identified for an individual, and which treatments are potentially offered at all levels of interaction. While many of these differences might be considered biologically based, a feminist perspective argues that gender and sexism instead are the key components of these differences. **Table 1-2** provides definitions of sex, gender, and biology so that the reader may gain an appreciation of the differences in the terms.

The significance of the social construction of gender is a critical consideration in the process of defining, providing, and receiving healthcare services. "The juxtaposition of gender and illness presents two major problems: sex differences versus gender differences and between group and within group differences" (Lorber, 1997, p. 5).

TABLE 1-2 Definitions of Sex, Gender, and Biology	
Sex	The classification of living things as man or woman according to their reproductive organs and functions assigned by chromosomal complement
Gender	A person's self-representation as man or woman or who that person is responded to by social institutions based on the individual's gender presentation. Gender is rooted in biology and shaped by the environment and experience.
Biology	The study of life and living organisms, including the genetic, molecular, biochemical, hormonal, cellular, physiological, behavioral, and psychosocial aspects of life

Source: Adapted from Wizemann & Pardue, as cited in Pinn, 2003a.

Social construction is the process by which societal expectations of behavior become interpreted or ascribed as innate characteristics that are biologically determined. Thus attributes associated with femininity—attributes that are socially expected and, therefore, performed in compliance with social expectations—become confused with innately determined behaviors rather than being recognized as socially constructed behaviors. As a result, health risks, treatments, and approaches to care are not necessarily scientifically or biologically based aspects of women's health, but rather are determined by social expectations that are based on assumptions about gender differences. In addition, diagnoses can be influenced by gendered assumptions regarding behavior or what is socially constructed as feminine behavior. There is significant documentation of such influences affecting the manner of diagnosis and treatment, particularly within the mental health arena (Tavris, 1992) and in the misdiagnosis of women's cardiovascular risk (Healy, 1991).

What becomes evident when the considerations of gender are explored within the context of health is that gender interacts with many of the other variables that are considered factors affecting health outcomes. Women tend to ask more questions, receive more information about their health, and have a more partnership-building relationship with their healthcare providers than men (Xu & Borders, 2003). At the same time, women are more likely to be affected by financial barriers to health care than men. In one study, "women who had lower incomes were consistently less likely to have visited a physician while men were more deterred by nonfinancial barriers to health care such as the length of time in a waiting room" (Xu & Borders, 2003, p. 1077). Women as a group experience greater barriers to obtaining healthcare services compared to their male counterparts.

Poor or low-income women and women who are members of disadvantaged racial or ethnic minorities often obtain fewer or receive different health services compared to more affluent women. Women from disadvantaged backgrounds often experience different risks to their health and have worse health statuses than their wealthier counterparts (Weisman, 1998). In fact, low income predicts who receives health care. Low socioeconomic status is the single most powerful contributor to illness and premature death (Lantz et al., 1998). Therefore, while understanding gender differences in the utilization of healthcare services is important, treating women as a homogeneous group has limitations, particularly when socioeconomic status and racial or ethnic identity are considered.

Nearly 40 million of the 140 million American women alive today are members of racial and ethnic minority groups (Satcher, 2001). Women of racial and ethnic minority groups experience many of the same health concerns as do white women; however, as a group, they are "in poorer health, use fewer health services, and continue to suffer disproportionately from premature death, disease, and disabilities" (Weisman, 1998, p. 11). Racial and ethnic health disparities have been explained by locating the differences in health outcomes in biologic explanations that presume homogeneity among racial and ethnic groups. Biologic explanations focus on biologic solutions rather than exploring the context in which health disparities occur. Today the use of race as a marker for capturing biologic divisions within the population has been challenged scientifically (Williams, 2002).

> Our racial categories are more alike than different in terms of biologic characteristics and genetics, and they do not capture patterns of genetic variation well. Thus it is not biologically plausible for genetic differences alone to play a major role in racial or ethnic differences in health. (Williams, 2002, p. 590)

It is not sufficient to explore differences in health issues simply by ethnic or racial identity or simply by gender. Gender interacts with many social causes of health and illness—in particular, age, socioeconomic status, race, and ethnicity (Weisman, 1998). As previously stated, low socioeconomic status is a significant contributor to poor health outcomes, but female gender further increases that risk. It is also evident that women from ethnic minority groups receive lower-quality health care and less health care overall than wealthier, better-educated, higher-status white women (Davis & Huber, 2004). What is missing from this consideration is how socioeconomic status is often used as a proxy to explain racial and ethnic health differences in women's health outcomes. When specific health conditions such as hypertension are explored, socioeconomic status is found to be strongly associated with its prevalence. There are also significant differences in the incidence of hypertension between black and white women, roughly as large as the difference in the incidence of hypertension found in poor black women compared to black women of higher incomes.

According to public health expert David Williams (2002), examples such as these demonstrate the complexity of trying to cast health disparities as being based solely on race or ethnic identity. The intersection of a variety of factors creates complexity when trying to research women's health issues such as health disparities. Williams argues for consideration of the social embeddedness of women's health and the need to attend to additional factors—such as types of medical care, geographic location, migration, acculturation, racism, exposure to stress, and access to resources—when exploring disparities in women's health. Only by incorporating these factors into the discussion can we fully and accurately appreciate the health disparities women experience.

Access to high-quality and culturally appropriate healthcare services is further limited by age and gendered assumptions. Social role differences between men and women are thought to affect health primarily by influencing access to health-producing resources such as nutrition, shelter, education, paid employment, supportive social networks, healthcare insurance, and healthcare services (Weisman, 1998). The manner in which women negotiate the healthcare system also reflects gendered assumptions that promote differential access to resources, resulting in power imbalances, as opposed to assumptions that would promote equally open and accessible health care across genders.

Gender has important health consequences that are intertwined with cultural values and considerations. An estimated 94 million girls and women are "missing" worldwide as a result of discriminatory treatment that ultimately increases their mortality rate (Klasen & Wink, 2002). To the extent that social and economic resources are differentially allocated by gender, or that gender conceptions vary by subcultural context, specific subgroups of women may have health experiences that are quite different from those of other women (Weisman, 1998). Gender-based cultural rituals or social role expectations can create undue burdens for women and may subsequently lead to increased health risks. For example, being denied access to contraceptive options may create reproductive health risks for some women. The practice of female circumcision carries significant health risks and has long-lasting health implications for some young women (see Chapter 6). Being denied access to education by virtue of gender can decrease economic opportunities, thereby limiting life choices for women. Extensive cultural preoccupation with dieting and thinness may lead to unsafe dieting practices and precipitate eating disorders. When various health conditions are explored, a number of disease states appear to be prevalent among women despite the lack of a clear biologic explanation for them, such as anorexia and bulimia.

Another example of a gender-based health risk is the disproportionate amount of gender-based violence that women experience. Gender-based violence was defined by the United Nations General Assembly in 1993 as follows:

> Any act of gender-based violence that results in or is likely to result in physical, sexual, or psychological harm or suffering to women, including threats of such acts, coercion, or arbitrary deprivations of liberty, whether occurring in public or private life. (As cited in Velzeboer, Ellsberg, Arcas, & Garcia-Moreno, 2003, p. 4)

The multiple health consequences of gender-based violence reveal the long-lasting layers of health consequences associated with a gender-based health risk. (Refer to Chapter 12 for further discussion of this topic.) "Gender-based violence is the most widespread human rights abuse and public health problem in the world today, affecting as many of one out of every three women" (Velzeboer et al., 2003, p. xi).

A Human Rights Perspective on Women's Health

The preceding examples provide evidence of the manner in which the social construction of gender creates undue health risks for women. This burden of risk that women endure has been the basis of addressing women's health disparities from a human rights perspective. A

TABLE 1-3 Human Rights Framework for Safe Motherhood
Rights relating to life, liberty, and security of the person
Rights relating to the foundation of families and of family life
Rights relating to the highest attainable standard of health and the benefits of scientific progress, including health information and education
Rights relating to equality and nondiscrimination on grounds such as sex, marital status, race, age, and class

human rights framework identifies a basic set of rights, regardless of gender, that members of a society should have access to or be guaranteed.

> Basic human rights generally refer to respect as a person of worth/value (human dignity), safety or security of one's person, food and nutrition, shelter, privacy, freedom from any form of discrimination, a right to information and education … and the right to health and equitable access to health and illness services of high quality. (Thompson, 2004, p. 177)

A feminist perspective is in concert with a human rights framework, but would argue that human rights are disproportionately denied to women.

While human rights have been defined within the World Health Organization (WHO) for many years, it is only in the last 20 years that reproductive rights were added to the basic human rights framework. More recently, a human rights framework has been advocated within the context of addressing maternal morbidity and mortality on a global level (Starrs, 1997; Thompson, 2004). Gender equity issues are a more recent consideration (Velzeboer et al., 2003). The goal of using a human rights framework is as follows:

> [To] characterize women's multiple disempowerments not just during pregnancy and childbirth but from their own births as a cumulative injustice that societies are obligated to remedy. The re-characterization of maternal mortality from a health disadvantage to a social injustice places governments under a legal obligation to remedy the injustice. (Starrs, p. 9)

Table 1-3 lists the four categories of basic human rights relating to safe motherhood.

Definitions of Health: Social Model Versus Biomedical Model

As the discussion of the social construction of gender and its relationship to health has unfolded, it has become evident that a broader model of health must be employed to address the health consequences of gender bias and sexism and the implications for the overall health and well-being of women. While the use of a human rights framework is congruent with the components of a feminist framework, again the acknowledgment of gender equity has been limited and less transparent in its application to models of health. Furthermore, our ability to hold governments accountable for a human rights framework remains in its infancy in regard to its application to the health rights of women (Starrs, 1997; Thompson, 2004; Velzeboer et al., 2003). A feminist framework encourages grassroots activism to promote acknowledgment of women's need for greater access to human rights and, therefore, provides an opportunity for increased awareness related to gender-based health disparities.

The first step in broadening the model of health requires redefining health. *Health* is biomedically defined as the absence of disease. Of course, this narrow definition does not address the context in which the absence of disease may occur. As feminist health advocates note, "No single or singular view of women's health will adequately reflect the complexities of women's lives, although dominant biomedical models are often taken to represent 'all of women's health'" (Ruzek, Olsen, & Clark, 1997, p. 12). It is argued that the dominance of the medical model must be challenged in an effort to broaden the opportunities to understand this complexity within the healthcare system, health research, and the experiences of health within the individual and the collective community. The biomedical model, however, does not address health beyond an individual perspective.

An alternative to the biomedical definition of health is the definition developed in 1946 by WHO: "Health is a state of complete physical, mental, and social well-being and not merely the absence of disease or infirmity." This broader definition is based on some assumptions of what must be present to secure health for individuals and the community in which they live. At least the following prerequisites must be in place before health can occur:

- Freedom from the fear of war
- Equal opportunity for all
- Satisfaction of basic needs for food, water and sanitation, education, and decent housing
- Secure work
- Useful role in society
- Political will
- Public support (Ruzek et al., 1997, p. 14)

Germaine to this definition is WHO's commitment to address social injustice, equity, economic development and opportunity, and accessibility of healthcare services as a basic human right for all individuals in any society (Tejada de Rivero, 2003). The WHO definition of health requires that the community and environment in which women live their lives must also be considered in the same context as a new medical procedure. The constraints of an individualistic, disease-only focused biomedical model of health become readily apparent when WHO's broader context and definition of health are considered.

An alternative to the biomedical model that is more congruent with a feminist perspective is the social model of health. The social model of health places the focus of health on the community, rather than on the individual. There is then an opportunity to focus on health disparities that are rooted in the social and cultural forces that affect how women live their lives. "Developing more inclusive models of health requires recognizing and dealing with complexities and differences in women's lives. Educational levels, income, culture, ethnicity, race and a host of other identities and experiences shape women's lives" (Ruzek et al., 1997, p. 20).

The interconnectedness of working and living conditions, environmental conditions, and access to community-based healthcare services becomes a focus when health and well-being are framed within a community context. Questions about health and well-being for an individual hone in on these factors as well as lifestyle decisions and health habits. The prevention of health problems becomes both a social burden and an individual responsibility. This wider emphasis forces greater consideration of the various social factors that can either create or destroy an individual's health (Ruzek et al., 1997).

A social model of health also requires asking questions about the health effects of socially situated factors such as racism, sexism, and other forms of oppression. Consideration of women as central to the health model, rather than marginal to it, is a requirement of the feminist social model of health care. The broader social models do not ignore biologic or genetic components of health, nor is the significance of individual lifestyle health habits denied. However, the broader social model frames these issues as important to health, but no more so than women's experiences within everyday life, their access to healthcare services, their socioeconomic status, their racial and ethnic identity, and their membership within a community (Schiebinger, 2003).

The health risks associated with the social construction of gender and the inequities associated with gender-based assumptions are essential components of the feminist social model of health. As links are forged between human rights, social models of health, women's health disparities, and opportunities to address those disparities, a feminist perspective offers new strategies and ways of thinking or asking questions that can promote expanded approaches to women's health issues.

Women's Health from a Feminist Perspective

Several aspects of analysis are important when considering women's health from a feminist perspective. The following strategies for analyzing women's health using a feminist framework are adapted from Franz and Stewart's (1994) strategies for conducting feminist research. Each of the strategies listed in **Table 1-4** can be used as a question to ask about women's health issues. Taken together, they constitute a feminist lens that allows for new considerations to arise as health issues are reframed. The following discussion highlights the manner in which some of the strategies can be applied.

Look for What Has Been Left Out or What We Do Not Know

This strategy is particularly applicable to investigations into the scientific basis of women's health. Much of what we know about women's health needs, outside of reproductive health, is historically based on androcentric models of men's health considerations (Rosser, 1994;

TABLE 1-4 Strategies for Analysis of Women's Health from a Feminist Perspective

Strategies	Questions
Look for what has been left out or what we do not know.	• What do we know, how do we know it, and who knows it? • Why don't we know? What do we want to know and why? • Who determines what is left out or who has access to what we want to know?
Analyze your own role or relationship to the issue or topic.	• Is it personal? Is it political? • Are you objective and removed, or engaged and subjective? • Are you invested in the outcome or topic or not? • Why do you care about the issue?
Identify women's agency in the midst of social constraint and the biomedical paradigm.	• Are woman really victims or are they acting with agency? • Are individuals making choices despite positions of powerlessness? Are the choices allowing individuals to remain in control or do they allow for some form of power in the context of the situation?
Consider the social construction of gender and how its assumptions may limit options or presume choices made within the context of health. This includes the social construction of health itself.	• What is defined as a health problem or concern? • Explore assumptions about the value of anatomy such as breasts or facial appearance. • Ask the question: "Would this health issue be defined or explored in the same manner if it primarily affected men or women?"
Explore the precise ways in which gender defines or affects power relationships and the implications of those power dynamics in terms of health.	• Physician/nurse • Parent/child • Clinician/patient • Father/daughter • Parent/adolescent • Married woman/single woman • Husband/wife • Lesbian/heterosexual
Identify other significant aspects of an individual's or group's social position, and explore the implications of that position as it relates to health issues.	• Consider examples such as an adolescent who is seeking reproductive healthcare services or a same-sex couple seeking fertility services. • Ask who has access to what forms of healthcare services and resources and who does not. • Consider the intersections of race, class, gender, sexuality, and socioeconomic status. • Who has a choice, what constitutes a choice, and who is able to exercise their right to choices within the context of health?
Consider the risks and benefits of generalizations and speaking in terms of groups versus individuals.	• Who are "we" or "all women"? Are "all women" the same? • When is coherence or consistency the goal compared to diversity in the healthcare consideration or experience? Which reflects reality most accurately? • When "grouping" occurs, who is missing from the group or who might not be reflected in the group process?

Source: Adapted from Franz & Stewart, 1994.

Tavris, 1992). For many years, almost all medical research that was not related to gynecology was conducted in male participants (human and animal), with the findings then being generalized to women. Large-scale investigations focusing on health promotion have been based primarily on study populations composed of only men. This practice persisted until well into the 1990s (Schiebinger, 2003).

According to feminist scientist Londa Schiebinger's analysis, many common health promotion measures have been assumed to be true for both men and women despite the fact that the evidence supporting the measures came from research in which the study populations were composed of only men. Examples of such studies include the Physician's Heart Study, in which the findings led to recommendations on the use of aspirin to prevent heart disease, and the Multiple Risk Factor Intervention Trial, which evaluated correlations between blood pressure, smoking, cholesterol, and heart disease. The research populations in these studies were composed of only men. In fact, one of the first studies to investigate the use of estrogen for heart disease was conducted on a study population consisting of only men (Schiebinger, 2003)!

Research agendas often reflect a societal bias that favors powerful, white, middle- to upper-class men in the United States (Rosser, 1994). Similarly, although most large-scale research trials have focused on or recruited primarily from this population for their research participants, most of the scientific members of the team would arguably claim lack of awareness of the inherent sexism in these study designs (Schiebinger, 1999). "Reforming certain aspects of how medical research is conducted with respect to females required new judgments of social worth and a new political will" (Schiebinger, 2003, p. 973).

The lack of representation of women in research trials extended through 1988, when clinical trials of new drugs were routinely conducted predominately on men—even though women consume approximately 80% of pharmaceuticals in the United States (Schiebinger, 2003; Wood, 2001). What was left out? Considerations of women's biologic variations in processing drugs! We now know that acetaminophen is eliminated in women at 60% of the rate at which this drug is eliminated in men. This finding obviously has gender-related implications for prescribing dosage regimens (Schiebinger).

Examples abound of the problematic manner in which the scientific base for women's health, beyond that of reproductive health, was initially developed. Even when positive study examples are cited, limitations were often present in the design of the studies. Many key women's health studies, such as the Framingham Heart Study and the Nurses Health Study I and II, were either observational or epidemiologic investigations instead of randomized clinical trials, even though the latter design has long been considered the gold standard for investigative research (Schiebinger, 2003). Clearly, women were being left out of the scientific understanding of many health issues that directly affected them.

Consumer health advocates, women's health activists, and members of the scientific community have been instrumental in coming together to address the many limitations concerning women's health care and scientific investigations of women's health issues. In 1993, the National Institutes of Health (NIH) Revitalization Act was considered a milestone in this regard:

[The act required that] women and minorities and their subpopulations be included in all NIH-supported biomedical and behavioral research, in phase III clinical trials in numbers adequate for valid analysis of differences, in intervention effects, and that cost not be the basis for exclusion, and that there needed to be support for outreach programs to recruit these individuals for clinical trials. (Schiebinger, 2003, p. 975)

As a result of this policy change, the next decade saw a significantly greater inclusion of women and minorities in research investigations. Asking "what had been left out" or "what was missing" provided an opportunity to alter what had been left out of women's health research. Even though much has been achieved, critics continue to call for continued innovation in medical theories and practice in this field (Ruzek et al., 1997; Schiebinger, 2003).

There is an ongoing need to employ this strategy to expose blind spots in what is being presented under the rubric of women's health. An example can be found in the current focus on heart disease in women. Heart disease is now the number one killer of women in the United States. It has been argued that at every step in the healthcare process related to cardiovascular disease, from identification of symptoms to diagnosis, treatment, and referral, gender differences abound. Johnson, Karvonen, Phelps, Nader, and Sanborn (2003) reviewed the literature regarding cardiovascular disease and found 30 systematic reviews. The limitations identified in the studies focusing on women and cardiovascular disease gave rise to the conclusion that there were not enough large-scale clinical trials or meta-analyses focusing on cardiovascular disease in women. The need to explore this disease process in women becomes even clearer when the question of "what has been left out of prior studies" is asked. The answer can help frame new ways to address this health condition. Rather than accepting the inappropriate misapplication of findings to women when the research was conducted only in men, researchers are being charged with exploring new avenues of research and new ways of asking the research question.

Analyze Your Own Role or Relationship to the Issue or Topic

Traditionally, the focus of women's health has been relegated to "between the breasts and the knees." Pregnancy and childbirth were long the focus when it came to health care of women, if only as a means of securing the survival of human society. The value of women was based on their role in procreation and continuation of the citizenry. Many historical examples can be cited to illustrate how a focus on reproductive health created opportunities to promote maternal and child health reforms in the public health arena. In such cases, women typically took advantage of the focus on reproductive health to advance an agenda that addressed both maternal and child health. At the same time, the practice of focusing solely on reproductive health carried risks, as it enabled normal physiological reproductive processes to be medicalized within a biomedical context.

In response to the practice of medicalizing aspects of women's health and traditional models of women's health care, consumer activism by women has been directed at reframing women's health and calling for reforms at even the most basic levels. The strategy of analyzing your own role or relationship to the issue may help reveal the role women play in relation to the process of rejecting medicalization of many of the normal healthy physiologic processes they experience. Over the years, various aspects of women's health have become topics of public debate and of organized social action; taken together, these episodes could be considered waves in a women's health mega-movement (Weisman, 1998).

In recent decades, two notable waves have occurred in the women's health mega-movement. One wave coincided with social action movements such as the civil rights and women's rights movements. A key feature of this wave was that it was grassroots oriented, with a key focus on access to information and expanded knowledge regarding health. One outcome of this movement was the creation of the Boston Women's Health Book Collective (BWHBC) and its publication of *Our Bodies, Ourselves* for consumers in 1974. The BWHBC is composed of women who are healthcare consumers. They developed a consumer-oriented women's health textbook through a process of conducting individual research related to women's health. During this period, primary access to health-related information was available only through medical textbooks.

Eventually, a second wave emerged from the first—namely, the opportunity for women to reclaim control of their health and to offer new definitions or ways of thinking about physiological processes. A key aspect of this process, which continues to this day, is demystifying health conditions and processes in an effort to empower women with knowledge so they can ask questions about their health and pose these questions to their healthcare providers. This change supported women in taking responsibility for their healthcare decision making rather than simply adhering to the biomedical model of the 1960s and 1970s, which placed authority for decision making under the control of the healthcare provider.

This wave of reclaiming control of health care from clinicians and focusing on women's role and authority over their own health was initially promoted by well-educated women from middle- and higher-income groups. A critique of this wave of the women's health movement reveals that it generalized women's health issues as a global consideration that included ethnic and cultural variation. In response, women's health groups were organized based on ethnic and cultural considerations related to women's health.

Consider the Risks and Benefits of Speaking in Terms of Groups Versus Individuals

The strategy of "considering the risks and benefits of speaking in terms of groups versus individuals" addressed a problematic aspect of the women's health movements of the1960s and 1970s. In an effort to be inclusive, many advocates of the women's health movement during this period claimed to be speaking collectively for all women—yet the primary focus and emphasis were on women who were privileged in society, rather than women who were marginalized. Schiebinger (2003) summarizes the progress of the women's health movement since then as follows: "Whereas the women's health movement of the 1970s sought to solidify sisterhood through the commonalities of female childbirth experiences, there is now an emphasis on the differing health needs of different racial and ethnic groups of women" (p. 974). Today, women's health activists demonstrate greater diversity and focus on a wider range of issues affecting the health of women and their families. This also includes attention to ageism, which was inherent in much of the earlier waves of the women's health movement (Pohl & Boyd, 1993).

Consider the Social Construction of Gender and How Its Assumptions May Limit Options or Presume Choices That Are Made Within the Context of Health

Earlier discussions regarding the social construction of gender highlighted the implications of this strategy. An additional aspect to consider is the manner in which women's health issues are described—that is, the terminology used. The language used for many of women's health concerns has been described by anthropologist Emily Martin (1992) as reflecting an androcentric bias—for example, the image of menstruation in medical texts is that of "failed reproduction" (p. 92).

Another example is the practice of referring to a woman who has experienced sexual assault as a victim rather than as a survivor of the process, implying inherent weakness rather than strength. Descriptions of childbirth usually invoke the term *delivery* or a woman being delivered rather than giving birth. The former terms focus on the actions of the healthcare provider and place the woman in a passive position, rather than seeing her as the central figure: the one giving birth.

Explore the Precise Ways in Which Gender Defines Power Relationships and the Implications of Those Power Dynamics on Health

Creating health care from a feminist perspective requires the elimination of power differentials between the individuals who are consuming health care and the individuals who are providing it. A partnership model more accurately reflects the manner in which healthcare interactions should occur. In this model, rather than invoking a level of authority by virtue of being a healthcare provider, the healthcare provider acknowledges the life experiences and knowledge that the individual brings to the interaction. What makes a practice "feminist" is not who provides the health care, but how that care is provided, how the clinician thinks about his or her work, and the populations with whom the clinician works (Brown, 1994).

While hierarchical relationships and structures are typically elements of the traditional healthcare delivery system, feminist practice requires an active process of action to eliminate asymmetrical relationships. Simple actions, such as not having a woman undress prior to meeting her clinician, allow the woman to greet the healthcare provider as an equal rather than from a vulnerable position, undressed and wrapped in an ill-fitting paper gown. Having a woman check her own weight and urine, as opposed to having someone else do this for her, places some accountability for health on the woman's shoulders. It gives the message that she can control aspects of her health. Although these simple changes can be readily made in the healthcare office setting, each demonstrates power sharing rather than placing the woman in a dependent position in relation to aspects of her health care that she should rightly control.

Each of the strategies discussed in this section provides an opportunity to consider the details as well as the global aspects of women's health care and women's health issues. The strategies can be applied both individually and collectively. They are not meant to be an exhaustive checklist to determine whether something is being considered from a feminist perspective, but rather are meant to serve as guidelines and considerations that allow for the identification of blind spots in how we are able to think about women's health issues when we are potentially constrained by the limitations of the biomedical model. Through the use of these strategies, healthcare providers, policy makers, and women themselves are able to reframe expectations, approaches, and the focus of women's health research, healthcare delivery, and even the receipt of healthcare services.

Why a Textbook on Gynecology?

Taking the same feminist strategies we use for analyzing women's health and applying them to this textbook on gynecologic aspects of women's health creates opportunities as well. Why, when a feminist perspective is being presented, along with the limitations of considering women's health as being equivalent to reproductive health, would a textbook purportedly using a feminist framework focus only on gynecologic aspects of women's health? The reason is that gynecologic health is still important. Focusing on gynecology for clinicians is important because reframing and expanding considerations of gynecologic health from a feminist perspective may more accurately reflect the experience for women in their everyday lives. By offering a feminist perspective throughout the chapters, we seek to dispel myths that pathologize normal gynecologic functioning, and we seek to support normality as opposed to medicalizing it. Rather than ignoring gynecologic health and allowing it to remain within the biomedical domain, this textbook seeks to reframe aspects of gynecologic health issues within a feminist framework. This perspective expands the opportunities for understanding gynecologic health from within a wellness-oriented, women-centered framework and encourages providers to look beyond the medical model and support normalcy instead of "manage" it.

References

Boston Women's Health Book Collective. (1974). *Our bodies, ourselves*. New York: Simon & Schuster.

Brown, L. (1994). *Subversive dialogues*. New York: Basic Books.

Conrad, P. (1992). Medicalization and social control. *Annual Review of Sociology, 18*, 209–232.

Davis, R., & Huber, K. (2004). Class, ethnicity, age, physical status, and sexual orientation: Implications for health and healthcare. In M. Condon (Ed.), *Women's health* (pp. 21–41). Upper Saddle River, NJ: Prentice Hall.

Franz, C., & Stewart, A. (Eds.). (1994). *Women creating lives: Identities, resilience, and resistance*. Boulder, CO: Westview Press.

Healy, B. (1991). The Yentil syndrome. *New England Journal of Medicine, 325*, 274–276.

hooks, b. (2000). *Feminism is for everybody.* Cambridge, MA: South End Press.

Johnson, S. M., Karvonen, C. A., Phelps, C. L., Nader, S., & Sanborn, B. M. (2003). Assessment of analysis by gender in the Cochrane reviews as related to treatment of cardiovascular disease. *Journal of Women's Health, 12*(5), 449–457.

Klasen, S., & Wink, C. (2002). A turning point in gender bias in mortality? An update on the number of missing women. *Population and Development Review, 28,* 285–312.

Lantz, P., House, J., Lepkowski, J., Williams, D., Mero, R., & Chen, J. (1998). Socioeconomic factors, health behaviors, and mortality: Results from a nationally representative prospective study of US adults. *Journal of the American Medical Association, 279*(21), 1703–1708.

Lorber, J. (1997). *Gender and the social construction of illness.* Thousand Oaks, CA: Sage.

Martin, E. (1992). *The woman in the body: A cultural analysis of reproduction.* Boston: Beacon Press.

Pinn, V. (2003a). Expanding the frontiers of women's health research—US style. *Medical Journal of Australia, 178*(16), 598–599.

Pinn, V. (2003b). Sex and gender factors in medical studies: Implications for health and clinical practice. *Journal of the American Medical Association, 289*(4), 397–400.

Pohl, J., & Boyd, C. (1993). Ageism within feminism. *Image, 25,* 200–203.

Rosser, S. V. (1994). Gender bias in clinical research: The difference it makes. In A. Dan (Ed.), *Reframing women's health* (pp. 253–265). Thousand Oaks, CA: Sage.

Ruzek, S., Olsen, V., & Clark, A. (1997). Social, biomedical and feminist models of women's health. In S. Ruzek, V. Olsen, & A. Clark (Eds.), *Women's health: Complexities and differences.* Columbus, OH: Ohio State University Press.

Satcher, D. (2001). American women and health disparities. *Journal of the American Medical Women's Association, 56*(4), 131–133.

Schiebinger, L. (1999). *Has feminism changed science?* Cambridge, MA: Harvard University Press.

Schiebinger, L. (2003). Women's health and clinical trials. *Journal of Clinical Investigation, 112*(7), 973–977.

Starrs, A. (1997). The Safe Motherhood Action Agenda: Report on the safe motherhood technical consultation. Sri Lanka: Family Care International.

Tavris, C. (1992). *The mismeasure of women.* New York: Simon & Schuster.

Tejada de Rivero, D. (2003). Alma-Ata revisited. *Perspectives in Health Magazine, 8*(2), 2–7.

Thompson, J. (2004) A human rights framework for midwifery care. *Journal of Midwifery and Women's Health, 49*(3), 175–181.

Velzeboer, M., Ellsberg, M., Arcas, C. C., & Garcia-Moreno, C. (2003). *Violence against women: The health sector responds.* Washington, DC: Pan American Health Organization.

Weisman, C. S. (1998). *Women's health care.* Baltimore: Johns Hopkins University Press.

Williams, D. (2002). Racial/ethnic variations in women's health: The social embeddedness of health. *American Journal of Public Health, 92*(4), 588–597.

Wood, S. (2001). Office of Women's Health, Food and Drug Administration: Future directions for women's health. *Journal of the American Medical Women's Association, 56*(4), 197–198.

Xu, K. T., & Borders, T. (2003). Gender health and physician visits among adults in the United States. *American Journal of Public Health, 93*(7), 1076–1078.

Zola, I. (1972). Medicine as an institution of social control. *Sociological Review, 20,* 487–504.

2

Women's Growth and Development Across the Life Span

Kerri Durnell Schuiling
Lisa Kane Low

Clinical textbooks typically describe what is considered normal growth and development; this description frames the upcoming chapters of this textbook's discussion of variations from what is considered normative. Although this approach may seem comprehensive, the dilemma is that the initial discussion of women's growth and development is often from a biomedical perspective. This representation deconstructs women's bodies into biologic parts and physiologic processes. While such an approach enables quantification of growth, it is known that qualitative aspects of women's lives also influence their growth.

The biomedical model of health is individualist and disease oriented. In Chapter 1, this model is contrasted with a feminist and social model of health. The latter model acknowledges the influence of the culture in which women live, their economic status, the social interactions they experience, and the context in which they access and receive health care. The feminist model acknowledges the many other factors beyond the physiologic functioning of women and the genetic inheritance that affect their growth and development. As a result, even the manner in which we understand and explain what normative growth and development includes changes in the expanded framework of a feminist perspective, thereby allowing for a clearer understanding of the complexity inherent in women's growth and development.

As a first step in considering women's development (cognitive, psychosocial, and functional behaviors), it is important to acknowledge that the traditional models that are used were developed from research about men. For example, psychoanalyst Erick Erikson (1950) expanded developmental theory beyond the years of adolescence to offer a grand theory of human development (**Table 2-1**). He identified eight general stages of development that included several within adulthood. The eight virtues that are the goals of the stages are trust, autonomy, initiative, industry, identity, intimacy, generativity, and integrity.

TABLE 2-1 Erikson's Eigenetic Model

Age Period for Crisis	1	2	3	4	5	6	7	8
					Stages			
Infancy	Trust vs. Mistrust							
Early childhood		Autonomy vs. Shame and Doubt						
Play age			Initiative vs. Guilt					
School age				Industry vs. Inferiority				
Adolescence					Identity vs. Identity Diffusion			
Young adult						Intimacy vs. Isolation		
Adulthood							Generativity vs. Self-absorption	
Mature age								Integrity vs. Despair

Source: Used with permission from Low, 2001.

Through a process of resolving eight developmental crises that are sequentially confronted, Erikson's theory offers a comprehensive account of individual development throughout the life span that until recently was applied to both males and females. It is important to understand that Erikson's stages of psychosocial development are based on studies of white, middle-class males (Erikson, 1968) and yet the model is universally applied to women with some gendered assumptions. The underlying gendered assumptions within Erickson's grand theory of development must be recognized because within this theory individuals are treated as a monolith, with minimal attention being paid to gender, socioeconomic, or ethnic variability (Gilligan, 1982; Taylor, 1994). Some of the gender-based assumptions include a normative linear pattern of identity, followed by marriage (intimacy), and then childbearing (generativity) in adulthood. Erikson's theory assumes the need for a female to first develop an intimate relationship with another before she can complete her sense of self as an individual. Interestingly, males (according to this theory) do not have the same requirement. Thus, while the larger context of the theory assumes the desirability of autonomy and distancing oneself from the family of origin, for females autonomy is defined as being dependent on another within the context of a relationship, with a primary focus on caretaking by females.

Other examples of grand theories that are misapplied to women include those developed by Kohlberg (1981) and Perry (1968). Kohlberg's levels of moral development are based on interviews with only men, and Perry actually discarded interviews he had with women, using only data from interviews with men to formulate his model of intellectual development. The difficulty that occurs when these scales are used to assess a woman's developmental level is that they assume universality in development and, again, treat all women as a monolith, not acknowledging the multiple variables that can affect progress through the stages (Belenky, Clinchy, Goldberger, & Tarule, 1986; Low, 2001). Tavris (1992) observes that "because of the (mis)measures we use, women fail to measure up to having the right body and fail to measure up to having the right life" (p. 36). The use of these androcentric models constrains the manner in which women's development is framed, such that women's development is presented as an aberration in comparison to white male development, which is held up as the standard.

This chapter discusses growth and development by contrasting traditional male-biased theoretical constructs with newer feminist theories that challenge some of the basic assumptions about women's growth and development. Alternative theories of female development were offered by feminist psychologists and researchers beginning in the 1970s (Taylor, 1994). Although there is substantial variation in the emphasis of feminist scholars, a primary focus is on the self-in-relation to others or in connection with others (family and peers) as a means of further development. Feminist theories of development emphasize the quality and nature of individual women's experiences. As a consequence, women's development is construed as broader than the traditional process of individualization and includes the value of maintaining connection and continuity within relationships (Gilchrist, 1997).

The definition of relationships within this model contains not just the self-in-relation to others but also inner constructions of relationships that form the sense of self of the female (Kaplan, Gleason, & Klein, 1991). These relationships progressively contain conflict, and it is through resolution of this conflict that the relationships become more complex, requiring flexibility that allows connections and relationships to be maintained (Baker Miller, 1991). This view stands in opposition to traditional theories of development that emphasize conflict resolution as entailing greater disconnection and the development of distinct boundaries around identity formation or the process of "becoming one's own man" (Baker Miller, 1991).

Feminist theories are primarily offered in contrast to Erikson's theory of psychosocial development. Gilligan (1982) and other feminist scholars have critiqued his work not only as being descriptive of male development in general, but also as descriptive of primarily white, privileged male development. Black-feminist scholarship has furthered this critique beyond that of the traditional male-based model to include limitations in contrasting models offered by early feminist theorists.

A key limitation of early feminist models is that they were developed by white middle-class Euro-American women who interpret relationships and connection as being similar across all women, regardless of ethnic identity or the influence of racism (Collins, 2000). Owing to this perspective, much of early feminist scholarship was limited by a lack of understanding of the role of ethnic identity and socioeconomic level on development.

The intention of newer feminist models is not to replace male generalist models of development with feminist generalist models of development, but rather to offer alternatives to the constrained models that were previously misapplied to all women. This chapter provides an overview of growth and development within the linear stages of adolescence through older age using a feminist perspective. Emphasis is placed on contrasting models of development outside the traditional biomedical focus.

Subscription to a model that delineates gender differences versus a model that identifies gender similarities and provides an explanation for differences based on gender is a key philosophical dilemma for developmental theorists. The emphasis on difference, rather than similarity, evokes a debate about the risk of essentializing women's development. The difficulty arises because gender differences described by these theories are ascribed as biologic or innate characteristics rather than considering the social and cultural context that can create these differences. Thus the differences described are consistent with social constructs of femininity rather than being biologically determined, but they are wrongly assumed to be biologic in origin (Gilligan, 1982; Martin, 1992). While lauding the work of Gilligan and other early feminist theorists who argue that women have a "different voice" through which they develop and speak, several feminist psychologists and theorists offer the critique that in recent developmental theories, what feminist theorists have described as being uniquely female is instead likely to be based in the social construction of gender roles and has been inadequately explored (Hare-Mustin & Marecek, 1998; Riger, 1998).

This perspective, which results in differing expectations at different times based on gender, is consistent with the model proposed by Erikson (1950). He argues that the particular developmental crisis is not necessarily chronologically driven but rather is driven by social expectations for behavior. Thus expectations for caregiving and consideration by females of themselves in relation to others may have more to do with socially prescribed gender roles of femininity than with biologically differing pathways for development. More similarities than differences between males and females may become evident when gender boundaries are broken down and males have a greater level of participation in caretaking for others rather than primarily for themselves. Until that time, however, contrasting developmental models with an emphasis on differences that are primarily socially constructed have prevailed and, therefore, will inform the perspectives presented in this chapter.

Adolescence

The adolescent years are generally described biologically as beginning with the onset of puberty and extending 8 to 10 years beyond this point (Murray & Zentner, 1997). In a chronological sense, these years encompass the ages of 11 to 21 (Condon, 2004). Often this period is described as the "stormy" years, a sobriquet reflecting the stress of puberty and the accompanying bodily changes. For most adolescents, however, the transition is quite smooth in spite of the myriad physical, developmental, emotional, and cognitive changes that occur during this time (Lewis & Bernstein, 1996). Stages of adolescence are commonly categorized into early adolescence (ages 11–13 years), mid-adolescence (ages 14–17 years), and late adolescence (ages 17–21 years) (Lewis & Bernstein; Slap, 1986). Although the changes that occur during this period are discussed here in the contexts of biology and physiology, it is important to remember from a healthcare standpoint that qualitative aspects must be considered. For example, an adolescent woman's sense of body image may be tied to her weight as much as it is to her past experiences (Leight, 2003).

Biology and Physiology

Significant physical changes occur during a young woman's adolescence. Adult height and weight are usually attained during this time, and probably most significant to the adolescent female are changes associated with the development of secondary sex characteristics. The usual sequence of female pubertal events begins with a growth spurt that occurs around the ages of 11 to 12. This growth spurt is followed by thelarche (breast development), adrenarche (growth of pubic hair due to androgen stimulation), and menarche (the onset of menses) (Skillman-Hull, 2003; Woods, 1995). Peak height usually occurs about two years after breast budding and about one year prior to menarche (Fritz & Speroff, 2011). On average, the growth spurt in girls begins around age 10, reaches its maximum rate at age 12, and subsides around age 16 (Bassey, Sayer, & Cooper, 2002).

Girls reach puberty earlier than boys. The timing of puberty and onset of menses is controlled primarily by the neuroendocrine system (Lewis & Bernstein, 1996) and genetic inheritance, although it is also believed to be affected by external factors such as general health and nutrition, race, geographic location, amount of exposure to light, and psychological makeup (Skillman-Hull, 2003). Girls who perceive themselves to be "on time" for puberty tend to have a better self-image and are more likely to view themselves as attractive than girls who believe themselves to be either early or late in relation to puberty (Woods, 1995).

Although the pubertal changes provoke perceptions about puberty, these perceptions are also shaped by the dominant culture (Woods). Lee (1998) observes that women often say their bodies become problematic at menarche—for example, women may state that their breasts are too big or too small, and their hips are an enemy because fat accumulates there.

The onset of puberty depends on a changing body accumulation of adipose tissue. As a consequence, this event marks the beginning of a tension between biologic development and the social context in which it occurs. Our culture today demands perfection, which causes many young women to suffer great anxiety about their bodies. The challenges that present for young women vary based on ethnicity, self-esteem, the social environment, and the contrast between the individual adolescent's sense of herself and society's perceived standard for beauty. In addition, many of the changes of puberty are framed within the social context of sexual development. As the physical sexual characteristics develop, many young women are challenged by a potential mismatch between their socially perceived sexual development and their interpersonal level of maturity and development. Clinicians can serve as an important source of support and information during what is often framed culturally as a tumultuous phase of development.

A commonly used scale for staging sexual maturity is the Tanner Scale, which relies on development of the breasts and growth of pubic hair. It divides sexual physical maturity into five stages that extend from preadolescence to the adult (**Figures 2-1, 2-2, and 2-3**). The Tanner model, although widely accepted for staging sexual maturity, is not appropriate to use for determining chronological age (Rosenbloom & Tanner, 1998). Additionally, Rosenbloom and Tanner note that because of the variability in timing of stages and of pubic hair growth, both of which are important elements of Tanner staging, the scale should not be used for staging individuals of Asian ethnicity.

Probably the most anticipated, feared, and socially misconstrued aspect of female adolescent development and puberty is the onset of menses. Menarche is an important milestone in a young girl's life. The median age for the onset of menstruation for adolescent girls in the United States is 12.8 years, with a range of ages 9 to 17 (Fritz & Speroff, 2011). The events of puberty trigger the onset of menses when a positive feedback of estrogen on the pituitary and hypothalamus stimulates a surge of luteinizing hormone at midcycle, which is critical to ovulation (Fritz

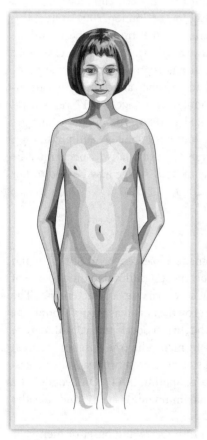

FIGURE 2-1 Tanner Stage I: Preadolescent (ages 10-14): Breasts have elevation of nipple only. There is no pubic hair except for vellus hair, which is fine body hair like that noted on the abdomen.

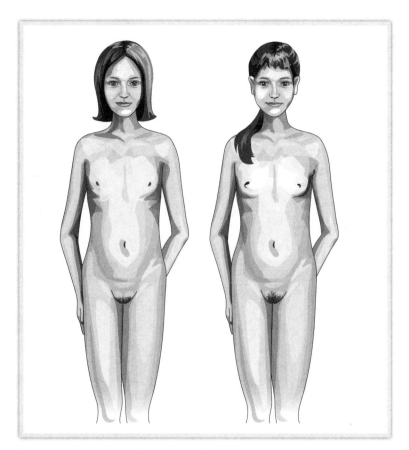

FIGURE 2-2 Tanner Stages 2 & 3: Tanner Stage 2 (left) is referred to as the breast bud stage. There is an elevation of the breast and nipple, and the areola widens. Pubic hair is sparse, long, and only slightly curly. It is observed mainly on the labia. Tanner Stage 3 (right) (ages 12–14 or middle adolescence): The breast and areola are enlarged further with increased elevation of the breast and nipple; however, there is no separation of their contours. The pubic hair growth begins to occur over the mons pubis, and hair is now darker, coarser, and curlier.

& Speroff). The first several menstrual cycles usually do not result in ovulation, and often a girl's first-year experience of menstruating is characterized by irregular anovulatory cycles, along with heavy bleeding (Fritz & Speroff).

Menarche is integrally linked to many layers of social meaning for girls and women. It is an event that symbolizes reproduction and sexual potential (Lee, 1998). Thus menarche is important both as a physiologic happening, albeit framed by biomedical metaphors of scientific knowledge, and because it is the social and cultural juncture at which girls become women and gender relations are reproduced (Lee). These relations deal with issues such as power and its absence, women's agency, and the ability to move through the world with credibility and respect (Lee).

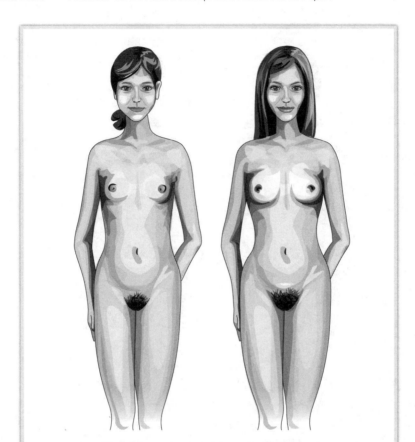

FIGURE 2-3 Tanner Stages 4 and 5: Tanner Stage 4 (left) reveals breasts with areola and nipple forming a secondary mound with projection of the nipple. Pubic hair is adult type but is observed over a smaller area with none noted on the thighs. Tanner Stage 5 (right) (ages 14–16 late adolescence): Breasts are fully mature and only the nipple protrudes as the areola is usually flush with the breast contour. However, a normal variation is for the areola to continue as a secondary mound. The pubic hair is normal adult type: thick, coarse, and curly, and spreads onto the medial surfaces of the thighs. Adult female hair pattern (inverted triangle) is observed.

Psychosocial Development

Adolescence, as previously described, focuses on changes associated with puberty in combination with preparation for the future (Goldharber, 1986). The traditional developmental task of adolescence is to develop a sense of identity and autonomy before progressing toward adulthood. There is a tendency to "try on" various roles as adolescents struggle with who they want to be and how they want to live (Crain, 1980). The role of peers becomes critical in this process, and a distancing from parents and other adults typically occurs (Goldharber). Within almost all cultures there is an acknowledgment that failure to successfully negotiate the developmental tasks of adolescence limits an individual's ability to function productively as an adult (Musick, 1993). The interaction between an adolescent's behavior and role performance may either promote or confuse his or her sense of identity depending on the social context in which it occurs. Through a process of trial and experimentation, individuals develop their own set of values and beliefs as well as a sense of themselves as they formalize or commit to their own identity. Initiation of sexual activity, pregnancy, childbearing, and parenting are all gendered roles and experiences that differ in their effects on any one individual adolescent based on the social, cultural, and historical definition that is associated with these behaviors and roles, as well as peers' and family's perceptions of these events.

In contrast, a feminist perspective of female adolescent development emphasizes the young girl's relationship with others instead of distancing from others in the process of individuation as described by Erikson (1950). Current theorists argue that the hallmark of healthy identity development is development of a sense of connection to others, with a primary task being the ability to participate in mutual relationships in which the individual feels active and effective, and is not "lost within" the relationship (Kaplan et al., 1991). The self-in-relation model of adolescent development proposed by Baker Miller (1991) and her colleagues at the Wellesley College Stone Center defines a woman's sense of self as emerging out of experience with a relational process that begins in infancy. From initial interactions with caregivers through the process of becoming a caretaker, the self-in-relation theory argues that women are socialized to care more and more about the development of relationships.

> Beginning with the earliest mother–daughter interactions, this relational sense of self develops out of women's involvement in progressively complex relationships, characterized by mutual identifications, attention to interplay between each other's emotions, and caring about the process and activity of relationship. (Kaplan et al., 1991, p. 123)

Development is delayed if the young girl's relationships are suppressive or oppressive (Woods, 1995). Unfortunately, all too often this is the case for many young women. The predominant culture in the United States discourages a young girl from acting with a sense of self when she is in a relationship. Acting as an autonomous agent is discouraged (Woods), and dependence is traditionally encouraged.

Girls usually interact closely with their mothers, a relationship that means girls, as compared to boys, are more apt to learn and appreciate the importance of empathy. Woods (1995) points out that this development may strengthen girls' sense of connection and being emotionally understood, which in turn provides an advantage to girls growing up in Western cultures because they will be carriers of aspects of human experience, including emotionality, vulnerability, and growth fostering.

Reasoning changes as a child grows to adolescence. Instead of just understanding a general rule governing the immediate and concrete, the thinking of the adolescent involves the use of symbols and opening up a world of possibilities (Strauss & Clark, 1996). This type of thinking influences and explains the risk-taking behaviors of adolescents. Strauss and

Clark point out that the adolescent girl might not be able to appreciate logical sequencing of events, such as pregnancy following an act of intercourse. Maturation in thinking behavior is supported by understanding family members, an emotionally stable environment, parental discipline, and positive life experiences.

Clinical Application

The health of adolescents is critically important to their health in later years (Woods, 1995). Almost from birth, females are socialized to be highly oriented to others, so it is not surprising that risk behaviors and conditions, such as depression or early sexual activity, are more likely to be influenced by the nature of an adolescent female's relational experiences with significant others, family, peers, and others (Baker Miller, 1991). In fact, the major health problems of adolescents relate to their risk-taking behaviors. In contrast to males, these behaviors in females are more often influenced by a desire to maintain important relationships than a desire to "take on" adult behaviors. Female adolescent morbidity is most likely to include pregnancy, sexually transmitted infections, running away, and suicide (Lee, 1998). Risk taking can also be a result of the young girl's environment or may be an expression of symptoms of depression.

The developmental self-in-relation model offered by feminist scholars can be extended into the healthcare visit for adolescents. Trust is a key component of any therapeutic relationship—a fact that cannot be emphasized enough for providers caring for adolescents. Additional time is often needed to establish a trusting relationship with an adolescent.

Sherwin (1998) suggests using a relational approach when providing adolescent females' healthcare services. This approach takes into consideration the full range of human relations that influence how adolescent females define their health (Sherwin). For example, "Tell me about your friends or who you hang out with" and "How would you describe yourself in relation to your friends?" are the types of questions that can be asked of an adolescent during a healthcare visit to assess who influences the adolescent and how she sees herself in relationship to others. The goal is not to isolate the behavior from the relational context in which it occurs, but rather to acknowledge the health implications of behaviors. This enables a more effective approach to risk reduction because the behavior is addressed along with the context in which it occurs. This relational model can be extended as a woman progresses in her healthcare needs across the life span.

Early Adulthood

Young adulthood is generally accepted as spanning the time from late adolescence (age 18) to the beginning of the perimenopausal years (ages 35–50). This period is often referred to as the *reproductive years*, reflecting a societal valuing of women primarily for their reproductive capacities (Olshansky, 1996). Health care during the young adulthood years traditionally focuses on health promotion and maintenance, with a primary emphasis on reproductive capacity rather than a broader, comprehensive focus on health promotion throughout the life span.

Biology and Physiology

The years between ages 18 and 35 are biomedically considered optimal for reproduction. Generally, most women experience regular menstrual cycles that are ovulatory, providing opportunity for pregnancy if unprotected intercourse occurs. The biologic changes that accompany a pregnancy and that affect motherhood and aging also have a psychological impact in our youth-oriented culture (Blakenship, 2003). Contraception is an important health consideration for heterosexual couples during these years.

Physical health in young adulthood is promoted by consumption of an adequate diet, exercise, and monitoring of overall well-being. These needs for health promotion and maintenance are best met when a woman lives within a social context that is conducive to health (Olshansky, 1996). Optimal health is more readily achievable when a woman does not have to confront racism, sexism, or classism, but instead has access to quality health care, economic stability, and other resources (Olshansky). In reality, however, most women have lives that incorporate multiple and competing demands related to work, economics, childbearing, and childrearing.

Women's changing roles—specifically, the transition from traditional homemaker to working outside the home—have come at a cost to their health, probably because women working outside the home continue to have significant responsibilities within the home. Balancing these competing demands increases the stress level of many women (Condon, 2004). As stress increases, many women have coped by developing unhealthy behaviors such as smoking, lack of exercise, and poor nutrition. As a result, women's health risks for some diseases are now similar to those of men. For example, cardiac disease is now the number one killer of women in the United States, whereas two decades ago the primary cause of illness and health risk for women was related to reproduction. Health problems that frequently occur during this stage of life include cardiac disease, arthritis, occupational injury and related illnesses, cancer, infections (sexually transmitted and otherwise), and reproductive disorders (Olshansky, 1996). Chapters 4 and 8 discuss health promotion and health maintenance in more specific detail.

Psychosocial Development

Erikson's (1968) model identifies two crises that occur during early adulthood. The first is the development of intimacy versus isolation: the process of entering into a life partnership with another individual. It is during this developmental phase that gender assumptions about behavior become more typically defined. As previously noted, women are assumed to require intimacy as a prerequisite for the completion of their identity development, whereas males may progress into this phase without any prior development related to their ability to participate in relationships.

It is this contrast of what is described as normative for both males and females that challenged Franz and White (1985) to offer an expansion of Erikson's theory of development. Using a feminist lens, Franz and White discourage the use of a single pathway of development that primarily focuses on individuation, and instead encourage the consideration of a two-pathway process that includes both individuation and a process of attachment. They argue that Erikson does not conceptualize being female as somehow inferior or lacking in purpose, nor simply as a vehicle for childbearing and caretaking. Instead, they describe his work as not attending to the process by which attachment occurs through intimacy and relationships with others. Franz and White argue that Erickson does not provide adequate opportunity in his traditional framework for male development of the capacity for intimacy and attachment.

The expanded model that Franz and White (1985) propose includes two processes of development: individuation combined with an attachment pathway in a double-helix model. The double-helix model allows for these two separate strands to be interconnected, depicting the relationship between psychological individuation and attachment as ascending in a spiral that represents the human life span. The strand representing individuation is essentially the same as it is in Erikson's model, but the attachment strand addresses the neglected relational dimension of human development. **Table 2-2** represents the individuation and attachment "strands" as described by Franz and White. The authors argue:

> With changing times and mores, [if] attachment processes were to undergo fuller development in men and individuation processes were to undergo fuller development in women, sex differences might become more elusive than ever, but individuation and attachment would retain their power as psychological variables associated with psychological value in important nomological nets. (Franz & White, 1985, p. 254)

The second crisis of early adulthood is acquiring the ability to become generative versus stagnation. Here *generative* is defined as acting on one's concern for the welfare of the next generation. Reproduction and parenting may accomplish this goal, as can service to others. Stagnation occurs when the person is unable to step outside of herself or himself and be generative. As stated earlier, Erikson's work is based on men and may not be an accurate model for assessing women's development. Newer models of women's development emphasize the relational aspects of women's lives. Understanding women's lives within their individual social context provides a women-oriented perspective for conceptualizing the degree to which a woman reaches a particular level of psychosocial development (Olshansky, 1996).

During the young adulthood years, women's psychosocial development may involve a variety of factors such as accepting responsibilities (parenting, caring for others), creating a career, forming enduring relationships, caring for elderly parents, and deciding whether to become a parent. Although all of these factors influence a woman's psychosocial development, they cannot be understood as generalities that are applied to all women, nor should each be assessed in isolation. Instead, each woman's relation to these factors—to herself and others, to the social context of her life, and to her lived experience—provides insight into her level of psychosocial development.

TABLE 2-2 Franz and White's Adaptation of Erikson's Theory of Development to a Two-Path Model

	Infancy	Early Childhood	Play Age	School Age	Adolescence	Young Adulthood	Adulthood	Old Age
Individuation pathway	Trust vs. mistrust	Autonomy vs. shame and doubt	Initiative vs. guilt	Industry vs. inferiority	Identity vs. identity diffusion	Career, lifestyle exploration vs. drifting	Lifestyle consolidation vs. emptiness	Integrity vs. despair
Attachment pathway	Trust vs. mistrust	Object and self-constancy vs. loneliness and helplessness	Playfulness vs. passivity or aggression	Empathy and collaboration vs. excessive caution or power	Mutuality interdependence vs. alienation	Intimacy vs. isolation	Generativity vs. self-absorption	Integrity vs. despair

Source: Used with permission from Low, 2001.

Clinical Application

A woman goes through many transitional periods from age 18 to 35. For women at risk of pregnancy, contraceptive decisions are of paramount importance, and it is critical to have access to and receive information and education about contraceptive options. Decisions related to childbearing (or not) are also prominent and frame much of the healthcare services that women traditionally receive during this phase of their lives. Many lifestyle-related health problems may become apparent during this time. Substance abuse, intimate partner violence, and stress related to her life or those she cares for can negatively affect a woman's health. Psychiatric illnesses that may become apparent during these years include bipolar disorder, schizophrenia, and psychosis, which may or may not be related to childbearing.

Although young adult women are primarily healthy, it is evident there are many opportunities for life events to negatively affect their health. Health promotion and maintenance during this period are critical to ensure optimal health in the later years of life.

Midlife

Midlife for women encompasses the perimenopausal years (ages 35–50) to menopause (ages 50–65) (Davis & Huber, 2004; Fogel & Woods, 1995). Midlife is actually a transition more than a phase of the human life cycle, and during this time many women experience a recognition that their lives are changing irrevocably. Some women will pursue goals and dreams they may have deferred while dealing with the greater life demands they faced in younger adulthood. If they were parenting during their earlier adulthood, then transitions into other aspects of their lives may be prompted by their children leaving home. Still others may be in the active phases of parenting as more women delay childbearing decisions until later into the early phases of midlife. During this phase of the life span, Erikson (1950) would continue to identify the phases of generativity versus stagnation as a continuing process.

Biology and Physiology

Perimenopause and menopause are biologic markers of the transition from young adult to midlife. Neither is a syndrome or disease, but instead demonstrates a natural maturing of the reproductive system. Social constructions of perimenopause and menopause abound. Martin (1992) encourages us to reframe perimenopause and menopause so that our ideas of a "single purpose" for the menstrual cycle can be reconstructed into images of healthy transitions.

During the perimenopausal years, women may experience physical changes associated with decreasing estrogen levels, such as the vasomotor symptoms of hot flashes and flushes. Other changes associated with aging include a decrease in the size of genitalia, changes in breast structure, and decreased skin elasticity. These changes are more fully described in Chapter 13.

Although for many years it was believed a preponderance of midlife women suffered mood changes caused by a deficiency of estrogen during this time of life, more recent studies suggest that psychosocial factors have a much greater effect on a midlife woman's mood than do the physiologic transitions of menopause. In fact, mood changes reported by women experiencing menopause may be caused by myriad factors including hormonal changes, normal aging processes, psychological transitions, and cultural beliefs and expectations (Fogel & Woods, 1995).

Psychosocial Development

Midlife is a dynamic period of development during which many complex changes occur (Fogel & Woods, 1995). Women during this time often experience a burst of new energy—termed *menopausal zest* by anthropologist Margaret Mead (Davis & Huber, 2004)—and pursue new interests, acquire new skills, and enjoy more time with friends and family (Boston Women's Health Collective, 1998). Conversely, Gilligan (1982) argues that midlife may be a time of risk for women precisely because of their embeddedness in relationships, orientation to interdependence, ability to subordinate achievement to care, and conflicts over competitive success. Women face midlife by making sense out of their experiences based on their relationships (Fogel & Woods).

Clinical Application

A common myth is that women lose their interest in sex when they reach middle age. Although aging decreases vaginal lubrication, use of vaginal lubricants aid comfortable intercourse. Women who engage in sexual intercourse with men and who are perimenopausal should be provided with information about contraception if they want to avoid pregnancy.

Some women experience changes in memory and cognition as they enter midlife. Research is sparse on this subject. Although some studies implicate decreasing estrogen as a possible cause (Phillips & Sherwin, 1992), others contradict these findings (Buckwalter, Crooks, Robins, & Petitti, 2004; Kang, Weuve, & Grodstein, 2004)

Ageism and bias due to age are common in Western society. As a clinician, it is important to provide supportive care throughout a woman's life span and not assume a woman's health concerns are entirely related to her age.

Older Women

The term *older women* refers to women who have completed menopause. The population of older adults in the United States is primarily female (Davis & Huber, 2004). Many of these women live in poverty and have health problems because they have outlived their support systems (Davis & Huber). Medicare reimbursement is either poor or nonexistent for many of the healthcare services needed by this population. Healthcare issues related to aging are primarily women's issues, because older women significantly outnumber older men (Davis & Huber).

Biology and Physiology

Aging changes are due to decrease or loss of functioning at the cellular and/or tissue level, diminished capacity of an organ or system, and a reduction in body capabilities (Pfister & Dougherty, 1996). Theories abound about the cause of aging and the biologic and physiologic impacts of aging, but more research is needed to produce definitive findings. Specifically, gender-related distinctions need more study.

Loss of lean muscle mass, diminished immune functioning, an increase in cardiovascular problems (coronary heart disease and hypertension), and osteoporosis and bone loss are all observed with advanced age (Dimond, 1995; Pfister & Dougherty, 1996).

Psychosocial Development

Research suggests that older women are often caregivers for ailing male spouses or partners, and many end up living alone (because they outlive their male partners), but they continue to maintain a connectedness to other family members. There is no research that looks at the caregiver issue when the partners or spouses are both female. Cognitive abilities involve a range of capacities including motivation, short- and long-term memory, intelligence, learning and retention, and many factors that either facilitate or impede cognitive functioning (Dimond, 1995). It is not possible to definitively attribute changes in cognitive functioning to aging because few studies have included repeated measures over time with the same subjects (Dimond). Theories suggest that as we age we begin to disengage from society, and that we make adjustments based on our lifelong patterns, likes, and dislikes. However, there are not enough studies to support these hypotheses.

Clinical Application

Health issues of older women are substantial. The elderly are commonly viewed as frail and vulnerable persons who consume a significant amount of healthcare time, space, and dollars (Pfister & Dougherty, 1996). Ageism—that is, stereotyping and discrimination of a person based on age—is even more common at this stage of life. Elderly women must contend not only with ageism, but also with sexism. Youth and beauty are highly valued in the United States. While older men may be viewed as attractive, the older woman is often pressured to ward off aging (Pfister & Dougherty). Pohl and Boyd (1993) suggest that a key area in which clinicians might begin to link feminist theory with aging women is in health policies and the inequities inherent in them. To promote health and wellness in older women, clinicians must provide them with adequate information about their health status, risks, and ways of improving health through diet and exercise commensurate with their age and capabilities.

Conclusion

The remainder of the chapters within this textbook present more detailed discussions of the clinical assessment and management of women's gynecologic health. Through the continued use of a feminist framework, an expanded model of gynecologic health is presented that includes great opportunity to both affect change and improve health outcomes for women.

References

Baker Miller, J. (1991). The development of women's sense of self. In J. Jordan, A. Kaplan, J. Miller, I. Stiver, & J. Surrey (Eds.), *Women's growth in connection: Writings from the Stone Center* (pp. 11–34). New York: Guilford Press.

Bassey, J., Sayer, A., & Cooper, C. (2002). A life course approach to musculoskeletal aging: Muscle strength, osteoporosis, and osteoarthritis. In D. Kuh & R. Hardy (Eds.), *A life course approach to women's health* (pp. 141–160). Oxford, UK: University Press.

Belenky, M., Clinchy, B., Goldberger, N., & Tarule, J. (1986). *Women's ways of knowing.* New York: Harper Collins.

Blakenship, V. (2003). Psychosocial development of women. In E. Breslin & V. Lucas (Eds.), *Women's health nursing: Toward evidence-based practice* (pp. 133–169). St. Louis, MO: Saunders.

Boston Women's Health Collective. (1998). *Our bodies, ourselves for the new century.* New York: Simon & Schuster.

Buckwalter, J., Crooks, V., Robins, S., & Petitti, D. (2004). Hormone use and cognitive performance in women of advanced age. *Journal of Advanced Geriatrics, 52,* 182–186.

Collins, P. (2000). *Black feminist thought: Knowledge, consciousness, and the politics of empowerment.* London: Harper Collins.

Condon, M. (Ed.). (2004). *Women's health.* New Jersey: Pearson Education.

Crain, W. (1980). *Theories of development: Concepts and application.* Upper Saddle River, NJ: Prentice Hall.

Davis, R., & Huber, K. (2004). Class, ethnicity, age, physical status, and sexual orientation: Implications for health and healthcare. In M. Condon (Ed.), *Women's health* (pp. 21–40). Upper Saddle River, NJ: Prentice Hall.

Dimond, M. (1995). Older women's health. In C. Fogel & N. Woods (Eds.), *Women's health care* (pp. 101–110). London: Sage.

Erikson, E. (1950). *Childhood and society.* New York: W. W. Norton.

Erikson, E. (1968). *Identity, youth and crisis.* New York: W. W. Norton.

Fogel, C., & Woods, N. (1995). Midlife women's health. In N. Fogel (Ed.), *Women's health* (pp. 79–100). London: Sage.

Franz, C., & White, K. (1985). Individuation and attachment in personality development: Extending Erikson's theory. *Journal of Personality, 53*(2), 224–256.

Fritz, M., & Speroff, L. (2011). *Clinical gynecologic endocrinology and infertility* (8th ed.). Baltimore, MD: Williams & Wilkins.

Gilchrist, V. (1997). Psychosocial development of girls and women. In J. Rosenfeld (Ed.), *Women's health in primary care* (pp. 21–28). Baltimore: Williams & Wilkins.

Gilligan, C. (1982). *In a different voice: Psychological theory and women's development.* Cambridge, MA: Harvard University Press.

Goldharber, D. (1986). *Lifespan and human development.* New York: Harcourt Brace Jovanovich.

Hare-Mustin, R. T., & Marecek, J. (1998). The meaning of difference: Gender theory, postmodernism and psychology. In B. McVicker Clinchy & J. K. Norem (Eds.), *The gender and psychology reader* (pp. 125–143). New York: New York University Press.

Kang, J., Weuve, J., & Grodstein, F. (2004). Postmenopausal hormone therapy and risks of cognitive decline in community-dwelling women. *Neurology, 63,* 101–107.

Kaplan, A., Gleason, N., & Klein, R. (1991). Women's self-development in late adolescence. In J. Jordan, A. Kaplan, J. Miller, I. Stiver, & J. Surrey (Eds.), *Women's growth in connection: Writings from the Stone Center* (pp. 122–140). New York: Guilford Press.

Kohlberg, L. (1981). *The philosophy of moral development.* San Francisco: Harper & Row.

Lee, J. (1998). Menarche and the (hetero) sexualization of the female body. In R. Weitz (Ed.), *The politics of women's bodies. Sexuality, appearance and behavior* (pp. 82–99). New York: Oxford University Press.

Leight, S. (2003). Health history. In E. Breslin & V. Lucas (Eds.), *Women's health nursing: Toward evidence-based practice* (pp. 251–274). Baltimore: Saunders.

Lewis, J., & Bernstein, J. (1996). *Women's health*. Sudbury, MA: Jones and Bartlett.

Low, L. K. (2001). *Adolescents' experiences of childbirth: Nothing is simple*. Unpublished doctoral dissertation, University of Michigan, Ann Arbor, MI.

Martin, E. (1992). *The woman in the body*. Boston: Beacon Press.

Murray, R., & Zentner, J. (1997). *Nursing assessment and health promotion* (6th ed.). Upper Saddle River, NJ: Prentice Hall.

Musick, J. (1993). Young, poor and pregnant: The psychology of teenage motherhood. New Haven, CT: Yale University Press.

Olshansky, E. (1996). The reproductive years. In J. Lewis & J. Bernstein (Eds.), *Women's health* (pp. 105–143). Sudbury, MA: Jones and Bartlett.

Perry, W. (1968). Forms of intellectual and ethical development in the college years. New York: Holt, Rinehart & Winston.

Pfister, S., & Dougherty, M. (1996). Growing older. In J. Lewis & J. Bernstein (Eds.), *Women's health: A relational perspective across the life cycle* (pp. 192–236). Sudbury, MA: Jones and Bartlett.

Phillips, S., & Sherwin, B. (1992). Effects of estrogen on memory function in surgically menopausal women. *Psychoneuroendocrinology, 17*, 485–495.

Pohl, J., & Boyd, C. (1993). Ageism within feminism. *Image, 25*, 200–203.

Riger, S. (1998). Epistemological debates, feminist voices: Science, social values and the study of women. In B. McVicker Clinchy & J. K. Norem (Eds.), *The gender and psychology reader* (pp. 34–53). New York: New York University Press.

Rosenbloom, A., & Tanner, M. (1998). Misuse of Tanner scale [Letter to the editor]. *Pediatrics, 102*, 1494.

Sherwin, S. (1998). A relational approach to autonomy in health care. In S. Sherwin, F. Baylis, M. Bell, M. DeKonick, J. Downie, & A. Lippmann (Eds.), *The politics of women's health: Exploring agency and autonomy* (pp. 19–47). Philadelphia: Temple University.

Skillman-Hull, L. (2003). Adolescent women's health care. In E. Breslin & V. Lucas (Eds.), *Women's health nursing: Toward evidence-based practice* (pp. 432–552). Baltimore: Saunders.

Slap, G. (1986). Normal physiological and psychological growth in the adolescent. *Journal of Adolescent Health Care, 7*, 13S–23S.

Strauss, S., & Clark, B. (1996). Adolescence. In J. Lewis & J. Bernstein (Eds.), *Women's health: A relational perspective across the lifespan* (pp. 65–106). Sudbury, MA: Jones and Bartlett.

Tavris, C. (1992). *Mismeasure of women*. New York: Simon & Schuster.

Taylor, C. (1994). Gender equity in research. *Journal of Women's Health, 3*, 143–153.

Woods, N. (1995). Young women's health. In C. Fogel & N. Woods (Eds.), *Women's health care* (pp. 61–78). London: Sage.

3

Using Evidence to Support Clinical Practice

Holly Powell Kennedy
Katherine Camacho Carr

What Is Evidence-Based Practice?

Sackett, Strauss, and colleagues (2000) define the elements of evidence-based practice (EBP) or medicine as "the integration of the best research evidence with clinical expertise and patient values" (p. 1). EBP demands a high level of scientific evidence at all decision-making points in a woman's care (Eisenberg, 2001; Sackett, Strauss, Richardson, Rosenberg, & Hayes, 2000). The influence of EBP is increasingly evident in clinical practice, in the education of clinicians, and in management and health policy (Buse, 2008; Eisenberg, 2001; Guyatt & Drummond, 2001; Sackett, Hayes, Guyatt, & Tugwell, 2000; Sackett, Strauss, et al., 2000; Walshe & Rundall, 2001; Wuff & Gotzsche, 2000).

EBP begins with a clinical question or query about best practice and proceeds to identifying and evaluating the best research available to find the answer. To comprehensively and accurately answer the question, there must be integration of clinical experience and patient preferences with the research evidence (See **Box 3-1**). Every clinician is a researcher on some level. As a consequence, each person in clinical practice must solve clinical problems. Sometimes we use evidence generated by other researchers; at other times we conduct research personally. For some clinicians, conducting research may entail a small study to develop a clinical protocol. For others, it may be supervising a clinical trial. Regardless of the scope of the research, the underlying principles are the same. The focus of this chapter is to review research principles, methods, and critique techniques to assist clinicians in developing skills in practice-based research so they can provide care that is truly evidence-based.

> **BOX 3-1** *Principles of Evidence-Based Practice*
>
> - Provides a foundation for practice guidelines, diagnostic testing, and changes in procedures or treatments
> - Forms the evidence base for pathways of care and helps to standardize care or eliminate wide variations in care that may not be efficacious, may not be safe, or may be superfluous
> - Assists with the development of clinical benchmarking and process- or outcome-based performance measures
> - Eliminates unnecessary processes or procedures
> - Sorts through research findings to find therapies that are effective or control costs

A Feminist Perspective on Research

This book is founded on a feminist framework that recognizes hierarchies are an oppressive reality in health care. These hierarchies are implicated in women's health disparities, as well as in the historical lack of research devoted to women's health issues (Doyal, 1995). Wuest (1994) notes that the major goal of feminist research is "seeing the world through the eyes of the other" (p. 578) to emancipate the world from systemic bias based on gender and class. By interpretatively studying social realities, we can move critically to change bias in our culture (Holland, 1990). Most feminists would agree that science is not acontextual or ahistorical—it must understand the woman's history and context of her life. Campbell and Bunting (1991) provide a helpful guide to critiquing research from a feminist perspective that we believe should be considered in the design and evaluation of research:

1. Research should be based on women's experiences.
2. Artificial dichotomies should be scrutinized.
3. The context and relationships of phenomena such as history and concurrent events should be considered.
4. The questions asked are as important as the questions answered.
5. Research should address questions women want answered.
6. The researcher's point of view should be described as part of the data to place the researcher on a plane with the researched.
7. Research should be nonhierarchal; participants and researchers should be partners.
8. Interpretations of observations should be validated and shared with participants.

The History of Evidence-Based Practice

Nursing science has a rich heritage of applying evidence to practice. Florence Nightingale (1859/1957) outlined the basic principles of nursing science in her best-known work, *Notes on Nursing*. The Nightingale method of nursing included rigorous monitoring of all treatments for their effectiveness, which was an early version of EBP. Authority for Nightingale's work in public health and hygiene was based on trial and error, intuition, clinical experience, careful observation, and discussion with patients (McDonald, 2004). This pioneer used statistical data to improve health, sanitation, administration of health services, and nursing education. Nightingale was not a romantic Victorian gentlewoman, but rather a bright, organized, tough feminist and mathematician. She applied statistics to the study of public health and mortality data and invented the polar diagram (pie chart) to display her research findings (Holliday & Parker, 1997; McDonald, 2002). Her work and that of other nurse theorists, researchers, and clinicians provided the foundation for a long tradition in nursing that combines careful scientific observation, sensitivity to the individual's needs, and recognition of the influence of context.

The initiation of the modern EBP movement in health care is attributed to a British epidemiologist, Dr. Archie Cochrane, who was concerned that clinicians often failed to evaluate the effectiveness of their own care and did not have widespread access to the scientific literature (Fullerton-Smith, 1995). His initial work in the 1970s led to the review of all randomized controlled trials in perinatal medicine and ultimately established the Cochrane Collaboration in 1992, which currently has a much wider scope covering reviews in many fields of health care. The Cochrane Database of Systematic Reviews (2004), an electronic database that is part of the Cochrane Library, remains one of the largest, most comprehensive reviews of evidence available.

The EBP movement is often described as a paradigm change in medicine, moving from reliance on expert opinion and experience to reliance on scientific evidence as the basis for practice (Eisenberg, 2001; Evidence-Based Medicine Working Group, 1992; Kuhn, 1970). The present paradigm shift to evidence-based care identifies the best drugs, clinical practices, and surgical procedures through rigorous study with randomized clinical trials (RCTs), meta-analyses, and systematic reviews of the scientific literature forming the primary evidence base for patient care (Sackett, Strauss, et al., 2000). In response to this shift away from expert opinion, there has been a proliferation of articles, books, and websites instructing clinicians how to conduct, evaluate, interpret, and apply the medical literature over the last decade (Guyatt & Drummond, 2001; Oxman, Cook, & Guyatt, 1994; Sackett, Hayes, et al., 2000; Sackett, Strauss, et al., 2000; Wuff & Gotzsche, 2000). (See also Appendix 3-A.) This compendium of resources on EBP supports a shift in the sort of evidence that is most valued for diagnosis, therapeutic decisions and interventions, and questions related to the patient's prognosis (see **Box 3-2**).

An examination of the state of the EBP movement, the philosophy of science, and the state of nursing science, however, suggests that the use of evidence is not a new or revolutionary paradigm shift and may explain only part of the science upon which the change is based (Sehon & Stanley, 2003). Quine (1952), another philosopher of science, describes the scientific worldview as a web of beliefs, like a spider web with an exterior edge or frame secured to an existing structure, and possessing an interconnecting interior of radii and connecting points. Using this metaphor, the web of scientific beliefs can encompass sensory information and new untested theories that now exist on the developing edge of the web. Foundational theories such as the laws of nature, logic, or mathematics form the center of the web. The interconnections between the center and the periphery are composed of well-

---

BOX 3-2 *Applications of Evidence-Based Practice*

- Many types of evidence are used in a variety of clinical decision-making scenarios (e.g., assessments, diagnostic tests, therapies, and treatments).

- The evidence is scrutinized for validity and applicability to the circumstances and the individual patient (i.e., What works? When, where, and why does it work? For whom does it work?).

- Lack of evidence about efficacy is not the same as evidence that something is ineffective. There will be missing evidence about some things.

- EBP uses information technology to make evidence available when needed by the clinician and often the woman herself.

- Clinicians need to have ready access to evidence to support clinical decision making in women's health care.

- While working toward a common goal of providing or receiving the highest-quality health care, clinicians and patients need information they can both understand.

---

proven hypotheses about health and clinical practice. According to the Quinian metaphor, we use a vast network or web of healthcare beliefs with logical and evidential relationships to determine best practices, including the findings of experimental research, primarily RCTs, intuition, and experience (Quine, 1952).

The sciences of medicine and nursing are composed of a vast network of beliefs, scientific observations, practices, hypothetical relationships, and theories. For example, in practice we include observations (blood pressure), hypotheses (how the blood pressure may need to be repeated before we accept that it is an accurate measurement), and theories (the psychophysiology of blood pressure regulation). Quine (1952) also suggests that scientific observations must be contextually examined as part of a whole, rather than being viewed in isolation from the rest of scientific knowledge. The concept of a web of knowledge, along with interconnected relationships between practices and underlying theories, supports a multiple-method approach to examining phenomena. The complexity of the human condition and human psychophysiology also demands multiple approaches to identify best clinical practices, interventions, and medications, and to identify basic scientific knowledge or antecedent plausibility (Goodman, 1999a, 1999b).

A more recent development in health care is the recognition that management of facilities and practices should also be evidence based—an approach termed *evidence-based management*. Managers of healthcare settings are beginning to realize that clinicians are not the only ones who should consider the importance of evidence in the provision of quality care. Walshe and Rundall (2001) note that management is obligated to oversee programs shown to be effective in terms of both quality and cost. Specifically, management has a key role in preventing the overuse of interventions not shown to be effective, the underuse of those interventions that are effective, and misuse when the evidence is unclear (Kohn, Corrigan,

& Donaldson, 1999). Managers must work in concert with clinicians and women to provide evidence-based programs and an environment of care that will be most conducive to quality outcomes, as well as prove efficient and cost-effective.

Decisions about which evidence and outcomes are most important should not be made in a vacuum. Studies have found that the clinical settings most effective in EBP implementation have a culture of adapting to change and encouraging strong nursing and obstetric leadership (Graham, Logan, Davies, & Nimrod, 2004). Main and colleagues (Main, Bloomfield, & Hunt, 2004; Main et al., 2006) found that using a multidisciplinary task force to choose benchmarks grounded in evidence and most accessible for measurement was the most helpful strategy for effecting change. Buse (2008) specifically calls for prospective policy analysis using research and best information relevant to stakeholders in care to provide effective and efficient healthcare systems.

Much of our existing science in medicine and nursing comes from a variety of sources, not all of which are evidence based. There is not always "one best way" to obtain scientific information about clinical practice. For this reason, we must remain open to and creative about research methods that will give us the best answer or will help us better define the interconnected web of knowledge related to the phenomena of interest. Nursing science values multiple ways of knowing because clinical practice is a complex and multidimensional process, and patients are unique human beings who each define health and illness differently (Mitchell, 1999).

Research and Clinical Decision Making

Research and practice are reciprocally linked in the web of healthcare knowledge (Lanuza, 1999). Clinical questions provide the basis for research; research provides a way to evaluate the safety and efficacy of practice. In other words, practice and science are mutually informative (Barrett, 2002). We also know that the knowledge needed for practice is based not only on research, but also on intuition, experience, tradition, and common sense (Ervin, 2002).

The educational preparation of clinicians usually includes core content on the research process. This can range from actual participation in research studies to general discussions about how to apply research findings to practice. Unfortunately, the word "research" can engender anxiety in many clinicians who are years removed from their educational experience. Research, like any skill, must be used on a regular basis to be effective.

One basic premise that helps clinicians shed their tentativeness in either considering conducting research or applying research to clinical practice is the need to reformulate how they think about the entire subject. Research follows the exact same principles that any good clinician follows in everyday clinical management. These principles are ongoing and often circular in nature. One step usually leads to another, but can also raise new questions that take you either back to the beginning or in a new direction. **Table 3-1** outlines the steps in the clinical management and research processes.

TABLE 3-1 Alignment of Clinical and Research Processes

The Clinical Management Process	The Research Process
Gathering the Data	
• Focused toward individual clinical scenario.	• Focused on a broader perspective of a health issue.
• Historical, physical, and laboratory data may be gathered.	• Historical data, review of literature, and pilot study may be involved.
Identifying the Problem	
• Assessment is made of the individual's clinical problem.	• A research question and/or hypothesis is generated.
Development of the Plan	
• An evidence-based clinical management plan is developed to meet the client's needs.	• A research design is constructed that will best answer the research question.
Implementation	
• The management plan is implemented.	• The research study is conducted.
Evaluation of the Results	
• Clinical follow-up is conducted to assess the effectiveness of the treatment plan.	• Data are analyzed to provide answers to the research questions.

Types of Research Evidence

Research evidence comes in many forms. We prefer to call them *types* of evidence, rather than *levels*, to dispel the notion that one is necessarily better than another, or to suggest linearity. As previously mentioned, clinical experience and patient preferences are two parts of the triad of clinical decision-making criteria. To complete the triad, they are combined with an evaluation of current clinical research.

The RCT is often held up as the "gold standard" in Western medicine, but not all clinical problems lend themselves to this kind of research. Whatever research method is used must serve the research question being asked, and the results should be evaluated in terms of the quality of the study and the potential benefit or harm to the patient. In the United States, the U.S. Preventive Services Task Force takes the lead on setting guidelines for evaluating healthcare research evidence (Harris et al., 2001). **Table 3-2** summarizes this approach.

Research Methods to Inform Clinical Practice

The historically defined parameters of science, particularly in the Western tradition, can create tension among researchers and clinicians as to what truly qualifies as scientific evidence.

TABLE 3-2 Recommendations for Using Research Evidence in Clinical Practice

U.S. Preventive Services Task Force Ratings—Strength of Recommendations

The U.S. Preventive Services Task Force grades its recommendations about specific health services or treatments according to one of five classifications, which reflect the strength of evidence and magnitude of net benefit (benefits minus harms).

A   Strongly recommended—There is good evidence that the service or treatment improves important health outcomes and benefits substantially outweigh harms.

B   Recommended—There is at least fair evidence that the service or treatment improves important health outcomes and benefits outweigh harms.

C   No recommendation for or against provision of the service or treatment—There is at least fair evidence that the service or treatment can improve health outcomes, but the balance of benefits and harms is too close to justify a general recommendation.

D   Recommends against—There is at least fair evidence that the service or treatment is ineffective and harms outweigh benefits.

I   Insufficient to recommend for or against—Evidence that the service or treatment is effective is lacking, of poor quality, or conflicting, and the balance of benefits and harms cannot be determined.

Quality of Evidence	Net Benefit			
	Substantial	Moderate	Small	Negative
Good: Evidence includes consistent results from well-designed, well-conducted studies in representative populations that directly assess effects on health outcomes.	A	B	C	D
Fair: Evidence is sufficient to determine effects on health outcomes, but the strength of the evidence is limited by the number, quality, or consistency of the individual studies, generalizability to routine practice, or indirect nature of the evidence on health outcomes.	B	B	C	D
Poor: Evidence is insufficient to assess the effects on health outcomes because of limited number or power of studies, important flaws in their design or conduct, gaps in the chain of evidence, or lack of information on important health outcomes.	Poor = I			

Hierarchy of Research Designs

I   Evidence obtained from at least one properly conducted, randomized controlled trial.

II-1   Evidence obtained from well-designed controlled trials without randomization.

II-2   Evidence obtained from well-designed cohort or case-control analytic studies, preferably from more than one center or research group.

II-3   Evidence obtained from multiple time series with or without the intervention. Dramatic results in uncontrolled experiments (such as the introduction of penicillin treatment in the 1940s) could be regarded as this type of evidence.

III   Opinions of respected authorities, based on clinical experience, descriptive studies and case reports, or reports of expert committees.

Source: Adapted from Harris et al., 2001.

Both quantitative and qualitative research approaches employ a variety of methods and techniques, and both aim to expand knowledge about a specific phenomenon. Attempting to pinpoint a defining difference between the two creates the possibility of oversimplifying the complexity of each. Our goal is to help you understand the differences, understand what is credible from both perspectives, and decide what is applicable to your practice and research. We do not seek to debate whether one approach is better than another, because such a judgment assumes one approach has more truth-value than the other. In reality, both approaches help us to fill in the "open spaces in the web of knowledge," according to Quine (1952).

Research often begins with a clinical problem or question that needs an answer. This problem or question usually arises from a broad topical area, so the first task of the researcher is to clearly define the problem. Research questions can be inspired by everyday practice or emerge from other research studies, especially where discrepancies, inconsistencies, or remaining questions about patient care practices, interventions, or products used exist. Social or policy issues, such as access to care, models of care, effects of racism or gender bias on health, health disparities, poverty, and violence, can also give rise to research questions.

The question is then translated into research aims, or what the study proposes to do. Minimally the aims should meet two criteria: reveal a gap in our current knowledge and be significant (National Institutes of Health, 2001). This means your exploration of the literature must reveal a lack of prior research in this area that could specifically address your questions. It also means that the results of the study could make a difference in the healthcare delivery or outcomes for the population being studied.

Quantitative Research

Quasi-experimental design is similar to experimental design but does not include random assignment of participants to an experimental or control group for practical, ethical, or other reasons. This weakness prohibits causal inference, because it can no longer be assumed that the two groups are equal. That is, the findings might be explained by differences between the groups or some other factor. Most researchers try to establish some control over these extraneous variables by matching groups or by establishing group equivalency with a variety of quasi-experimental designs and statistical analyses (Polit & Beck, 2008). The strength of the quasi-experimental design lies in its practicality and feasibility in the real world of health care and informed choice, where subjects often cannot be randomly assigned to groups.

Nonexperimental research answers questions that do not lend themselves to manipulation of a variable. For example, if we want to study the effects of the death of a child on the mother, the independent variable (the death of a child) is clearly not something that can be manipulated or controlled. Nevertheless, control and experimental groups could be identified, consisting of those mothers who did not experience the death of a child and those who did (as the death naturally occurs), respectively. Psychological and physical well-being could still be described and measured and compared in both groups, but cause and effect cannot be determined. In this kind of study, a vast array of human factors cannot be manipulated and, therefore, cannot be studied experimentally (Polit & Beck, 2008). They can, however, be described and interrelationships can be examined with nonexperimental research.

Meta-analyses and systematic reviews are considered to be highly reliable forms of evidence. Meta-analysis uses the single study as the unit of analysis and statistically combines the findings of several similarly designed studies on the same topic. This method provides a standardized way to compare findings across studies, adding together larger numbers to observe patterns and relationships that might not have otherwise been observed in a single study (Polit & Beck, 2008). A well-conducted meta-analysis allows for a more objective assessment of the evidence obtained in RCTs, especially where findings from multiple studies have produced disagreement or uncertainty. This consideration might be important when testing a new drug, procedure, or intervention that may have different effects in subgroups or varying results in different studies.

Systematic review is the method used to analyze a general body of scientific data using clearly defined criteria. Systematic reviews can include meta-analyses, appraisals of single trials, and other sources of evidence. Great care is taken to find all relevant published and unpublished studies, assess each study, synthesize the findings, present a balanced and unbiased summary of the findings, and consider any flaws that may be present in the evidence. Many high-quality systematic reviews are available in journals and online, most notably the Cochrane Library. The need for rigor in systematic review has led to a formal process for their conduct. Although meta-analysis always uses a quantitative statistical analysis of the findings, systematic review may include a quantitative meta-analytic combination of study results, or a more qualitative summary of the aggregated data (Davies & Crombie, 2001).

Rigor in Quantitative Research

Just like clinical practice, quality research depends on adherence to standards to ensure that it is conducted accurately and ethically. The description of the research design must be clear so the reader can fully assess what took place and could replicate the study if desired. Errors in any step of the process will invalidate the results. This possibility can be minimized through careful attention to the accuracy of the instruments used for measurement, appropriate sample selection, and understanding of how to apply the findings in the acceptance or rejection of the research hypotheses.

Variables must be well defined—you must be sure you understand what is being tested and measured. Validity indicates how well the measurement actually measures the variable. For example, a sphygmomanometer must accurately reflect a blood pressure measurement. The reliability of the measure indicates how consistently it performs. For machines operated by humans, reliability includes how well the operator conducts the measurement (e.g., using the correct size cuff and positioning each time a measurement is obtained).

A research sample must reflect the population it is meant to represent. Error is minimized by use of appropriate sampling techniques and random assignment to study groups. For example, if you were measuring the reporting of menopausal symptoms, you might find a difference in prevalence if you obtained your sample from a women's clinic (where women might be seeking therapy) versus shoppers at a local supermarket (where there might be a more representative population). In addition, where the supermarket is located might affect the outcome because of socioeconomic or cultural differences that may bias the results. These issues can potentially affect the generalizability of the study findings—that is, the ability to apply the results to populations other than the sample group studied. The size of the sample reflects its "power" and also affects the research findings. A sample that is too small will not have enough power to detect a significant difference between study groups. Likewise, a too-large sample may provide significant results related to size only, rather than producing meaningful findings (Munro, 2001).

There are two commonly cited types of errors in research—Type I and Type II (Polit & Beck, 2008). A Type I error is made when the researcher concludes that a relationship exists—Drug A is effective in treating Disease X—when it actually does not (a "false positive" in clinical terms). The differences observed between the groups are often due to a sampling error such as self-selection bias. Random assignment to groups controls for sampling error and associated Type I error. The level of significance, referred to as *alpha* (α) and reported as a *p* value, will also influence a Type I error. The most frequently used levels of significance (i.e., alpha levels) are .05 and .01. With a .05 alpha, the researcher accepts the probability that out of 100 samples, a true hypothesis will be falsely rejected only 5 times, and in 95 out of 100 samples a true hypothesis will be correctly accepted. With a .01 alpha, there is only 1 chance out of 100 that the true hypothesis will be falsely rejected, so this level of significance makes the incidence of Type I error lower. Usually, the minimal acceptable level of significance in quantitative research is .05.

A Type II error, also called *beta* (β), is made when the researcher concludes that no relationship exists when it actually does (a "false negative" in clinical terms). As the risk of a Type I error decreases, the risk of a Type II error increases. Researchers try to avoid both Type I and Type II errors. To do so, they frequently conduct a power analysis of a sample size, while taking into account the desired level of significance (alpha level) and the probability of Type II error (beta). Random sampling, random assignment to groups to avoid selection bias, and adequate sample size are all steps that can help researchers avoid these kinds of errors.

Confidence intervals provide more information than *p* values because they give a range of values and allow inference of the true placement of a parameter applied to the population (Munro, 2001). The range specifies where the parameter (e.g., the mean) is most likely to lie (Polit & Beck, 2008). Most confidence ranges are set at 95%; they provide a statement of the level of confidence the researcher has about the findings.

Qualitative Research

Qualitative research methods use different techniques and answer different questions than quantitative research methods. Guba and Lincoln (1998) propose that how we perceive reality provides the backdrop for how we conduct science. This sets the stage for understanding the nature between the knower (researcher) and what can be known, commonly called epistemology. Together they form the question asked about method: How does one choose a way to learn about the world?

A person's view of the world shapes the answer to this question and influences his or her entire approach to science. Denzin and Lincoln (1998) suggest that scientists who value qualitative research believe that reality is relative and never completely apprehended. They believe there are many ways to tell and hear a story. The richness and details of the individual story provide the data we need to extend our knowledge of the world. The individual's point of view within the constraints of everyday life can only be known from the specifics of each case and cannot be controlled. Scientists using qualitative methods believe the researcher cannot be fully removed from the participants. For this reason, they sometimes call this type of research "naturalistic" because the testing usually takes place in a setting that is not controlled.

These perspectives differ in fundamental ways from the more objectivist stance of traditional Western science, in which quantitative methods—and particularly the RCT—are highly valued. Ultimately, however, the key features are the different language used and the different perspective assumed. Each has its place and role; each can inform the other. One induces why something happens, and the other deduces the reason or explanation of why it happens. A simple example is the development of a hypothesis from clinical observations and discussions with women that a specific method of contraception causes weight gain (qualitative findings). To support this hypothesis, a study using quantitative methods can be designed to examine whether this actually does occur.

The research questions most appropriate for qualitative methods are often exploratory. Why do things happen? What does it feel like? What does it mean? How should I interpret this result? All of these questions are excellent candidates for the use of qualitative methods. Such questions can arise from either clinical problems or specific gaps in clinical evidence.

A variety of lenses serve as the underlying basis for the traditions of qualitative research. The term *bricoleur* is often applied to a scientist who can navigate these traditions and lenses to answer the original research question and those that emerge as the study progresses. A bricoleur is characterized by his or her ability to "put together a complex array of data, derived from a variety of sources, and using a variety of methods" (Polit & Beck, 2008, p. 219). Skills required to accomplish this feat include astute observation, reflection, interpretation, and introspection.

Qualitative Research Design and Methods

Qualitative research explores a problem by induction and often moves toward hypothesis or theory development. Data are derived from multiple sources, such as interviews, fieldwork, observations, videotapes, art, media, and other documents, but are usually textual in composition rather than numerical. The researcher is considered to be the "instrument," and his or her role is closely tied to the collection and interpretation of the data. Sometimes the researcher is also a participant, such as in fieldwork where observations of specific clinical practices are being conducted. This can lead to an increase in trust between the participants being observed and the researcher.

Qualitative studies are descriptive from the perspective of those who have experienced a particular phenomenon; therefore, samples are not random, but rather "purposive" (Speziale & Carpenter, 2003). This means specific research participants are sought who can shed the most light on the research problem. For example, if you wanted to learn about the experience of postpartum depression, it would be fruitless to interview people who had never been exposed to the phenomenon.

To refine ideas based on emerging findings in the data analysis, the researcher may "theoretically sample" to answer specific questions (Charmaz, 2000). Sample size is usually not predetermined, and the power of the samples used in qualitative studies reflects the robust richness of the textual data. Data collection usually continues until the researcher observes saturation or redundancy, or until nothing new is coming to light or being observed. Data analysis is conducted in a variety of ways, but usually produces findings that are richly descriptive in textual or thematic language.

Choosing from among the many qualitative methods requires that the researcher have an understanding of his or her disciplinary focus. Each area has its own complexity and methodology (a topic that goes beyond the scope of this chapter). For an easier understanding of some of the basic methods, the various qualitative research approaches have been organized here using general categories adapted from Polit and Beck (2008) to reflect the area of knowledge they explore.

Understanding the Experiences and Processes of Health and Illness

Many of our research questions address what it is like to go through a certain health event, for the purpose of helping us find ways to improve life for others who have similar experiences. These approaches focus on understanding the basic experiences and processes of how a person moves through the event. The methods come from the traditions of philosophy and sociology.

Phenomenology is derived from a philosophical tradition that provides a "textual reflection on the lived experiences and practical actions of everyday life with the intent to increase one's thoughtfulness and practical resourcefulness or tact" (van Manen, 1990, p. 4). The focus is on understanding what it is like for this person to be in this experience within the context of his or her life. The work is interpretative or hermeneutical. The findings are often presented as paradigm cases or exemplars, creating "a dialogue between practical concerns and lived experience through engaged reasoning and imaginative dwelling in the immediacy of the participant's worlds" (Benner, 1994, p. 99). The results provide a vivid description that can help us to better understand the social, political, or historical context of the individual's experience (Polit & Beck, 2008).

Asking questions from the tradition of sociology assists us in understanding how social structures and human interactions affect people's experience of health and illness (Polit & Beck, 2008; Speziale & Carpenter, 2003). These approaches range from understanding how people make sense of their social interactions (symbolic interaction) to discovering how social processes are structured and developed (grounded theory). Charon (1992) describes four central foci of symbolic interactionism:

- The nature of the social interaction
- Human action that both causes and results from social interaction
- Present rather than past focus
- Actions of the person who is unpredictable and active in his or her world

Grounded theory was developed by Glaser and Strauss in the 1960s as a research method that addresses both the chief concern or problem for people and the basic processes available to address that concern (Glaser, 1978, 1992; Strauss & Corbin, 1998). The goal of this approach is to develop theory in a substantive area that is grounded directly from the data. Grounded theories "are likely to offer insight, enhance understanding, and provide a meaningful guide to action" (Strauss & Corbin, 1998, p. 12). One example is Quinn's (1991) work on the process women go through during perimenopause.

Understanding Human Behavior

The tradition of psychology focuses specifically on how and why people act; its aim is to describe behavior. Studying human behavior can help us understand how behaviors are related to health and illness. Ethology examines the evolution of human behavior in its natural context (Polit & Beck, 2008); observations of human behavior are used to expose structures essential to life. One example is the observation of attachment behaviors as necessary and instinctive to survival (Ardovini, 2002; Sable, 2004). This observational approach can also be used from an environmental perspective, as in ecological psychology. Ecological models examine the relationship of environmental influences with specific human attributes (Humpel et al., 2004). For example, immigration status (acculturation into a new environment) has been demonstrated to be a risk factor for psychological distress and unhealthy eating behaviors (Skreblin & Sujoldzic, 2003).

Learning how people communicate is another approach to learning about human behavior. Human communication has many processes and forms. Scientists explore the construction of meaning in the nuances of these processes. To do so, they use methods derived from both sociology and linguistics. Sociolinguistics is the examination of the forms and rules of conversation through discourse analysis (Polit & Beck, 2008). Mishler (1984) proposes that by examining the talk between clinicians and patients, we can encourage the development of noncoercive discourse and humane clinical practice.

Understanding Cultural Traditions and Influences

One of the oldest qualitative traditions comes from the field of anthropology, where scientists strive to understand cultural variations among the many peoples of the world. Although several approaches are used in this disciplinary area, ethnography is the most common.

An ethnographer's goal is to carefully describe a specific culture. Historically, grand ethnographies often explored indigenous peoples. In health-related research, smaller specific subsets are often the focus of study. For example, Ka'opua and Mueller (2004) studied how cultural values and social support practices relate to adherence to highly active antiretroviral therapy for HIV among Native Hawaiians, a group with historic difficulty in using Western healthcare services because of cultural conflict.

Synthesizing Qualitative Research Findings

Meta-synthesis is another qualitative method. This research method analyzes, synthesizes, and interprets a specified body of research and holds the potential to provide valuable insight and knowledge about the distinctive aspects of a phenomenon (Kennedy, Rousseau, & Kane Low, 2003). It shares some commonalties with the type of meta-analysis conducted in quantitative research, but is distinguished by some important differences. Meta-synthesis provides an organized, yet interpretive approach to a specific group of qualitative studies (Noblit & Hare, 1988). Sandelowski and her colleagues (1997) note that it is essential to systematically examine qualitative findings about a specific phenomenon to keep from repeating ourselves if we are to change practice and policy making. The meta-synthesis method involves identifying similar qualitative studies about a particular phenomenon, determining how they are related, and synthesizing the findings. This analysis entails more than a systematic review; it becomes an interpretative study itself.

Rigor in Qualitative Research

Just as in quantitative research, a clearly articulated study design is essential to understanding the purpose and results of any qualitative project. Because qualitative research uses textual rather than numerical data, relative terms such as *trustworthiness* or *dependability* are used to describe results, whereas *error* is used as the corresponding term with quantitative study results (Speziale & Carpenter, 2003). Specific terminology associated with qualitative research can help you assess whether the results of such studies are valid and reliable.

Credibility reflects how much confidence you have in the study results (Polit & Beck, 2008). It is enhanced by complete descriptions of the sample and setting, data collection, analytic procedures, the way in which decisions were made, and the researcher's role in the study. Preparation and experience with the methods and acknowledgment of preconceived ideas, sometimes called bracketing, are helpful in understanding the researcher's perspective and influence on the study. This practice is similar to evaluating whether a specific statistical test is appropriate in a quantitative study.

A qualitative study should provide enough documentation for the results to be confirmed—a characteristic sometimes called *confirmability* (Polit & Beck, 2008). Confirmability helps to ensure that later researchers can follow the analysis and understand how decisions were made. The findings are enhanced when there is evidence that a team of researchers was involved with peer debriefing and searches for negative cases (Polit & Beck). These procedures allow the research team to reflect on their analysis and to check for bias and interpretative errors. Another approach, called *member checking*, has study participants read and react to the researchers' analytic decisions to see if their findings reflect their personal experience with the phenomenon under investigation.

All research findings should make conceptual sense. The investigators should provide enough thick, rich description to prove that the results clearly fit with the data presented. *Transferability* refers to how well the findings can be applied to another setting and is similar to the concept of *generalizability* in quantitative research (Polit & Beck, 2008). A study should provide enough evidence in the description of the study to help you assess whether the findings could apply to your setting.

Mixed Research Methods

Sometimes the research questions beg for a mixed method approach—that is, a combination of quantitative and qualitative methods. There are multiple ways to combine methods. Perhaps one method is more dominant than the other, or perhaps research is conducted sequentially using the various methods (Tashakkori & Teddlie, 1998). A helpful way to think about this issue is to consider how different lenses help you see different things. You might design a study that examines how a specific intervention affects a woman's perinatal outcomes and health behaviors (quantitative measures). Yet, within the same study, you could also interview women (qualitative methods) about the experience of the intervention—how it affected their lives.

Another term appropriate to this discussion is triangulation, which refers to the use of multiple referents to capture a more complete and contextualized picture of the phenomenon under investigation (Polit & Beck, 2008). This approach may involve the use of multiple sources of data, time collection points, sites, and samples, all providing different perspectives on the same research question.

Moving from Best Evidence to Best Practice

Research can improve practice by providing answers to clinical questions; evaluating the safety, effectiveness, or cost of therapeutics; refining practice guidelines; or testing theories relevant to practice (Lanuza, 1999). Increased access to research evidence that has been reviewed, compiled, and analyzed by a variety of credible resources enhances our ability to obtain and apply research findings. Resources that help us fulfill this goal include the Cochrane Collaboration, professional organizations, and government agencies. A comprehensive list of resources is included in Appendix 3-A. This information has been made available via the Internet so it is readily available to the busy clinician. Yet clinicians continue to struggle with the issue how to apply the results of research to practice: How do you actually make it happen?

As clinicians, we must be able to use the computer and must be familiar with the EBP resources in all fields of health. We must also be cognizant of the criticisms and limitations of EBP, including over-reliance on RCT-derived results and systematic reviews, an emphasis on the routinization of practice, and the daunting effort required to stay current, as today's evidence may be tomorrow's inappropriate practice (Kim, 2000).

Clinicians must be able to critically appraise individual studies to determine how much faith should be put into their findings. The strengths and weaknesses of each study must be readily identifiable. Evidence hierarchies rank studies according to the strength of the evidence they provide (Polit & Beck, 2008). Most such hierarchies put meta-analyses of RCTs at the top and opinions of experts at the bottom. Owing to this tendency, there is some concern that using such hierarchies inevitably emphasizes a scientific and rational focus and assumes causation (the design of the tightly woven web structure) can be identified only by rigorous quantitative study. This approach fails to recognize the gaps in the web of knowledge and discounts qualitative research or naturalistic observations that focus on the understanding of the human experience. EBP attempts to escape this reductionist approach by integrating information from a variety of well-designed studies, clinical experience, existing resources, and the woman's preference. When developing clinical practice guidelines, protocols, or clinical pathways, all of these elements should be included (Camacho Carr, 2000). No single study or group of studies can provide an infallible answer to a clinical question.

The Stetler (2001) model of research utilization was designed to help individual clinicians, as well as organizations, move the best evidence into the practice setting. Individual clinicians or organizations can use this model to critically analyze the research evidence and apply the findings to real-world practice (see **Figure 3-1**).

The current model includes five sequential phases:

1. The preparation phase includes the identification of the purpose of the project and the searching, sorting, and selection of the research evidence.
2. The validation phase involves a critique of the evidence.
3. If the evidence is found to be sound, then the process continues to the comparative evaluation and decision-making stage. The evidence is synthesized, and four criteria—fit of the setting, feasibility, current practice, and substantiating evidence—are used to assess the applicability of the evidence. Fit with the setting examines the similarity of the study's environment with the one in which the findings will be applied and compares the characteristics of the study population with the client population where the evidence will be applied. Feasibility implies that potential benefits outweigh any risk to patients, resources for implementation are available, and the involved persons are ready for change. Congruency with current practice philosophy and values must also be considered.
4. The translation application phase is when a dissemination plan is developed and strategies that need to be changed are revised.
5. In the evaluation phase, the level of successful integration of the evidence into practice must be assessed.

Using a model such as the one proposed by Stetler (2001) can make EBP more focused and acceptable to those clinicians who assert, "This is the way we've always done it." Integrat-

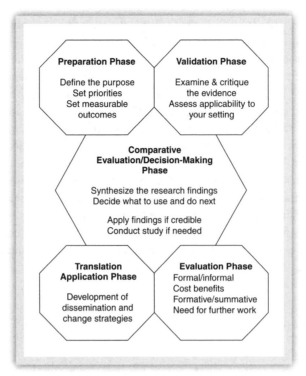

FIGURE 3-1 Conceptual adaptation of the Stetler model for applying research findings into clinical practice.

ing a methodical approach to applying evidence to practice can be effective in overcoming this all too frequently encountered mantra.

Barriers to Using Research Evidence in Clinical Practice

The two most common reasons clinicians and students cite for their failure to apply the latest research evidence are (1) lack of confidence in critiquing research studies and (2) lack of time to find the studies. We empathize with both concerns, and offer some practical strategies to overcome them in this section.

Critiquing Research Studies

Critiquing research studies takes practice and some basic knowledge about how research is conducted. We suggest that all clinicians have a basic research text on their bookshelf to look up unfamiliar terms and statistics. We have used Polit and Beck's (2008) *Nursing Research: Generating and Assessing Evidence for Nursing Practice* to provide some structure for this chapter and find it easy to read and practically written; however, many other good basic texts are available. *The Journal of the American Medical Association* has also compiled an extensive set of *Users' Guides to the Medical Literature* that are both instructive and illustrative (Giacomini, 2000a, 2000b; Guyatt & Drummond, 2001).

To assess applicability of any research findings to patient care, clinicians must evaluate the validity of the research; determine the practicality of implementing the findings; weigh any associated risks and benefits to the patient; and consider the ethical issues, available resources, and cost. Clinicians applying EBP guidelines must be able to recognize the limitations of the available databases as well as the limitations of scientific evidence. They must also know how to integrate clinical expertise, ethical considerations, patient individuality, and choice into the decision-making process. Additional objectives of EBP may include cost reduction, a desire to reduce wide variation in healthcare practices, and the desire to include clients as partners in their own care (Agency for Healthcare Research and Quality, 2004b; Gray, Hayes, Sackett, Cook, & Guyatt, 1997). None of these ideas is novel to clinicians.

Table 3-3 provides a brief summary of important points to consider when evaluating the quality of a research study and determining whether you should apply the findings to your practice.

TABLE 3-3 Practical Points in Critiquing Research Studies

Title

Does the title of the article accurately describe the study? Is the language that is used in the title understandable and informative?

Abstract

Does the abstract accurately present the study? It should state the purpose of the study, the problems that were investigated, the research question or hypotheses, a description of the study design and the methodology used, the sample, instruments used, other data collection procedures, and the results or findings.

Research Questions and Purpose of the Study

What are the research questions? Are these questions researchable in the sense that they can be carried out by the investigators? What is the significance of the study in terms of practice, adding to the body of scientific knowledge, etc.? Are the research questions stated in a concise and precise manner?

Research Variables

Can you delineate the independent and dependent variables if it is a quantitative study? Is the phenomenon of study clear if it is a qualitative study?

Review of the Literature and Conceptual Frameworks/Model

Is the literature review relevant to the study? Does it include timely as well as classic articles that pertain to the study? Does the review provide adequate background information? Do the authors state how this review provides support for their study (i.e., give background information for the identified research problem/question)?

TABLE 3-3 Practical Points in Critiquing Research Studies *(Continued)*

Sample and Setting

Is there a description of how the sample was selected and the location of the study? What are the sources of bias, if any, that are associated with the sample selection process. Were power and effect size calculated for this study? In qualitative studies was the sample purposive, and when was sampling stopped?

Ethical Considerations

Do the authors address protection of human study participants? Did they obtain permission to conduct this study in the setting?

Method: The Design

Is the design appropriate for the research questions? Is it described? What extraneous variables are associated with the design, if any? Are they identified? Is the description adequate enough to allow replication of the entire study?

The Instrumentation and Data Collection Procedures

How are issues of scientific rigor addressed? Are validity and reliability of the instruments described? Was collection of data conducted in a standardized manner? In qualitative research, is the "researcher as instrument" described?

Data Analysis

Are the analytic techniques supportive and appropriate for the research design? Does the article include supportive graphs, tables, or charts? Do these help to describe the results? Are they easily understood?

Results

Do the results follow logically from the design and method? Do the authors describe the results in a way that is understandable and clear? Do the results answer the research question(s) or hypotheses?

Summary and Conclusions

What is your overall impression of the study? Does the author convince you about the conclusions that are drawn? Do the conclusions seem logical in light of the method and procedures, etc.?

Source: Adapted from lectures and presentations by Judith Fullerton, CNM, PhD, FACNM at the American College of Nurse-Midwives Annual Meeting 2002, Atlanta, GA.

Finding the Relevant Research

Today's information-rich world places the most recent research virtually at your fingertips. It is important to realize, however, that published findings are inevitably outdated the minute they hit the press. Journal articles can take one to two years from first submission to printed page, and textbooks take even longer to hit the market. The advent of the Internet, however, has substantially improved our ability to keep up with the most recently published research.

Several excellent sources provide the best evidence in a succinct format for the busy clinician, including the Cochrane Database of Systematic Reviews from the Cochrane Collaboration, an organization that makes up-to-date, accurate information about the effects of health care readily available worldwide. It produces and disseminates systematic reviews of healthcare interventions and promotes the search for evidence in the form of clinical trials and other well-controlled studies (Cochrane Database of Systematic Reviews, 2004). MEDLINE, the National Library of Medicine's database of more than 4500 peer-reviewed biomedical journals, is another excellent source for research findings, although the reader must evaluate most of the studies to determine their scientific merit and clinical applicability. The Agency for Healthcare Research and Quality (2004a) provides evidence reports and technology assessments, consisting of technical reviews on many clinical topics. The Database of Abstracts of Reviews of Effectiveness (2004) is another healthcare-related database, produced at the University of York in England; it provides quality-assessed evidence reviews. Many other agencies and organizations prepare evidence-based guidelines and protocols, which can usually be accessed conveniently on the Internet. Additional resources for EBP are listed in Appendix 3-A.

Conclusion

As a clinician, when considering the issue of research, it is helpful to look at what using evidence in practice actually means. Examples of applying evidence to clinical practice abound—from the choice of pharmaceutical versus alternative therapies for vaginitis, to whether women need continuous electronic fetal monitoring during labor. Every clinical scenario faced will need to be addressed from the perspective of your personal experience, the woman's desires, and the best evidence to support your recommendations. Your first challenge is to blend these considerations artfully in everyday practice. Your second challenge is to work within the healthcare system to influence management and policy makers to use the best information and evidence possible to provide the highest quality of care.

If you walk away with anything from this chapter, it should be the following lesson: Question everything. These questions need not immobilize you, but should set the stage for thinking critically about the causes of clinical problems and ways to search for the best evidence available. Women will be your partners on this path of discovery, as they access the Internet and come to you with questions about different strategies in their health care.

For example, a recent study by Johnson and colleagues (2004) surmises that the theory that women are born with a finite number of oocytes is questionable. If the results of their research on mice are extrapolated, they propose that we may actually use stem cells to continue reproducing oocytes—a finding that could significantly affect the way we look at fertility in the future. Dr. Allen Spradling of the Carnegie Institution in Washington was interviewed about this study on National Public Radio (Hamilton, 2004). His personal reaction to this rather stunning paradigm shift was chagrin with himself for never questioning the original theory of a finite set of oocytes: "I shouldn't have believed that. Why wasn't I more skeptical?" As clinicians and researchers, we should never be caught wondering, "Why didn't I ask the question?" We owe it to women and to ourselves to search for the best evidence to support our healthcare practices.

References

Agency for Healthcare Research and Quality. (2004a). *Evidence Reports and Technology Assessments*. Retrieved from http://www.ahcpr.gov/clinic

Agency for Healthcare Research and Quality. (2004b). *National Guideline Clearinghouse fact sheet: Clinical practice guidelines*. Retrieved from http://www.ahcpr.gov/clinic/cpgsix.htm

Ardovini, C. (2002). Attachment theory, metacognitive functions and the therapeutic relationship in eating disorders. *Eating and Weight Disorders, 7*(4), 328–331.

Barrett, E. A. (2002). What is nursing science? *Nursing Science Quarterly, 15*(1), 51–60.

Benner, P. (1994). The tradition and skill of interpretive phenomenology in studying health, illness, and caring practices. In P. Benner (Ed.), *Interpretive phenomenology: Embodiment, caring, and ethics in health and illness* (pp. 99–127). Thousand Oaks, CA: Sage.

Buse, K. (2008). Addressing the theoretical, practical, and ethical challenges inherent in prospective health policy analysis. *Health Policy and Planning, 23*(5), 351–360. Retrieved from http://heapol.oxfordjournals.org/content/23/5/351.full

Camacho Carr, K. (2000). Developing an evidence-based practice protocol: Implications for midwifery practice. *Journal of Midwifery & Women's Health, 45*(6), 544–551.

Campbell, J. C., & Bunting, S. (1991). Voices and paradigms: Perspectives on critical and feminist theory in nursing. *Advances in Nursing Science, 13*(3), 1–15.

Charmaz, K. (2000). Grounded theory: Objectivist and constructivist methods. In N. K. Denzin & Y. S. Lincoln (Eds.), *Handbook of qualitative research* (2nd ed., pp. 509–535). Thousand Oaks, CA: Sage.

Charon, J. M. (1992). *Symbolic interactionism: An introduction, an interpretation, an integration* (4th ed.). Englewood Cliffs, NJ: Prentice Hall.

Cochrane Database of Systematic Reviews. (2004). London: BMJ Publishing Group. Retrieved from http://www.update-software.com/cochrane

Database of Abstracts of Reviews of Effectiveness. (2004). Retrieved from http://agatha.york.ac.uk/darehp.htm

Davies, H. T. O., & Crombie, I. K. (2001). *What is a systematic review?* Retrieved from http://www.evidence-based-medicine.co.uk

Denzin, N. K., & Lincoln, Y. S. (Eds.). (1998). *The landscape of qualitative research: Theories and issues*. Thousand Oaks, CA: Sage.

Doyal, L. (1995). *What makes women sick? Gender and the political economy of health*. New Brunswick, NJ: Rutgers University Press.

Eisenberg, J. M. (2001). *Evidence-based medicine: Expert voices*. Washington, DC: Agency for Healthcare Research and Quality.

Ervin, C. E. (2002). Evidence-based nursing practice: Are we there yet? *Journal of the New York State Nurses Association, 33*(2), 11–16.

Evidence-Based Medicine Working Group. (1992). Evidence-based medicine: A new approach to teaching the practice of medicine. *Journal of the American Medical Association, 268*(17), 2420–2425.

Fullerton-Smith, I. (1995). How members of the Cochrane Collaboration prepare and maintain systematic reviews of the effects of health care. *Evidence-Based Medicine, 1*, 7–8.

Giacomini, M. K. (2000a). Users guide to the medical literature: XXIII. Qualitative research in health care. A. Are the results of the study valid? *Journal of the American Medical Association, 284*(3), 357–362.

Giacomini, M. K. (2000b). Users guide to the medical literature: XXIII. Qualitative research in health care. B. What are the results and how do they help me care for my patients? *Journal of the American Medical Association, 284*(4), 478–482.

Glaser, B. G. (1978). *Theoretical sensitivity*. Mill Valley, CA: Sociology Press.

Glaser, B. G. (1992). *Basics of grounded theory analysis*. Mill Valley, CA: Sociology Press.

Goodman, S. N. (1999a). Toward evidence-based medical statistics, 1. The *p* value fallacy. *Annals of Internal Medicine, 130*, 995–1004.

Goodman, S. N. (1999b). Toward evidence-based medical statistics, 2. The Bayes factor. *Annals of Internal Medicine, 130*, 1005–1013.

Graham, I. D., Logan, J., Davies, B., & Nimrod, C. (2004). Changing the use of electronic fetal monitoring and labor support: A case study of barriers and facilitators. *Birth, 31*(4), 293–301.

Gray, J., Hayes, R. B., Sackett, D., Cook, D., & Guyatt, G. H. (1997). Transferring evidence from research into practice: 3. Developing evidence-based clinical policy. *American College of Physicians Journal Club, 126*(2), A14–A16.

Guba, E. G., & Lincoln, N. K. (1998). Competing paradigms in qualitative research. In N. K. Denzin & Y. S. Lincoln (Eds.), *The landscape of qualitative research: Theories and issues* (pp. 195–220). Thousand Oaks, CA: Sage.

Guyatt, G. H., & Drummond, R. (Eds.). (2001). *Users' guide to the medical literature: A manual for evidence-based practice.* Chicago: American Medical Association.

Hamilton, J. [Interviewer]. (2004, March 11). Study: Ovaries may replenish eggs. [Morning Edition broadcast]. National Public Radio, Washington, DC. Retrieved from http://www.npr.org/rundowns/rundown.php?prgId=3&prgDate=11-Mar-2004

Harris, R. P., Helfand, M., Woolf, S. H., Lohr, K. N., Mulrow, C. D., Teutsch, S. M., & Atkins, D. (2001). Current methods of the U.S. Preventive Services Task Force: A review of the process. *American Journal of Preventive Medicine, 20*(suppl 3), 21–35.

Holland, N. J. (1990). *Is women's philosophy possible?* Savage, MD: Rowman and Little.

Holliday, M. E., & Parker, D. L. (1997). Florence Nightingale, feminism and nursing. *Journal of Advanced Nursing, 26,* 483–488.

Humpel, N., Owen, N., Leslie, E., Marshall, A. L., Bauman, A. E., & Sallis, J. F. (2004). Associations of location and perceived environmental attributes with walking in neighborhoods. *American Journal of Health Promotion, 18*(3), 239–242.

Johnson, J., Canning, J., Kaneko, T., Pru, J. K., & Tilly, J. L. (2004). Germline stem cells and follicular renewal in the postnatal mammalian ovary. *Nature, 428*(6979), 145–150.

Ka'opua, L. S. I., & Mueller, C. W. (2004). Treatment adherence among native Hawaiians living with HIV. *Social Work, 49*(1), 55–63.

Kennedy, H. P., Rousseau, A. L., & Kane Low, L. (2003). An exploratory metasynthesis of midwifery care. *Midwifery, 19*(3), 203–214.

Kim, M. (2000). Evidence-based nursing: Connecting knowledge to practice. *Chart, 97*(9), 1, 4–6.

Kohn, L. T., Corrigan, J. M., & Donaldson, M. S. (Eds.). (1999). *To err is human: Building a safer health system.* Washington, DC: Committee on Quality of Health Care in America, Institute of Medicine.

Kuhn, T. S. (1970). *The structure of scientific revolutions.* Chicago: University of Chicago Press.

Lanuza, D. M. (1999). Research and practice. In M. A. Mateo & K. T. Kirchoff (Eds.), *Using and conducting nursing research in the clinical setting* (2nd ed., pp. 2–12). Philadelphia: Saunders.

Main, E. K., Bloomfield, L., & Hunt, G. (2004). Development of a large-scale obstetric quality-improvement program that focused on the nulliparous patient at term. *American Journal of Obstetrics & Gynecology, 190,* 1747–1758.

Main, E. K., Moore, D., Farrell, B., Schimmel, L. D., Altman, R. J., Abrahams, C., Campbell Bliss, M., ... Sterling, J. (2006). Is there a useful cesarean birth measure? Assessment of the nulliparous term singleton vertex cesarean birth rate as a tool for obstetric quality improvement. *American Journal of Obstetrics & Gynecology, 194,* 1644–1652.

McDonald, L. (Ed.). (2002). *Collected works of Florence Nightingale: Vol. 1. Florence Nightingale: An introduction to her life and family.* Ontario, Canada: Wilfred Laurier University Press.

McDonald, L. (Ed.). (2004). *Florence Nightingale and the foundations of public health care, as seen through her collected works.* Retrieved from http://www.sociology.uoguelph.ca/fnightingale/Public%20Health%20Care

Mishler, E. G. (1984). *The discourse of medicine: Dialectics of medical interviews.* Norwood, NJ: Ablex.

Mitchell, G. J. (1999). Evidence-based practice: Critique and alternative view. *Nursing Science Quarterly, 12*(1), 30–35.

Munro, B. H. (2001). *Statistical methods for health care research* (4th ed.). New York: Lippincott.

National Institutes of Health (NIH). (2001). *Qualitative methods in health research.* NIH Publication No. 02-5046. Bethesda, MD: Office of Behavioral and Social Sciences Research, NIH.

Nightingale, F. (1859/1957). *Notes on nursing: What it is and what it is not.* Philadelphia: Lippincott.

Noblit, D. W., & Hare, R. D. (1988). *Meta-ethnography: Synthesizing qualitative studies.* Newbury Park, CA: Sage.

Oxman, A. D., Cook, D. J., & Guyatt, G. H. (1994). Users' guides to the medical literature: VI. How to use an overview. *Journal of the American Medical Association, 272*(17), 1367–1371.

Polit, D. F., & Beck, C. T. (2008). *Nursing research: Generating and assessing evidence for nursing practice* (8th ed.). New York: Lippincott Williams & Wilkins.

Quine, W. V. (1952). *From a logical point of view* (2nd ed.). Cambridge, MA: Harvard University Press.

Quinn, A. A. (1991). A theoretical model of the perimenopausal process. *Journal of Nurse-Midwifery, 36*(1), 25–29.

Sable, P. (2004). Attachment, ethology and adult psychotherapy. *Attachment and Human Development, 6*(1), 3–19.

Sackett, D. L., Hayes, R. B., Guyatt, G. H., & Tugwell, P. (2000). *Clinical epidemiology and science for clinical medicine* (2nd ed.). Boston: Little Brown.

Sackett, D. L., Strauss, S. E., Richardson, W. S., Rosenberg, W., & Hayes, R. B. (2000). *Evidence-based medicine: How to practice and teach EBM.* New York: Churchill Livingstone.

Sandelowski, M., Docherty, S., & Emden, C. (1997). Qualitative metasynthesis: Issues and techniques. *Research in Nursing & Health, 20*, 365–371.

Sehon, S. R., & Stanley, D. E. (2003). A philosophical analysis of the evidence-based medicine debate. *BMC Health Services Research, 3*(14). Retrieved from http://www.biomedcentral.com/1472-6963/3/14

Skreblin, L., & Sujoldzic, A. (2003). Acculturation process and its effect on dietary habits, nutrition behavior and body-image in adolescents. *Collegium antropologicum, 27*(2), 469–477.

Speziale, H. J. S., & Carpenter, D. R. (2003). *Qualitative research in nursing: Advancing the humanistic imperative* (3rd ed.). New York: Lippincott Williams & Wilkins.

Stetler, C. B. (2001). Updating the Stetler model of research utilization to facilitate evidence-based practice. *Nursing Outlook, 49*, 272–279.

Strauss, A., & Corbin, J. (1998). *Basics of qualitative research: Techniques and procedures for developing grounded theory* (2nd ed.). Thousand Oaks, CA: Sage.

Tashakkori, A., & Teddlie, C. (1998). *Mixed methodology: Combining qualitative and quantitative approaches.* Thousand Oaks, CA: Sage.

van Manen, M. (1990). *Researching lived experience: Human science for an action sensitive pedagogy.* Ontario, Canada: State University of New York Press.

Walshe, K., & Rundall, T. G. (2001). Evidence-based management: From theory to practice in health care. *Milbank Quarterly, 79*(3), 429–457.

Wuest, J. (1994). A feminist approach to concept analysis. *Western Journal of Nursing Research, 16*(5), 577–586.

Wuff, H. R., & Gotzsche, P. C. (2000). *Rational diagnosis and treatment: Evidence-based clinical decision-making* (3rd ed.). Boston: Blackwell.

Sources of Research Evidence

Agency for Healthcare Research and Quality, Evidence Reports and Technology Assessments

http://www.ahcpr.gov/clinic

American College of Physicians, ACP Journal Club (CD-ROM)

http://www.acponline.org

BMJ Best Practice (online database)

http://bestpractice.bmj.com/best-practice/welcome.html

Cochrane Database of Systematic Reviews

http://www.cochrane.org

Core Library for Evidence-Based Practice

Comprehensive website that is a virtual library with many links to full-text documents on all aspects of evidence-based practice, including texts, the Users' Guides to the Medical Literature (*Journal of the American Medical Association* articles), basic statistics for clinicians, systematic reviews from the *Annals of Internal Medicine*, and instructions for how to read various kinds of scientific papers series from the *British Medical Journal*.

http://www.shef.ac.uk/~scharr/ir/core.html

Database of Abstracts of Reviews of Effectiveness (DARE)

http://agatha.york.ac.uk/darehp.htm

MEDLINE

The peer-reviewed biomedical literature and review articles on the state of the science.

http://www.ncbi.nlm.nih.gov/entrez/query/static/overview.html

Useful Websites for Systematic Reviews

Bandolier: http://www.medicine.ox.ac.uk/bandolier

Center for Evidence-Based Medicine at Oxford: http://www.cebm.net

Cochrane Collaboration: http://www.cochrane.org/cochrane-reviews

NHS Centre for Reviews and Dissemination: http://www.york.ac.uk/inst/crd/welcome.htm

Systematic Reviews Training Unit: http://www.ich.ucl.ac.uk/srtu

Health Assessment and Promotion

CHAPTER 4

Health Promotion

Kathryn Osborne

The leading causes of death for women in the United States are related to modifiable, behavioral risk factors (Centers for Disease Control and Prevention [CDC], 2007c). Smoking-related illnesses kill an average of 178,311 women each year (CDC, 2005). An increasing number of women are also experiencing morbidity and mortality as a result of being overweight or obese. More than 61% of all American women were overweight in the period 2001 to 2004, and more than half of these women were obese (National Center for Health Statistics [NCHS], 2007). In addition to causing premature death and disability, illnesses related to just these modifiable behavioral risk factors lead to annual medical expenditures of more than $160 billion in the United States (CDC, 2007a). Health promotion and disease prevention must be priorities to improve the overall health of the nation and to reduce the spending of our limited healthcare dollars on illnesses related to modifiable risk factors.

Health Promotion: A National Initiative

The 1979 Surgeon General's report *Healthy People* set the stage for the development of a national initiative that is founded on scientific evidence and focuses on disease prevention. One year after the *Healthy People* report *Promoting Health/Preventing Disease: Objectives for the Nation* and *Healthy People 2000: National Health Promotion and Disease Prevention Objectives* established health objectives for use by state and local agencies and private organizations in the development of plans to move the population toward improved levels of wellness. *Healthy People* is designed to measure changes in health status over time and identifies 10-year national objectives for improving the health of all Americans (*Healthy People 2020*, 2010).

Healthy People 2010 expanded the content found in the aforementioned documents and established a set of health-related objectives for the nation to achieve in the new millennium. The primary goals of *Healthy People 2010* were to "increase quality and years of healthy life and to eliminate health disparities" (*Healthy People 2010*, 2004, p. 2). During the last 10 years the nation has either met or moved forward toward the targets for 71 percent of the *Healthy People 2010* goals (Koh, 2010).

In December 2010, the U.S. Department of Health and Human Services announced the *Healthy People 2020* goals and objectives for the nation. The overarching goals of *Healthy People 2020* are:

- Attain high-quality, longer lives free of preventable disease, disability, injury, and premature death.
- Achieve health equity, eliminate disparities, and improve the health of all groups.
- Create social and physical environments that promote good health for all.
- Promote quality of life, healthy development, and healthy behaviors across all lifestyles (*Healthy People 2020*, 2010).

Healthy People 2020 uses a social determinants of health approach (Koh, 2010). Determinants of health is a range of personal, social, economic, and environmental factors that influence health status and which fall under several broad categories including policymaking, social factors, health services, individual behavior, biology, and genetics (*Healthy People 2020*, 2010). Four foundation health measures will be used to monitor the progress of *Healthy People 2020* initiatives: (1) general health status, (2) health-related quality of life and well-being, (3) determinants of health, and (4) disparities (*Healthy People 2020*). Currently *Health People 2020* identifies 39 topic areas, and others are evolving (see **Table 4-1**).

The membership of the *Healthy People* initiative is made up of private and public sector groups, including the U.S. Department of Health and Human Services, state and local health departments, and hundreds of private-sector groups and organizations. Members of the initiative periodically assess the health status of the nation and evaluate the effectiveness of specific interventions (*Healthy People 2010*, 2004; *Healthy People 2020*, 2010).

Healthy People 2010 identified multiple objectives that were associated with each of the indicators that reflect the major health concerns in the United States. *Healthy People 2020* maintained some of these as focus areas and added new focus areas for the 2020 program (see Table 4-1).

Clinicians are encouraged to utilize the objectives in establishing local programs focused on the improvement of the health of communities. More information about these objectives—and specifically ways in which they may be applied to the delivery of women's health care—can be found at http://www.healthypeople.gov.

As the United States continues to deal with the financial realities of health care, it is becoming increasingly clear to policy makers, clinicians, and insurance underwriters that there are benefits from allocating healthcare dollars for health promotion and disease prevention. The United States spent $2 trillion on health care in 2005, or 16% of the nation's gross domestic product (NCHS, 2007). In 2002, almost half of the total U.S. healthcare

TABLE 4-1 *Healthy People 2020* Focus Areas

Access to quality health services	HIV
Adolescent health*	Immunization and infectious disease
Arthritis, osteoporosis, and chronic back conditions	Injury and violence prevention
Blood disorders and blood safety	Lesbian, gay, bisexual, and transgender health*
Cancer	Maternal, infant, and child health
Chronic kidney disease	Medical product safety
Dementias, including Alzheimer's disease*	Mental health and mental disorders
Diabetes*	Nutrition and weight status
Disability and health	Occupational safety and health
Early and middle childhood*	Older adults*
Educational and community-based programs	Oral health
Environmental health	Physical activity
Family planning	Preparedness*
Food safety	Public health infrastructure
Genomics*	Respiratory diseases
Global health*	Sexually transmitted infections
Health communication and health information technology	Sleep health*
Health-related quality of life and wellbeing*	Social determinants of health*
Healthcare-associated infections*	Substance abuse
Hearing and other sensory or communication disorders	Tobacco use
Heart disease and stroke	Vision

*Identifies new focus area for *Healthy People 2020*
Source: *Healthy People 2020*, 2010.

budget was spent on just 5% of the population: individuals whose healthcare expenses were primarily related to expensive chronic conditions, many of which are preventable (Agency for Healthcare Research and Quality, 2006). Healthcare costs have continued to rise and in 2008 the United States surpassed $2.3 trillion in expenditures on health care. The dollar amount per U.S. resident was about $7,681. This was more than three times the $714 billion spent in 1990 (Centers for Medicare & Medicaid Services, 2010).

Moving away from the traditional medical focus on the treatment of illness to health care that includes health promotion and disease prevention is an important step in the quest for cost containment (Meunier, 2009). The looming question is, "How can a healthcare delivery system that is illness centered undergo a paradigm shift to focus on wellness?" Clinicians are taking initial steps by clarifying the definitions of *health* and *prevention*. The multidisciplinary nature of healthcare delivery creates an opportunity for variations in these definitions.

Defining Health

Many organizations and specialty groups have their own standard definition of health. Perhaps the broadest of these definitions is that established by the World Health Organization (WHO) in 1948: "Health is a state of complete physical, mental and social well-being and not merely the absence of disease or infirmity." To some, this definition may appear to make health unattainable. Yet, when health is viewed through a holistic lens, this definition begins to make sense. A holistic view of health includes its assessment in the context of physical, mental, and social well-being. Health, as defined in various contexts, can be achieved even in the presence of illness. For example, a young woman who has been HIV positive for 5 years may feel a sense of physical, mental, and social well-being if she is being cared for in a healthcare delivery system that addresses her healthcare needs in a holistic fashion. The presence of a disease state does not exclude her from being considered healthy according to the WHO definition of health.

The American Medical Association (2003) defines health as a "state of physical and mental well-being." The medical model's perspective of health has historically assumed the clinician's point of view. However, as the practice of medicine evolves to focus more on cost-effectiveness and respect for patient autonomy, this perspective will necessarily shift and become patient oriented. Subjective information from the patient will determine his or her relative health, not just the clinician's viewpoint. Changing to a patient-oriented perspective of health will encourage clinicians to shift from evaluating and assessing patient's bodies to assessing the complete lives of their patients (Sullivan, 2003).

Nursing is a discipline that focuses on health and wellness. Numerous nursing theorists have proposed definitions of health. Perhaps one of the most well known is that developed by Martha Rogers (1970), who theorized that the study of human beings would yield meaningful theories and concepts only when their wholeness is perceived. Rogers' perception has served as a springboard for the development of myriad nursing definitions of health, each of which uses a holistic lens, viewing human beings as whole persons, encompassing mind, body, and spirit.

Madeleine Leininger, expanding on the work of earlier nurse theorists, provides a conceptual framework for nursing care. She proposes that caring is the essence of nursing and theorizes that while it may be expressed in different ways, caring is universal across cultures (Leininger, 1985). Supporting this theory are reports that the cultural beliefs of patients influence their perceptions of health, and outcomes of care are improved when the patient's definition of health is considered and care is provided within the patient's cultural context (Fisher & Owen, 2008). Applying Leininger's theory of transcultural caring to earlier definitions of health, one could conclude that proper health care requires a consideration of the whole person and must include knowledge and appreciation for the cultural context of the individual. This view provides a definition of health that is patient specific and includes the individual patient's cultural perceptions of health. Health promotion then encompasses a wide range of services that are delivered within the cultural context of the patient and that promote the general health and well-being of individuals and the communities in which they live.

Defining Prevention

The delivery of healthcare services aimed at the prevention of physical and mental illness and disease is defined on three levels:

- Primary prevention: These services focus on preventing disease in susceptible populations (Meunier, 2009). Examples of primary preventive efforts include health education and counseling, and targeted immunization.
- Secondary prevention: These services focus on the early detection of disease states and subsequent prompt treatment that will reduce the severity and limit the short- and long-term sequelae of the disease (Shi & Singh, 2004). Routine laboratory screening is an example of secondary prevention.
- Tertiary prevention: These services limit disability and promote rehabilitation from clinical disease states (Shi & Singh).

The rest of this chapter focuses on primary preventive efforts in healthcare delivery.

Counseling and Education as Preventive Strategies

Clinicians are in a prime position to offer information that provides their patients with the tools needed to maintain a healthy lifestyle and assist in altering behaviors that may cause harm or illness. Women often seek information during their yearly physical examination that can guide them in making lifestyle changes and confirm that their current practices are an effective means of maintaining health. However, episodic visits may offer more frequent opportunities for providing health promotion and disease prevention information. Statistics reveal that during 2006, more than 60% of ambulatory healthcare visits by women were made for chronic or acute problems (including injuries), while only 21.5% were made for preventive care (Cherry, Burt, & Woodwell, 2003).

In 1984, the U.S. Public Health Service convened the U.S. Preventive Service Task Force (USPSTF). One of the goals of the USPSTF was to examine the evidence regarding the effective use of preventive services to reduce morbidity and mortality rates. After examining the use and effectiveness of hundreds of preventive services, the USPSTF identified four categories—counseling interventions, screening tests, immunizations, and chemoprophylaxis—for which there was evidence of significant health benefits. In 2003, the Institute of Medicine

(IOM) issued a report mandating that "all health professionals should be educated to deliver patient-centered care as members of an interdisciplinary team, emphasizing evidence-based practice, quality improvement approaches and informatics" (p. 3). Further, Sackett, Strauss, and colleagues (2000) define the elements of evidence-based practice as "the integration of the best research evidence with clinical expertise and patient values" (p. 1).

Consistent with this definition of evidence-based practice, and in keeping with the basic tenets of evidence-based practice, the USPSTF continues to seek out and appraise the evidence regarding effective counseling interventions using well-established rating schemas. It provides recommendations that are intended to be integrated with the clinician's own expertise and experience, as well as the patient's preference and values, to guide professional decision making and practice (USPSTF, 2007a). USPSTF guidelines recommend that clinicians use every patient interaction as an opportunity to participate in counseling and education (see Chapter 8 for a detailed discussion of the USPSTF).

Effective Counseling Interventions for Healthy, Asymptomatic Women

Dental Health

The USPSTF guidelines recommend that, in combination with regular oral hygiene practices, all women should be counseled to seek regular care from a dentist. Regular oral hygiene practices include daily brushing with fluoride-containing toothpaste and daily flossing between the teeth (USPSTF, 1996).

Diet and Exercise

In the second edition of *Guide to Clinical Preventive Services*, the USPSTF (1996) recommends that all women be counseled to limit the amount of fat and cholesterol in their diet. Plans for diet and regular exercise should be designed so that caloric intake is balanced with energy expenditures. Women's diets should contain a variety of foods, particularly whole grains, fruits, and vegetables. In addition, efforts should be taken to limit consumption of foods containing saturated fats, *trans*-fatty acids, and cholesterol. Studies reviewed by the USPSTF reveal that individuals who follow these guidelines have lower rates of morbidity and mortality from coronary artery disease and certain forms of cancer.

All women are advised to consume the recommended daily allowance of calcium (1200–1500 mg/day for adolescents and young adults, 1000 mg/day for women aged 25 to 50 years, and 1000–1500 mg/day for postmenopausal women) and to participate in regular physical activity to reduce both bone mineral loss and the risk of osteoporosis. In addition to slowing bone mineral loss, regular exercise reduces the risk of developing diabetes, obesity, heart disease, and hypertension. The USPSTF (1996) recommends that clinicians encourage patients to implement exercise programs that gradually increase their activity levels over time, and emphasizes the importance of engaging in regular physical activity rather than sporadic exercise practices.

During 2002 and 2003, the USPSTF amended these recommendations after reviewing more recent research and concluded that there was insufficient evidence to advise either for or against routine dietary counseling or behavioral counseling to promote physical activity for unselected patients in the primary care setting. The evidence does, however, support intensive dietary counseling provided by a clinician for adult women with hyperlipidemia or other known risk factors for cardiovascular or other diet-related chronic diseases. Clinicians who choose to provide dietary counseling to women who are not at increased risk should follow the recommendations published in the second edition of *Guide to Clinical Preventive Services* (USPSTF, 2003, 2004).

Injury Prevention

Motor vehicle accidents (MVAs) are the leading cause of death for people ages 1 to 34 and result in more than 5 million emergency department visits and approximately 500,000 hospitalizations each year in the United States (NCHS, 2009). Male deaths from MVAs declined 11% from 1975 to 2007 in this country, while female deaths increased 1% over the same period (Insurance Institute for Highway Safety [IIHS], 2007). Consequently, the USPSTF (2007b) recommends that all women be encouraged to use lap and shoulder restraints, and that passengers in the cars they drive also use restraints (including age-appropriate restraints for infants and young children). The guidelines also urge the appropriate use of bicycle, all-terrain vehicle, and motorcycle helmets. All women should be counseled on the dangers of operating a motor vehicle while under the influence of alcohol or other drugs, as well as the risks associated with riding in the vehicle of an impaired driver. In particular, adolescents and young adults should be counseled on the importance of not combining driving and substance use, with an emphasis on making arrangements for alternative forms of transportation at times when alcohol and other drugs have been used (USPSTF, 1996).

In 2007, the USPSTF updated the recommendations for counseling patients about proper use of motor vehicle occupant restraints to prevent motor vehicle occupant injuries. Legislative efforts and community-based interventions over the past decade have resulted in high rates of seatbelt use among patients of all ages; an estimated 80% of all adults in the United States currently use seatbelts (USPSTF, 2007b). The USPSTF found no well-conducted research that evaluated the effect of counseling in the primary care setting on seatbelt use. It also did not find any research addressing the impact of counseling in the primary care setting on driving while under the influence of alcohol or riding with an impaired driver. Nevertheless, strong evidence suggests that seatbelt laws and enforcement strategies have resulted in increased use of these restraints. Consequently, the USPSTF finds that current evidence is insufficient to recommend for or against counseling patients in the primary care setting about seatbelt use, noting the potential harms of such counseling are estimated to be none or of minimal magnitude (USPSTF, 2007b). The American College of Obstetricians and Gynecologists recommends that clinicians counsel all women about the proper use of seatbelts (including pregnant women), and all adolescent women on the dangers of driving under the influence of alcohol or riding with an impaired driver.

Household Safety

The USPSTF recommends counseling women about several aspects of household safety. Smoke detectors should be installed in appropriate places in all homes and tested regularly for proper functioning. Infants and children should be dressed in flame-resistant bedclothes for sleeping. Water heaters should be set at 120–130°F.

All homes with children should have a 1-ounce bottle of syrup of ipecac, and phone numbers to poison control centers and emergency departments should be available in an easily accessible location (USPSTF, 1996). The American Association of Poison Control Centers (2009) advises that in the event of a poisoning, the first line of action should be to call the local poison control center. Individuals suspected of poisoning should not take anything by mouth or be forced to vomit unless so directed by the poison control center. Medications and toxic substances should be placed out of the reach of children.

Installing gates or barriers in front of stairways can prevent falls. A 4-foot enclosed fence should surround swimming pools, and swimming pool owners should be encouraged to learn to perform cardiopulmonary resuscitation. Window guards should be placed in buildings that pose a high risk for falls. Firearms should either be removed from the home or stored, unloaded, in locked compartments (USPSTF, 1996).

Recreational Safety

The USPSTF (1996) recommends counseling women about recreational safety. In addition, it recommends wearing bright orange clothing when hunting, and following safe boating practices, including the wearing of approved flotation devices. Accidental injury is the leading cause of death for women ages 15 to 34 in the United States, and the cause of death for more than 15,000 women ages 15 to 65 each year (NCHS, 2011). Although the number of recreational accidents may be small, clinicians should counsel women about safety with regard to all aspects of their lives.

Prevention for Elderly Women

The USPSTF (1996) advises counseling older women about preventing falls. Counseling should include recommendations for exercise, learning safety-related skills and behaviors, reducing environmental hazards, and monitoring and adjusting medications under the direction of their clinician.

Sexual Behavior

The USPSTF recommends high-intensity behavioral counseling to prevent sexually transmitted infections (STIs) for all sexually active adolescents and all sexually active adult women at increased risk for STIs. Adult women at increased risk for STIs include those with current STIs or infections within the past year, and women with multiple current sexual partners.

Counseling should be based on individual risk factors, which can be assessed during a careful drug and sexual history (see Chapters 6 and 21), as well as based on local information about the epidemiologic risks for STIs. Clinicians who work in practices located in high-prevalence areas should consider all sexually active women in nonmonogamous relationships to be at increased risk.

Patients identified as being at increased risk for the acquisition of an STI need to receive information about risk factors and ways to reduce the likelihood of infection. Such measures include abstinence, maintaining a mutually monogamous sexual relationship with a partner who is not infected, regular use of latex condoms, and avoiding sexual interaction with individuals who are at increased risk for STIs (USPSTF, 2008). The USPSTF found little evidence to support the effectiveness of brief, individual counseling sessions in the primary care setting and no evidence supporting abstinence-only education. In contrast, strong evidence suggests that moderate- to high-intensity counseling, delivered in multiple individual or group sessions (with a total duration of 3–9 hours), results in a statistically significant reduction in STIs (USPSTF, 2008).

Women who are at increased risk for STIs should be advised to use a condom with every sexual encounter and to avoid anal intercourse. Those who use condoms should be advised to use them in accordance with the manufacturer's recommendations. Measures to reduce the chance of infection when a partner will not use a condom should also be discussed—for example, use of the female condom. All women who are at increased risk for STIs should be offered screening and should be counseled to receive the hepatitis B vaccine. Finally, the USPSTF (1996) recommends advising, as appropriate, that the use of alcohol or drugs can lead to high-risk sexual behavior.

In light of the fact that more than half of the pregnancies in the United States each year are unintended, the USPSTF (1996) recommends counseling all women who are sexually active with male partners about effective contraceptive methods (see Chapter 12). Counseling should be based on information obtained from a detailed sexual history, as discussed in Chapters 6 and 21.

Some researchers have suggested that preconception counseling should be integrated into the routine women's health visit (Elzinga, de Jong-Potjer, van der Pal-de Bruin, le Cessie, Assendelft, & Buitendiijk, 2008). Certainly, there is strong evidence to support the idea that general wellness counseling serves to improve pregnancy outcomes (Elzinga et al.). However, clinicians should demonstrate sensitivity and an understanding and respect for an individual's preferences when initiating preconception counseling. It is important to keep in mind that some women will choose not to conceive, and not all women who conceive will choose to continue the pregnancy.

Tobacco Use

Tobacco use is the leading preventable cause of death in the United States. Recent morbidity and mortality figures reveal that an average of 178,311 women die from smoking-related illnesses each year (CDC, 2005), and lung cancer is the leading cause of cancer death among women (CDC, 2006). The USPSTF strongly recommends that clinicians offer counseling on interventions that aid in smoking cessation to patients who use tobacco. Evidence demonstrates that interventions such as screening, brief behavioral counseling, and the use of pharmacotherapeutics can increase the number of patients who attempt to quit and remain abstinent for one year (USPSTF, 2003). A framework provided by the "five As" is an effective way in which to engage women who smoke in discussion about cessation:

- Asking about tobacco use
- Advising to quit through clear personalized messages
- Assessing willingness to quit
- Assisting to quit
- Arranging follow-up and support

The USPSTF found insufficient evidence to recommend either for or against counseling children and adolescents about tobacco use or efforts to discontinue use by children and adolescents who already use tobacco. There currently is insufficient evidence to suggest that efforts directed at preventing use and assisting in cessation among children and adolescents are effective in the primary care setting. Decisions to initiate such counseling are left to the discretion of the individual clinician (USPSTF, 2003).

Immunization Guidelines and Recommendations

In addition to counseling interventions to assist patients in making healthy lifestyle choices and changes, primary prevention includes the delivery of targeted immunizations. Immunizations play an important role in the prevention of infectious diseases, many of which are debilitating and, in some cases, may prove fatal. Recognizing the effectiveness of immunizations as a strategy to significantly reduce the incidence of vaccine-preventable disease, *Healthy People 2010* identified immunization status as one of the 10 leading health indicators by which to measure the health of the nation. The USPSTF also acknowledges the importance of immunizations as a primary preventive measure. Since 1996, it has deferred to the CDC's Advisory Committee on Immunization Practices regarding evidence-based recommendations and guidelines for clinicians (USPSTF, n.d.).

Primary care clinicians are in a key position to implement policies to improve the immunization status of women in the United States. However, evidence suggests many of these clinicians fail to provide appropriate preventive care services, including the administration of immunizations, to women in the outpatient setting. In a recent study examining the preventive health services delivered to 4683 women age 65 and older, researchers found that almost half of the participants had not receive the recommended immunizations for their age group. Conversely, many of the women in the sample population had received cervical cancer screening well past the age at which such screening is considered to be beneficial (Schonberg, Leveille, & Marcantonio, 2008). The authors concluded that few older women receive the appropriate preventive health measures; cancer screening, from which older women likely do not benefit, is often provided, whereas immunizations, from which they may benefit, are not.

Similar findings were obtained in a study that examined the level of unmet preventive healthcare needs of patients presenting for acute care in the emergency room. The researchers found that most adults seen in the emergency room had unmet preventive healthcare needs, and one of the most frequently unmet needs was the provision of age-appropriate immunizations. This was true despite that fact that 60% of the sample population had a primary care physician and more than 78% of the population was insured (Zun & Downey, 2006). The findings from this study reinforce the recommendations of the U.S. Public Health Service to use every patient contact as an opportunity to provide preventive health services, including immunizations (Zun & Downey, 2006).

The reasons women present for health care are many, but include contraceptive counseling, yearly physical examinations, prenatal care, preconception care, and urgent care. Each of these encounters should be considered an opportunity to provide preventive health services for women. **Table 4-2** gives the current immunization guidelines for women, As the human papillomavirus (HPV) vaccine is relatively new, issues surrounding its use remain somewhat controversial and are discussed further in Chapter 21. When considering appropriate vaccination schedules for women, it is important to note that the measles, mumps, and rubella (MMR); herpes zoster; and varicella vaccines are contraindicated for women who are pregnant or who are immunocompromised, including some women with HIV infection (CDC, 2009). Decisions regarding the administration of vaccines other than these, to women who are pregnant, should be made on a risk–benefit basis (CDC, 2007b).

TABLE 4-2 Recommended Vaccination Schedule for Women

Vaccine	Age-Related Recommendations						
	11–12 Years	13–18 Years	19–26 Years	27–49 Years	50–59 Years	60–64 Years	≥ 65 Years
Hepatitis A	2 doses for children at increased risk for infection	2 doses for women with chronic liver disease or who receive clotting factor concentrates, women who use illegal drugs, and women who have occupational or travel exposure to hepatitis A					
Hepatitis B	3 doses beginning at birth; ages 11–18 if not previously immunized	3 doses for women with risk factors for infection: end stage renal disease, HIV infection, chronic renal disease, occupational and/or household exposure, travel exposure, IV drug use, increased STI risk					
Human papillomavirus (HPV)	3 doses	3 doses for all women age 13–26 not previously immunized		Not recommended			
Influenza	1 dose annually to all females age 6 months to 18 years		1 dose annually for those at increased risk for infection and all healthcare workers		1 dose annually for all women over age 50		

TABLE 4-2   Recommended Vaccination Schedule for Women *(Continued)*

Vaccine	Age-Related Recommendations						
	11–12 Years	**13–18 Years**	**19–26 Years**	**27–49 Years**	**50–59 Years**	**60–64 Years**	**≥ 65 Years**
Meningococcal	1 dose if not previously immunized	1 dose for women over 18 at increased risk for infection: first-year college students living in dormitories, military recruits, microbiologists exposed to *N. meningitidis*, travel to epidemic areas					
Measles, mumps, and rubella (MMR)*	2 doses for those not previously immunized			1 or 2 doses for certain populations at increased risk*			
Pneumococcal (polysaccharide)	1 dose for women with risk factors for infection: chronic lung and cardiovascular diseases, diabetes mellitus, chronic renal and liver disease, asplenia, chronic alcoholism, cochlear implant, immunocompromised					1 dose for all women ≥ 65	
Tetanus, diphtheria (Td)/ tentanus, diphtheria, pertussis (Tdap)	1 time dose of Tdap for those who have received the primary immunization series followed by Td booster every 10 years					Td booster every 10 years	
Varicella	2 doses for all women and girls without evidence of immunity (previous infection or vaccination)						
Zoster (herpes)	Not recommended					1 dose for all women ≥ age 60	

*In the absence of a contraindication, women born during or after 1957 should receive 1 dose of MMR unless there is documented evidence of receipt of one or more previous doses; a history or measles, mumps and/or rubella based on healthcare provider diagnosis; or laboratory evidence of immunity. A second dose of MMR is recommended for women who (1) have been exposed to measles or mumps, or who live in an outbreak area; (2) are students in postsecondary education institutions; (3) work in a healthcare facility; (4) plan international travel; or (5) were vaccinated previously with killed or unknown measles vaccine. Unvaccinated women born before 1957 without evidence of mumps immunity and who work in healthcare settings should receive one dose of MMR; administering a second dose during an outbreak should be strongly considered. Rubella immunity should be determined for all women of childbearing age; those without evidence of immunity should receive MMR vaccine upon completion or termination of pregnancy and before discharge from the healthcare facility. MMR vaccine is contraindicated in pregnancy.
Source: Centers for Disease Control and Prevention, 2009.

Conclusion

This chapter has examined definitions of health and the utilization of those definitions in the provision of primary preventive services, both as a national initiative and for individual clinicians. Secondary prevention is discussed in Chapter 8. Readers are encouraged to use this information, in conjunction with frequently updated guidelines available from the USPSTF,

CDC, and other organizations (which can often be found online), in the development of management plans addressing the total healthcare needs of women across the life span.

References

Agency for Healthcare Research and Quality. (2006). *The high concentration of U.S. healthcare expenditures.* Retrieved from http://www.ahrq.gov/research/ria19/expendria.htm#diff1

American Association of Poison Control Centers. (2009). *Prevention tips.* Retrieved from http://www.aapcc.org/dnn/PoisoningPrevention/tabid/116/Default.aspx

American Medical Association. (2003). *H-160.997 AMA Program.* Retrieved from: http://www.ama-assn.org/apps/pf_new/pf_online

Centers for Disease Control and Prevention (CDC). (2005). Cigarette smoking among adults—United States, 2004. *Morbidity and Mortality Weekly Report, 54*(44), 1121–1124. Retrieved from http://www.cdc.gov/tobacco/data_statistics/fact_sheets/populations/women/index.htm

Centers for Disease Control and Prevention (CDC). (2006). *Women's health: Smoking and tobacco.* Retrieved from http://www.cdc.gov/women/natstat/smoking.htm#stats

Centers for Disease Control and Prevention (CDC). (2007a). *Economic facts about U.S. tobacco use and tobacco production.* Retrieved from http://www.cdc.gov/tobacco/data_statistics/fact_sheets/economics/economic_facts.htm.

Centers for Disease Control and Prevention (CDC). (2007b). *Guidelines for vaccinating pregnant women.* Retrieved from http://www.cdc.gov/vaccines/pubs/preg-guide.htm

Centers for Disease Control and Prevention (CDC). (2007c). *Leading causes of death in females United States, 2004.* Retrieved from http://www.cdc.gov/women/lcod.htm

Centers for Disease Control and Prevention (CDC). (2008). *Data 2010: The* Healthy People 2010 *database.* Retrieved from http://wonder.cdc.gov/data2010

Centers for Disease Control and Prevention (CDC). (2009). *Vaccines and immunizations.* Retrieved from http://www.cdc.gov/vaccines

Centers for Medicare and Medicaid Services, Office of the Actuary, National Health Statistics Group. (2010). *National health care expenditures data, January 2010.* Retrieved from https://www.cms.gov/NationalHealthExpendData

Cherry, D., Burt, C., & Woodwell, D. (2003). *National ambulatory medical care survey: 2001 summary* (NCHS Publication No. 337). Washington, DC: U.S. Department of Health and Human Services.

Elzinga, J., de Jong-Potjer, L., van der Pal-de Bruin, K., le Cessie, S., Assendelft, W., & Buitendiijk, S. (2008). The effect of preconception counseling on lifestyle and other behavior before and during pregnancy. *Women's Health Issues, 18,* S117–S125. doi:10.1016/j.whi.2008.09.003

Fisher, P., & Owen, J. (2008). Empowering interventions in health and social care: Recognition through "ecologies of practice." *Social Science & Medicine, 67,* 2063–2071.

Healthy People 2010. (2004). About *Healthy People.* Retrieved from http://www.healthy people. gov/About

Healthy People 2020 (2010). About *Healthy People.* Retrieved from http://www.healthypeople.gov/about/default.aspx

Institute of Medicine (IOM). (2003). *Health professions education: A bridge to quality.* Washington, DC: National Academies Press.

Insurance Institute for Highway Safety (IIHS). (2007). *Fatality facts: Gender.* Retrieved from http://www.iihs.org/research/fatality_facts_2007/gender.html

Koh, H. (2010). Healthy People 2020: *A roadmap for health.* Retrieved from http://www.healthcare.gov/news/blog/healthypeople.html

Leininger, M. M. (1985). Transcultural care diversity and universality: A theory of nursing. *Nursing and Health Care, 6,* 209–212.

Meunier, Y. A. (2009). Healthcare: The case for the urgent need and widespread use of preventive medicine in the U.S. [Report]. *Internet Journal of Healthcare Administration, 6.2.* Retrieved from http://find.galegroup.com/gtx/start.do?prodId=HRCA

National Center for Health Statistics (NCHS). (2007). *Health, United States, 2007: With chartbook on trends in the health of Americans.* Hyattsville, MD: Author.

National Center for Health Statistics (NCHS). (2009). *Motor vehicle safety.* Retrieved from http://www.cdc .gov/Motorvehiclesafety/index.html

National Center for Health Statistics (NCHS). (2011). *Deaths, percent of total deaths, and death rates for the 15 leading causes of death in selected age groups, by race and sex: United States, 1999–2007* [Data file]. Retrieved from http://www.cdc.gov/nchs/nvss/ mortality/lcwk3.htm

Rogers, M. E. (1970). *An introduction to the theoretical basis of nursing.* Philadelphia, PA: Davis.

Sackett, D. L., Strauss, S. E., Richardson, W. S., Rosenberg, W., & Hayes, R. B. (2000). *Evidence-based medicine: How to practice and teach EBM.* New York, NY: Churchill Livingston.

Schonberg, M., Leveille, S., & Marcantonio, E. (2008). Preventive health care among older women: Missed opportunities and poor targeting. *American Journal of Medicine, 121*(11), 974–981.

Shi, L., & Singh, D. (2004). *Delivering health care in America: A systems approach* (3rd ed.). Sudbury, MA: Jones and Bartlett.

Sullivan, M. (2003). The new subjective medicine: Taking the patient's point of view on health care and health. *Social Science and Medicine, 56*(7), 1595–1605.

U.S. Department of Health and Human Services. (2008). Healthy People 2020: *The road ahead.* Retrieved from http://www.healthypeople.gov/hp2020

U.S. Preventive Services Task Force (USPSTF). (n.d.). *Immunizations for adults.* Retrieved from http://www .ahrq.gov/clinic/uspstf/uspsadim.htm

U.S. Preventive Services Task Force (USPSTF). (1996). *Guide to clinical preventive services* (2nd ed.). Baltimore, MD: Williams & Wilkins. Retrieved from http://www.ahrq.gov/clinic/cps3dix.htm

U.S. Preventive Services Task Force (USPSTF). (2003, 2004). *Guide to clinical preventive service, third edition: Periodic updates.* Retrieved from http://www .ahcpr.gov/clinic/gcpspu.htm

U.S. Preventive Services Task Force (USPSTF). (2007a). *About USPSTF.* Retrieved from http://www.ahrq.gov/ clinic/uspstfab.htm

U.S. Preventive Services Task Force (USPSTF). (2007b). *Counseling about motor vehicle occupant restraints and avoidance of alcohol use while driving.* Retrieved from http://www.ahrq.gov/clinic/uspstf07/mvoi/ mvoirs.htm

U.S. Preventive Services Task Force (USPSTF). (2008). *Behavioral counseling to prevent sexually transmitted infections.* Retrieved from http://www.ahrq.gov/ clinic/uspstf08/sti/stirs.htm

World Health Organization (WHO). (1948). *WHO definition of health.* Retrieved from http://www.who.int/ about/definition/en/print.html

Zun, L., & Downey, L. (2006). Adult health screening and referral in the emergency department. *Southern Medical Journal, 99*(9), 940–948.

CHAPTER 5

Gynecologic Anatomy and Physiology

Nancy J. Hughes
Nancy M. Steele
Suzanne M. Leclaire

The women's health movement encourages women to be knowledgeable about their bodies, to appreciate the unique form and function of the female body, and to take responsibility for caring and making decisions about their bodies that will positively affect their health. This chapter reviews female anatomy and physiology in terms of how it directly affects gynecologic health and well-being. Female anatomy and physiology is often referred to as reproductive anatomy and physiology, and gynecology is defined as the branch of medicine dealing with the study of diseases and treatment of the female reproductive system. Regardless of whether a woman is pregnant or ever intends to reproduce, her gynecologic care has historically focused on reproduction. This example of naming provides insight as to why women often continue to be essentialized to reproductive functions by clinicians.

The authors of this chapter assume the reader has had basic human anatomy and physiology content. Readers requiring a more in-depth discussion are referred to general anatomy and physiology references.

Pelvic Anatomy

Pelvic Bones and Pelvic Joints

The pelvis is composed of: (1) two hip bones called the innominate bones (also known as *ox coxae*); (2) the sacrum; and (3) the coccyx. The innominate bones consist of the pubis, the ischium, and the ilium, all of which fuse at the acetabulum (Corton, 2008). The ilium comprises the posterior and upper portion of the innominate bone, forming what is known as the iliac crest. It articulates with the sacroiliac joint posteriorly and together with its ligaments is the major contributor to pelvic stability. The pubic bones articulate anteriorly with the symphysis pubis and, with their inferior angles from the descending rami, form the important bony landmark of the pubic arch (**Figure 5-1**). The ischial spines are bony prominences that are clinically important because they are used as landmarks when performing pudendal blocks, and other medical procedures such as sacrospinous ligament suspension (Anderson & Gendry, 2007). The ischial spines are also used to assess progression of fetal descent during childbirth.

The sacrum and the coccyx shape the posterior portion of the pelvis. The sacrum is formed by the fusion of the five sacral vertebrae, includes the important bony landmark of the sacral promontory, and joins the coccyx at the sacrococcygeal symphysis. The coccyx is formed by the fusion of four rudimentary vertebrae, is usually movable, and is itself a key bony landmark. The true pelvis constitutes the bony passageway through which the fetus must maneuver to be born vaginally.

The Caldwell–Moloy (1933) classification includes four basic pelvic types: gynecoid, android, anthropoid, and platypelloid (**Figure 5-2**). Each pelvic type is classified in accordance with the characteristics of the posterior segment of the inlet. Most pelves are not pure types but rather a mixture of types.

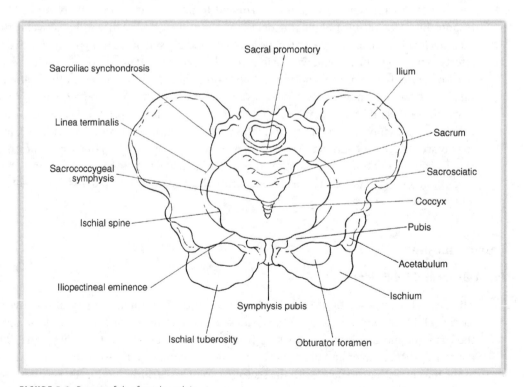

FIGURE 5-1 Bones of the female pelvis.

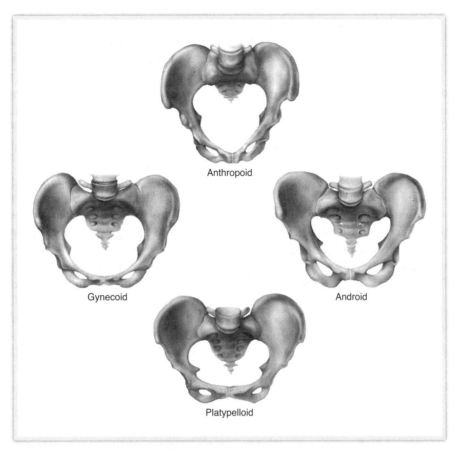

Anthropoid

Gynecoid

Android

Platypelloid

FIGURE 5-2 Caldwell-Moloy classification of pelves.

Pelvic Support

Pelvic support structures include not only the muscles and connective tissue of the pelvic floor, but also the fibromuscular tissue of the vaginal wall and endopelvic connective tissue (Richter & Varner, 2007). The piriformis and obturator internus muscles and their fasciae form part of the walls of the pelvic cavity. The piriformis muscle originates at the front of the sacrum, near the third and fourth sacral foramina. This muscle leaves the pelvis by passing laterally through the greater sciatic foramen and inserts on the upper border of the greater trochanter of the femur. The origin of the obturator internus muscle includes the pelvic surfaces of the ilium and ischium and the obturator membrane. It exits the pelvis through the lesser sciatic foramen, where it attaches to the greater trochanter of the hip enabling it to function in external hip rotation (Anderson & Gendry, 2007; Corton, 2008).

The deep perineal space is a pouch that lies superiorly to the perineal membrane (**Figure 5-3**). This deep space is continuous with the pelvic cavity and contains the compressor urethrae and urethrovaginal sphincter muscles, the external urethral sphincter, parts of the urethra and vagina, branches of the pudendal artery, and the dorsal nerve and vein of the clitoris (Corton, 2008). The perineal membrane (also known as the urogenital diaphragm, although this label is a misnomer) is a sheet made up of dense fibrous tissue that spans the opening of the anterior pelvic outlet. The perineal membrane attaches to the side walls of the vagina and provides support to the distal vagina and urethra by attaching these structures to the bony pelvis (Corton, 2008).

The levator ani muscle is a critical component of pelvic support; indeed, it is often considered the most important muscle of the pelvic floor (Corton, 2008). Normally this muscle is in a constant state of contraction, providing support for all of the abdominopelvic contents against intra-abdominal pressures (Corton, 2008). The levator ani muscle is actually a complex unit of several muscles with different origins, insertions, and functions. The pubococcygeus, puborectalis, and iliococcygeus are the primary components making up this muscle. The pubococcygeus is further divided into the pubovaginalis, puboperinealis, and puboanalis (Corton, 2008).

The levator ani and coccygeus muscles form the pelvic floor, and the related fascia form a supportive sling for the pelvic contents. The muscle fibers insert at various points in the

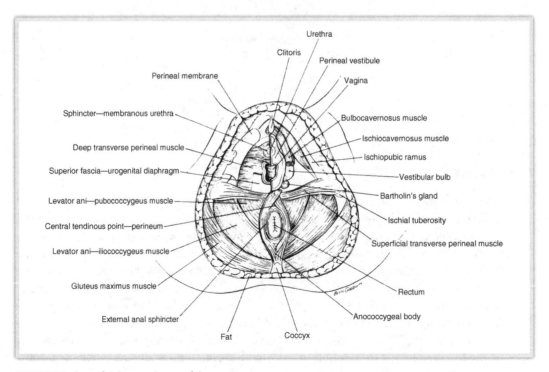

FIGURE 5-3 Superficial musculature of the perineum.

bony pelvis and form functional sphincters for the vagina, rectum, and urethra. The origin of the levator ani muscle is the pubic bone and the adjacent fascia of the obturator internus muscle. Various portions of this muscular sheet insert on the coccyx (the anococcygeal rapine) and the perineal body, which is a fibrous band lying between the vagina and the rectum. The different sections of the levator ani muscular sheet are subdivided based on the exact origin and insertion of the fibers:

- The levator prostatae or sphincter vaginae fibers form the sling around the vagina and originate from the posterior surface of the pubis; they insert in the perineal body.
- The puborectalis fibers are considered important in maintaining fecal continence; they originate from the posterior surface of the pubis and form a sling around the rectum.
- The pubococcygeus fibers originate from the posterior surface of the pubis and insert into the anococcygeal rapine.
- The iliococcygeus fibers originate from the obturator internus fascia and the ischium and insert into the anococcygeal rapine.

The fan-shaped coccygeus muscle lies anterior to the sacrospinous ligament, originates from the ischial spine, inserts onto the lower part of the sacrum and coccyx, and works synergistically to aid the levator ani muscle. The transverse perinei are small straplike muscles that help support the pelvic viscera. They originate from the ischial tuberosity, pass by the genitalia, and insert on the central tendon at the midline. The bulbocavernosus muscles aid in strengthening the pelvic diaphragm and in constricting the urinary and vaginal openings. Their muscle fibers originate in the perineal body and surround the vaginal openings as the muscle fibers pass forward to insert into the pubis. The ischiocavernous muscle contracts to cause erection of the clitoris during sexual arousal. Its muscle fibers originate in the tuberosities of the ischium and continue at an angle to insert next to the bulbocavernosus muscle (Anderson & Gendry, 2007).

Female Genitalia

Dr. Nelson Soucasaux, a Brazilian gynecologist, has devoted much of her writing to the traditionally typical and symbolic aspects of women's sexual organs, and the importance these views have in influencing our understanding of women's nature. She found that historically it was believed the key to understanding the female psyche was related to a deeper understanding of woman's genital functions (Soucasaux, 1993a, 1993b). By tradition, a woman's uterus was considered "the fundamental organ" and was synonymous with her genital organs. This conception depicted a woman's wholeness to be totally related to her genitals, of which the most important was her uterus. Consequently, there was little appreciation for female genitalia.

This section describes the multiple organs and anatomic structures that constitute a woman's gynecologic anatomy, which are shown in a midsagittal view in **Figure** 5-4 and **Color Plate 1**. Equally important to the discussion of women's gynecologic anatomy are the multiple nongenital peripheral anatomic structures involved in female sexual responses, such as salivary and sweat glands, cutaneous blood vessels, and breasts.

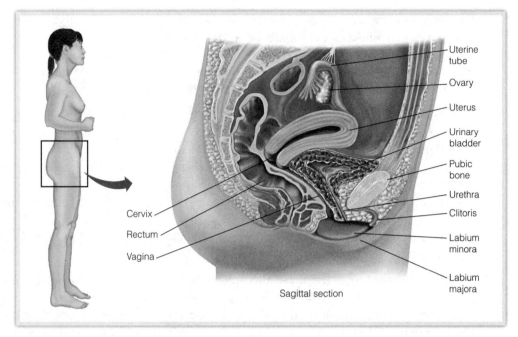

FIGURE 5-4 Midsagittal view of a woman's pelvic organs.

External Genital Anatomy

The Vulva The vulva is the externally visible outer genitalia (**Figure 5-5** and **Color Plate 2**). It includes the mons pubis, labia minora, labia majora, clitoris, urinary meatus, vaginal opening, and corpus spongiosum erectile tissue (vestibular bulbs) of the labia minora and perineum. The vestibule is inside the labia minora and outside the hymen. On each side of the vestibule is a Bartholin's gland, which secretes lubricating mucus into the introitus during sexual excitement. The mons pubis is the mound-like fatty tissue that covers and protects the symphysis pubis. During puberty, genital hair growth covers this pad of tissue.

The labia majora are fused anteriorly with the mons veneris, or anterior prominence of the symphysis pubis, and posteriorly with the perineal body or posterior commissure. They assist in keeping the vaginal introitus closed, which in turn helps prevent infection. The labia minora are surrounded by the labia majora and are smaller, non-fatty folds covered by non-hair-bearing skin laterally and by vaginal mucosa on the medial aspect. The anterior aspect of the labia minora forms the prepuce of the clitoris and also assists in enclosing the opening of the urethra and the vagina.

Women's vulva vary in size, related to the amount of adipose tissue, length, and pigment color of the labia minora or majora, which may be light pink, dark pink, shades of gray, peach, brown, or black. There is also considerable variation in the size of the labia minora in women of reproductive age (Katz, 2007). The labia minora are usually more prominent in children and women who are postmenopausal (Katz).

Clitoris The clitoris is a sensitive organ that is typically described as the female homologue of the penis in the male, particularly in its erogenous function (Federation of Women's Health Centers, 1981). During the early 1800s, a respected English gynecologist, Isaac Baker Brown, theorized that habitual clitoral stimulation was the cause of the majority of women's diseases because it caused an overexcitement of a woman's nervous system. As a result, clitorectomy came into favor as a means to rid women of ailments believed to be caused by clitoral stimulation (Duffy, 1963; Hall, 1998). Fortunately, this theory and practice has long been refuted, and the practice of clitorectomy in the Western world is rare.

Anatomically, the clitoris is formed from the genital tubercle (Bradshaw, 2008; Martini, Timmons, & Tallitsch, 2011). It is 1.5 to 2 cm in length, consists of two crura and two corpora cavernosa, and is covered by a sensitive rounded tubercle known as the glans (Anderson & Gendry, 2007; Katz, 2007). The clitoris is a small, sensitive organ consisting of two paired erectile chambers and is located at the superior portion of the vestibule (Katz). These chambers are composed of endothelial-lined lacunar spaces, trabecular smooth muscle, and trabecular connective tissue; they are surrounded by a fibrous sheath, the tunica albuginea. The paired corpus spongiosum (bilateral vestibular bulbs) unite ventrally to the urethral orifice to form a thin strand of spongiosus erectile tissue connection (pars intermedia) that ends in the clitoris as the glans (Martini et al.). The clitoris is capped externally by the glans, which is covered by a clitoral hood formed in part by the fusion of the upper part of the two labia minora. The clitoris has numerous nerve endings and contains tissue that fills with blood when sexually aroused. The blood supply to this organ includes the dorsal and clitoral cavernosal arteries, which arise from the iliohypogastric pudendal bed. The autonomic efferent motor innervation occurs via the cavernosal nerve of the clitoris arising from the pelvic and hypogastric plexus (Bradshaw; Katz).

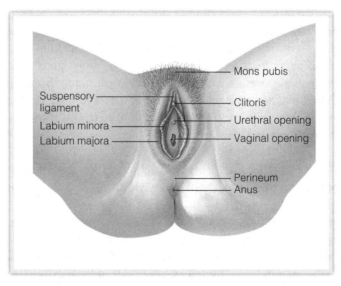

FIGURE 5-5 Female external genitalia.

The labia minora, together with the clitoris, play a critical role in sexual activity. Because of their rich nerve and vascular supply, they are easily sensitized and become engorged with blood during sexual arousal. This vascular erectile tissue is capable of becoming significantly enlarged and tense during sexual excitement. In addition to the great quantity of erectile tissue in the clitoris, erectile tissue is found inside the labia majora and minora, around the vulvovaginal opening, and along the lower third of the vagina. A very small quantity of this tissue can also be found in the vaginal walls and along the urethra. Age-associated female sexual dysfunction from decreased clitoral sensitivity may be associated with histologic changes in clitoral cavernosal erectile tissue (Katz, 2007).

Periurethral Glands Two Skene's (paraurethral) glands open directly into the vulva and are adjacent to the distal urethra (Katz, 2007). The Skene's glands, which release mucus, form a triangular area of mucous membrane surrounding the urethral meatus from the clitoral glans to the vaginal upper rim or caruncle (Martini et al., 2011).

Bartholin's or Greater Vestibular Glands The pea-sized Bartholin's glands are located at about the 4 and 8 o'clock positions in the vulvovaginal area, just beneath the fascia. Each gland has an approximately 2-cm duct that opens into a groove between the labia minora and hymen. The glands, which are made of columnar cells that secrete clear or whitish mucus, are stimulated during sexual arousal (Corton, 2008). If the Bartholin's ducts are blocked, infection can occur, resulting in cyst formation that can lead to the development of an abscess requiring surgical incision and drainage.

Internal Genital Anatomy

Urethra The urethra is a short conduit, approximately 3 to 5 cm long, extending from the base of the bladder and exiting externally in the periurethral glans area (Katz, 2007). The urethral mucosa is composed of stratified transitional epithelium near the urinary bladder; the rest of this structure is lined by a stratified squamous epithelium (Katz; Martini et al., 2011). In women, the urethra passes through the urogenital diaphragm, which is a circular band of skeletal muscle that forms the sphincter urethrae, better known as the external urethral sphincter (Martini et al.) For a woman to urinate, this sphincter must be voluntarily relaxed—its typical state is contraction.

Ovaries The paired ovaries resemble a large almond in terms of their size and configuration; they are located near the lateral walls of the pelvic cavity (Katz, 2007; Martini et al., 2011) Each ovary measures approximately 1.5 cm × 2.5 cm × 4 cm and weighs 3 to 6 gm (Katz).

The ovaries produce gametes (also known as ova) and the sex hormones estrogen and progesterone. The color and texture of these organs change with a woman's age and reproductive stage. The ovaries in a nulliparous woman are situated on a shallow depression called the ovarian fossa, located on either side of the uterus in the upper pelvic cavity. Several ligaments support the ovaries. The broad ligament is the principal supporting membrane of a woman's internal genital organs, including the fallopian tubes and uterus. The remaining ligaments include the mesovarium, a posterior extension of the broad ligament; the ovarian ligament, which is anchored to the uterus; and a suspensory ligament, which is attached to the pelvic wall. The outermost layer of the ovary is composed of a thin layer of cuboidal epithelial cells called the germinal epithelium. Immediately below this epithelial layer is the tunica albuginea, which is made up of collagenous tissue (Katz, 2007).

The ovaries comprise three parts:

- An outer cortical region (cortex), which contains germinal epithelium with oogonia and ovarian follicles that number about 400,000 at the initiation of puberty (Halvorson, 2008a)
- The medullary region (medulla), which consists of connective tissue, myoid-like contractile cells, and interstitial cells
- A hilum, which is the point of entrance for all of the ovarian vessels and nerves (Halvorson, 2008a; Katz, 2007)

Two ovarian arteries that arise from the aorta descend in the retroperitoneal space and cross in front of the psoas muscles and internal iliac vessels (Katz, 2007). They enter the infundibulopelvic ligaments, finally reaching the mesovarium found in the broad ligament (Katz). The ovarian blood supply enters through the hilum, and venous return occurs through a venous plexus, which collects blood from the adnexal region and drains into the vena cava on the right and the renal vein on the left (Katz).

Innervation of the ovaries is accomplished by sympathetic and parasympathetic fibers of the ovarian plexus that descend along the ovarian vessels. These nerves supply the ovaries, broad ligaments, and uterine tube. The parasympathetic fibers in the ovarian plexus arise from the vagus nerves. The nerve fibers to the ovaries innervate only the vascular networks, and not the stroma (Katz, 2007). Because the ovaries and surrounding peritoneum are sensitive to pain and pressure, it is important to take great care when examining the ovaries during the bimanual examination.

Fallopian Tubes The fallopian tubes (also known as the oviducts) are paired narrow muscular tubes that extend approximately 10 cm from each cornu of the body of the uterus, outward to their openings near the ovaries. Each fallopian tube includes four segments:

- The pars interstitialis (intramural portion) penetrates the uterine wall. It contains the fewest mucosal folds with the myometrium contributing to its muscularis.
- The isthmus, the narrow segment adjacent to the uterine wall, contains few mucosal folds.
- The middle segment known as the ampulla is the widest and longest segment, contains extensive branched mucosal folds, and is the most common site of fertilization.
- The infundibulum, the funnel-shaped distal segment, opens near the ovary but is not attached (Katz, 2007). Very fine fingerlike fronds of its mucosal folds, the fimbriae, project from the opening toward the ovary to help direct the oocyte into the lumen of the fallopian tube.

The inner surface of each fallopian tubes is covered by fine hairlike structures called cilia that help to move ova, released from the ovaries, along the tube and into the cavity of the uterus. The fallopian tube extends medially and inferiorly from the infundibulum into the superior-lateral cavity of the uterine opening (Katz, 2007).

The wall of the fallopian tube is composed of three layers: mucosa, muscularis, and serosa. The internal mucosa includes the lamina propria and ciliated columnar epithelium, consisting primarily of two main cell types. On the surface, the abundant ciliated columnar cells beat in waves toward the uterus, aiding in egg transport. Shorter, mucus-secreting peg cells are interspersed among the ciliated cells. These cilia propel the film they produce toward the uterus, help transport the ovum, and hinder bacterial access to the peritoneal cavity. The muscularis—the middle layer—contains both inner circular and outer longitudinal smooth muscle layers. Its wavelike contractions move the ovum toward the uterus. The outer covering of the fallopian tubes is the serosa; this lubricative layer is part of the visceral peritoneum (Corton, 2008; Katz, 2007).

The ovarian and uterine arteries supply blood to the fallopian tubes. The uterine veins, which parallel the path of the arteries, provide the venous drainage. Sympathetic and parasympathetic innervation to the fallopian tubes from the hypogastric plexus and pelvic splanchnic nerves regulates the activity of the smooth muscles and blood vessels (Corton, 2008).

Uterus   The uterus is a muscular, inverted, pear-shaped, hollow, thick-walled organ that opens to the vagina at the cervix and then widens toward the top where the uterine tubes enter. Its anatomic regions include the fundus, body, and cervix (**Figure 5-6** and **Color Plate 3**). The fundus is the uppermost dome-shaped extension of the uterine body, located above the point of entry of the fallopian tubes. The body is the enlarged main portion. The cervix is the downward constricted extension of the uterus that opens into the vagina.

The uterus is located anteriorly between the urinary bladder and posteriorly between the sigmoid colon and rectum. When the bladder is empty, the uterus angles forward over the bladder. As the bladder fills, the uterus is lifted dorsally and may become retroflexed, pressing against the rectum. The nulliparous uterus is approximately 8 cm long, 5 cm wide, and 2.5 cm thick, and weighs approximately 40 to 50 gm (Katz, 2007).

The uterine wall of the fundus and body consists of three layers: the endometrium, the myometrium, and the serosa (also known as the adventitia). The uterine mucosa layer consists of simple columnar epithelium supported by a lamina propria. Simple tubular glands extend from the luminal surface into the lamina propria. The stratum functionale is the temporary layer at the luminal surface that responds to ovarian hormones by undergoing cyclic thickening and shedding. The stratum basale is the deeper, thinner, permanent layer that contains the basal portions of the endometrial glands; this layer is retained during menstruation. The epithelial cells lining these glands divide and cover the raw surface of exposed endometrium that occurs during menstruation.

The endometrium receives a double blood supply. In the middle of the myometrium, a pair of uterine arteries branch to form the arcuate arteries. These arteries bifurcate into two sets of arteries: straight arteries to the stratum basale and coiled arteries to the functionalis.

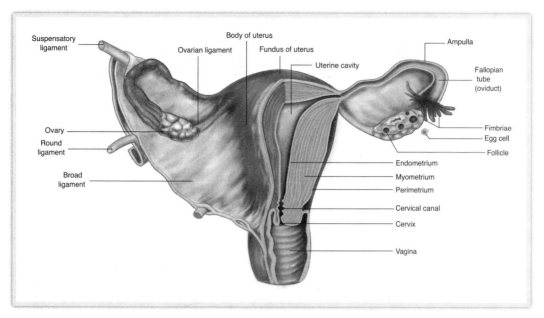

FIGURE 5-6 An anterior view of the female internal genital anatomy showing the relationships of the ovaries, fallopian tubes, uterus, cervix, and vagina.

The double blood supply to the endometrium is important in the cyclic shedding of the functionalis; the straight arteries are retained as the coiled arteries are lost (Anderson & Gendry, 2007).

The myometrium is composed of four poorly defined layers of smooth muscle that are thickest at the top of the uterus. The middle layers contain the abundant arcuate arteries. The outer layer of the uterus consists of two types of outer coverings: A cap of serosa covers the fundus, and the body is surrounded by an adventitia of loose connective tissue (Anderson & Gendry, 2007).

Structurally, the cervix is made mostly of dense connective tissue, is about 2.5 cm in length, and is covered interiorly by a mucus-secreting ciliated epithelium at the upper regions and by stratified squamous epithelium at the vaginal end. The opening of the cervix into the vagina occurs at almost a right angle to the long axis of the vagina. Uterine blood supply is provided via the uterine and ovarian arteries, with venous return traveling via the uterine veins. The hypogastric and ovarian nerve plexuses supply sympathetic and parasympathetic fibers as well as carry uterine afferent sensory fibers on their way to the spinal cord at T11 and T12 (Anderson & Gendry, 2007; Faiz & Moffat, 2002).

Vagina The vagina is a thin-walled tube extending from the external vulva to the cervix. Its walls are normally in apposition and flattened, but can extend (stretch) greatly, as observed during childbirth. The length of the vaginal walls varies greatly but on average the anterior vaginal length is 6 to 9 cm and the posterior vaginal length is 8 to 12 cm (Corton, 2008;

Katz, 2007). The upper portion of the vagina encircles the vaginal portion of the cervix. The vagina touches the empty bladder on the ventral and superior surface. Inferiorly, it adheres to the posterior wall of the urethra and opens adjacent to the labia minora.

The internal mucosal layer of the vagina contains traverse folds, known as rugae. This muscular canal extends from the midpoint of the cervix to its opening located between the urethra and rectum. The mucous membrane lining the vagina and musculature is continuous with the uterus. The vaginal walls can be easily separated because their surfaces are normally moist, lubricated by a basal vaginal fluid.

The vaginal wall is composed of three layers: mucosa, muscle, and adventitia. Vaginal epithelium is stratified squamous epithelium supported by a thick lamina propria. The lamina propria has many thin-walled blood vessels that contribute to diffusion of vaginal fluid across the epithelium. The lamina propria of the mucosa contains many elastic fibers as well as a dense network of blood vessels, lymph nodes, and nerve supply. To a much lesser degree than seen in the skin, this epithelium undergoes hormone-related cyclic changes, including slight keratinization of the superficial cells during the menstrual cycle (Corton, 2008). The epithelium has no glands, and therefore it does not secrete mucus. Estrogen causes the epithelium to thicken, differentiate, and accumulate glycogen. Vaginal bacteria metabolize the glycogen to lactic acid, causing the typically low pH of the vaginal environment.

Loose connective tissue containing many elastic fibers is found underneath the vaginal epithelium, which has a subdermal layer rich in capillaries. This rich vascular supply is the source for vaginal moisture during sexual stimulation (Soper, 2007).

Within the epithelium lie the smooth muscles of the muscularis oriented longitudinally on the outer layer, and circular bundles on the inner layer. The outer layer—the adventitia—consists of dense connective tissue with many elastic fibers, which provides structural support for the vagina. It also contains an extensive nerve supply and venous capillaries. The adventitia is elastic and rich in collagen, provides structural support to the vagina, and allows for expansion of the vagina during intercourse and childbirth.

The upper two-thirds of the vagina receives efferent innervation through the uterovaginal plexus, which contains both sympathetic and parasympathetic fibers. The pelvic splanchnic nerves provide the parasympathetic efferent input to the uterovaginal plexus. The proximal two-thirds of the vagina is innervated via the uterovaginal plexus. The lower vagina receives autonomic efferent innervation from the pudendal nerve. The distal one-third of the vagina has primarily somatic sensation; this innervation arises from the pudendal nerve and is carried to the sacral spinal cord (Katz, 2007).

Breast Anatomy and Physiology

In Western society, it often seems that a woman's breasts have two functions or roles: one that is sexual, and one that is maternal. The breasts are visible social sex symbols, and they are often a key source of a woman's anxiety about her body. Breasts often define women in both the public and private eye.

The breasts—that is, the mammary glands—are large, modified sebaceous glands contained within the superficial fascia of the chest wall located over the pectoral muscles (Valea & Katz, 2007). Each consists of a nipple, lobes, ducts, and fibrous and fatty tissue (**Color Plate 4**). Each breast is composed of 15 to 20 lobes of glandular tissue. The number of lobes is not related to the size of the breast. The lobes branch to form 20 to 40 lobules, which are subdivided into many secretory alveoli. These glands are connected together by a series of ducts. The alveoli produce milk and other substances during lactation. Each lobe empties into a single lactiferous duct that travels out through the nipple. As a result, there are 15 to 20 passages through the nipple, resulting in just as many openings in the nipple. Behind the nipple, the lactiferous ducts enlarge slightly to form small reservoirs called lactiferous sinuses. Each sinus is 2 to 4 mm in diameter.

Fatty and connective tissues surround the lobes of glandular tissue. The amount of fatty tissue depends on many factors including age, percentage of body fat, and heredity. Cooper's ligaments connect the chest wall to the skin of the breast, giving the breast its shape and elasticity (Valea & Katz, 2007). The size of the nonpregnant breasts reflects the amount of adipose tissue in the breast rather than the amount of glandular tissue. The secretory nature of the breasts develops during pregnancy.

The nipple and areola are located near the center of each breast; the areola is the pigmented area surrounding the nipple. These areas usually have a color and texture that differs from that of the adjacent skin. The color varies and darkens during pregnancy and lactation. The consistency of the nipple and areola may range from very smooth to wrinkled and bumpy. The size of the nipples and areolae also varies a great deal from woman to woman, and some size variation between a woman's breasts is normal. The nipple and areola are made of smooth muscle fibers and feature a thick network of nerve endings.

The areola is populated by numerous oil-producing Montgomery's glands. These glands may form raised bumps and be responsive to a woman's menstrual cycle. They protect and lubricate the nipple during lactation.

The nipple usually protrudes out from the surface of the breast. Some nipples project inward or are flat with the surface of the breast. Neither flat nor inverted nipples appear to negatively affect a woman's ability to breastfeed.

Reproductive hormones are vital to the development of the breast during puberty and lactation. Prolactin (PRL) and growth hormone (GH) from the anterior lobe of the pituitary stimulate mammary gland development. These hormones are aided by human placental lactogen from the placenta, which stimulates the mammary gland ducts to become active during pregnancy. Estrogen promotes the growth of the gland and ducts, while progesterone stimulates the development of milk-producing cells. Prolactin, which is released from the anterior pituitary, stimulates milk production. Oxytocin, which is released from the posterior pituitary in response to suckling, causes milk ejection from the lactating breast.

The lymphatic system in the breast is abundant and empties the breast tissue of excess fluid. Lymph nodes along the pathway of drainage monitor for foreign bodies such as bacteria or viruses. Although the main flow moves toward the axilla and anterior axillary nodes, lymph drainage has been shown to pass in all directions from the breast (Martini et al., 2011).

Menstrual Cycle Physiology

The initiation of menstruation, called menarche, usually happens between the ages of 12 and 15. Menstrual cycles typically continue to age 45 to 55, when menopause occurs. Many women find themselves reluctant to discuss the existence and normality of menstruation. The word "menstruation" has been replaced by a variety of euphemisms, such as "the curse," "my period," "my monthly," "my friend," "the red flag," or "on the rag."

Most women experience deviations from the average menstrual cycle during their reproductive years. As a result, it is not uncommon for women to display certain preoccupations regarding their menstrual bleeding, not only in relation to the regularity of its occurrence, but also in regard to the characteristics of the flow, such as volume, duration, and associated signs and symptoms. Unfortunately, society has encouraged the notion that a woman's normalcy is based on her ability to bear children. This misperception has understandably forced women to perseverate over the most miniscule changes in their menstrual cycles. Changes in menstruation are one of the most frequent reasons why women visit their clinician.

Numerous patterns in the secretion of estrogens and progesterone are possible; in fact, it is difficult to find two cycles that are exactly the same. Studies that include women of different ethnicities, occupations, nutritional status, and age have demonstrated that the length and duration of different menstrual cycles are as variable as the cycles themselves (Koff, Rierdan, & Stubbs, 1990; Robert, 1992).

Menarche is the most readily evident external event that indicates the end of one developmental stage and the beginning of a new one. It is now believed that body composition is critically important in determining the onset of puberty and menstruation in young women (Lobo, 2007). The ratio of total body weight to lean body weight is probably the most relevant factor, and individuals who are moderately obese (20% to 30% above their ideal body weight) have an earlier onset of menarche (Lobo). Widely accepted standards for distinguishing what are regular versus irregular, or normal versus abnormal menses, are generally based on what is considered average and not necessarily typical for every woman. According to these standards, the normal menstrual cycle is 21 to 35 days with a menstrual flow lasting 4 to 6 days, although a flow for as few as 2 days or as many as 8 days is still considered normal (Olive & Palter, 2007).

The amount of menstrual flow varies, with the average being 50 mL; nevertheless, the amount of flow may be as little as 20 mL or as much as 80 mL. Generally, women are not aware that anovulatory cycles and abnormal uterine bleeding (changes in bleeding outside of normal; see Chapter 25) are common after menarche and just prior to menopause (Fritz & Speroff, 2011; Olive & Palter, 2007). Menstrual cycles that occur during the first year to year and a half after menarche are frequently irregular due to the immaturity of the hypothalamic–pituitary–ovarian axes (Fritz & Speroff).

The Hypothalamic–Pituitary–Ovarian Axis

Hypothalamus The hypothalamus controls anterior pituitary functions via the secretion of releasing and inhibiting factors. Together with the pituitary, it manages the production of hormones that serve as chemical messengers for the regulation of the gynecologic system. The hypothalamus initially releases gonadotropin-releasing hormone (GnRH) in a pulsatile manner. On average, the frequency of GnRH secretion is once per 90 minutes during the early follicular phase, increases to once per 60 to 70 minutes, and then decreases during the luteal phase (Halvorson, 2008b). The release of GnRH stimulates the pituitary gland to produce follicle-stimulating hormone (FSH) and luteinizing hormone (LH). Estrogen and progesterone are secreted by the ovaries at the command of FSH and LH and complete the hormonal group necessary for gynecologic health.

Pituitary Gland The oval-shaped, pea-sized pituitary gland is located in a small depression in the sphenoid bone of the skull. It is controlled by the hypothalamus, which secretes releasing factors into a special blood vessel network (hypothalamic–hypophyseal portal system) that feeds the pituicytes (Olive & Palter, 2007). These releasing factors either stimulate or inhibit the release of pituitary hormones that travel via the circulatory system to target organs.

The anterior pituitary synthesizes seven hormones:

- Growth hormone (GH)
- Thyroid-stimulating hormone (TSH)
- Adrenocorticotropin (ACTH)
- Melanocyte-stimulating hormone (MSH)
- Prolactin (PRL)
- Follicle-stimulating hormone (FSH)
- Luteinizing hormone (LH)

FSH and LH (both gonadotropins), are responsible for regulating gynecologic organ activities. FSH targets the ovaries, where it stimulates the growth and development of the primary follicles and results in the production of estrogen and progesterone. The release of FSH from the pituitary is governed by a negative feedback mechanism involving these steroids. The target for LH is the developing follicle within the ovary. LH is responsible for ovulation, corpus luteum formation, and hormone production in the ovaries. Prolactin is responsible for preparing the mammary gland for lactation and brings about the synthesis of milk (Olive & Palter, 2007).

Ovaries and Uterus Complex changes occur in the ovaries and the endometrium as a result of the rhythmic fluctuations of gonadotropic hormones. The endometrium emulates the activities of the ovaries; thus whatever happens in the uterus during the cycle is precisely correlated with whatever is occurring in the ovaries. The objective of the ovarian cycle is to produce an ovum, while the objective of the endometrial cycle is to prepare a site to nourish and maintain the ovum if it becomes fertilized. The ovarian cycle includes three distinct phases:

the follicular phase, ovulation, and the luteal phase. The endometrial cycle can be divided into the proliferative phase, the secretory phase, and menstruation (Fritz & Speroff, 2011).

Hormonal Feedback System

The menstrual cycle is determined by a complex interaction of hormones. The monthly rhythmic functioning of the menstrual cycle depends on the changing concentrations of gonadotropic hormones. The release of LH and FSH from the pituitary depends on the secretion of GnRH from the hypothalamus, which is modulated by the feedback effects of estrogen and progesterone. The hormones LH and FSH, in turn, play important roles in stimulating secretion of estrogen and progesterone. Virtually all hormones are released in short pulses at intervals of 60 to 90 minutes throughout most of the cycle, with these pulses decreasing in frequency closer to menstruation. Steroid hormones modulate the frequency and amplitude of the pulse, which varies throughout the cycle (Fritz & Speroff, 2011) (see **Color Plate 5**).

Under normal physiologic conditions, GnRH pulses stimulate the release of FSH and LH. Under the influence of gonadotropic hormone stimulation, the ovarian follicles develop and produce estrogen. As the amount of estrogen in the circulation increases and reaches the pituitary gland, it affects the amount of FSH and LH secreted, albeit without significantly affecting the pulse frequency (negative feedback). When the estrogen level becomes high enough, the negative feedback effect on the pituitary is reversed. Now estrogen causes a mid-cycle positive feedback effect on the pituitary, which results in a surge of LH and FSH and causes ovulation. Under LH influence, the ruptured follicle becomes the corpus luteum and secretes progesterone. Although the presence of progesterone reduces the frequency of the hypothalamic GnRH pulses, the amount of LH released from the pituitary is proportionally increased to sustain the corpus luteum and the production of progesterone. In the absence of pregnancy, the corpus luteum degenerates, progesterone levels decline, and menstruation occurs. The GnRH pulses return to the frequency associated with the beginning of the follicular phase and a new cycle begins (Olive & Palter, 2007).

The Ovarian Cycle

The ovarian cycle has three phases: follicular, ovulatory, and luteal.

Follicular Phase The follicular phase is characterized by the development of ovarian follicles and usually lasts from day 1 (first day of menses) to day 14 of the ovarian cycle. Folliculogenesis begins during the last few days of the previous menstrual cycle and continues until the release of the mature follicle at ovulation. The decrease in estrogen production by the corpus luteum and the dramatic fall of inhibin levels allow the FSH level to rise during the last few days of the menstrual cycle. During days 1 through 4 of the menstrual cycle, a cohort of primary follicles is recruited from a pool of nonproliferating follicles in response to the increased concentration of FSH (Fritz & Speroff, 2011). Follicles that have enough granulosa cells will develop receptors for estrogen and FSH on the cells of the granulosa layers, and LH receptors on the theca cells. The primary role of FSH is to induce the development of increased receptors on the granulosa cells to produce estrogen. The preliminary role of LH is to stimulate the cells' production of androgen that will be converted to estrogen by the granulosa layers.

Between cycle days 5 and 7, only one dominant follicle from the cohort of recruited follicles is destined to ovulate during the next menstrual cycle. As menses progresses, FSH levels decline due to the negative feedback of estrogen and the negative effects of the peptide hormone inhibin, which is secreted by the granulosa and theca cells of the developing follicle (Fritz & Speroff, 2011; Olive & Palter, 2007). The decrease in FSH level promotes a more androgenic microenvironment within adjacent follicles. By the eighth day of the cycle, the dominant follicle (Graafian follicle) is producing more estrogen than the total amount produced by the other developing follicles. In response to the dominant follicle's combined production of estrogen and FSH, LH receptors develop on its outermost granulosa layers. The dominant follicle continues to flourish and gradually moves toward the surface of the ovary (see **Color Plate 6**). The Graafian follicle contains the ovum and is surrounded by a layer of granulosa cells, which are further surrounded by the specialized theca interna and theca externa cells. An oocyte maturation inhibitor (OMI) in the follicular fluid suppresses the final maturation of the dominant follicle until the time of ovulation. The OMI's suppressive effects will end hours before the LH surge that causes ovulation (Olive & Palter).

Ovulatory Phase Ovulation is the process whereby the mature ovum is released from the follicle (Olive & Palter, 2007). It occurs approximately 10 to 12 hours after the LH peak—that is, when the highest level of LH is attained. Ovulation and the subsequent conversion of the follicle to the corpus luteum are dependent on an increased level of estrogen and the LH surge, which marks the beginning of the rapid rise of LH. During the mid-follicular phase, the dominant follicle's FSH levels diminish, but estrogen levels continue to increase. At the end of the follicular phase, estrogen reaches a blood level of approximately 200 picograms per milliliter (pg/mL); this concentration may be maintained for as long as 50 hours (Fritz & Speroff, 2011; Olive & Palter). At this critical time, the high estrogen level initiates a positive feedback of LH, generating the preovulatory LH surge. The LH surge begins 34 to 36 hours prior to ovulation and provides a relatively accurate predictor for timing ovulation. The LH surge is responsible for many changes in the follicle selected for rupture.

Initially the nuclear membrane around the oocyte breaks down, the chromosomes progress through the rest of the first meiotic division, and the egg moves on to the secondary stage. Meiosis ceases at this time and will be initiated again only if the ovum is fertilized. The LH surge stimulates luteinization of the granulosa cells as well as synthesis of progesterone. Progesterone, in turn, enhances the positive feedback effect of estrogen on the LH surge and is responsible for promoting enzyme activity in the follicular fluid capable of digesting the follicle wall. High levels of LH and progesterone cause the synthesis of prostaglandins and proteolytic enzymes such as collagenase and plasmin. Although the exact mechanism at work is unknown, the activated proteolytic enzymes and prostaglandins digest collagen in the follicular wall, leading to an explosive release of the ovum (oocyte), along with the zona pellucida and corona radiata surrounding it. At ovulation, the ovum is expelled and drawn up by the ciliated fimbriae of the fallopian tube to initiate its migration through the oviduct (Fritz & Speroff, 2011; Olive & Palter, 2007).

New information about the timing of the LH surge and ovulation is available now because of the amount of data collected by many clinicians during in vitro fertilization. The LH surge has a tendency to occur around 3 a.m. in more than two-thirds of women, and ovulation has been found to occur primarily in the morning during the spring months and primarily during the evening during autumn and winter (Fritz & Speroff, 2011). In the Northern Hemisphere, from July to February, around 90% of women will ovulate between 4 and 7 p.m. During the spring, 50% of women will ovulate between midnight and 11 a.m. (Fritz & Speroff, p. 228).

Luteal Phase Under the influence of LH, the follicle's granulosa cells that are left in the ruptured follicle become enlarged, undergo luteinization, and form the corpus luteum. The corpus luteum continues to function for approximately 8 days after ovulation. It secretes increased progesterone and some estrogen that start the negative feedback loop to the hypothalamus and pituitary gland, preventing further ovulation within the current cycle. In the absence of a fertilized ovum, luteal cells degenerate, causing a decline in estrogen and progesterone levels, and the corpus luteum regresses to become the corpus albicans. As a result of the regression of the corpus luteum, estrogen and progesterone levels decrease rapidly, removing the negative feedback effect. FSH and LH then begin to increase once again to initiate the next menstrual cycle (Fritz & Speroff, 2011; Olive & Palter, 2007).

The Endometrial Cycle

The endometrial cycle has three phases: proliferative, secretory, and menstrual.

Proliferative Phase The proliferative phase is influenced by estrogen and entails the regrowth of endometrium after the menstrual bleed. It starts on about the fourth or fifth day of the cycle and usually lasts about 10 days, ending with the release of the ovum. The proliferative phase involves changes in the endometrium, myometrium, and ovaries. These cyclic changes, which result from fluctuations in gonadotropin and estrogen levels, are characterized by progressive mitotic growth of the deciduas functionalis in response to increasing levels of estrogen secreted by the ovary. The changes occur in preparation for implantation of the fertilized ovum.

At the beginning of the proliferative phase, the endometrium is relatively thin and the endometrial glands are straight, narrow, and short. As the phase progresses, the glands become long and tortuous. The endometrium becomes thicker as a result of the glandular hyperplasia and growth of the stroma. The endometrium proliferates from 0.5 to 5 mm in height and increases eightfold in thickness in preparation for implantation of the fertilized ovum (Olive & Palter, 2007).

Secretory Phase The secretory phase begins at ovulation. When part of a 28-day cycle, it usually lasts from day 15 (the day after ovulation—the exact cycle day will vary with cycle length) to day 28. This phase does not take place if ovulation has not occurred. It tends to be the most constant phase, in terms of time.

During the secretory phase, the glands of the endometrium become more tortuous and dilated and fill with secretions, primarily as a result of increased progesterone production. The endometrium becomes thick, cushiony, and nutritive in preparation for implantation of the fertilized ovum. In the absence of implantation, the corpus luteum shrinks, and progesterone and estrogen levels subsequently fall. The endometrium begins to regress toward the end of the secretory phase. By days 25 to 26, progesterone and estrogen withdrawal results in increased tortuous coiling and constriction of the spiral arterioles in the thinning layer.

Until the last decade, it was believed that decreased blood flow to the superficial endometrial layers resulted in tissue ischemia and resulting menses. The end of menses was believed to be caused "by longer and more intense waves of vasoconstriction, combined with coagulation mechanisms activated by vascular stasis and endometrial collapse, aided by rapid re-epitheliazation mediated by estrogen from the emerging new follicular cohort" (Fritz & Speroff, 2011, p. 595). Newer studies do not support the theory that menstruation results due to vascular events. The current theory about the initiation of the menstruation is that it is due to enzymatic autodigestion of the functional layer of the endometrium, which is triggered by estrogen–progesterone withdrawal (Fritz & Speroff). As estrogen and progesterone levels fall during the days prior to menses, lysosomal membranes become destabilized, such that the enzymes within them are released into the cytoplasm of the epithelial, stromal, and endothelial cells and into the intercellular space. These enzymes are proteolytic: They digest the cells surrounding them as well as surface membranes. Their actions result in platelet deposition, release of prostaglandins, vascular thrombosis, extravasation of red blood cells, and tissue necrosis in the vascular endothelium (Olive & Palter, 2007). Enzymatic action progressively degrades the endometrium and eventually disrupts the capillaries and venous system just under the endometrial surface, causing interstitial hemorrhage and dissolution of the surface membrane and allowing blood to escape into the endometrial cavity (Fritz & Speroff). This degeneration continues and extends to the functional layer of the endometrium, where rupture of the basal arterioles contributes to the bleeding. The concepts about how the menstrual flow ceases remain unchanged.

Menstrual Phase The menstrual phase begins with the initiation of menses and lasts four to six days. Prostaglandins initiate contractions of the uterine smooth muscle and sloughing of the degraded endometrial tissue, leading to menstruation. The composition of menstrual fluid comprises desquamated endometrial tissue, red blood cells, inflammatory exudates, and proteolytic enzymes. Because some of the clotting factors ordinarily found in blood are lysed by lysosomal enzymes in the uterus, menstrual blood does not clot (Fritz & Speroff, 2011; Olive & Palter, 2007). For three to five days, 20 to 80 mL (on average) of blood loss occurs. Approximately two days after the start of menstruation, estrogen stimulates the regeneration of the surface endometrial epithelium, while concurrent simultaneous endometrial shedding is occurring.

Changes in Organs Due to Cyclic Changes

Cervix After menstruation, the cervical mucus is scant and viscous. During the late follicular phase, it becomes clear, copious, and elastic. The quantity of cervical mucus increases 30-fold compared to the early follicular phase (Fritz & Speroff, 2011; Halvorson, 2008b). The cervical mucus during this time is clear and stretchable (spinnbarkeit). It displays a characteristic ferning appearance during the ovulatory period if observed under a microscope.

After ovulation, when progesterone levels are high, the cervical mucus once again becomes thick, viscous, opaque, and decreased in amount. This thick mucus is hostile and impenetrable to the sperm. The increased viscosity also reduces the risk of ascending infection at the time of possible implantation.

Increased estrogen levels promote stromal vascularization and edema and relax the myometrial fibers that supply the cervix. Activated collagenase causes the tightly bound collagen bundles to become a loose matrix, triggering the cervix to become softer a few days prior to and at ovulation. The external cervical os everts prior to ovulation. Progesterone causes the cervical muscle to retract, the collagen matrix to tighten, and the cervix to become firmer (Fritz & Speroff, 2011; Halvorson, 2008b).

Fallopian Tube Mobility Estrogen stimulates epithelial cell activity, resulting in increased cilia movement and secretions in the uterine tubes. These special effects assist ovum mobility along the fallopian tube following ovulation. Progesterone reverses these effects, thereby inhibiting the peristaltic activity of the fallopian tube smooth muscle.

Vagina The changes in hormonal levels of estrogen and progesterone have characteristic effects on the vaginal epithelium. This information becomes important when cervical cells are examined under the microscope, as their morphological differences can be related to specific stages of the menstrual cycle. During the early follicular phase, exfoliated vaginal epithelial cells have vesicular nuclei and are basophilic. They appear flatter than those in the later phases under the influence of progesterone, when they are folded and clumped. The pH of the vagina responds to cyclical changes as estrogen stimulates the growth of lactobacilli. Lactobacilli metabolize glycogen from cervical secretions, producing lactic acid that decreases the vaginal pH to a level that assists in protecting the gynecologic tract against opportunistic pathogens (Fritz & Speroff, 2011; Halvorson, 2008b).

References

Anderson, J., & Gendry, R. (2007). Anatomy and embryology. In J. Berek (Ed.), *Berek and Novak's gynecology* (14th ed., pp. 75–127). Philadelphia: Lippincott Williams & Wilkins.

Bradshaw, K. (2008). Anatomic disorders. In J. Schorge, J. Schaffer, L. Halvorson, B. Hoffman, K. Bradshaw, & F. G. Cunningham (Eds.), *Williams gynecology* (pp. 402–425). New York: McGraw Hill.

Caldwell, W. E., & Moloy, H. C. (1933). Anatomical variations in female pelvic bones and their effect on labor with a suggested classification. *American Journal of Obstetrics and Gynecology, 26,* 479–482.

Corton, M. (2008). Anatomy. In J. Schorge, J. Schaffer, L. Halvorson, B. Hoffman, K. Bradshaw, & F. G. Cunningham (Eds.), *Williams gynecology* (pp. 773–802). New York: McGraw Hill.

Duffy, J. (1963, October 19). Masturbation and clitoridectomy. *Journal of the American Medical Association, 186,* 246–248.

Faize, O., & Moffat, D. (2002). *Anatomy at a glance.* Oxford, UK: Blackwell.

Federation of Women's Health Centers. (1981). *A new view of a woman's body: A fully illustrated guide.* New York: Simon & Schuster.

Fritz, M., & Speroff, L. (2011). *Clinical gynecologic endocrinology and infertility.* Philadelphia: Lippincott Williams & Wilkins.

Hall, L. A. (1998). *The other in the mirror: Sex, Victorians, and historians.* Retrieved from http://homepages.primex.co.uk/~lesleyah/sexvict.htm

Halvorson, L. (2008a). Amenorrhea. In J. Schorge, J. Schaffer, L. Halvorson, B. Hoffman, K. Bradshaw, & F. G. Cunningham (Eds.), *Williams gynecology* (pp. 365–382). New York: McGraw Hill.

Halvorson, L. M. (2008b). Reproductive endocrinology. In J. Schorge, J. Schaffer, L. Halvorson, B. Hoffman, K. Bradshaw, & F. G. Cunningham (Eds.), *Williams gynecology* (pp. 330–364). New York: McGraw Hill.

Katz, V. (2007). Reproductive anatomy. In V. Katz, G. Lentz, R. Lobob, & D. Gershenson (Eds.), *Comprehensive gynecology* (5th ed., pp. 43–71). Philadelphia: Mosby Elsevier.

Koff, E., Rierdan, J., & Stubbs, M. I. (1990). Conceptions and misconceptions of the menstrual cycle. *Women and Health, 16*(3–4), 119–136.

Lobo, R. (2007). Primary and secondary amenorrhea and precocious puberty. In V. Katz, G. Lentz, R. Lobo, & D. Gershenson (Eds.), *Comprehensive gynecology* (5th ed., pp. 933–961). Philadelphia: Mosby Elsevier.

Martini, F., Timmons, M. J., & Tallitsch, R. (2011). *Human anatomy* (7th ed.). San Francisco: Benjamin Cummings.

Olive, D., & Palter, S. (2007). Reproductive physiology. In J. Berek (Ed.), *Berek and Novak's gynecology* (14th ed., pp. 171–184). Philadelphia: Lippincott Williams & Wilkins.

Richter, H., & Varner, R. (2007). Pelvic organ prolapse. In J. Berek (Ed.), *Berek and Novak's gynecology* (14th ed., pp. 897–934). Philadelphia: Lippincott Williams & Wilkins.

Robert, D. (1992). Cultural change and the reproductive cycle. *Social Science & Medicine, 34,* 485–490.

Soper, D. (2007). Genitourinary infections and sexually transmitted diseases. In J. Berek (Ed.), *Berek and Novak's gynecology* (14th ed., pp. 541–559). Philadelphia: Lippincott Williams & Wilkins.

Soucasaux, N. (1993a). *Archetypal aspects of the female genitals.* Retrieved, from http://www.mum.org/sougenit.htm

Soucasaux, N. (1993b). *Psychosomatic and symbolic aspects of menstruation.* Retrieved from http://www158.pair.com/hfinley/psychos

Valea, F., & Katz, V. (2007). Breast diseases. In V. Katz, G. Lentz, R. Lobo, & D. Gershenson (Eds.), *Comprehensive gynecology* (5th ed., pp. 327–357). Philadelphia: Mosby Elsevier.

CHAPTER 6

Gynecologic History and Physical Examination

Deborah Narrigan

The word *gynecology* is derived from the Greek term *gyne*, meaning "woman—more as queen" and is defined as "a branch of medicine that deals with the diseases and routine physical care of the reproductive system of women" (*Merriam-Webster Online Dictionary*, 2009). If clinicians apply this definition of gynecology in practice, then women will be cared for as royalty. Elevated to a high place, each woman will hold the center of the clinician's attention and receive expert, respectful care.

Gynecologic care occurs for two main reasons: to enhance or maintain health and to identify and treat a problem of the gynecologic system. This chapter presents the core knowledge and skill base for the gynecologic health history and physical examination. Often this examination is embedded within a clinical visit that has a wider focus on primary care screening and counseling (see Chapter 8).

Health History

The purpose of the health history is to establish a relationship with a woman while learning about her health. To a great extent, taking a health history means listening to her story. Both the content and the manner of what she conveys provide important information for a clinician's understanding of what an individual woman wants and needs. To optimize health history taking, several environmental and logistical arrangements should be consistently in place. These include providing a comfortable and private setting, scheduling an appropriate amount of time, and choosing the optimal format and staff member for obtaining the health history.

Privacy is an essential condition for obtaining the health history. Ideally, the room or office where the history is taken will have a door that can be closed so no noise or traffic interrupts the interview. A closed door ensures confidentiality and conveys the clinician's intent to offer the woman undivided attention. The woman should remain fully clothed. The clinician and the woman should be seated a comfortable distance from each other, preferably at a 45° angle, without furniture between them. This seating arrangement promotes a conversational, rather than a confrontational or hierarchical, approach. If an interpreter is present, he or she should be seated so that all three persons can see and hear one another.

Generally, the optimal way to gather the health history is to interview the woman alone, because distractions are minimized and privacy is ensured. If the woman prefers to have a spouse, friend, or other person with her, however, she should have this choice. If young children are present, a second adult should be available to attend to them.

If the woman has another person present during the health history, it is essential that at some point the woman be given the opportunity to speak privately with the clinician. This practice is advisable for handling topics that either clinician or woman find sensitive, such as the sexual health history. It also allows the clinician to ensure that the choice to have the other adult present was made freely by the woman. For adolescents accompanied by parents or guardians, this policy is particularly important.

Try to listen intently.

> Learn how to listen while being still, achieving "intellectual repose." This will help the listener be open to all the messages in the patient's words and body talk. ... Every one of the interviewer's behaviors should contribute to the communication of empathy and the building of trust essential to a therapeutic partnership. (Seidel, Ball, Dains, & Benedict, 2006, p. 5)

Schedule an appropriate amount of time to allow a woman being seen for an initial visit to tell her story in an unhurried manner. This approach generally yields a rich and pertinent database. Structure the interview around standard questions (**Boxes 6-1** and **6-2**), but encourage responses to be open ended. The reality of time pressure in ambulatory care settings may make an allocation of 20 to 30 minutes for obtaining a health history seem like a luxury, but it should be considered a key to excellent care. Many clinicians posit that 90% of the information needed for accurate diagnosis comes directly from the health history.

A variety of formats may be used for obtaining the health history, ranging from a self-administered questionnaire to a conversation between the clinician and the woman, with information recorded on a prepared form. The trade-offs required for each of these alternatives are obvious. Disadvantages to self-administered health questionnaires include the possibilities that answers to items may be omitted, questions may be misunderstood, or terms may be unfamiliar to the respondent. In addition, the entire questionnaire will require visual and verbal review by a nurse or the clinician to fill in missing information and clarify answers. Advantages include that some persons may disclose information more freely on sensitive topics in writing than if asked verbally, and the total time for this procedure may be less than if all information is obtained in an interview. Regardless of which staff person is responsible for obtaining the health history, whoever conducts the interview should be skilled at putting the woman at ease, and in conveying respectful attention through his or her verbal style and behavior.

BOX 6-1 *General Health History*

Reason the woman desires care (chief concern)
History of present illness
General medical history
 Current illnesses and diseases
 Past hospitalizations
 Prior surgical procedures
 Immunization status
 Previous serious illnesses
Medications and allergies
 Current medications
 Medication and other allergies
Substance use
 Tobacco
 Alcohol
 Illicit substances
Family health history
 Illnesses and causes of death of first-degree
  relatives
 Congenital malformations and unexplained
  intellectual and developmental disabilities
Social and occupational history
Safety
Personal habits

General Health History

Initially the interviewer briefly introduces herself or himself, states the purposes of the interview, and invites questions from the woman at any point during the visit. The interviewer proceeds next to checking basic demographic information, which is less personal and helps to put the woman at ease.

Reason the Woman Desires Care/Chief Concern Asking, "How may I help you today?" or "What has brought you here today?" are good ways to begin determining what is traditionally referred to as the chief complaint. The woman should be encouraged to describe the problem or reason for the visit in her own words. For example, "I think I want to change from pills to an IUD." She should be interrupted only for specific clarification or to bring her back to the topic if she seems to be digressing too far (Katz, Lentz, Lobo, & Gershenson, 2007).

History of Present Illness When the woman has finished describing the reason for her visit, the interviewer will need to "give structure to the present problem … giving it a chronologic and sequential framework … probing for the underlying concerns" (Seidel et al., 2006, p. 15). To maximize understanding of the woman's problem, the clinician should be sure he or she has answers to the following relevant questions:

1. What were the circumstances at the time the problem started?
2. What has been the sequence of events for symptoms?
3. Has the problem occurred before? If so, what were the circumstances of the previous occurrence and what led to its disappearance?
4. To what extent is the problem interfering with daily life or relationships?
5. Which questions does the woman want answered today? What is the woman expecting from today's visit?
6. Have other steps been taken to solve the problem? If so, what were they and how effective have they been?

General Medical History The woman will need to list any significant health problems she has had in her lifetime, including all hospitalizations and surgical procedures. In addition, the interviewer should ask about specific illnesses that occur frequently, such as diabetes, hypertension, respiratory illnesses, infectious diseases, and mental health problems. A review of adult immunizations is also necessary.

Medications and Allergies Review all medications the woman is currently taking, including over-the-counter preparations and complementary therapies, and reasons for their use. If the woman cannot recall the name of a medication she is using, encourage her to bring the package to the next visit. Describe allergic responses to medications, foods, or other substances.

Substance Use Perhaps the easiest way to proceed with this topic is to inquire about each substance separately, beginning with the legal and most commonly used substance—tobacco—continuing to alcohol, and ending with illicit substances. When inquiring about tobacco use, find out if the woman has smoked or is currently smoking, the daily number of cigarettes, the length of time smoked, the number of attempts at quitting, and interest in quitting now. Then ask about alcohol use, again determining the amount and type used per day or week, and any binge drinking habits. For illicit substances, inquire about types, amount, route, and frequency of use. For interviewers new to the process, positive answers to these questions may elicit surprise or concern, but this is not the time to intervene with counseling. The interviewer needs to stay focused on gathering information. See Chapter 8 for further discussion of screening for substance use.

Family Health History Gather information about first-degree relatives: parents, grandparents, siblings, and children. A family tree or narrative can be recorded, and information on serious illnesses and causes of death for each of these individuals should be obtained. In addition, occurrences of congenital malformations, unexplained intellectual and developmental disabilities, or other disabilities should be covered to offer clues to possible inherited diseases.

Social and Occupational History Ask the woman about her highest educational level attained, marital status/significant relationships, and employment or vocational history. Information about housing, financial status, family relationships, and potential and actual stressors or social problems should also be elicited.

Safety Safety issues—primarily the use of seat belts in motor vehicles, and helmets with bicycle or motorcycle use—should be checked, as well as presence of firearms in the woman's household. Inquiries about current or past intimate partner violence are often included at this point, but at present it is not clear whether gathering this information from all women should be standard practice (see Chapters 4, 8, and 14).

Personal Habits Ask the woman about her exercise, sleep, and nutrition patterns.

Gynecologic Health History

The gynecologic health history elicits significant details that provide the essential background for the problem-oriented encounter, as well as for a health maintenance visit for a well woman. The standard topics for this health history are listed in Box 6-2. Specific points that should be included about each topic follow.

Menstrual History The menstrual history is usually the first topic in the gynecologic history, and should cover the following information: age at menarche; date of last normal menstrual period (LMP); length of the cycle, counting from the first day of one menstrual flow until the first day of the next menstrual flow; average number of days of menses; characteristics of the menstrual flow; regularity of cycles; and description of any irregularities and/or accompanying symptoms. In general, cycles range from 21 to 35 days, and menses last from 4 to 7 days.

Pregnancy History Begin by asking the woman the total number of times she has been pregnant. Then ask her to describe each pregnancy in chronologic order. As the woman explains her pregnancy history, the interviewer will not only make written notes, but will also complete the GTPAL five-digit numeric summary description of pregnancies (**Box 6-3**).

Specific information to obtain for each pregnancy includes the year it occurred; its duration; the type of birth (spontaneous vaginal birth, assisted vaginal birth, or cesarean); sex and weight of the newborn; complications; and whether the child is currently alive and well. The category of abortion includes information about induced abortions, spontaneous abortions, ectopic pregnancies, and molar pregnancies. For these pregnancies, details of gestational age, procedure, complications, and outcome should be recorded.

History of Vaginal and Pelvic Infections Ask which types of infections, if any, the woman has had; which treatments she has received; how frequently each infection has occurred; and what, if any, complications have occurred. Screening for human immunodeficiency virus (HIV) risk can be done at this point. Ask the woman the number of sexual partners she has at present and has had during her lifetime. Inquire if she is sexually active with persons who present high risk for HIV transmission and whether she uses condoms. Detailed assessment of sexual risk is described in Chapter 21.

Douching Ask the woman about frequency, medication or solutions used, and reasons for douching.

Gynecologic Surgical Procedures Include information on minor procedures such as endometrial biopsies and laparoscopic examinations, as well as major procedures including female genital mutilation (see **Box 6-4** and **Figure 6-1**). The information needed includes the year in which the procedure was performed, the indication necessitating the surgery, significant

BOX 6-2 *Gynecologic Health History*

Menstrual History

- Age at menarche
- Date of last normal menstrual period (LMP)
- Cycle length, duration, and flow
- Any menstrual irregularities or symptoms associated with menses

Pregnancy History

- Gravida and para (See Box 6-3)
- Course of pregnancies: date, duration, type of birth, complications, newborn's sex and weight, and whether the child is currently alive and well
- For induced and/or spontaneous abortions: gestational age, procedure, and complications

History of Vaginal and Pelvic Infections

- Types of infections, treatments received, frequency of infections, and complications
- Previous vaginal infections and sexually transmitted infections

Douching

- Frequency, medication or solutions used, reasons for douching

Gynecologic Surgical Procedures

- Type of surgery, date, indication, complications, and outcome

Urologic Health

- Occurrence and frequency of infections
- Incontinence or other abnormal symptoms (e.g., frequency, dysuria)

Cervical Cancer Screening

- Date of last testing
- History of an abnormal result, and if so, follow-up and results since then

Sexual Health

- Sexual orientation
- Current sexual relationship(s)—number of partners, sexual practices, safer sex practices
- Sexual satisfaction
- Sexual concerns or problems

Contraceptive Use

- Present contraceptive method: type, duration used, satisfaction, side effects, and consistency of use
- Previous contraceptive use: method(s), duration of use, satisfaction, side effects, and reasons for discontinuing

Abnormal Symptoms

- Pelvic pain, bleeding unrelated to menstrual flow, etc.

BOX 6-3 *GTPAL System for Recording Pregnancy History*

G—Gravida or pregnancy, the total number of pregnancies the woman has had
T—Term births, those occurring from 37–42 weeks' gestation
P—Preterm births, those occurring after the point of viability, which is usually interpreted as gestational age greater than 20 weeks and less than 37 weeks and/or fetal weight greater than 500 gm
A—Abortions, spontaneous and induced prior to 20 weeks gestation
L—Living children

BOX 6-4 *Female Genital Mutilation*

Female genital mutilation, also called female circumcision and genital cutting, comprises "all procedures that involve partial or total removal of the external female genitalia, or other injury to the female genital organs for nonmedical reasons" (World Health Organization, 2008, p. 1). There are four major types of female genital mutilation:

- *Type I*—Partial or total removal of the clitoris and/or the prepuce (clitoridectomy)

- *Type II*—Partial or total removal of the clitoris and the labia minora, with or without excision of the labia majora (excision)

- *Type III*—Narrowing of the vaginal orifice with creation of a covering seal by cutting and appositioning the labia minora and/or the labia majora, with or without excision of the clitoris (infibulation)

- *Type IV*—All other harmful procedures to the female genitalia for nonmedical purposes, e.g., pricking, piercing, incising, scraping, and cauterization (World Health Organization, 2008, p. 4)

Long-term sequelae of female circumcision include urinary and menstrual problems, scarring, pain, infections, reduced quality of sexual life, infertility, obstetric complications, and psychological consequences (World Health Organization, 2008).

Women may not disclose during the health history that they have been circumcised for a variety of reasons, including fear that the clinician will disapprove or respond negatively to this information. If a woman does disclose that she is circumcised, it may be in describing associated complications noted previously. A woman may also provide this information in response to an open-ended question such as, "Is there anything else you would like me to know about your health background before we begin your examination?" It is important for the clinician to ask when the circumcision occurred, whether the woman has previously had a pelvic examination, and if she is experiencing symptoms of long-term sequelae.

The extent of circumcision will be determined during the inspection of the external genitalia. A pediatric speculum and single digit bimanual examination may be necessary for pelvic examination. A special form for recording health history and physical findings relevant to female circumcision can be helpful (see Campbell, 2004 for a sample form).

complications, and outcome. Obtaining pertinent medical records may also be useful if the woman cannot supply sufficient information.

Urologic Health   Topics include the occurrence and frequency of bladder infections, renal infections, incontinence, or other abnormal symptoms.

Cervical Cancer Screening   Determine whether the woman has had previous cervical cytology screening. If so, find out the approximate date of the last test and if the results were abnormal. For a woman who has had an abnormal cervical cancer screening result, ask what follow-up occurred, and whether subsequent screening results have been normal.

Sexual Health   Ask if the woman is sexually active. If so, determine whether this activity occurs with men, women, or both; whether she is satisfied with her sexual function; and whether she or her partner or partners have any concerns or problems. Further information about assessment of sexual health can be found in Chapter 11.

Contraceptive Use   The contraceptive history is obtained from heterosexual women. Determine whether the woman or her partner is currently using a contraceptive method, whether she is satisfied with the method or desires a change, or if she has questions about her current

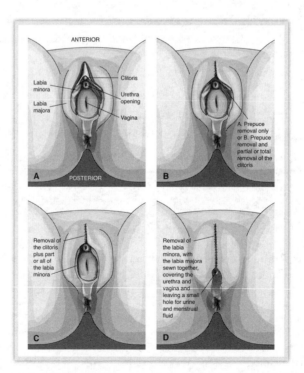

FIGURE 6-1 Female genital mutilation. A. Normal anatomy; B. Type I; C. Type II; D. Type III.

method. Discussing past methods used may be relevant depending on the woman's reason for the visit.

Abnormal Symptoms Problems such as pelvic pain should be fully described, noting their relationship in time with the menstrual cycle, and any association with coitus, tampon use, or other factors. Additionally, any vaginal bleeding not related to menstrual flow should be fully described. See Chapters 25 and 29 for detailed information about the assessment of bleeding and pelvic pain.

Final Steps

Closure of the health history should include offering the woman the chance to add comments or ask questions. One approach is simply to say, "I have finished with my questions about your health. Is there anything I have omitted or not covered, or that you would like to add to help me better understand your health or problem today?"

Once the clinician has completed taking the health history, the next step is to begin to examine, sort, and prioritize the information gathered; and to decide which further assessment measures, such as laboratory tests, are needed. It is often helpful at this time to summarize the findings and offer tentative answers to questions or concerns posed by the woman about her health. An example would be to say, "At this point I think you would be a good candidate for an intrauterine device (IUD), but I'd like to wait to discuss this further after I do your physical examination." This type of statement emphasizes the woman and clinician's partnership in her care.

Physical Examination for a Gynecologic Visit

Evaluating a new patient usually includes performing a physical examination. The details and description of the techniques, such as auscultation, are beyond the scope of this chapter. Readers are referred to textbooks on physical examination for a review of maneuvers, equipment, and organization of the examination (Bickley & Szilagyi, 2008; Seidel et al., 2006). This text assumes that the age range for patients will extend from adolescence through the older adult, or from about 12 to 70 years of age. Care outside this age range requires specialized pediatric or geriatric skills that go beyond the scope of this chapter.

What constitutes a complete physical examination in the ambulatory gynecology or primary care setting is not standardized. It is customary to evaluate major organ systems briefly and carefully, but not exhaustively. For example, the cardiovascular examination would include complete auscultation of the heart and evaluation of circulation by noting skin color, but would usually omit other maneuvers, such as checking carotid bruits or palpation of the precordium. When deciding what to include in the physical examination, novice clinicians may want to use the following principle as a guideline: Be able to state the rationale for including or excluding any assessment maneuver or particular feature of any organ system. If a rationale for performing any maneuver and obtaining the specific information that maneuver provides can be stated, then including it would be justified.

General Physical Examination

The order of the examination presented here assumes the woman is sitting up to begin the examination. This description proceeds from head to toe, rather than by system.

1. *Physical measurements.* Obtain and review height, weight, blood pressure, pulse, and temperature (if indicated), before performing the physical examination. Height and weight are most useful when converted to the body mass index (BMI) using **Table 6-1**. Both BMI and blood pressure should be considered screening tools (see Chapter 8 for further discussion).
2. *General appearance.* Observe the woman for posture; striking or obvious characteristics or limitations; general emotional state; and appropriateness of dress, speech pattern, and social interaction during the visit.
3. *Eyes, ears, nose, and throat.* Inspect the physical health of eyes, nose, and ears. Examination of the ears with the otoscope and examination of the eyes with the ophthalmoscope may be performed as indicated. The oropharynx examination includes inspection of the lips, teeth, and gums for dental health, and visualization of the oral cavity for mucosal color, lesions, and tonsillar edema or exudates.
4. *Neck.* Note range of motion and palpate lymph nodes in the neck and clavicular area.
5. *Thyroid.* Palpate the gland and isthmus.
6. *Chest and lungs.* Auscultate the posterior, lateral, and anterior lobes.
7. *Spine.* Palpate vertebral column, inspect skin.
8. *Kidneys.* Check costovertebral tenderness.
9. *Reflexes.* Elicit patellar and additional reflexes as indicated.
10. *Peripheral circulation and varicosities.* Inspect legs and feet.

The woman then reclines and the examination continues:

11. *Heart.* Auscultate.
12. *Breasts and axillary lymph nodes.* See the next section.
13. *Abdomen.* Inspect the skin, palpate superficially and deeply in all quadrants, and palpate inguinal lymph nodes.

Breast Examination

Despite ongoing controversy regarding the efficacy of breast self-examination (BSE), clinical breast examination performed by health professionals remains a part of the general physical examination (see Chapter 8 for further discussion of breast cancer screening). It is relatively simple and quick, and involves only two types of maneuvers: inspection and palpation. Conditions that promote ease and accuracy in findings are also simple. Adequate

TABLE 6-1 Body Mass Index Table

	Normal						Overweight					Obese										Extreme Obesity														
BMI	19	20	21	22	23	24	25	26	27	28	29	30	31	32	33	34	35	36	37	38	39	40	41	42	43	44	45	46	47	48	49	50	51	52	53	54
Height (inches)												Body Weight (pounds)																								
58	91	96	100	105	110	115	119	124	129	134	138	143	148	153	158	162	167	172	177	181	186	191	196	201	205	210	215	220	224	229	234	239	244	248	253	258
59	94	99	104	109	114	119	124	128	133	138	143	148	153	158	163	168	173	178	183	188	193	198	203	208	212	217	222	227	232	237	242	247	252	257	262	267
60	97	102	107	112	118	123	128	133	138	143	148	153	158	163	168	174	179	184	189	194	199	204	209	215	220	225	230	235	240	245	250	255	261	266	271	276
61	100	106	111	116	122	127	132	137	143	148	153	158	164	169	174	180	185	190	195	201	206	211	217	222	227	232	238	243	248	254	259	264	269	275	280	285
62	104	109	115	120	126	131	136	142	147	153	158	164	169	175	180	186	191	196	202	207	213	218	224	229	235	240	246	251	256	262	267	273	278	284	289	295
63	107	113	118	124	130	135	141	146	152	158	163	169	175	180	186	191	197	203	208	214	220	225	231	237	242	248	254	259	265	270	278	282	287	293	299	304
64	110	116	122	128	134	140	145	151	157	163	169	174	180	186	192	197	204	209	215	221	227	232	238	244	250	256	262	267	273	279	285	291	296	302	308	314
65	114	120	126	132	138	144	150	156	162	168	174	180	186	192	198	204	210	216	222	228	234	240	246	252	258	264	270	276	282	288	294	300	306	312	318	324
66	118	124	130	136	142	148	155	161	167	173	179	186	192	198	204	210	216	223	229	235	241	247	253	260	266	272	278	284	291	297	303	309	315	322	328	334
67	121	127	134	140	146	153	159	166	172	178	185	191	198	204	211	217	223	230	236	242	249	255	261	268	274	280	287	293	299	306	312	319	325	331	338	344
68	125	131	138	144	151	158	164	171	177	184	190	197	203	210	216	223	230	236	243	249	256	262	269	276	282	289	295	302	308	315	322	328	335	341	348	354
69	128	135	142	149	155	162	169	176	182	189	196	203	209	216	223	230	236	243	250	257	263	270	277	284	291	297	304	311	318	324	331	338	345	351	358	365
70	132	139	146	153	160	167	174	181	188	195	202	209	216	222	229	236	243	250	257	264	271	278	285	292	299	306	313	320	327	334	341	348	355	362	369	376
71	136	143	150	157	165	172	179	186	193	200	208	215	222	229	236	243	250	257	265	272	279	286	293	301	308	315	322	329	338	343	351	358	365	372	379	386
72	140	147	154	162	169	177	184	191	199	206	213	221	228	235	242	250	258	265	272	279	287	294	302	309	316	324	331	338	346	353	361	368	375	383	390	397
73	144	151	159	166	174	182	189	197	204	212	219	227	235	242	250	257	265	272	280	288	295	302	310	318	325	333	340	348	355	363	371	378	386	393	401	408
74	148	155	163	171	179	186	194	202	210	218	225	233	241	249	256	264	272	280	287	295	303	311	319	326	334	342	350	358	365	373	381	389	396	404	412	420
75	152	160	168	176	184	192	200	208	216	224	232	240	248	256	264	272	279	287	295	303	311	319	327	335	343	351	359	367	375	383	391	399	407	415	423	431
76	156	164	172	180	189	197	205	213	221	230	238	246	254	263	271	279	287	295	304	312	320	328	336	344	353	361	369	377	385	394	402	410	418	426	435	443

lighting helps to reveal subtle variations in skin texture and color. Adequate exposure, or having the woman disrobe to the waist, allows simultaneous observation and comparison of both breasts. Modesty may be a concern for some women. Explaining why this exposure is needed and employing an approach that is gentle but focused on the examination convey the clinician's concern and respect.

Breast Inspection This maneuver begins with the woman sitting, usually on the examining table, with arms relaxed at her sides, and the examiner standing facing her. Look at each breast and compare them for size, symmetry, contour, skin color, texture, venous patterns, and lesions. Lift the breast with fingertips to inspect the lower and lateral aspects. Breasts vary in shape, and frequently one will be slightly larger than the other. Skin texture should be smooth, contours uninterrupted bilaterally, and venous patterning similar in both breasts. Benign lesions, such as nevi, if long-standing, unchanged, and nontender, are considered normal findings.

Next, inspect the nipples and areolae. The areolae should be round or oval, and bilaterally nearly equal in configuration with a smooth surface. Color ranges from pink to black. Montgomery's tubercles—very small sebaceous glands—may be seen as slightly raised fleshy protuberances, and are a common finding. The nipples also should be equal or nearly equal in size. Most nipples are everted. If one or both are inverted, ask if inversion has been a lifelong characteristic. A newly inverted nipple suggests pathology. A second abnormal finding to note is nipple retraction, or a flattening of the nipple. Look also at the orientation of the nipples. If one points in a different direction from the other, this may be caused by the presence of malignant tissue in the breast. The color of the nipples should be the same as the areolae, while the surface may be smooth or wrinkled and should be without discharge. Supernumerary or extra nipples may also be seen. They are benign and usually small, and are commonly mistaken as moles. They may occur anywhere along a vertical line from the axilla to the inner thigh and are usually unilateral.

The last step in inspection in the sitting position is to have the woman change positions slightly so that the contour and symmetry of the breasts can be assessed completely. The three positions for examination while seated are arms over the head, hands pressed against the hips, and leaning forward at the waist.

Breast Palpation The woman remains sitting with arms resting freely at her sides. The examiner remains standing facing her. Palpate all four quadrants for nodules and lumps. Use the finger pads because they are more sensitive to touch than the fingertips. Press firmly enough to get a good sense of underlying tissue but not so firmly that the tissue is compressed against the rib cage. Rotate the fingers in a clockwise or counterclockwise direction. Palpating systematically is key to performing a complete examination. Two patterns commonly used for breast palpation are concentric circles starting from the outer edge and spiraling inward to the nipple, and top to bottom in vertical strips. For this latter pattern begin at the top, palpate downward and then upward, working gradually over the entire breast. Either pattern is acceptable as long as the entire breast is palpated.

Do a complete light palpation followed by a deep palpation. Be aware that a firm transverse ridge of compressed tissue is often found along the lower edge of the breast. It comprises the inframammary ridge and is a normal finding. For large breasts, it may be helpful to place one hand beneath the breast to stabilize it while palpating with the other hand (**Figure 6-2**).

Breast tissue in adult women feels dense, firm, and elastic. Prior to and during menstruation, some women experience cyclical tenderness, swelling, and nodularity. If a mass is felt, note the location, size, shape, consistency, tenderness, mobility, and demarcation of borders.

The tail of Spence—breast tissue that extends from the upper outer quadrant toward the axilla—must also be palpated because most malignancies develop in the upper outer quadrant (Seidel et al., 2006). This is best done

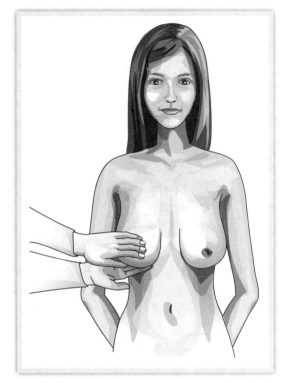

FIGURE 6-2 Palpating large breasts.

by having the woman raise her arms over her head while the examiner gently compresses the tissue where it enters the axilla between thumb and fingers (**Figure 6-3**).

Palpation now continues with the woman supine. Place a small pillow or folded towel under the shoulder before beginning the examination of the breast on that side. Use the same palpation technique and pattern for the supine position as for the sitting position. Repeat the examination with the woman's arm at her side. This repetition aids in a complete palpation because breast tissue shifts with different positions. After the entire breast is palpated, the nipple should also be gently palpated. Compress the nipple between thumb and index finger to inspect for discharge. This usually causes the nipple to become erect, and may be momentarily painful.

Examination of Lymph Nodes Have the woman sit with arms flexed at the elbow. The examiner stands facing the woman, but slightly off center. If beginning with the right axilla, use the left hand. Reach deeply into the axillary hollow and press firmly upward with the palmar surfaces of the fingers. Then bring the fingers downward to gently roll the soft tissue against the chest wall. Be sure to examine not only the apex, but also the central and medial aspects along the rib cage, the lateral aspect along the medial surface of the arm, the anterior wall along the pectoral muscles, and the posterior wall along the border of the

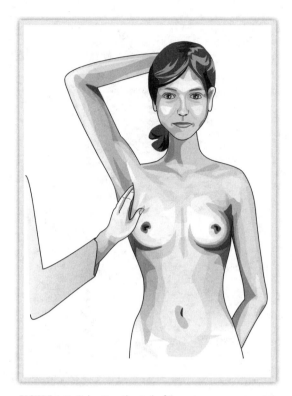

FIGURE 6-3 Palpating the tail of Spence.

scapula. Repeat this procedure with the other axilla. Axillary lymph nodes are usually not palpable in adults. The supraclavicular area should also be palpated. Hook the fingers over the clavicle and rotate them over the entire supraclavicular area.

The Pelvic Examination

The pelvic examination customarily concludes the physical examination. The description offered here assumes the reader is familiar with the anatomy of the pelvic structures, and particularly the anatomy of the gynecologic organs, both internal and external (see Chapter 5). A few features of these structures, such as their size and relative locations, are particularly pertinent to performing this examination easily and successfully.

Few experiences that women encounter in the evaluation of their health are as intimate and thus potentially anxiety producing as the pelvic examination. All clinicians who perform this type of examination have the professional responsibility to carry it out proficiently, promptly, and respectfully. Each woman brings her own past experiences and her own needs to the present examination. Specific conditions that generally enhance the experience include the following:

1. Before starting the examination, and at several points during it, explain in general what you are going to do before you do it.
2. Use language that can be understood by the woman. Use common words, not medical terms.
3. Ask the woman if she has any special concerns or questions.
4. Never talk lightly or make jokes about genitalia or the examination. This is entirely inappropriate.
5. Maintain eye contact during the examination as much as is possible, recognizing that women from many cultural groups may not return eye contact. In addition, if the examiner encounters an unexpected finding, conscious attempts should be made to avoid expressing surprise in facial expression or voice, as this will usually raise anxiety. If it is feasible, wait until the examination is completed to discuss the finding. If assistance is needed from another health professional to evaluate an abnormal or unexpected finding, briefly explain the finding and the reason for a second examiner's assessment.

6. Assure the woman that the examination will proceed as gently as possible and ask her to indicate if and when she feels discomfort.

7. Be sure the examination room is a comfortable temperature.

8. Ensure privacy for this examination. Close, or preferably lock, the door to the room.

9. Invite the woman to have someone accompany her for support during the examination if she desires.

10. The clinician may or may not have an assistant. If the clinician is male, it is often policy to have a female assistant present as a legal protection for both woman and clinician.

Preparing and Beginning the Pelvic Examination

1. Encourage the woman to empty her bladder for two reasons. First, bimanual examination can be very uncomfortable with a full bladder. Second, a full bladder makes palpation of pelvic organs difficult.

2. Offer the woman the option of a drape. It provides some privacy and warmth and may facilitate her relaxing, but some women may find it intrusive or unnecessary. Its use is optional.

3. Raise the top portion of the examination table to at least 30° and have a pillow at the head of the table. These measures add to the woman's comfort and make it easier for the clinician to maintain eye contact with her once the examination is in progress.

4. Assist the woman into the lithotomy position, first helping stabilize her feet in the footrests. Place one hand at the edge of the table and instruct her to move down, being sure her buttocks are slightly beyond the edge of the examination table. This detail is important to allow correct positioning of the speculum.

5. After making sure that all examination materials are prepared and within easy reach, wash your hands. Seat yourself on a stool so you are at eye level with the perineum. Don latex or nonlatex gloves (depending on clinician or patient allergy) and start the examination.

6. Ask the woman to separate her legs. Never try to spread her legs, even gently. It is sometimes helpful to touch the outside of the woman's knees or thighs and ask her to open her legs toward the examiner's hands. Adjust the light so it illuminates the perineal and vaginal area.

7. The examination is intrusive. Wait a moment until both the examiner and the woman are ready, and then tell the woman that the examination will begin. Start with a firm touch of one gloved hand on one of the woman's lower thighs, and then move the examining hand along the thigh toward the external genitalia.

8. If the woman becomes tense or upset during the examination, stop and find out what the problem is. Tell her the examination will not continue until she is at ease. Then make any adjustments that will enable her to cope with the examination before continuing.

Inspection and Palpation of External Genitalia, Vaginal Orifice, and Accessory Glands

1. Inspect, and then palpate the mons pubis, labia majora, and perineum, noting pattern of hair distribution, size and shape of the labia, presence of lesions, scars, rashes, erythema, discharge, or discoloration.

2. Separate the labia majora, inspect and palpate the labia minora, and inspect the urethral orifice and clitoris.

3. Inspect and palpate the vaginal introitus (opening) for presence or absence of the hymen and shape of the opening; note swelling, discharge, or lesions.

4. Insert the index and third fingers to the second joint into the vagina, and press down gently against the posterior vaginal wall. To assess for cystocele, ask the woman to cough or bear down. If she has a cystocele (**Figure 6-4**), the anterior vaginal wall will bulge with this maneuver. Many parous women have a first-degree cystocele. Observe also for rectocele (**Figure 6-5**), or bulging of the posterior vaginal wall. This is an abnormal and far less common finding.

5. To assess the tone of the perineal muscles, ask the woman to tighten her muscles around your vaginal examining fingers.

6. Palpate the Bartholin's glands by inserting the index finger of the examining hand about 2 cm into the vagina, turn the hand laterally and gently palpate the tissue behind the vaginal wall between the thumb and index finger on one side, and then, rotating the examining hand, palpate in the same manner on the other side of the vagina. Healthy Bartholin's glands are not palpable, but if they are inflamed this maneuver will elicit notable pain. If a cyst is present, a fluctuant, nontender mass will be palpable.

7. Palpation of the Skene's glands, which lie immediately lateral to the urethral meatus, is rapidly performed by turning the examining hand upward and then inserting the index

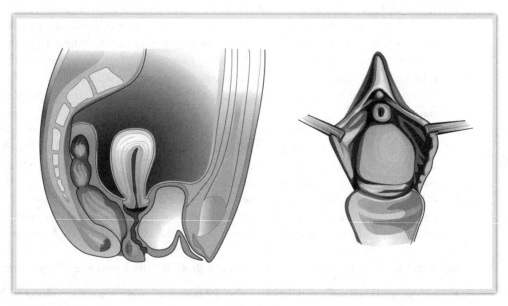

FIGURE 6-4 Cystocele.

finger into the vagina to the second knuckle and pressing gently upward, then sliding this finger outward. Discharge at the urethral meatus with palpation of the Skene's glands usually indicates infection. This examination lasts only about 10 seconds, but usually causes pain. Some clinicians think it is necessary to perform this palpation only if gonorrheal infection is suspected (Seidel et al., 2006).

Note that steps 4–7 may be performed with the bimanual examination, according to the clinician's preference.

Speculum Examination It is essential that clinicians become familiar with how the speculum operates before performing this examination. This preparation ensures women do not experience inadvertent pain caused by its incorrect use. Each clinician must also decide which hand to use for holding the speculum—a decision that is based entirely on personal preference.

1. Select the appropriate type (Graves or Pederson) and size (pediatric, small, medium or standard, or large) of speculum (**Figure 6-6**). For most parous women, the standard Graves speculum is used. For very obese women with significant perineal adipose tissue or for grand multiparas, the large Graves speculum will not only allow the best visualization but will also be more comfortable. The wider blade size of the large Graves speculum more effectively holds the lax vaginal walls open, permitting visualization of the cervix.

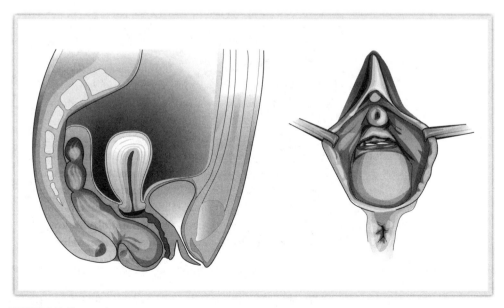

FIGURE 6-5 Rectocele.

For nulliparous women, the Pederson speculum is the usual choice. Its blades are the same length as the Graves, but are narrower and flat rather than curved. This shape and size minimizes pressure on the anterior and posterior vaginal walls, promoting a more comfortable examination. Use either a plastic or metal speculum (Figure 6-6).

2. Warm the speculum by running it under warm tap water, or equip the examination table drawer with a heating pad where speculums can be stored. Lubricate the end of the speculum blades with water or a small amount (one teaspoon) of water-soluble gel. Wetting the speculum with water instead of lubricating it with water-soluble gel has been thought to be necessary to ensure optimal collection of specimens for cervical cytology. Multiple studies examining this practice have found that using a small amount of gel on the speculum does not interfere with cervical cytology specimens or results, and decreases discomfort of the speculum insertion (Amies, Miller, Lee, & Koutsky, 2002; Griffith, Stuart, Gluck, & Heartwell, 2005; Harer, Valenzuela, & Lebo, 2002).

3. With the index and third fingers of one hand, separate the labia majora and slide these fingers slightly inside the vagina. Tell the woman she is going to feel some pressure, then press these two fingers downward. The very close proximity of the urethra to the anterior vaginal wall can lead to distinct discomfort when the speculum or examining fingers enter and exit the vagina. This maneuver allows for good visualization of the opening

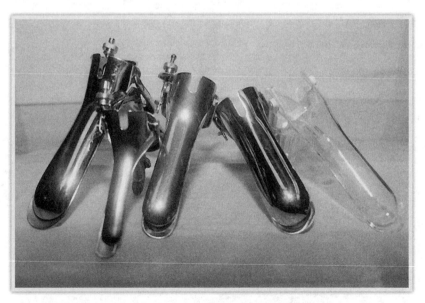

FIGURE 6-6 Types of specula. From left to right: metal Graves (large size), pediatric, Pederson, Graves (standard size), and plastic (regular size).

Source: Reprinted with permission from Varney, H., Kriebs, J. M., & Gegor, C. L. (2004). *Varney's midwifery* (4th ed.). Sudbury, MA: Jones and Bartlett Publishers.

of the vagina. With the other hand, grasp the speculum with index finger over the top of the proximal end of the anterior blade and the other fingers around the handle. This position allows control of the blades as the speculum is inserted.

4. Insert the speculum into the vagina at an oblique angle. Keeping the blades closed, let them slide into the vagina following the direction of the vagina until the blades are all the way in the vagina (**Figure 6-7**). The length of the blades is 6 to 7 inches, which matches the length of the vagina. Remember that when lying supine, a woman's vagina inclines posteriorly about 45° downward from the vaginal opening toward the sacrum. Keeping the blades at this angle also avoids pressure on the urethra, thereby minimizing discomfort.

5. Rotate the speculum horizontally and open the blades by pressing firmly and steadily on the thumbpiece. The cervix should come into view between the blades at the end of the vagina. If it is not immediately visible with the blades wide open, relax the pressure on the thumbpiece, allowing the blades to close. Then reposition the speculum. Slide the speculum partially out of the vagina, redirect the blades at a slightly different angle, and reinsert it obliquely. Open the blades; the cervix should now come into view. Adequate cervical visualization is essential for obtaining any specimens from the cervix.

6. Once the cervix is visualized, manipulate the speculum a little farther into the vagina so that the cervix is well exposed. If using a metal speculum, tighten the screw on the thumbpiece. If using a plastic speculum, click the upper blade onto the notch of the handle. The speculum should remain in place so that both hands can be taken off the speculum, making it possible for the examiner to handle other equipment.

Inspect the cervix for color, position, size, surface characteristics, shape of the os, and discharge. The cervix is remarkable for the vast variety of shapes, sizes, and appearances that are within the range of health. The color should be pink. Symmetric, circumscribed erythema around the os is a normal finding caused by exposing, or everting, the columnar epithelium lining of the endocervical canal. This eversion results from pressure of the speculum blades against the anterior and posterior fornices.

The position of the cervix correlates to the position of the uterus. The most common position of the cervix is posterior, indicating an anteflexed uterus. The cervix should be located in the midline; deviation may indicate a pelvic mass or adhesions. The diameter of the cervix is about 2 to 3 cm, and its length is about 3 cm. The os of a nulliparous woman is small and round, while a multiparous os is usually a horizontal slit or may be irregular or stellate (**Figure 6-8**). The surface should be smooth. Nabothian cysts may be seen as small white or yellow, raised areas; these retention cysts of endocervical glands are a normal variation (see Chapter 27). Note any friable tissue, granular areas, or red or white patchy areas. Note any discharge, and determine if its source is vaginal, which is far more common than a cervical origin. Note the color and consistency of the discharge. Normal vaginal discharge is odorless, creamy or clear, and thick or thin, depending on time in the menstrual cycle.

Three types of specimens are frequently collected at this point in the speculum examination: cervical cells for cytology screening, a vaginal or endocervical sample for

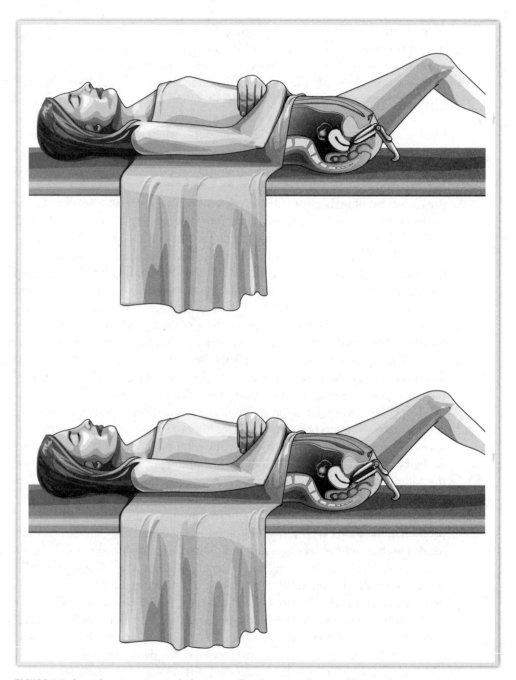

FIGURE 6-7 Speculum insertion and placement. Top: Insertion; Bottom: Placement.

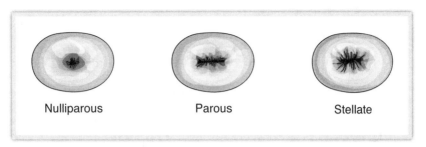

FIGURE 6-8 Variations of the cervical os.

gonorrhea and chlamydia testing, and vaginal secretions for microscopy (see the chapter appendices for information on these procedures). In some laboratories, the same cervical sample is used for cytology screening and gonorrhea and chlamydia testing. If separate cervical samples are collected for these tests, the optimal order for collecting these specimens is unknown because no evidence exists to guide this choice. Recently, vaginal swabs were identified as the preferred specimen type for gonorrhea and chlamydia testing, even if a full pelvic examination is performed (Association of Public Health Laboratories, 2009).

7. To begin removing a metal speculum, loosen the screw on the thumbpiece, but press on it to keep the blades open as the speculum is withdrawn from around the cervix. If using a plastic speculum, press on the thumbpiece to release it from the notch that has kept the anterior blade open. Once the cervix is no longer within the speculum blades, release most of the pressure on the thumbpiece, and rotate the speculum back to the oblique angle. As the speculum is withdrawn, inspect the vaginal walls. Note color, surface characteristics, and secretions. Vaginal mucosa should be almost the same color as the cervix, and the surface should be moist and smooth or rugated. Normal discharge will appear thin, clear or cloudy, and odorless. After inspection, continue to remove the speculum. Release all pressure on the thumbpiece and the blades will close themselves. Taking care not to pinch the vaginal mucosa, quickly and completely withdraw the speculum in an upward direction, but with downward pressure. This maneuver provides the most comfort for the woman.

8. Deposit the speculum in an appropriate container.

Bimanual Examination Inform the woman that the next step is examining her gynecologic organs internally with your fingers (**Figure 6-9**). This examination is most easily done with the examiner standing.

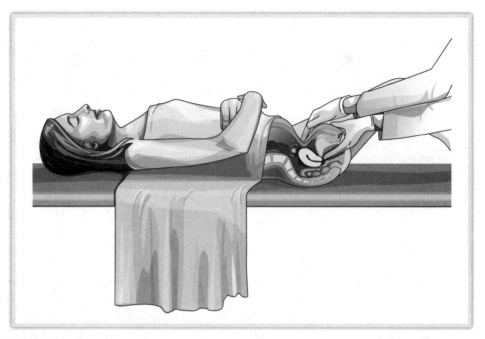

FIGURE 6-9 Bimanual examination.

1. Remove the glove from one hand, and lubricate the index and middle fingers of the gloved hand. Generally the dominant hand is gloved and used for the internal examination, but this is a clinician preference. Place these two fingers just inside the vaginal orifice, press downward, and gently insert them their full length into the vagina.
2. As the examination continues, be careful of where the thumb of the examining hand is resting. Try to avoid touching the clitoris, which is usually very sensitive.
3. Locate and touch the end of the cervix with the palmar surface of the examining fingers, then run the examining fingers around the circumference of the cervix to feel the size, length, shape, and consistency. A nonpregnant cervix will be firm, like the tip of the nose, while during pregnancy it is softer. Note nodules, surface texture, and position.
4. Assess for cervical motion tenderness by grasping the cervix gently between the examining fingers, moving it from side to side once, and observing the woman for any expression of pain or discomfort. The cervix should move 1 to 2 cm laterally without discomfort. Painful cervical movement suggests a pelvic inflammatory process.
5. Begin palpation of the uterus by placing the ungloved hand on the abdomen, halfway between the umbilicus and the pubis at the midline. Place the intravaginal fingers in front of the cervix in the anterior fornix. Slowly slide the abdominal hand down toward

the pubis, pressing downward and forward with the flat surface of all four fingers. At the same time, press upward with the vaginal fingers. This combination of abdominal and vaginal pressure will feel as if the two hands are pressing against each other. The uterus is relatively mobile, usually inclines forward at about 45°, and is essentially flat. It measures about 5–8 cm long, 3.5–5 cm wide, and 2–3 cm thick. If the uterus is anteflexed or anteverted (**Figure 6-10**), the fundus will be palpable between the fingers of the two hands at the level of the pubis.

6. If the uterus cannot be palpated with the maneuver described in step 5, place the vaginal fingers together in the posterior fornix with the abdominal hand at the pubis. Press firmly downward with the abdominal fingers. With the vaginal fingers turned upward, press up against the cervix moving it inward. If the uterus is retroverted (Figure 6-10), the fundus should be palpable with this maneuver.

7. If the uterus still is not palpated, move the vaginal fingers to the sides of the cervix, pressing the cervix inward as far as possible. Then move one finger on top and the other beneath the cervix, continuing to press inward, while pressing down with the abdominal fingers. If the uterus is in the midposition (Figure 6-10), it is not possible to palpate the fundus with the abdominal hand. Confirm the location of the uterus as midline, regardless of its anterior, midposition, or posterior position. Also palpate the uterus for size, contour, and consistency. It should feel smooth, firm, round, and flat. It should be mobile in the anterior–posterior plane. This examination should not cause pain, although a sensation of pressure is common.

8. Continue the bimanual examination by palpating the ovaries and surrounding area, called the adnexae. This term refers to the areas lateral to the uterus, which are taken up by the broad ligaments, as well as to the structures located there. Move the abdominal hand to the right lower quadrant. The vaginal fingers remain facing upward. Now put both fingers in the right lateral fornix. Press deeply inward and upward toward the abdominal hand. At the same time, with the abdominal hand, sweep the flat surface of the fingers deeply inward and obliquely down toward the pubis. Palpate the entire area in this manner, repeating this sweeping movement, while at the same time the vaginal fingers press upward, inward, and slide downward (**Figure 6-11**). This maneuver is then repeated on the left side.

    Often normal ovaries are difficult to palpate because they are small, sometimes positioned deep in the pelvis, or obscured by the presence of abdominal adipose tissue or tense abdominal muscles. If palpable, they are about $3 \times 2 \times 1$ cm, smooth and firm. If the ovaries are palpable, this examination usually causes momentary moderate pain when the ovaries are located. Usually no other adnexal structures are palpable. However, palpable ovaries in postmenopausal women are reason for concern and require follow-up. If the ovaries are not felt after thorough palpation, the examination is normal in the absence of any clinical signs or symptoms.

9. Once the adnexal examination is completed, remove the intravaginal fingers, and take off and discard the examination glove.

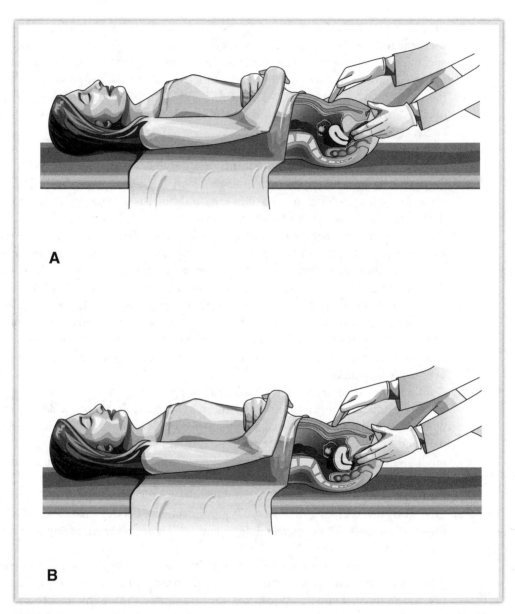

FIGURE 6-10 Variations in uterine position. A: Anteverted; B: Anteflexed; C: Retroverted; D: Retroflexed; E: Midposition of the uterus.

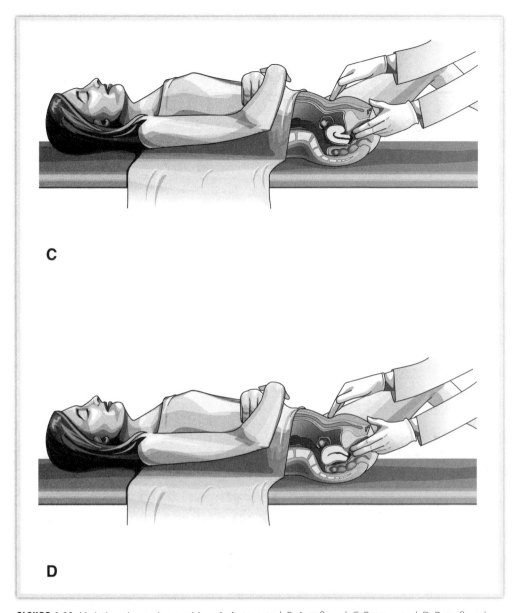

C

D

FIGURE 6-10 Variations in uterine position. A: Anteverted; B: Anteflexed; C: Retroverted; D: Retroflexed; E: Midposition of the uterus. (Continued)

(continues)

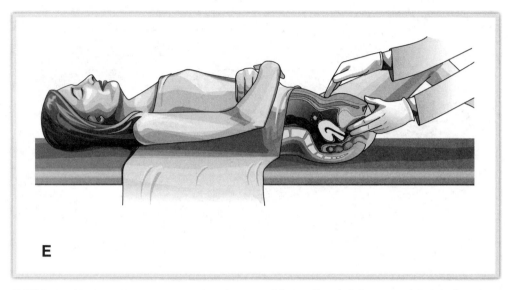

E

FIGURE 6-10 Variations in uterine position. A: Anteverted; B: Anteflexed; C: Retroverted; D: Retroflexed; E: Midposition of the uterus. (Continued)

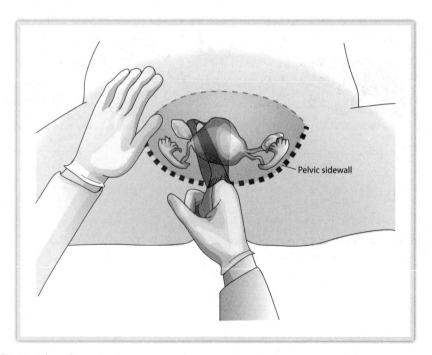

Pelvic sidewall

FIGURE 6-11 Adnexal examination.

Rectovaginal Examination This part of the pelvic examination allows palpation to a depth of an additional 2.5 cm, facilitating a more complete evaluation of some pelvic structures (**Figure 6-12**). Such an examination is perhaps most useful if the uterus is retroflexed or retroverted. It is usually an uncomfortable examination, but once mastered, can be very rapidly completed. Many clinicians omit this examination because the vaginal examination has allowed for sufficient palpation of gynecologic organs and because digital rectal examination to collect a stool sample for fecal occult blood testing is an unacceptable screening strategy for colorectal cancer screening (Levin et al., 2008).

1. Before beginning, tell the woman that the rectum and vagina will be briefly examined. Inform her that this may be uncomfortable and may also cause a sensation similar to that of having a bowel movement. Assure her that she will not have one.
2. Put an examination glove on one hand, and lubricate the index and third fingertips with water-soluble gel. Place the third finger against the anus, ask the woman to bear down, and insert this finger into the rectum just past the sphincter. Palpate the anorectal junction and rotate the examining finger to sweep over the anterior and then posterior rectum that can be reached above the sphincter. Note sphincter tone. The mucosal surfaces should feel smooth and uninterrupted.
3. Now also insert the index finger of the examining hand into the vagina as far as it will go. Palpate the septum between the rectum and posterior vaginal wall for thickness. Ask

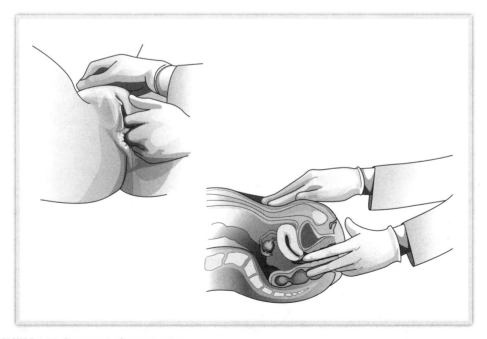

FIGURE 6-12 Rectovaginal examination.

the woman to bear down, which will bring the uterus about 1 cm closer to your examining finger. Place the vaginal finger in the posterior fornix. With the other hand, press firmly on the abdomen just above the pubis. The posterior surface of the uterus should be palpable, especially if it is retroverted. If the findings of the adnexal examination were questionable, repeat that examination as described previously.

4. Gently remove the examining fingers, inspect for secretions, and prepare a specimen for fecal occult blood testing if indicated. Remove and discard gloves, and help the woman to sit up. Give her a moment to regain her composure, and then offer her tissues to wipe secretions and lubricant from her perineal area. Leave the examining room to allow her privacy and time to dress. Tell her you will discuss your findings with her after she is clothed.

Conclusion: Summing Up and Documenting Findings

Having a conversation that summarizes findings from the full physical examination takes little time but is very important. If findings are uniformly normal, describing the examination as "healthy," "fine," or "what is expected" is preferable to characterizing the examination as "normal." If any abnormal findings occurred, they should be explained appropriately. The clinician should gauge how much detailed explanation, description, and thoughts on a therapeutic plan should be presented based on the individual woman's desire for information and the degree of severity of the finding. If the clinician is not sure of the implications of the finding, it is reasonable to say so, but also assure the woman that consultation with another health professional will be sought promptly, and that a more complete explanation and therapeutic plan will be forthcoming.

Women also need to be encouraged to voice their concerns, questions, and reactions to the examination. Attention to these issues demonstrates the clinician's commitment to understanding and responding to the individual woman.

The final clinical responsibility for this step in management is concise and accurate documentation of findings in the woman's record. Try "to give the patient records a vibrancy that might otherwise be lost" (Seidel et al., 2006, p. 15) by balancing technical documentation with descriptions that highlight the woman's substance and uniqueness.

References

Amies, A. E., Miller, L., Lee, S., & Koutsky, L. (2002). The effect of vaginal speculum lubrication on the rate of unsatisfactory cervical cytology diagnosis. *Obstetrics & Gynecology, 100*, 899–892.

Association of Public Health Laboratories. (2009). Laboratory diagnostic testing for *Chlamydia trachomatis* and *Neisseria gonorrhoeae*. *Expert Consultation Meeting Summary Report*, January 13–15, 2009, Atlanta, GA. Retrieved from http://www.aphl.org/aphl programs/infectious/std/documents/ctgclabguide-linesmeetingreport.pdf

Bickley, L. S., & Szilagyi, P. G. (2008). *Bates' guide to physical examination and history taking* (10th ed.). Baltimore: Lippincott Williams & Wilkins.

Campbell, C. C. (2004). Care of women with female circumcision. *Journal of Midwifery & Women's Health, 49*, 364–365.

Griffith, W. F., Stuart, G. S., Gluck, K. L., & Heartwell, S.F. (2005). Vaginal speculum lubrication and its effects on cervical cytology and microbiology. *Contraception, 72*(1), 60–64.

Harer, W. B., Valenzuela, G., & Lebo, D. (2002). Lubrication of the vaginal introitus and speculum does not affect Papanicolaou smears. *Obstetrics & Gynecology, 100*(5), 887–888.

Katz, V. L., Lentz, G. M., Lobo, R. A., & Gershenson, D. M. (2007). *Comprehensive gynecology* (5th ed.). St Louis, MO: Mosby.

Levin, B., Lieberman, D. A., McFarland, B., Smith, R. A., Brooks, D., Andrews, K. S., … Winawer, S. J. (2008). Screening and surveillance for the early detection of colorectal cancer and adenomatous polyps, 2008: A joint guideline from the American Cancer Society, the US Multi-Society Task Force on Colorectal Cancer, and the American College of Radiology. *Gastroenterology, 134*(5), 1570–1595.

Merriam-Webster online dictionary. (2009). Retrieved from http://www.merriam-webster.com/dictionary/gynecology

Seidel, H. M., Ball, J. W., Dains, J. E., & Benedict, W. G. (2006). *Mosby's guide to physical examination* (6th ed.). St Louis, MO: Mosby.

World Health Organization. (2008). *Eliminating female genital mutilation: An interagency statement: OHCHR, UNAIDS, UNDP, UNECA, UNESCO, UNFPA, UNHCR, UNICEF, UNIFEM, WHO*. Geneva, Switzerland: Author. Retrieved from http://whqlibdoc.who.int/publications/2008/9789241596442_eng.pdf

6-A

Cervical Cytology Screening

The goal of this test is to obtain adequate cells from the cervical squamocolumnar junction (SCJ) for cytology screening. The SCJ, or transformation zone, where columnar endocervical epithelium and squamous ectocervical epithelium meet, is where most cervical cancers arise. For many years, specimens were collected using a special wooden spatula (Ayer spatula), sometimes in conjunction with a cotton-tipped swab. The conventional method of preparing the sample for cytology is the Papanicolaou (Pap) smear, which entails applying the specimen to a glass slide. Limitations of this method of specimen collection and preparation are well documented. They include not obtaining sufficient endocervical cells for adequate laboratory cytologic evaluation; unavoidably leaving much of the cellular sample on the collection device when transferring the materials to the glass slide; and obscured detection of abnormal cells due to the presence of blood, mucus, air-drying, or other artifacts on the slide. Newer specimen collection devices and liquid-based preparation methods have been developed to try to overcome these limitations and improve cervical cytology screening.

More recent specimen collection devices include the endocervical brush (Cytobrush), a broom-like device that can simultaneously sample the ectocervix and endocervix, and extended-tip spatulas (**Figure 6A-1**). The use of cotton-tipped swabs is no longer recommended. Plastic spatulas are preferable to wooden spatulas, because they retain more cervical cells, and extended-tip spatulas are better than the rounded Ayer spatula. Using an extended-tip spatula and an endocervical brush for specimen collection results in the highest rate of detection of endocervical cells by cytologic examination (Martin-Hirsch, Jarvis, Kitchener, & Lilford, 2000).

Liquid-based methods for cervical cytology screening (ThinPrep, SurePath) allow for more complete removal of cellular material by rinsing the sampling devices in a liq-

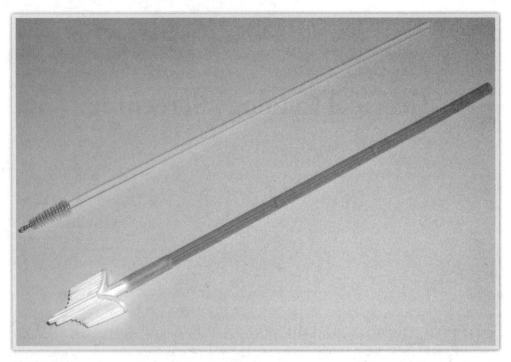

FIGURE 6A-1 Specimen collection devices for cervical cytology screening: Endocervical brush (left) and broom (right).

uid medium. Cells for cytologic examination are removed from the medium via a filtering process that minimizes the presence of obscuring artifacts. A survey of obstetricians and gynecologists revealed that almost 90% of them use liquid-based cytology (Noller, Bettes, & Schulkin, 2003). However, liquid-based methods are neither more sensitive nor more specific than the conventional Pap test for detecting high-grade cervical intraepithelial neoplasia (American College of Obstetricians and Gynecologists, 2009a, 2009b; Arbyn et al., 2008). An advantage of liquid-based cytology methods is that the sample can also be used to test for human papillomavirus deoxyribonucleic acid (HPV DNA), chlamydia, and gonorrhea. This eliminates the need for a second visit for a woman who has a cytologic abnormality that warrants HPV DNA testing. A disadvantage of liquid-based methods is their higher cost compared to the conventional (Pap) cytology method. These considerations, and the failure of scientific evidence to establish clear superiority of one method over the other, have led to differing recommendations about the use of liquid-based cervical cytology (American College of Obstetricians and Gynecologists, 2009a, 2009b; Saslow et al., 2002; United States Preventive Services Task Force, 2003). See Chapter 8 for recommendations.

Procedures for both conventional and liquid-based methods for cervical cytology screening using the different specimen collection devices are described in the next section.

Conventional Method for Cervical Cytology Screening

1. Assemble the necessary materials: a labeled container for one or two standard microscope slides, slides, spatula, endocervical brush, and canister of fixative.
2. Tell the woman the Pap smear will be performed and she may feel slight pressure or discomfort, which is caused primarily from the contact of the sampling devices with the endocervix.
3. Visualize the cervix, using the speculum examination procedure described in this chapter.
4. Pick up the spatula, and insert the longer end into the cervical os. Press and rotate the spatula 360°, making sure it stays in direct contact with the inner surface of the cervical os (**Figure 6A-2**).
5. Pick up the glass slide, press the spatula flat against the surface, and smear the spatula across the slide (**Figure 6A-3**). Turn the spatula over, and spread the secretions from the second side of the spatula onto the slide. Discard the spatula. Some clinicians prefer to proceed to step 6 and place samples from the spatula and endocervical brush onto the slide after both specimens have been collected.

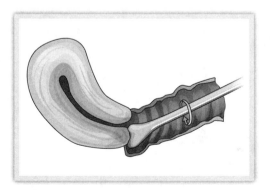

FIGURE 6A-2 Obtaining cervical cells with a spatula.

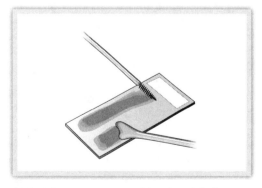

FIGURE 6A-3 Preparation of the glass slide for cervical cytology screening.

6. Insert the endocervical brush so that the bristles are fully in the cervical os and rotate the brush 180° to 360°, which is one-half to one turn (**Figure 6A-4**).
7. Pick up the glass slide (or the second glass slide if using two) and, with firm pressure, roll the bristles of the endocervical brush across the slide surface (Figure 6A-3). If using one slide, recommendations vary as to whether to keep the spatula and endocervical brush samples separate (placing one on each half of the slide), or to place the endocervical brush sample over the spatula sample. Clinicians should consult their laboratory for the preferred preparation method. Discard the endocervical brush.
8. Spray fixative promptly onto the slide, holding the container about 12 inches away from the slide. Allow the sample to air-dry for a few minutes before placing the slide in the transport container.
9. Continue the speculum examination or prepare to collect additional specimens.

Note that an assistant, if present, can hold the slides for the clinician and apply the fixative.

Liquid-Based Methods for Cervical Cytology Screening

Specimen Collection with the Spatula and Endocervical Brush

1. Assemble the necessary materials: labeled vial of liquid medium, spatula, and endocervical brush. Take the lid off the vial.
2. Prepare the woman as described in step 2 for the conventional method.
3. Visualize the cervix as described in step 3 for the conventional method.
4. Collect a specimen with the spatula as described in step 4 for the conventional method.

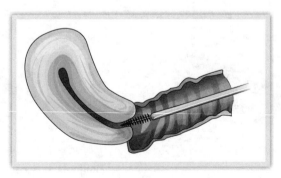

FIGURE 6A-4 Obtaining cells with an endocervical brush.

5. Place the spatula into the vial and swirl vigorously 10 times to mix the specimen and the medium (**Figure 6A-5**). Remove and discard the spatula.
6. Collect the specimen with the endocervical brush as described in step 6 for the conventional method.
7. Place the endocervical brush into the vial and swirl vigorously 10 times to mix the specimen and the medium (Figure 6A-5). Discard the endocervical brush.
8. Screw the lid tightly and securely onto the vial.
9. Proceed as described in step 9 for the conventional method.

Specimen Collection with the Broom-like Device

1. Assemble the necessary materials: labeled vial of liquid medium and broom-like device. Take the lid off the vial.
2. Prepare the woman as described in step 2 for the conventional method.
3. Visualize the cervix as described in step 3 for the conventional method.
4. Insert the central bristles of the broom into the endocervical canal deep enough to allow the shorter bristles to fully contact the ectocervix (**Figure 6A-6**). Push gently, and rotate the broom in a clockwise direction five times.
5. Place the broom into the vial and press firmly to the bottom of the vial so that the bristles of the broom are forced apart. Swirl vigorously 10 times to mix the specimen and the medium (Figure 6A-5). Remove and discard the broom.
6. Screw the lid tightly and securely onto the vial.
7. Proceed as described in step 9 for the conventional method.

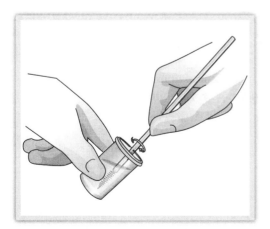

FIGURE 6A-5 Placing cervical cell sample into liquid medium.

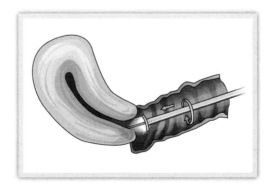

FIGURE 6A-6 Obtaining cervical cells with a broom-like device.

References

American College of Obstetricians and Gynecologists. (2009a). Cervical cytology screening. *ACOG Practice Bulletin No. 109*. Retrieved from: http://www.acog .org/publications/educational_bulletins/pb109.cfm

American College of Obstetricians and Gynecologists. (2009b). Routine pelvic examination and cervical cytology screening. ACOG Committee Opinion Number 431. *Obstetrics & Gynecology, 113*(5), 1190–1193.

Arbyn, M., Bergeron, C., Klinkhamer, P., Martin-Hirsch, P., Siebers, A. G., & Bulten, J. (2008). Liquid compared with conventional cervical cytology: A systematic review and meta-analysis. *Obstetrics & Gynecology, 111*(1), 167–177.

Martin-Hirsch, P., Jarvis, G., Kitchener, J., & Lilford, R. (2000, most recent substantative amendment). Collection devices for obtaining cervical cytology samples (Cochrane Review). In *The Cochrane library*. Chichester, UK: John Wiley & Sons.

Noller, K. L., Bettes, B., Zinberg, S., & Schulkin, J. (2003). Cervical cytology screening practices among obstetrician-gynecologists. *Obstetrics & Gynecology, 102*, 259–265.

Saslow, D., Runowicz, C. D., Solomon, D., Moscicki, A., Smith, R. A., Eyre, H. J., & Cohen, C. (2002). American Cancer Society guideline for the early detection of cervical neoplasia and cancer. *CA: Cancer Journal for Clinicians, 52*, 342–362.

United States Preventive Services Task Force. (2003). *Screening for cervical cancer: Recommendations and rationale*. Retrieved from http://www.ahcpr.gov/ clinic/3rduspstf/cervcan/cervcanrr.pdf

6-B

Screening for *Chlamydia trachomatis* and *Neisseria gonorrhoeae* Infections

The nucleic acid amplification test (NAAT) is the recommended method for detecting gynecologic tract infections with *Chlamydia trachomatis* and *Neisseria gonorrhoeae* (Association of Public Health Laboratories, 2009). Chlamydia and gonorrhea cultures should be reserved for specific indications, such as supporting research activities and monitoring resistance to treatment regimens. The preferred specimen type for NAATs for women is vaginal swabs, and cervical samples are also acceptable (Association of Public Health Laboratories, 2009). Several commercial NAAT products are available, including some that test for *C. trachomatis* and *N. gonorrhoeae* from the same sample. Clinicians should follow the manufacturer's instructions when using these products.

To collect a vaginal swab specimen, the swab is inserted into the vagina about 2 inches past the introitus and gently rotated for 10 to 30 seconds (**Figure 6B-1**). The swab should touch the walls of the vagina to absorb moisture. The swab is then withdrawn and placed into the transport medium (Gen-Probe Incorporated, 2007). The sample may be self-collected by the woman or obtained by the clinician (Hobbs et al., 2008).

The Centers for Disease Control and Prevention (2002) provides the following general guidelines for the endocervical specimen collection procedure:

1. Prepare materials by opening the test kit, labeling the medium container, and placing the swabs provided in the test kit within easy reach.
2. Visualize the cervix using the speculum examination procedure described in Chapter 6.
3. Remove all secretions and discharge from the cervix with a large swab.
4. Insert the swab supplied by the manufacturer 1 to 2 cm into the cervical os, rotate it firmly at least twice against the walls of the canal, and allow it to remain in the os for the time recommended by the manufacturer.

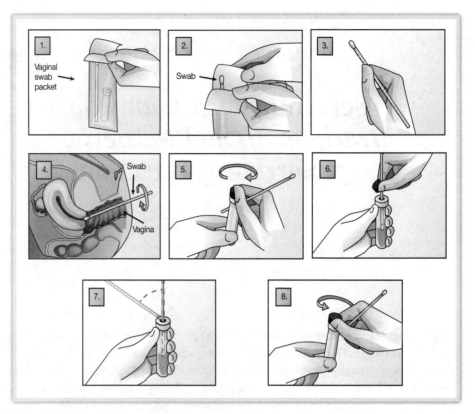

FIGURE 6B-1 Vaginal swab collection.

5. Withdraw the swab without touching any vaginal surfaces.
6. Place the swab in the appropriate transport medium, or follow the manufacturer's directions provided with the medium collection kit.

References

Association of Public Health Laboratories. (2009). Laboratory diagnostic testing for *Chlamydia trachomatis* and *Neisseria gonorrhoeae*. *Expert Consultation Meeting Summary Report*, January 13–15, 2009, Atlanta, GA. Retrieved from http://www.aphl.org/aphlprograms/infectious/std/documents/ctgclabguidelinesmeetingreport.pdf

Centers for Disease Control and Prevention (CDC). (2002). Screening tests to detect *Chlamydia trachomatis* and *Neisseria gonorrhoeae* infection. *Morbidity and Mortality Weekly Review, 51*(RR-15), 1–27. Retrieved from http://www.cdc.gov/mmwr/Preview/mmwrhtml/rr5115a1.htm

Gen-Probe Incorporated. (2007). *APTIMA® vaginal swab specimen collection kit*. San Diego, CA: Author. Retrieved from http://www.gen-probe.com/pdfs/pi/BX0155-ARTRevC.pdf

Hobbs, M. M., van der Pol, B., Totten, P., Gaydos, C. A., Wald, A., Warren., ... Martin, D. H. (2008). From the NIH: Proceedings of a workshop on the importance of self-obtained vaginal specimens for detection of sexually transmitted infections. *Sexually Transmitted Diseases, 35*(1), 8–13.

APPENDIX **6-C**

Preparing a Sample of Vaginal Secretions for Microscopic Examination

Vaginal secretions and exudates can be directly examined with a microscope to aid in the diagnosis of vaginal and sexually transmitted infections (see Chapters 20 and 21). Immediately after obtaining the vaginal secretions, mix one sample with normal saline solution, and a second sample with a 10% solution of potassium hydroxide (KOH). *Candida albicans, Trichomonas vaginalis,* clue cells (epithelial cells with indistinct borders due to adherent bacteria) associated with bacterial vaginosis, and white blood cells can be seen in normal saline solution. Potassium hydroxide lyses trichomonads, white blood cells, and most bacteria, making visualization of *Candida* species easier. The presence of an amine or fishy odor with the addition of KOH to the vaginal secretions should be noted (whiff test), and is associated with, but not diagnostic for, bacterial vaginosis and trichonomiasis.

The CDC (2001) offers the following directions for collecting and preparing these specimens for microscopic examination:

1. Assemble the necessary materials: one or two standard glass microscope slides and cover slips, nonsterile cotton-tipped swabs, saline solution, and potassium hydroxide (KOH) solution. Some clinicians also use a small test tube.
2. Using a dropper or single-use blister pack of the solutions, place two to three large drops of saline on one slide and KOH on the second slide. Alternatives include the use of one slide (put drops of both solutions separately on it), or the test tube method (place drops of saline in a test tube and drops of KOH on a slide).
3. Obtain a specimen of vaginal discharge by either swabbing the vaginal walls and posterior fornix with a cotton-tipped swab or by sampling from the concave surfaces of the speculum blade after the speculum has been removed.

4. Mix the sample of discharge with the drops of saline and KOH on the slides. Be sure to put the sample in the saline before the KOH and to keep the saline and KOH solutions separate. If using the test tube method, immerse the swab in the test tube, and then use the swab to apply the premixed specimen onto a dry slide.
5. Cover each specimen with a glass cover slip. Avoid trapping air bubbles under the cover slip, which makes the microscopic examination more difficult. Put one edge of the cover slip into the mixed specimen, and then lower the cover slip onto the specimen. Proceed as soon as possible to microscopic examination of the slide.

Reference

Centers for Disease Control and Prevention (CDC). (2001). *Program operations guidelines for STD prevention: Appendix ML-B*. Retrieved from http://www.cdc.gov/std/program/medlab/ApB-PGmedlab.htm

CHAPTER 7

Diagnosis of Pregnancy at the Gynecologic Visit

Robin G. Jordan

Introduction

There are 4.3 million births per year in the United States, making pregnancy care one of the leading reasons for ambulatory care visits (Sakala & Corry, 2008). More than 50% of all pregnancies in the United States are unintended (Finer & Henshaw, 2006); therefore, it is not uncommon to diagnose a pregnancy during a healthcare visit for other conditions. Pregnancy is the most common cause of secondary amenorrhea (Master-Hunter & Heiman, 2006). Of 474 reproductive-age women coming to the emergency department for other health issues, 2.3% were found to be unexpectedly pregnant on routine testing (Strote & Chen, 2006).

The focus of this chapter is the care of the woman who presents for gynecologic or episodic health care, and in whom a diagnosis of pregnancy is made. This chapter is provided primarily for those clinicians who typically provide only gynecologic care and not prenatal care. Women seeking pregnancy care would schedule a visit with a clinician who provides antepartum care. For more in-depth information on antepartum care, the reader is referred to midwifery and obstetric books such as *Varney's Midwifery* (Varney, Kriebs, & Gegor, 2004) and *Obstetrics: Normal and Problem Pregnancy* (Gabbe, Niebyl, & Simpson, 2007).

Diagnosis of Pregnancy

Pregnancy discovery occurs most often during the first trimester, or the first 12 weeks of gestation. An unanticipated diagnosis of pregnancy may be either welcome or devastating news for a woman. The emotional impact of learning of a pregnancy should be addressed immediately after diagnosis and before the history taking and physical examination, because a

BOX 7-1 *Conditions That Cause Symptoms Similar to Pregnancy*

- Gastrointestinal problems
- Gastroenteritis
- Hepatitis
- Bloating
- Uterine fibroids
- Ovarian cysts
- Menopause-related menstrual changes
- Endocrine causes of amenorrhea

diagnosis of pregnancy often becomes the priority issue for a woman upon hearing that she is pregnant. Refer to Chapter 18 on unintended pregnancy for more information on assisting women to explore their feelings about the pregnancy and the options available to them. Taking cues from the woman's response should guide the clinician in determining what to include with regard to pregnancy continuation in the remainder of the visit.

While some other conditions mimic pregnancy signs and symptoms (see **Box 7-1**), most pregnancies can be reliably detected by assessment of clinical signs, symptoms, and physical examination. Presumptive signs are those body changes perceived by the woman. Amenorrhea is often the first clue to possible pregnancy. Overwhelming fatigue due to a rise in basal metabolic rate often occurs at 6 weeks after the last menstrual period (LMP) and is often out of proportion to common tiredness. Breast tenderness generally occurs 4 to 6 weeks post LMP, reflecting increased estrogen levels in the body. Urinary frequency may increase 6 to 8 weeks post LMP owing to uterine enlargement that compresses the bladder. Nausea and vomiting occur in more than half of pregnant women beginning at approximately 5 to 6 weeks post LMP; they are thought to be the result of increased human chorionic gonadotropin (hCG) and estrogen levels. If a woman is more than 16 weeks' gestation, she may feel fetal movement, which may sometimes be misinterpreted as intestinal activity.

When there is a clinical suspicion of pregnancy, laboratory tests can be conducted to confirm (or disprove) the diagnosis. Pregnancy tests determine the presence of hCG in the urine or blood. Human chorionic gonadotropin is released in the maternal blood at the time of implantation of the fertilized egg (blastocyst) and is detectable in the serum within 24 to 48 hours, or approximately 8 days after conception (Gabbe et al., 2007). Urine pregnancy testing is often positive around the time of the first missed menses, which is approximately 4 weeks after the first day of the LMP. False-positive hCG test results are rare and can be caused by medications such as anticonvulsants, anti-Parkinson drugs, hypnotics, and tranquilizers; multiple myeloma; or trophoblastic disease (hydatidiform mole) (Stanback, Raymond, & Janowitz, 2002).

Qualitative urine testing for hCG is readily available in clinical office settings and is commonly used to diagnose pregnancy. Quantitative serum testing involves obtaining blood to detect the β subunit of hCG. This test is positive in pregnant women 7 to 9 days after implantation of the blastocyst. Serum tests can detect hCG levels in the range of 5 to 10 mIU/mL. A qualitative urine hCG test is sufficient for pregnancy diagnosis. Serum hCG testing is unnecessary for pregnancy diagnosis and should be reserved for specific indications, such as serial measurement in suspected ectopic pregnancy.

Risk Assessment

Risk assessment is the process by which clinicians screen for conditions that, if unmanaged, may increase chance of pregnancy complications or adverse outcome. Risk assessment occurs throughout the history taking and physical examination and includes interpreting the meaning of the results of laboratory tests.

Initial risk assessment reveals lifestyle or physical issues that need modification or intervention to promote the optimal pregnancy outcome.

History

Screening by health history is an important component of the initial prenatal visit. Refer to Chapter 6 for elements of the gynecologic history. Additional areas to cover when taking the history of a pregnant woman are identified here.

Menstrual History Data about a woman's last normal menses are needed to make a determination of gestational age and to determine an estimated date of birth (EDB). To determine if the date of the LMP can be used to accurately date the pregnancy, the woman should be certain of the date of onset, it should be a normal flow and duration, and she should have a history of regular 28- to 30-day cycles (Phelan, 2008). Gestational age refers to the length of pregnancy after the first day of the LMP and is usually expressed in weeks and days; it is also known as menstrual age. Women are considered pregnant from the first day of the last menstrual period, because this is a known date, unlike the unknown date of conception.

The EDB can be determined by using Nägele's rule: Add 7 days to the first day of the LMP, then subtract 3 months (**Box 7-2**). This mathematical model assumes 28-day menstrual cycles and a length of gestation of 266 days. With this information, estimation of the current gestational age can be made. Gestational age wheels are commonly used to simplify this calculation. These devices consist of an outer wheel that has markings for the calendar and an inner, sliding wheel with weeks and days of gestation. They facilitate the estimation of gestational age and the calculation of the EDB, but their quality varies. More accurate results can be obtained by using computer software or Web-based online calculators.

If the LMP date is unknown and the uterus is below the level of the symphysis pubis, then a transvaginal ultrasound is needed to date the pregnancy. However, if the uterus is above this landmark, an abdominal ultrasound can be used to date the pregnancy.

Prior Obstetric History In addition to recording data about her gravid and parity

> **BOX 7-2** *Calculating an Estimated Date of Birth (EDB) from the Date of the Last Menstrual Period (LMP) Using Nägele's Rule*
>
> 4/23 LMP of April 23
> + 7 days
> 4/30
> – 3 months
> 1/30 January 30 (of following year)

status (Chapter 6), information on prior pregnancy complications such as presence of infection, preeclampsia, gestational diabetes, episodes of bleeding, preterm birth, and genetic issues should be obtained by the clinician.

Infectious Disease History Prior history of genital herpes, Group B *Streptococcus* (GBS) infection, sexually transmitted infection (STI), and hepatitis B is obtained, because all of these infections can influence pregnancy care and outcome.

Environmental History Some substances found in workplaces and homes have the potential to cause reproductive harm. An early environmental risk assessment should be done for all pregnant women. Occupational health history includes—at a minimum—the following three questions:

- Describe your current job/career environment.
- Are you currently exposed to chemicals/pesticides, solvents, metals, fumes, gas, dust, noise, radiation, infectious disease, body fluids, emotional stress, or other hazards?
- Have you had any prior symptoms or illness due to work?

If substance exposure is noted, then a more detailed history covering the route, timing, and duration of exposure, as well as any protective measures taken, is essential. Many women do not know the names of chemicals used in their workplace. The Occupational Health and Safety Administration (OSHA) mandates that the names and health effects of all work-related chemicals be available to employees in the workplace via material safety data sheets (MSDSs). Asking the woman to obtain the relevant MSDSs is the clinician's starting point in learning more about many workplace exposures.

Home assessment is an integral part of an environmental exposure assessment. Although one's home is considered safe, it can contain many potentially harmful gardening and household chemicals, lead, mercury, pesticides, poor air quality due to wood stove use, and other potentially toxic substances. **Table 7-1** summarizes specific substances to be included in initial data gathering and discussion.

Social History Pregnancy is not only a physical event for a woman, but also a change in family constellation requiring role readjustment in other family members. Lack of social support has been associated with poor pregnancy outcomes such as preterm birth and fetal growth abnormalities (Elsenbruch et al., 2007). Assessing family structure and support available allows for early referral to social services for financial and family assistance programs as needed.

Substance History Substance use raises particular concerns during pregnancy. Approximately 11% to 20% of pregnant women smoke cigarettes during pregnancy (Centers for Disease Control and Prevention [CDC], 2004). Smoking during pregnancy increases risk for multiple adverse reproductive and perinatal outcomes, including difficulty conceiving, infertility, spontaneous abortion, premature rupture of membranes, low birth weight, neonatal

TABLE 7-1 Potentially Fetotoxic Environmental Exposures

Substance	Potential Exposure	Potential Problem	Recommendations
Lead	Older homes with lead pipes, lead paint, hobbies using lead (stained glass, furniture restoration, pottery making), Mexican pottery	Neurotoxin: learning deficits, developmental delays	Do not disturb pre-1970 paint. Run water 30 seconds in lead pipes. Drink bottled water
Mercury	Fish: swordfish, king mackerel, tilefish, shark, albacore tuna	Neurotoxin: learning deficits, developmental delays	Avoid high mercury fish. Check local fresh water fish safety advisories
Organic solvents	Occupations or hobbies involving adhesives, cleaning solvents, paints, resins, plastics, dyeing and printing materials	Birth defects	Eliminate substance contact. Ensure adequate ventilation. Wear personal protection devices, such as gloves and masks

mortality, stillbirth, preterm birth, and sudden infant death syndrome (SIDS). According to the CDC, approximately 16% of pregnant women continue to drink alcohol during their pregnancies, with 2% of pregnant women reporting binge drinking (CDC, 2004). Prenatal exposure to alcohol can cause a range of disorders, collectively known as fetal alcohol spectrum disorder (FASD). The most severe effect of alcohol consumption during pregnancy is fetal alcohol syndrome (FAS), one of the leading known preventable causes of mental retardation and birth defects. Chapter 8 describes substance abuse screening methods.

Present Pregnancy History Information about physical pregnancy symptoms, illness, fever, environmental exposures, and significant family or social changes since the LMP should be obtained.

Physical Examination

The physical examination of a pregnant woman includes additional assessments as well as the routine gynecologic examination (see Chapter 6). Uterine size should be assessed by pelvic examination prior to 11 weeks' gestation, when the uterus is still a pelvic organ, and by abdominal palpation after 12 weeks' gestation when the uterus rises out of the pelvis. The uterine fundus, or top of the uterus, is felt at the level of the symphysis pubis at 12 weeks' gestation. By 16 weeks' gestation, the fundus is midway between the symphysis and the umbilicus (**Figure 7-1**). Fetal heart tones can be heard with a handheld Doppler (**Figure 7-2**) as early as 10 to 12 weeks from the LMP. Normal range for fetal heart tones is 120 to 160 beats per minute.

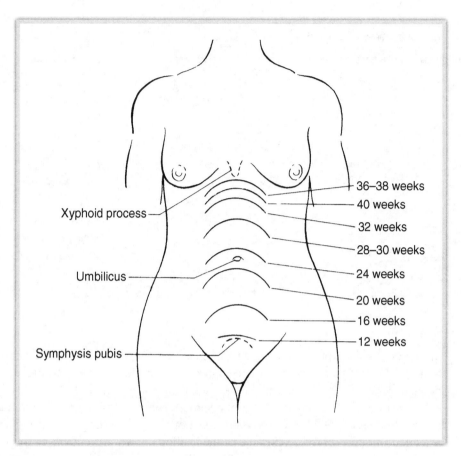

Xyphoid process

36–38 weeks
40 weeks
32 weeks
28–30 weeks

Umbilicus

24 weeks
20 weeks

Symphysis pubis

16 weeks
12 weeks

FIGURE 7-1 Approximate normal fundal heights during pregnancy.

Source: Varney, H., Kriebs, J. M., & Gegor, C. L. (2004). *Varney's midwifery* (4th ed.). Sudbury, MA: Jones and Bartlett Publishers.

A speculum examination is done to visualize the cervix, and to obtain a Pap test if the woman is due to receive one (see Chapter 8 for recommended screening intervals). Specimens for chlamydia and gonorrhea testing are collected (see Chapter 6 for techniques). The cervix is often friable (bleeds easily) in early pregnancy due to increased cervical vascularization that causes the cervix to appear blue in color. The bluish hue is known as Chadwick's sign. The increased vascularization may cause occasional spotting after a gentle speculum examination. If spotting occurs after the speculum examination, reassurance of normalcy is appropriate. A bimanual pelvic examination is done to assess uterine size and position.

If bleeding or pain is noted during the pelvic examination, spontaneous abortion and ectopic pregnancy should be considered. See the section on first-trimester bleeding for additional information about these conditions.

Laboratory Testing

Specific laboratory tests are also performed during the initial prenatal visit (**Box 7-3**). The CDC now recommends testing all healthcare patients for HIV regardless of their reported risk behaviors using an "opt-out" approach in which patients are informed that an HIV test will be conducted unless they explicitly decline to be tested (CDC, 2006).

Management

Patient Education

Education is an essential component of prenatal care. Priorities for the first visit teaching include lifestyle modification. Women should be apprised of risks associated with prenatal alcohol consumption and advised to abstain

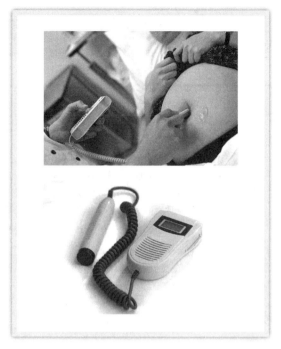

FIGURE 7-2 Handheld Doppler.

Source: (top) © iStockphoto/Thinkstock; (bottom) © Science Photo Library/Alamy.

BOX 7-3 *Laboratory Testing at the First Prenatal Visit*

- Complete blood count or hemoglobin and hematocrit
- Blood type
- Rh factor
- Rh antibody screen
- Rubella titer
- Varicella antibody screen
- Hepatitis B surface antigen
- HIV
- Venereal disease research laboratory (VDRL) or rapid plasma reagin (RPR) testing for syphilis
- Urine culture
- Chlamydia and gonorrhea
- Pap test
- Sickle cell trait screening, if indicated and desired (offer to all African American women)

during pregnancy. Instruction on the pregnancy health risks associated with smoking and strategies for cessation should be provided. Some drugs, such as isotretinoin, valproic acid, and certain angiotensin-converting enzyme (ACE) inhibitors, are contraindicated in pregnancy because of their potential to be fetotoxic. Pregnant women should be advised to contact their clinician prior to taking any nonprescription medication. At the initial visit, general information on topics such as sexuality during pregnancy, continuing exercise habits, wearing a seat belt, and avoidance of hot tubs and saunas due to hyperthermia risk are also typically covered.

Nutritional assessment and counseling are critical components of a comprehensive prenatal care program. Body mass index (BMI; see Chapter 6) should be calculated at the first visit to determine weight gain parameters for each woman. A diet history is then taken to determine adequacy of food groups and nutrients. Weight gain guidelines established by the Institute of Medicine (IOM, 2009) and recommended ranges for weight are as follows:

BMI < 18.5 (underweight): 28 to 40 lb
BMI 18.5 to 24.9 (normal): 25 to 35 lb
BMI 25 to 29.9 (overweight): 15 to 25 lb
BMI > 30 (obese): should gain 11 to 20 lb

Women who begin pregnancy with a BMI in the underweight, overweight, or obese category can benefit from a referral to a dietician skilled in pregnancy nutrition.

A balanced diet with an increase of approximately 350 calories per day after the first trimester, spread over three meals and two snacks daily, should be advised. Pregnant women should be encouraged to consume foods rich in docosahexaenoic acid (DHA) to meet the needs of the rapidly growing fetal brain and nervous system. Pregnancy-related DHA needs can be met with two servings of fatty low-mercury-content fish per week, such as salmon, trout, or herring (Greenburg, Bell, & Van Ausdal, 2008). In general, pregnancy nutrition needs can be met with 6 to 11 servings of breads and grains, 2 to 4 servings of fruit, 4 or more servings of vegetables, and 3 servings of protein. Pregnant women need between 3 and 4 servings of dairy products to meet the 1000 mg calcium daily requirement for fetal bone growth. A prenatal vitamin supplement should be prescribed to meet daily iron and folic acid needs in pregnancy.

Caffeine intake during pregnancy should be limited to approximately 200 mg daily, which is equivalent to one 12-ounce serving of coffee. High doses of caffeine are associated with an increased risk of first-trimester miscarriage (Weng, Odouli, & Li, 2008). Foods to avoid during pregnancy are listed in **Table 7-2**.

Common Discomforts

Many women experience pregnancy-related discomforts that are normal and not due to pathology. An explanation for the physiologic basis of these commonly occurring symptoms, and information on relief measures, should be provided as part of prenatal care. Nausea and vomiting are the most common symptoms experienced in early pregnancy, with nausea

TABLE 7-2 Foods to Avoid During Pregnancy

Food to Avoid	Increased Risk For:	To Reduce Risk:
Unpasteurized milk, soft cheeses (e.g., Camembert), gorgonzola, Mexican cheeses (e.g., queso fresco)	Listeriosis	Avoid
Prepackaged lunch meat, hot dogs, pâté and meat spreads	Listeriosis	Heat until steaming
Unpasteurized juices	*E. coli* infection, *Salmonella* enteritis	Avoid
Unwashed fruits and vegetables	Toxoplasmosis	Wash well prior to eating
Raw alfalfa sprouts	*E. coli* infection, *Salmonella* enteritis	Avoid
Raw eggs	*Salmonella* enteritis	Avoid
Rare meat	Toxoplasmosis	Cook meat to medium doneness
Raw fish and shellfish	Coliform bacteria and algae-related infection	Avoid

Source: Adapted from March of Dimes. (2009). *Food-borne risks in pregnancy.* Retrieved from http://www.marchofdimes.com/professionals/14332_1152.asp

affecting between 50% and 80% of all pregnant women (Davis, 2004). The effectiveness of relief measures varies from woman to woman, so it is appropriate to offer a variety of strategies. Lifestyle changes to reduce nausea and vomiting can be quickly incorporated until this discomfort passes, which is typically around 12 weeks' gestation.

Women experiencing nausea and vomiting should be advised to eat five to six small meals daily to avoid blood glucose spikes, eat carbohydrates just before going to bed and upon arising, avoid strong odors, and eliminate fatty and spicy foods. Increasing the amount of sleep at night and not brushing the teeth right after meals to avoid triggering the gag reflex may be helpful. Other effective remedies to offer include vitamin B_6 (pyridoxine) 25 mg orally twice daily. One-half to one full Unisom (doxylamine succinate) tablet can be added to the vitamin B_6 at night if the latter alone is ineffective. This method is documented to be safe and provides relief for many women (Davis, 2004). Ginger, in the form of candy, ginger ale, or 250-mg capsules orally four times per day, and acupressure with the use of Sea Bands are effective and safe measures to relieve nausea and vomiting for many pregnant women (Davis, 2004). Reassurance of symptom normalcy and that relief can be expected by approximately 12 to 14 weeks' gestation should be part of the treatment for nausea and vomiting.

Extreme fatigue is another common early pregnancy symptom. This is due to the sleep-inducing effects of increased levels of progesterone that initially maintain the pregnancy. Early pregnancy fatigue reaches a peak between 9 and 12 weeks' gestation (Varney et al.,

2004). Women should be encouraged to increase rest periods as able, and reassured that they should feel marked improvement in energy level by 12 to 14 weeks' gestation.

Breast tenderness is one of the most common pregnancy symptoms reported by women, often occurring as early as 2 weeks after fertilization. Increase in the breast size and deepening of areolar pigment are also present early in the first trimester. By 12 to 14 weeks' gestation, some women may leak colostrum. These breast changes are caused by increased levels of progesterone and estrogen that prepare the breasts for lactation. Women experiencing breast discomfort should be encouraged to wear a well-fitting and supportive bra, and reassured that the discomfort diminishes in the second trimester.

Genetic Screening

Genetic screening tests for Down syndrome and neural tube defects (NTDs) are offered to all pregnant women. The screening tests are time dependent; thus it is essential to provide information about testing options at the first prenatal visit. In addition to a discussion about the screening tests that are available, written information should be provided because the risks for certain genetic problems and testing options can be complex. Testing options are presented in **Table 7-3**.

The false-positive rate for the genetic screening tests is 5%. In other words, for every 100 women who have the test, 5 will have an abnormal result. However, only 2% to 3% of those women with an abnormal result will actually have a baby affected by one of the detectable chromosomal anomalies. If a screening test is positive, an invasive test, such as amniocentesis, is offered for diagnosis.

TABLE 7-3 Genetic Screening Tests for Down Syndrome, Trisomy 18, and Neural Tube Defects

Screening Test	Components	Anomalies Detected	Detection Rate	Timing
First trimester combined	Ultrasound evaluation of the nuchal translucency (NT) and serum screen	Down syndrome, trisomy 18	85–90%	11–13 weeks' gestation
Quad screen	Serum screen	Neural tube defects (NTDs), down syndrome, trisomy 18	80–85%	15–22 weeks' gestation
Integrated screening	Ultrasound evaluation of the NT and serum screen in both first and second trimesters	NTDs, down syndrome, trisomy 18	85–90%	11–13 and 15–22 weeks' gestation

Screening for maternal sickle cell trait is also offered at the first visit. In the United States, most cases of sickle cell disease occur among African Americans (1 in every 500 births) and Hispanic Americans (1 in every 1000–1400 births) (American College of Obstetricians and Gynecologists, 2007).

Key points to consider when discussing genetic screening with pregnant women are presented in **Box 7-4**.

First-Trimester Bleeding

Approximately one in four women experiences bleeding during the first trimester of pregnancy (Deutchman, Tubay, & Turok, 2009). Bleeding can vary from light spotting to heavy bleeding with clots. Implantation of the zygote in the uterine lining can cause spotting around the time the first missed period is due and is light and transient. This bleeding is not uncommon and is of no clinical significance. Another common etiology of bleeding is postcoital spotting due to the normal hyperemia of pregnancy. Preexisting cervical or genital infection, such as chlamydia or trichomoniasis, can also cause cervical friability with bleeding, and may be noted during the speculum examination. If cervical causes of first-trimester bleeding are ruled out after visualization of the cervix, early pregnancy loss and ectopic pregnancy should be considered.

Early Pregnancy Loss

The most common diagnosis in a woman experiencing first-trimester bleeding is spontaneous abortion, also known as miscarriage. Approximately 15% to 20% of all clinically recognized pregnancies are lost, and most losses occur in the first trimester (Chen & Creinin, 2007). The majority of early pregnancy losses are due to chromosomal abnormalities, which occur more often as maternal age increases (Gabbe et al., 2007).

The pattern, severity, duration, and pain associated with threatened pregnancy loss are highly variable. The bleeding can be pink, red (fresh), or brown (old), and may last from a few hours to several days and be continual or intermittent. Uterine cramping is a typical symptom of active miscarriage and may present in varying degrees with increasing severity as bleeding increases.

BOX 7-4 *Key Points in Offering Genetic Screening*

- All women should be offered screening tests for neural tube defects (NTDs) and Down syndrome up to 20 weeks' gestation.
- The risk for Down syndrome, trisomy 18, and NTDs is quite small for most women.
- Screening does not diagnose chromosomal anomalies; it indicates increased risk.
- Nondirective counseling and informed consent principles should be used when discussing testing options.
- Women can freely decline genetic screening and diagnostic tests.

A transvaginal ultrasound should be done, as the gestational sac should be able to be visualized by 5.5 weeks' gestation, with the fetal heartbeat often seen by 6 weeks' gestation (Gabbe et al., 2007). An initial quantitative serum hCG to evaluate serial measures for expected increase in hCG levels will aid in differentiating between viable pregnancy and early pregnancy loss or ectopic pregnancy (Chen & Creinin, 2007). Most first-trimester losses do not require intervention. For the woman who is uncomfortable with expectant management, treatment options include medical management with misoprostol, manual vacuum aspiration, and dilatation and curettage (Deutchman et al., 2009). Information regarding potential diagnoses, testing, and management options should be explained with sensitivity to the woman's reaction to learning that she is pregnant and to the possibility of losing the pregnancy.

Ectopic Pregnancy

Ectopic pregnancy is a potentially life-threatening form of pregnancy in which implantation of the fertilized egg occurs outside the uterus. With a prevalence of approximately 1.9% of reported pregnancies (Lozeau & Potter, 2005), ectopic pregnancy must be considered with early pregnancy bleeding between 4 and 10 weeks' gestation. This type of pregnancy is the leading cause of first-trimester maternal death. Risk factors for ectopic pregnancy include anything that causes tubal damage, such as a history of tubal surgery, prior ectopic pregnancy, history of pelvic inflammatory disease (PID) and STIs, and previous tubal ligation (American Society for Reproductive Medicine, 2008). Additional risk factors are current use of an intrauterine device (IUD), smoking, and history of infertility.

Symptoms typically present between 5 and 8 weeks' gestation and include amenorrhea, unilateral lower quadrant pain, and vaginal spotting. Approximately 60% to 85% of women with an ectopic pregnancy do not experience any bleeding (Mukul & Teal, 2007). When bleeding does occur, it is often lighter than normal menses and irregular, is rarely profuse, and can occur over a period of several weeks. On pelvic examination, findings may include uterine enlargement due to pregnancy hormones, significant abdominal tenderness, and, occasionally, exquisite cervical motion tenderness (Lozeau & Potter, 2005). An adnexal mass may or may not be palpated.

Rapid diagnosis of ectopic pregnancy may prevent surgical emergency and loss of future fertility. The first step in the evaluation and management of a pregnant woman experiencing first-trimester bleeding with risk factors for an ectopic pregnancy is identifying pregnancy location. A transvaginal ultrasound should be performed immediately. Determining serum ß-hCG level is useful, as levels greater than 2000 IU/L with an absent gestational sac are strong indicators of ectopic pregnancy. A woman with an ectopic pregnancy should be referred for a follow-up appointment within 24 hours with an obstetrician or perinatologist. Ectopic pregnancy may be managed medically, with medications, or surgically.

Referral for Routine Prenatal Care

Several types of pregnancy care, based on differing philosophical foundations, are available to women. The midwifery model of care views pregnancy as a healthy event, and places value on supporting normal pregnancy processes and family formation (Rooks, 1999; Varney, Kriebs, & Gegor, 2004). Medical care typically focuses on pathology detection and management, and is especially well suited for women experiencing pregnancy complications such as preeclampsia, continuous bleeding, or fetal growth abnormalities.

Optimal pregnancy care requires a holistic approach to a woman's physical, social, and emotional needs. A contemporary model of prenatal care delivery called CenteringPregnancy has become more widely available in the last decade. In this model, women have their first visit with one provider as in the traditional care model, but all subsequent visits are held in a group setting. Groups are formed with women of similar gestational age, and each session lasts 90 to 120 minutes. Elements of routine care, such as assessment of maternal and fetal health, are included; however, discussion of pertinent pregnancy topics such as nutrition, sexuality, smoking cessation, and family role adjustment are covered in facilitated group discussions. Benefits include developing social support networks, improved infant birth weights, higher rates of breastfeeding, reduced preterm births, and increased patient satisfaction (Ickovics et al., 2007).

Pregnancy is not only a normal physiologic process; it is a transformative process encompassing profound emotions and role change. Referrals and recommendations for prenatal care providers who will promote holistic pregnancy health should be made intentionally.

References

American College of Obstetricians and Gynecologists. (2007). Hemoglobinopathies in pregnancy. *ACOG Practice Bulletin N. 78*, January 2007. *Obstetrics & Gynecology, 109*(1), 229–237.

American Society for Reproductive Medicine. (2008). Medical treatment of ectopic pregnancy (ASRM Technical Bulletin). *Fertility and Sterility, 90*(3), S206–S212.

Centers for Disease Control and Prevention (CDC). (2004). Alcohol consumption among women who are pregnant or who might become pregnant—United States, 2002. *Morbidity and Mortality Weekly Report, 53*(50), 1178–1181.

Centers for Disease Control and Prevention (CDC). (2006). Revised recommendation for HIV testing in adults, adolescents and pregnant women in health care settings. *Morbidity and Mortality Weekly Report, 55*(RR14), 1–17.

Chen B., & Creinin, M. (2007). Contemporary management of early pregnancy loss. *Clinical Obstetrics & Gynecology, 50*(1), 67–88.

Davis, M. (2004). Nausea and vomiting of pregnancy: An evidence based review. *Journal of Perinatal and Neonatal Nursing, 18*(4), 312–328.

Deutchman, M., Tubay, A. T., & Turok, D. K. (2009). First trimester bleeding. *American Family Physician, 79*(11), 985–994.

Elsenbruch, S., Bensen, S., Rucke, M., Rose, M., Dudenhausen, J., Pincus-Knaackstedt, M., . . . , & Arck, P. (2007). Social support during pregnancy: Effects on maternal depressive symptoms, smoking and pregnancy outcome. *Human Reproduction, 22*(3), 869–877.

Finer, L., & Henshaw, S. (2006). Disparities in the rates of unintended pregnancies, 1994 and 2001. *Perspectives on Sexual Reproductive Health, 38*, 90–96.

Gabbe, S., Niebyl, J., & Simpson, J. (2007). *Obstetrics: Normal and problem pregnancy* (5th ed). New York: Churchill Livingstone.

Greenburg, J. A., Bell, S. J., & Van Ausdal, W. (2008). Omega-3 supplementation during pregnancy. *Review in Obstetrics & Gynecology, 1*(4), 162–169.

Ickovics, J., Kershaw, T., Westdahl, C., Massey, Z., Reynolds, Z. & Rising, S. S. (2007). Group prenatal care and perinatal outcomes. *Obstetrics & Gynecology, 110*(2), 330–339.

Institute of Medicine (IOM). (2009). *Weight gain during pregnancy: Reexamining the guidelines.* Retrieved July 30, 2009, from www.nap.edu.

Lozeau, A. M., & Potter, B. (2005). Diagnosis and management of ectopic pregnancy. *American Family Physician, 72*(9), 1707–1714.

Master-Hunter, T., & Heiman, D. L. (2006). Amenorrhea: Evaluation and treatment. *American Family Physician, 73*(8), 1374–1382.

Mukul, L., & Teal, S. (2007). Current management of ectopic pregnancy. *Obstetric and Gynecologic Clinics of North America, 24*(3), 403–419.

Phelan, S. (2008). Components and timing of prenatal care. *Obstetric and Gynecologic Clinical of North America, 35*(1), 339–353.

Rooks, J. (1999). The midwifery model of care. *Journal of Nurse Midwifery, 44*(4), 370–374.

Sakala, C., & Corry, M. (2008). *Evidence-based maternity care: What it is and what it can achieve.* Retrieved from http://www.childbirthconnection.org/article .asp?ck=10575

Stanback, J., Raymond, E., & Janowitz, B. (2002). Hormonal pregnancy test redux. *Contraception, 66*(4), 295–296.

Strote, J., & Chen, G. (2006). Patient self-assessment of pregnancy status in the emergency department. *Emergency Medicine Journal, 23*, 554–557. Retrieved from http://emj.bmj.com/cgi/content/abstract/23/7/554

Varney, H., Kriebs, J., & Gegor, C. (2004) *Varney's midwifery* (4th ed.). Sudbury, MA: Jones and Bartlett.

Weng, X., Odouli, R., & Li, D. K. (2008). Maternal caffeine consumption during pregnancy and risk of miscarriage: A prospective cohort study. *American Journal of Obstetrics and Gynecology, 198*(3), 1–8.

CHAPTER 8

Periodic Screening and Health Maintenance

Kathryn Osborne

Secondary preventive services are those services that enable early identification of risk factors or diagnosis of disease conditions in asymptomatic patients. The initial step in secondary prevention is assessment, which includes obtaining the patient's medical history, performing a physical examination, and evaluating data from laboratory tests. A comprehensive patient history is one of the most valuable screening tools available to the clinician. It affords the clinician an opportunity to receive detailed information about the patient and an opportunity to establish a therapeutic relationship with the patient. A patient's health history forms the basis for determining disease entities for which the patient is at risk and, therefore, requires further screening. A management plan is developed once risk factors are identified and should include measures that focus on reducing the short- and long-term consequences of identified risks.

Cost containment continues to be critically important in today's healthcare environment, so it is imperative that clinicians make decisions about testing and treatment that are based on current evidence. Only tests and treatments having proven benefits should be utilized. The yearly performance of routine laboratory tests has not proven to be the most effective tool in the process of delivering preventive health services (U.S. Preventive Services Task Force [USPSTF], 1996. It is the professional responsibility of every clinician to contain healthcare costs.

The U.S. Public Health Service gathered together a panel of experts to examine the efficacy of preventive health services including screening tests, counseling, immunizations, and chemoprevention. That panel—the Task Force—remains active today and presently has 15 experts from various private-sector specialty groups. It has the following mission:

- "Evaluate the benefits of individual services based on age, gender, and risk factors for disease

- Make recommendations about which preventive services should routinely be incorporated into primary medical care and for which populations
- Identify a research agenda for clinical preventive care" (Agency for Healthcare Research and Quality, 2009, para 2)

The initial findings of the Task Force were published in 1989 as *Guide to Clinical Preventive Services*. These findings were updated in 1996 and include the evaluation of more than 200 clinical services. The current edition (2008c) is available as a pocket guide for clinicians and can be downloaded from the following website: http://www.ahrq.gov/clinic/pocketgd.htm. The Task Force also posts periodic updates on its website: http://www.ahcpr.gov/clinic/uspstfix.htm. The initial recommendations from this panel were not based on cost-effectiveness, but the Task Force now recommends that cost-effectiveness be considered in all decision making about preventive health services. The intent of the Task Force is to provide clinicians with a framework for decision making about patient management plans that result in improved patient outcomes. It recognizes the importance of involving the patient in the decision-making process and acknowledges that some patients will prefer to use interventions for which there is no scientific evidence (Sheridan, Harris, & Woolf, 2004).

The current recommendation scheme assigns each recommendation to a grade that serves as a guide for informed and shared decision making. "A" and "B" designated services are those for which the Task Force found sufficient evidence to recommend them. The use of services designated as "C" or "I" should be based on the clinical judgment of the clinician, in conjunction with patient education and counseling. Many of the "C" and "I" services are services for which the Task Force found insufficient evidence to either recommend for or against, leaving open the opportunity for clinicians and patients to individualize a management plan. Services with a "D" recommendation are those that the Task Force found to be either of no benefit or potentially harmful. The Task Force updated its definitions and recommendation grades in 2007 and began including "suggestions for practice" (**Table 8-1**). This change came about because of a change in methods that occurred in May 2007. The grade definitions in use prior to 2007 are in Appendix A and are included because they apply to recommendations voted on prior to 2007. Clarification regarding the level of certainty relative to net benefits of testing is described in **Table 8-2**.

These screening recommendations are intended for the general population of individuals who do not have risk factors for specific disease entities. Lopez, Mathers, Ezzati, Jamison, and Murray (2006) define a risk factor as "an attribute or exposure which is causally associated with an increased probability of a disease or injury" (p. 467). When no risk factors are found for a particular disease, a woman is considered not at risk for that disease. However, women experience change throughout their lives, and occasionally change is accompanied by developing risk factors. When that happens, there is a subsequent change in their risk status. For example, a 30-year-old woman who is not at increased risk for breast cancer experiences a change in risk status when she turns 40. The clinician must be aware of the various risk factors that may alter the risk status of individual women so that additional screening is obtained when needed.

TABLE 8-1 U.S. Preventive Services Task Force (USPSTF) Grade Definitions After May 2007

Grade	Definition	Suggestions for Practice
A	The USPSTF recommends the service. There is high certainty that the net benefit is substantial.	Offer or provide this service.
B	The USPSTF recommends the service. There is high certainty that the net benefit is moderate or there is moderate certainty that the net benefit is moderate to substantial.	Offer or provide this service.
C	The USPSTF recommends against routinely providing the service. There may be considerations that support providing the service in an individual patient. There is at least moderate certainty that the net benefit is small.	Offer or provide this service only if other considerations support the offering or providing the service in an individual patient.
D	The USPSTF recommends against the service. There is moderate or high certainty that the service has no net benefit or that the harms outweigh the benefits.	Discourage the use of this service.
I Statement	The USPSTF concludes that the current evidence is insufficient to assess the balance of benefits and harms of the service. Evidence is lacking, of poor quality, or conflicting, and the balance of benefits and harms cannot be determined.	Read the clinical considerations section of USPSTF Recommendation Statement. If the service is offered, patients should understand the uncertainty about the balance of benefits and harms.

Source: U.S. Preventive Services Task Force, 2008a.

This chapter focuses on the recommendations of the Task Force and provides a brief summary of its evidence-based recommendations. The Task Force recommendations and guidelines developed by other professional groups are provided so that clinicians may compare and contrast the recommendations from each group (**Table 8-3**). The Task Force's *Guide to Clinical Preventive Services* provides a more detailed description of the research underlying these recommendations, and highlights the implications that the recommendations have for clinical practice.

TABLE 8-2 Levels of Certainty Regarding Net Benefit

Level of Certainty*	Description
High	The available evidence usually includes consistent results from well-designed, well-conducted studies in representative primary care populations. These studies assess the effects of the preventive service on health outcomes. This conclusion is therefore unlikely to be strongly affected by the results of future studies.
Moderate	The available evidence is sufficient to determine the effects of the preventive service on health outcomes, but confidence in the estimate is constrained by such factors as: • The number, size, or quality of individual studies. • Inconsistency of findings across individual studies. • Limited generalizability of findings to routine primary care practice. • Lack of coherence in the chain of evidence. As more information becomes available, the magnitude or direction of the observed effect could change, and this change may be large enough to alter the conclusion.
Low	The available evidence is insufficient to assess effects on health outcomes. Evidence is insufficient because of: • The limited number or size of studies. • Important flaws in study design or methods. • Inconsistency of findings across individual studies. • Gaps in the chain of evidence. • Findings not generalizable to routine primary care practice. • Lack of information on important health outcomes. More information may allow estimation of effects on health outcomes.

*The USPSTF defines certainty as "likelihood that the USPSTF assessment of the net benefit of a preventive service is correct." The net benefit is defined as benefit minus harm of the preventive service as implemented in a general, primary care population. The USPSTF assigns a certainty level based on the nature of the overall evidence available to assess the net benefit of a preventive service.

Source: U.S. Preventive Services Task Force, 2008a.

TABLE 8-3 A Comparison of Screening Recommendations

	U.S. Preventive Services Task Force (USPSTF)	American College of Obstetricians and Gynecologists	American Cancer Society (ACS)	Other Groups
Cervical cancer	Pap smear every 1–3 years for all women within 3 years of beginning sexual activity or by age 21, whichever comes first. Recommends against screening women over 65 if they have had normal Pap smears and are otherwise not at risk for cervical cancer. Recommends against screening women who have had a total hysterectomy for benign disease. Finds that there is insufficient evidence to recommend for or against the use of new technologies to screen for cervical cancer.	Yearly cervical cytology within 3 years of the onset of sexual activity or by age 21, continue to age 30. May decrease testing to every 2–3 years after 3 consecutive negative test results if age 30 or older with no history of cervical intraepithelial neoplasia (CIN) 2 or CIN 3, not immune suppressed, not infected with HIV, and have no history of in utero exposure to diethylstilbestrol. Women with any of the aforementioned need to continue annual screening. Women who are HIV positive should have cervical cytology testing every 6 months after diagnosis and then annually after two consecutive normal results. Women with a history of hysterectomy for reasons other than carcinoma may discontinue screening. Women with a history of CIN 2 or 3 should be screened yearly until they have 3 consecutive negative vaginal cytology tests.	Yearly Pap smear (using conventional Pap tests) for women within 3 years of beginning vaginal sexual activity or by age 21. Screening may be done every 2 years if liquid-based tests are used. Testing may be extended to every 2–3 years for women at age 30 who have had 3 normal screens. Screening can be discontinued at age 70 if women have had 3 consecutive normal screens and no abnormal test results in the prior 10 years, and is not necessary following total hysterectomy for reasons other than cervical cancer.	

(continues)

TABLE 8-3 A Comparison of Screening Recommendations *(Continued)*

	U.S. Preventive Services Task Force (USPSTF)	American College of Obstetricians and Gynecologists	American Cancer Society (ACS)	Other Groups
Breast cancer	Mammogram (with or without clinical breast examination [CBE]) every 1–2 years beginning at age 40. Insufficient evidence to recommend for or against breast self-examination (BSE) or CBE alone at any age.	Mammogram and CBE every 1–2 years for women age 40–49 and yearly for women age 50 and older. Annual CBE for all women. BSE for women of all ages can be recommended.	Mammogram and CBE every year beginning at age 40. CBE every 2–3 years and the performance of monthly BSE for women age 20–39.	
Elevated cholesterol	Strongly recommends routinely screening women age 45 and older who are at increased risk for coronary heart disease. Also recommends screening women age 20–45 who are at increased risk for coronary artery disease. Makes no recommendation for or against screening women age 20 and older without known risk factors for coronary artery disease.	Nonfasting total cholesterol and high-density lipoprotein (HDL) every 5 years beginning at age 45. Screening is recommended for women age 19–44 based on risk factors.		The National Cholesterol Education Program (sponsored by NIH) recommends screening all adults over age 20 with total cholesterol, low-density lipoprotein (LDL), HDL, and triglycerides (TG) every 5 years.
Osteoporosis	Recommends routine screening for osteoporosis with bone density measurements for all women age 65 and older, and screening for women at increased risk beginning at age 60.	Concurs with the National Osteoporosis Foundation.		The National Osteoporosis Foundation recommends screening all women age 65 and older, and younger postmenopausal women who have had a fracture or who have one or more risk factors for osteoporosis.

TABLE 8-3 A Comparison of Screening Recommendations *(Continued)*

	U.S. Preventive Services Task Force (USPSTF)	American College of Obstetricians and Gynecologists	American Cancer Society (ACS)	Other Groups
Colo-rectal cancer	Strongly recommends screening women age 50–75 for colorectal cancer. Recommends against routine screening for colorectal cancer in adults age 76–85; screening women age 76–85 should be based on risk factors. Recommends against screening adults older than 85 years of age. Found insufficient evidence to determine which strategy is best in terms of the balance of benefits and potential harms or cost-effectiveness.	Concurs with ACS recommendations. As of 2007, ACOG recognizes colonoscopy every 10 years for all women starting at age 50 as the preferred method of screening.	Fecal occult blood testing every year beginning at age 50 and flexible sigmoidoscopy every 5 years. The combination of these is preferable to either one alone. ACS also recommends double contrast barium enema every five years and a colonoscopy every 10 years.	The American Academy of Family Physicians has recommendations similar to ACS.
Ovarian cancer	Recommends against routine screening with tumor markers, ultrasound, or pelvic examination. Insufficient evidence to recommend for or against routinely screening asymptomatic women at increased risk of developing ovarian cancer.	No techniques have proven to be effective in the routine screening of asymptomatic low-risk women for ovarian cancer. Clinicians should remain vigilant for signs and symptoms of disease.	During periodic health examinations, a cancer check-up should include health counseling and may include examinations for ovarian cancer. Clinicians should remain alert for signs and symptoms of ovarian cancer which may include: • bloating • pelvic or abdominal pain • trouble eating or feeling full quickly • urinary symptoms such as urgency • fatigue • upset stomach • back pain • painful intercourse • constipation	

(continues)

TABLE 8-3 A Comparison of Screening Recommendations *(Continued)*

	U.S. Preventive Services Task Force (USPSTF)	American College of Obstetricians and Gynecologists	American Cancer Society (ACS)	Other Groups
Intimate partner violence (IPV)	Insufficient evidence to recommend for or against routine screening.	Routinely ask all women direct, specific questions about abuse. Refer to community-based services when identified.		The American Academy of Family Physicians advises to remain alert for signs of family violence at every patient encounter.

Source: Data from American Cancer Society, 2008; American College of Obstetricians and Gynecologists, 2007; U.S. Preventive Services Task Force, 2008b.

Screening Recommendations for All Women

Alcohol Misuse

The Task Force assigns a "B" recommendation to screening all adults (including pregnant women) for alcohol misuse (Task Force, 2008b). Historically, research regarding the effects of alcohol on humans and animals has been conducted on males. Only recently has the research focus changed in an attempt to discover the effects of alcohol on females. An initial finding of these studies is that smaller quantities of alcohol can result in more severe damage to women (National Institute on Alcohol Abuse and Alcoholism [NIAAA], 2008). Alcohol consumption is considered hazardous for a woman who has either seven or more drinks in one week or three drinks per occasion. This is considerably less than the threshold allowable for males. Alcohol abuse causes physical, social, or emotional harm to the drinker or is defined as drinking that causes harm to others, but falls short of dependence and addiction (NIAAA). A variety of effective alcohol screening tools are available, and many of these can be found at the NIAAA website at http://www.niaaa.nih.gov.

The Task Force (2008b) suggests using the CAGE questionnaire for alcohol screening. This instrument is short and effective and consists of a series of four questions that can be asked during a health history:

- Do you ever feel the need to **C**ut down your drinking?
- Are you ever **A**nnoyed by people's criticism of your drinking?
- Do you ever feel **G**uilty about drinking?
- Do you ever feel the need for an "**E**ye-opener" in the morning?

Brief questions about the quantity and the frequency of alcohol consumption are also helpful. The CAGE questionnaire can be administered to women who are found to consume hazardous amounts of alcohol. Women who answer "yes" to three or four CAGE questions may be alcohol dependent. Those who answer "yes" to one or two may have alcohol-related problems. Those who answer "no" to all questions may still be considered at risk for alcohol misuse if they indicate that they consume hazardous amounts of alcohol. The Task Force further recommends that patients who misuse alcohol undergo counseling, either in the primary care setting or with clinicians specialized in the treatment of alcohol misuse. All pregnant women should be counseled about the harmful effects alcohol has on the developing fetus (Task Force, 2008b).

Cervical Cancer

The Task Force assigns an "A" recommendation to screening for cervical cancer. Screening should begin within 3 years of the onset of sexual activity or by age 21. The recommended screening test is the Papanicolaou smear, commonly called a Pap smear. There currently is no evidence to support annual Pap smear screening. Annual Pap smears have not demonstrated any improvement in health outcomes. However, the Task Force also recognizes that because of the sensitivity of the Pap smear, many specialty organizations in the United States continue to recommend yearly screening until a minimum number of tests are found to be cytologically normal. Women who are at increased risk for cervical cancer include those infected with human papillomavirus (HPV), those who engage in sexual activity at an early age, those who have had multiple sexual partners, and those women who smoke cigarettes (Task Force, 2008b). The Task Force recommends against screening ("D" recommendation) women older than 65 years who are not at increased risk for cervical cancer, and who have a history of cytologically normal screens. The same recommendation against screening is made for women who have had a hysterectomy for reasons other than carcinoma (Task Force, 2008b).

Depression

The Task Force assigns a "B" recommendation to screening all adults for depression in settings where there is a mechanism in place for follow-up testing and treatment. It assigns an "I" recommendation to routinely screening adolescents for depression, although clinicians should be alert for signs of depression in young girls and teens (Task Force, 2008b). Screening for depression is an important aspect of women's health care because they are at an increased risk for developing clinical depression (National Mental Health Association [NMHA], 2009). Notably, women are two times more likely than men to develop clinical depression (Mental Health America, 2009).

A variety of depression screening tools are available, but perhaps the easiest screening tool is to simply ask a few questions about the woman's mood and her ability to find pleasure in activities she usually enjoys. There is no recommended frequency for this type of screening. Patients who elicit a positive screen should be referred to clinicians who are skilled in the diagnosis and treatment of depressive disorders for further testing and management. The Task Force found little benefit in routinely screening patients for whom follow-up care is unavailable (Task Force, 2008b). It is currently in the process of updating the recommendations regarding routine screening for depression. Clinicians are advised to check the online periodic updates for changes in the recommendations.

Height and Weight

The Task Force assigns a "B" recommendation to screening all patients for obesity. The body mass index (BMI) is the recommended method of identifying women at increased risk for morbidity and mortality from excessive weight. It is calculated by dividing a woman's weight in kilograms by her height in meters squared (see Chapter 6). Overweight is defined as having a BMI in the range of 25 to 29.9. Anyone with a BMI of 30 or greater is classified as obese. Patients should be counseled on the importance of maintaining a healthy diet and regular exercise (Task Force, 2008b).

Hypertension

The Task Force assigns an "A" recommendation to screening adults 18 years and older for hypertension; the routine screening of children and adolescents is an "I" recommendation. The recommended screening test for hypertension is a blood pressure measurement using a sphygmomanometer. Based on the findings of the Joint National Committee on Prevention, Detection, Evaluation, and Treatment of High Blood Pressure (JNC7), the recommended frequency of screening is every 2 years for women with blood pressure readings of less than 120/80 mm Hg, and more frequently for those with higher readings (Task Force, 2008b). The JNC7 recommends a restructuring of traditional blood pressure classifications. The report classifies systolic pressures of 120 to 139 mm Hg or diastolic pressures of 80 to 89 mm Hg as prehypertensive and recommends clinicians consider drug therapy for certain individuals who fall within this classification (JNC7, 2004).

Intimate Partner Violence

The Task Force assigns an "I" recommendation to screening patients for intimate partner violence (IPV). There are currently no studies that confirm the accuracy of specific screening tools, or indicate that the use of such tools decreases disability or premature death as a result of IPV. Nor are there studies that have examined the harmful effects of screening for IPV. Consequently, the Task Force (2008b) is unable to recommend for or against the use of specific tools to screen for IPV.

According to the Centers for Disease Control and Prevention (CDC, 2006), in the United States almost 5 million women each year experience IPV. The Task Force (2008b) recommends that all clinicians remain alert for signs and symptoms of IPV. Women presenting with symptoms or injuries should receive detailed documentation of the injuries, medical treatment, counseling referrals, and a list of community resources that provide shelter and protection. See Chapter 14 for more information on IPV and Chapter 15 for more information on sexual assault.

Ovarian Cancer

Routinely screening women for ovarian cancer by measuring serum tumor markers, ultrasound, or pelvic examination receives a "D" recommendation from the Task Force. There is no evidence to demonstrate that such screening leads to improvement in overall health outcomes, and the best available evidence suggests that the risks associated with routine screening for ovarian cancer outweigh the benefits. The Task Force (2008b) does not recommend routine screening for ovarian cancer for the general population because of the risks, inconvenience, and cost of follow-up.

In addition, the Task Force recommends against ("D" recommendation) routinely referring women without specific family history patterns, which place women at increased risk for ovarian or breast cancer, for genetic counseling or *BRCA*1 and/or *BRCA2* testing. However, the Task Force does recommend that women whose family history is suggestive of an increased risk for *BRCA1* and *BRCA2* mutations be referred for genetic counseling ("B" recommendation) to allow for informed decision making about further testing and prophylactic treatment. The Task Force (2008b) recommends that genetic counseling be conducted by a suitably trained clinician.

See Chapter 28 for a more in-depth discussion of gynecologic cancers.

Rubella Immunity

Based on the findings and recommendations of the CDC with regard to immunizations, the Task Force recommends screening all women of childbearing age for rubella immunity at the time of their first clinical contact. Screening is accomplished either by obtaining a history of vaccination or by ordering serologic studies. The Task Force further recommends that all nonpregnant women of childbearing age receive vaccinations, and those who are pregnant should be vaccinated immediately postpartum (CDC, 2009; Task Force, 2008b). It recommends against the routine screening of postmenopausal women for rubella (Task Force, 1996).

Tobacco Use

The Task Force assigns an "A" recommendation to screening all adults for tobacco use. The recommended screening tool is careful questioning by the clinician about the patient's tobacco use during the routine health history. The most recent data indicate that 18% of U.S. women smoke cigarettes (CDC, 2007). The CDC analyzed U.S. data from the 2006 National Health Interview Survey (NHIS) and found the prevalence of smoking among adults has changed very little since 2004, which suggests tobacco use has plateaued since 1997 to 2004, when cigarette smoking among adults declined (CDC, 2007). As discussed in Chapter 4, the Task Force recommends implementation of interventions to promote smoking cessation in all patients who use tobacco. Scientific evidence demonstrates that patients who quit using tobacco are likely to have substantial overall health benefits, regardless of the number of years of tobacco use (Task Force, 2008b).

Special Populations

Screening Recommendations for Adolescents

Chlamydia The Task Force assigns an "A" recommendation to screening all sexually active women age 24 years and younger, and women older than 24 who are at an increased risk for a sexually transmitted infection for chlamydia. It recommends against routinely screening women age 25 and older who are not at increased risk for chlamydia. The most significant risk factor for infection is age. Adolescents and women through 24 years of age are at highest risk. Additionally, women at increased risk of infection include African American and Hispanic women, women with a history of sexually transmitted infections, those with new or multiple sexual partners, women who exchange sex for money or drugs, and those who inconsistently use barrier methods of contraception. In addition to individual risk factors, chlamydia infection is seen more frequently in particular communities. Clinicians should be aware of prevalence rates of infection in the communities in which they practice (Task Force, 2008b).

A number of screening tests for chlamydia are available (see Chapter 6). The choice of screening test is based on cost, convenience, and feasibility.

Screening Recommendations for Older Women

Breast Cancer The Task Force updated its recommendations regarding screening for breast cancer in 2009. The most recent recommendations are provided here (Task Force, 2009). Screening mammography every 2 years for women age 50 to 74 years receives a "B" recommendation from the Task Force. There is insufficient evidence to weigh the benefits or harms of screening mammograms after the age of 74 (Grade: I statement). Recommending a biennial screening mammogram prior to age 50 should be made on an individual basis, and the clinician should take into account the patient's beliefs and values about benefits and harms (Grade: C recommendation). The Task Force recommends against teaching BSE because there is no evidence to support it (Grade: D recommendation). Additionally, the Task Force concluded that there is a lack of evidence that CBE has any effect on breast cancer mortality and that there is not enough evidence to assess its benefits and harms beyond a screening mammography in women age 40 years and older (Grade: I Statement). Furthermore, the Task Force states that there is not enough evidence to assess benefits and risks of either digital mammography or magnetic resonance imaging (MRI) versus the standard film mammography as to which provides the best screen for disease (Grade: I Statement). Some evidence further suggests that CBE and BSE may actually increase the likelihood of further testing and biopsy while doing little to improve outcomes (Task Force, 2009).

Women at an increased risk for developing breast cancer should begin having mammograms at an earlier age and benefit from the increased frequency of screening. The following factors place a woman at an increased risk for breast cancer: age, history of breast cancer in her mother or sister, having her first child after age 30, and a previous breast biopsy that revealed atypical hyperplasia (Task Force, 2008b, 2009). Refer to Chapter 16 for a more in-depth discussion of breast cancer.

Colorectal Cancer The Task Force recommends screening all adults age 50 years and older for colorectal cancer ("A" classification). Individuals with existing risk factors for colon cancer have approximately a 20% occurrence rate of disease. In light of the fact that colon cancer occurs frequently in individuals who are considered at average risk, the Task Force suggests that earlier initiation of screening for women at higher risk of colorectal cancer is reasonable. Risk factors for colorectal cancer include the following:

- History of colorectal cancer in a first-degree relative
- Rare genetic disorders such as familial adenomatous polyposis or hereditary nonpolyposis colorectal cancer
- Chronic ulcerative colitis
- History of polyps or colorectal cancer
- A family history of adenomatous polyps that were diagnosed before the age of 60 years

Screening tests include home fecal occult blood testing (FOBT), flexible sigmoidoscopy, FOBT combined with flexible sigmoidoscopy, colonoscopy, and double-contrast barium enema. Each of these options has advantages and disadvantages for the patient and the practice setting. Clinicians should discuss the risks and benefits of each screening test, and include patient preference in choosing a screening method. The optimal interval for screening depends on the screening test used and can vary from yearly FOBT to colonoscopy every 10 years (Task Force, 2008b). Clinicians who provide health care for women who require screening should familiarize themselves with the risks, costs, and benefits of the various screening options.

Elevated Cholesterol Levels The Task Force assigns an "A" recommendation to routinely screening women 45 years of age and older for lipid disorders only if they are at increased risk for coronary heart disease (CHD). Screening cholesterol levels in women aged between the years 20 and 44 with preexisting risk factors for coronary artery disease receives a "B" recommendation. The Task Force makes no recommendation—either for or against—routinely screening women age 20 and older who are not at increased risk for coronary heart disease (Task Force, 2008c). Increased risk is defined by the Task Force as the presence of any one of the following risk factors:

- Diabetes
- Previous personal history of CHD or noncoronary atherosclerosis
- Family history of cardiovascular disease before age 50 in male relatives or age 60 in female relatives

- Tobacco use
- Hypertension
- Obesity (BMI ≥ 30)

The recommended screening tool is a serum measurement of total cholesterol and high-density lipoprotein (HDL) cholesterol with the patient either fasting or nonfasting. The optimal frequency of screening is unknown; however, the Task Force recommends screening every 5 years for the general population, and more frequently for individuals with high normal lipid levels, and less frequently for women with repeatedly low levels. All women should receive counseling about the benefits of a healthy diet (low in saturated fats and high in fruits and vegetables), regular exercise, and maintaining a healthy weight (Task Force, 2008d).

Hearing Impairment The Task Force assigns a "B" recommendation to screening all older adults for hearing impairment. The recommended screening method is to ask the patient about her perception of changes in hearing. Patients should be informed that although changes in hearing often occur with aging, they are not considered a normal aging process, and utilization of hearing devices often can improve hearing. Women in whom hearing loss is suspected should be referred to specialists for further testing. Traditional hearing screens involve the use of audiometry—a series of auditory tones that, upon recognition, elicit an affirmative response from the patient. There is insufficient evidence to recommend for or against the use of audiometry, so audiometry is a "C" recommendation. There is no recommended frequency of testing; this decision is left to the discretion of the clinician (Task Force, 1996).

Osteoporosis Screening women older than age 65 for osteoporosis receives a "B" recommendation. The Task Force recommends routine screening beginning at age 60 for women who are at increased risk of osteoporosis. Some evidence indicates that earlier screening may prevent some fractures; however, there is not enough evidence to definitively demonstrate that early screening outweighs the risk associated with screening and treatment.

The Task Force assigns a "C" recommendation to routinely screening women younger than 60 years of age for osteoporosis. Factors associated with increased risk for the development of osteoporosis include low body weight (less than 70 kg/154 lb), cigarette smoking, sedentary lifestyle, family history, decreased lifetime calcium intake, increased alcohol and caffeine intake, and white or Asian ethnicity. Low body weight appears to be the best predictor of risk for developing osteoporosis. The best predictor of hip fracture is bone density testing using dual-energy X-ray absorptiometry of the head of the femur. The Task Force recognizes that bone density testing of peripheral sites using other modalities can also be effective in predicting increased risk of fracture. Optimal frequency of screening has not been studied, but evidence suggests it may take up to 2 years to identify changes in bone density. More frequent screening may be appropriate in women with low baseline bone density measurements. Women in whom osteoporosis is identified should be counseled on the risks and benefits of various treatment options (Task Force, 2008b). See Chapter 13 for further information about osteoporosis.

Visual Changes The Task Force assigns a "B" recommendation to screening older adults for visual impairment. Visual changes leading to accidental injury are more prevalent after the age of 65 years (Task Force, 1996). The Task Force also concluded that while the effect of routine screening for visual changes in the elderly has not been assessed, there is fair evidence that routine screening can result in overall improvements in acuity and offers little likelihood of serious harm as a result of the screening. The recommended screening tool is the Snellen Acuity Chart.

The Task Force leaves the determination of frequency to the discretion of the clinician; there is no recommended frequency for visual screening. Further, the Task Force found insufficient evidence to recommend for or against screening adults for glaucoma (Task Force, 2008b).

Additional Recommendations for Women with Hypertension

Type 2 Diabetes Mellitus Approximately 9% of the adult population in the United States has type 2 diabetes mellitus (DM), and the prevalence of this disease is increasing. The Task Force has recently revised its recommendations for screening women for type 2 DM and now assigns a "B" recommendation to screening asymptomatic women who have a sustained blood pressure (treated or untreated) of greater than 135/80 mm Hg. It found insufficient evidence to recommend for or against routinely screening asymptomatic adults with blood pressures of 135/80 mm Hg or lower ("I" recommendation). Screening tests for DM include fasting plasma glucose, 2-hour postload plasma glucose, and hemoglobin A1C. The optimal screening interval is unknown, although based on expert opinion the American Diabetes Association recommends screening every 3 years (Task Force, 2008e)

Additional Observations

It is important to remember that the screening recommendations discussed in this chapter are intended for healthy, asymptomatic women unless otherwise specified. In addition to these screening recommendations, the Task Force recommends that clinicians remain alert for findings that are suggestive of conditions listed in **Table 8-4**. As noted in Chapter 6, the gynecologic history and physical examination provide excellent opportunities to gather important screening information about the patient. Answers to a few direct questions and close attention during the physical examination can give the clinician important information and should always be part of a routine patient encounter.

TABLE 8-4 Additional Observations

Condition	Population
Symptoms of peripheral arterial disease	Older women, smokers, women with diabetes
Skin lesions with malignant features	All women, especially those with increased risk factors (white race; presence of atypical moles; increased number of common moles or freckles; family or personal history of skin cancer; history of severe sunburns in childhood; light skin, hair, and eye color)
Signs and symptoms of oral cancer or premalignancy	Women who use tobacco and older women who drink alcohol regularly
Subtle or nonspecific signs and symptoms of thyroid dysfunction	Older women, postpartum women, and women with Down syndrome
Signs and symptoms of hearing impairment	All women
Spinal curvatures	Adolescents
Change in functional performance	Older women
Suicidal ideation	Women with established risk factors for suicide (history of previous attempts or threats, previous psychiatric diagnosis or treatment, substance abuse, recent loss)
Family violence	All women
Drug abuse	All women
Untreated tooth and gum disease	All women

Source: Adapted from U.S. Preventive Services Task Force, 2008b.

References

Agency for Healthcare Research and Quality. (2009). *About the USPSTF.* Rockville, MD: U.S. Preventive Services Task Force. Retrieved from http://www.ahrq.gov/clinic/uspstfab.htm

American Cancer Society (ACS). (2008). *Cancer facts and figures.* Retrieved from http://www.cancer.org/Research/CancerFactsFigures/CancerFactsFigures/cancer-facts-figures-2008

American College of Obstetricians and Gynecologists. (2007). *Primary and preventive care: Periodic assessments.* Committee Opinion No. 357. Washington, DC: Author.

Centers for Disease Control and Prevention (CDC). (2006). *Fact sheet: Understanding intimate partner violence.* Retrieved from http://www.cdc.gov/ncipc/dvp/ipv_factsheet.pdf

Centers for Disease Control and Prevention (CDC). (2007). Cigarette smoking among adults—United States, 2006. *Morbidity and Mortality Weekly Report, 56*(44), 1157–1161. Retrieved from http://www.cdc.gov/mmwr/preview/mmwrhtml/mm5644a2.htm

Centers for Disease Control and Prevention (CDC). (2009). Recommended adult immunization schedule—United States, 2009. *Morbidity and Mortality Weekly Report, 57*, 53.

Joint National Committee on Prevention. (2004). *The complete report: The science behind the new guidelines: Prevention, detection, evaluation and treat-*

ment of high blood pressure (NIH Publication No. 04-5230). Retrieved from http://www.nhlbi.nih.gov/guidelines/hypertension/jnc7full.pdf

Lopez, A., Mathers, C., Ezzati, M., Jamison, D., & Murray, C. (2006). *Global burden of disease and risk factors.* Washington, DC: Oxford University Press & World Bank.

Mental Health America. (2009). *Fact sheet: Depression in women.* Retrieved from http://www.mentalhealthamerica.net/index.cfm?objectid=C7DF952E-1372-4D20-C8A3DDCD5459D07B

National Institute on Alcohol Abuse and Alcoholism (NIAAA). (2008). *Alcohol: A woman's health issue* (NIH Publication No. 03–4956, revised 2008). Retrieved from http://pubs.niaaa.nih.gov/publications/brochurewomen/women.htm#drinking nih.gov/extramural/gendiff.htm

National Mental Health Association. (2009). W*omen and depression: Discovering hope.* Retrieved from http://www.nimh.nih.gov/health/publications/women-and-depression-discovering-hope/complete-index.shtml

Sheridan, S., Harris, R., & Woolf, S. (2004). *Shared decision making about screening and chemoprevention: A suggested approach from the U.S. Preventive Services Task Force.* Retrieved from http://www.ahrq.gov/clinic/3rduspstf/shared/sharedba.htm

United States Preventive Services Task Force (Task Force). (1996). *Guide to clinical preventive services* (2nd ed.). Baltimore: Williams & Wilkins.

United States Preventive Services Task Force (Task Force). (2008a). *Grade definitions after May 2007.* Retrieved from http://www.uspreventiveservicestaskforce.org/uspstf/gradespost.htm

United States Preventive Services Task Force (Task Force). (2008b). *Guide to clinical preventive services 2008.* Retrieved from http://www.ahrq.gov/clinic/pocketgd.htm

United States Preventive Services Task Force (Task Force). (2008c). *Pocket guide to clinical preventive services.* Retrieved from http://www.ahrq.gov/clinic/pocketgd.htm

United States Preventive Services Task Force (Task Force). (2008d). *Screening for lipid disorders in adults.* Retrieved from http://www.ahrq.gov/clinic/uspstf08/lipid/lipidrs.htm

United States Preventive Services Task Force (Task Force). (2008e). *Screening for type 2 diabetes mellitus in adults.* Retrieved from http://www.ahrq.gov/clinic/uspstf08/type2/type2rs.htm

United States Preventive Services Task Force (Task Force). (2009). *Screening for breast cancer.* Retrieved from http://www.uspreventiveservicestaskforce.org/uspstf09/breastcancer/brcanrs.htm

9

Women's Health After Bariatric Surgery

Janet Graham

Introduction

Obesity in the United States is a major health concern that is reaching epidemic proportions (Centers for Disease Control and Prevention [CDC], 2006). The incidence of obesity has doubled in the past 20 years, with an estimated 61.3 million Americans currently classified as obese (Barth & Jenson, 2006). Clinicians are confronted with the consequences of a society that is becoming increasingly more obese (Norman et al., 2004).

Diet and exercise—the traditional approaches to treating obesity—have met with only limited success in treating morbid obesity (Landsberger & Gurewitsch, 2007). Consequently, bariatric (weight loss) surgery, an invasive procedure, is now recognized as the treatment of choice for many individuals who are extremely obese (Firment & Morrison, 2006; Landsberger & Gurewitsch; Virij & Murr, 2006). The number of weight-loss surgeries performed in the United States between 1994 and 2004 increased more than 10-fold, and the number continues to rise. It is predicted that more than 250,000 weight-loss surgeries occur each year (Zhao & Encinosa, 2007). More than 80% of the adults aged 18 to 44 who undergo bariatric surgery are women (Zhao & Encinosa). Thus clinicians providing health care for women will likely encounter women who have had or are contemplating bariatric surgical procedures.

Definitions

Obesity is defined in terms of body mass index (BMI), and individuals are considered obese if they have a BMI between 30 and 40 (Firment & Morrison, 2006). Body mass index is calculated as weight in kilograms divided by height in meters squared. Individuals with a BMI greater than 40 are considered extremely obese and meet the criteria for weight loss surgery (Firment & Morrison, 2006). If a person's BMI is between 35 and 40 and is accompanied by a high-risk comorbid disease such as hypertension, bariatric surgery is considered a valid treatment (see Chapter 6 for a BMI chart).

Bariatric surgical procedures fall into two broad categories: malabsorptive and restrictive surgeries. Both types can be performed by laparoscopy or laparotomy. Malabsorptive surgeries (e.g., the Roux-en-Y procedure [see **Color Plate 7**]) bypass parts of the digestive system and also reduce the size of the stomach pouch to limit the amount eaten as well as the nutrients the body is able to absorb. Restrictive bariatric surgeries (e.g., gastric banding [see **Color Plate 8**]) produce a small stomach pouch, so that the individual feels full after ingesting very little food. The reduced size of the stomach pouch also slows digestion, producing a longer feeling of satiation. Both types of surgery necessitate a change in eating habits, the consistency and amounts of food that can be ingested, and the need for supplementation of nutrients with vitamins or minerals. Clinicians who provide care to women who have had bariatric surgery should be knowledgeable about the types of surgery available, the possible complications from each type of surgery, and the care that each woman may require.

Assessment

History

When a woman who has had bariatric surgery presents for gynecologic or maternity care, a careful and thorough history should be obtained. Obesity has been shown to evoke negative responses from clinicians. Some clinicians may also attribute negative personal characteristics to women who are or have been obese, simply because they are obese (Anderson et al., 2001; Drury, 2002). This attitude could manifest itself in a subtle, unintentional bias against women who struggle with obesity. Clinicians need to strive to be nonjudgmental and accepting of their patients, regardless of the patient's current or past body habitus.

In addition to the routine health history information (see Chapter 6), the health history of a woman who has had bariatric surgery should include the following elements:

- Date of bariatric surgery
- Type of bariatric surgery
- Maximum amount of weight lost and current weight
- Dietary habits and restrictions
- Medications and supplementations
- Menstrual history, including any problems or irregularities before or after the bariatric surgery
- Contraception
- Psychological history

Physical Examination

The initial physical examination should include a complete assessment. If it has been several years since the bariatric surgery or logistical problems (e.g., long distances, lack of health insurance) have prevented follow-up, presentation to the clinician may be the woman's only interaction with the healthcare system. Vital clues to the woman's overall health may be observed during the assessment of body systems that are not usually included during a gynecologic visit. For example, a neurologic assessment may reveal abnormalities commonly associated with a vitamin B_{12} deficiency; assessment of the integumentary system may reveal symptoms of anemia or deficiencies in fat-soluble vitamins; and the abdominal examination may alert the clinician to hernia formation near the surgical site or cholelithiasis, which are both frequent complications following bariatric surgery (Barth & Jenson, 2006). A physical examination of a woman who has had bariatric surgery may also take longer, so it is important to allow enough time for the clinician to complete the initial assessment.

General Diagnostic Testing

Monitoring nutritional status through laboratory studies should be considered. If the woman has not continued follow-up with her bariatric surgeon, it is prudent for the clinician to monitor laboratory results. Important laboratory tests to include as part of an annual gynecologic visit include a complete blood count, albumin, serum vitamin B_{12}, iron, ferritin level, phosphorus, calcium, folic acid, homocysteine level, and 15-hydroxyvitamin D level (Boan, 2005; Smith, 2005). If an abnormality is noted in any of these laboratory tests, treatment needs to be initiated along with follow-up at more frequent intervals (see the discussion of treatment later in this chapter).

Iron and calcium absorption occurs primarily in the duodenum. Therefore, women who have had most of the stomach, duodenum, and upper intestine bypassed with Roux-en-Y gastric bypass surgery are not able to absorb much of the iron and calcium they ingest. For this reason, iron deficiency is of particular concern for menstruating women who have undergone bariatric surgery. These deficiencies can usually be controlled with proper diet and vitamin and mineral supplementation. Adequate fluid intake—especially water intake—should be emphasized because of the constipating properties of iron and calcium supplements.

Bone density studies should be done for all women who have had bariatric surgery, especially after menopause, to assess for bone loss. Malabsorptive surgeries alter bone metabolism and can lead to osteomalacia and osteoporosis (Fujioka, 2005). Daily supplementation with calcium (1200–1500 mg) and vitamin D (up to 2000 IU) is crucial for these women. Weight-bearing exercise for both the upper and lower extremities can also help reduce the severity of bone loss. Bisphosphonates, which are frequently prescribed for osteoporosis, may not be well tolerated after bariatric surgeries because of the smaller, surgically altered stomach pouch. The clinician needs to assess the risks and benefits and decide whether a woman who is post bariatric surgery and has osteoporosis will benefit more from the available intravenous or subcutaneous medications to treat her osteoporosis.

Fertility and Pregnancy

Infertility related to ovarian dysfunction and anovulation is a common problem among women who are obese (Deitel, 1998; McCook, Reame, & Thatcher, 2005; Raymond, 2005). One-third to one-half of women who are obese have irregular menstrual cycles, and this condition worsens in direct proportion to increased weight (Nelson & Fleming, 2006). Weight loss is considered first-line therapy for treatment of infertility in women who are obese and, in fact, infertility and a desire for pregnancy may be the impetus for weight-loss surgery.

A waiting period of 12 to 24 months between bariatric surgery and pregnancy is recommended (Dao, Kuhn, Ehmer, Fisher, & McCarty, 2006; Jacques, 2005; Shuster & Vasquez, 2005). A woman experiences rapid weight loss following weight-loss surgery and is in a relative catabolic state during the first 12 to 18 months after surgery which increases the potential for nutritional deficits in both the mother and the fetus. The early post-bariatric adjustment phase often is characterized by rapid weight loss, frequent vomiting, and inability to ingest appropriate calories or nutrients, all of which may threaten the sustainability of a pregnancy.

A woman who experienced infertility prior to surgery may resume ovulation with a relatively small weight loss, which can lead to an unplanned pregnancy soon after bariatric surgery. Pregnancy rates for adolescents who have had bariatric surgery are double the rate in the general adolescent population, making this population particularly in need of contraceptive counseling (Roehrig, Xanthakos, Sweeney, Zeller, & Inge, 2007).

Ideally, all women who have had bariatric surgery and are potentially fertile should be placed on folic acid supplements, regardless of whether the woman chooses to use contraception. The usual dose of folic acid for supplementation is 2 mg daily.

The clinician should offer appropriate contraceptive options, especially if gynecologic care is provided within the first 18 months after bariatric surgery and there is a potential for pregnancy. There is still some controversy about the efficacy of combined oral contraceptives (COCs) for women who have undergone gastric bypass surgery. If the bariatric surgery has a malabsorptive component, non-oral administration of contraceptive hormones should be considered (Merhi, 2007), as the limited size of the stomach and lack of enzymes or stomach digestive acids may limit the absorption of COCs. Backup of COCs with barrier methods should be discussed with women who are fertile or who may become fertile soon after weight loss begins. If a woman who has had bariatric surgery has a comorbid condition such as hypertension, COC use may also exacerbate blood pressure elevations. Estrogen-containing contraceptive pills are known to increase the incidence of gallstones—also a frequent complication after bariatric surgery (Barth & Jenson, 2006).

Intrauterine contraception (IUC) can provide long-term contraceptive benefits without potential digestive problems. Other contraceptive options that bypass the digestive system include progestin-based methods such as the depot medroxyprogesterone injection (DMPA, Depo-Provera) and the subdermal progestin implant (Implanon). However, DMPA may promote weight gain, making it an unpopular choice for women who are trying to lose weight. The implant has not been studied in women who are significantly overweight, so its efficacy is unknown in this population. The combined estrogen and progestin vaginal ring may also provide contraception while bypassing the digestive system. Although the cervical cap and diaphragm do not affect the digestive system, rapid weight loss could alter the efficacy of these methods when the cervix or vaginal walls change size. This would necessitate frequent fittings to adapt to the weight changes.

Consideration of the woman's cultural and religious background as well as current or potential health problems is necessary when discussing contraception. See Chapter 12 for additional information about contraceptive options.

Pregnancy presents some distinct challenges for women who have undergone bariatric surgery. For example, malabsorption related to the bypassing of segments of the bowel where nutrients are absorbed may put both mother and fetus at risk of nutrient deficiencies (Landsberger & Gurewitsch, 2007). Also, the increased nausea and vomiting experienced by many pregnant women may cause disruption of the adjustable gastric band placement or place the pregnant woman at an even higher risk for protein malnutrition (Patel, Colella, Esaka, Patel, & Thomas, 2007; Weiss et al., 2001). In addition, because of the relatively recent surge in numbers of bariatric surgeries performed, best practice clinical guidelines for directing the care of women who become pregnant after bariatric surgery have yet to be developed. Therefore, clinicians need to gather the most recent evidence and use it as a guide when providing prenatal care for women who have had bariatric surgery.

Tables 9-1, **9-2** and **9-3** provide guidelines that are evidenced-based interpretations of the currently available literature for nutritional counseling, laboratory testing, and weight management for women who are pregnant after having bariatric surgery (Graham, 2007). Using Stetler et al.'s (1998) criteria and taking into consideration the level of evidence found in the studies reviewed, only reasonable recommendations (in light of low risk) or pragmatic recommendations (in light of high need and/or based on national experts' opinions) can be made. The recommendations used to support the use of a practice deemed reasonable are based on limited but suggestive research-based evidence combined with low risk for the persons using that recommendation. Pragmatic recommendations are based on national expert opinion, local expert opinion, and/or high need for recommendations in a given area (Stetler et al., 1998).

Close nutritional and supplementation monitoring of the woman who has had bariatric surgery should continue into the postpartum period. Several case reports have described infants who developed nutritional deficiencies after being breastfed by women who have had bariatric surgery (Campbell, Ganesh, & Ficicioglu, 2005; Grange & Finlay, 1994).

Mental Health

A relationship between obesity and psychological disorders is thought to exist, but it is uncertain whether psychopathology is a cause or a consequence of extreme obesity (Sarwer, Wadden, & Fabricatore, 2005). Some research suggests that patients who have bariatric surgery have high rates of psychiatric disorders at the time of surgery (Kalarchian et al., 2007).

TABLE 9-1 Recommendations for Nutritional Management

Nutrition Need	R/P*	Recommendation
Protein	R	70 gm or 1.5 gm per kg weight
Vitamin B_{12}	R	500–1000 mcg crystalline per day
Folic acid	R	2–4 mg per day
Vitamin A	R	No more than 10,000 international units per day
Vitamin D	R	1000 international units per day
Prenatal vitamins	R	One daily, check vitamin A content
Calcium	R	1200–1500 mg calcium citrate per day
Carbohydrates	P	No more than 130 gm per day Avoid high sugar and simple carbohydrates
Iron	R	40 to 65 mg ferrous fumerate daily
Vitamin C	P	Usual RDA, take with iron to increase iron's absorption
Fluids	R	Minimum of 64 oz per day, no fluids 15 min before or 90 min after meals
Thiamine	R	50 mg per day
Fats	P	Polyunsaturated, omega-3

*R = reasonable; P = pragmatic
RDA = recommended daily allowance

The *Harvard Mental Health Letter* (2008) further elaborates that people eligible for weight-loss surgery have high rates of depression and anxiety. Researchers have also documented that a large number of patients who present for bariatric surgery have a preexisting eating disorder such as binge eating (Boan, 2005). Some epidemiologic studies have shown that mood disorders antedate weight problems. Often mood disorders tend to be recurrent, such

TABLE 9-2 Recommended Laboratory Studies to Evaluate Nutritional Status

Timing	R/P*	Laboratory Testing
Initial prenatal visit	P	Complete blood count, albumin, serum B_{12}, serum iron, ferritin level, phosphorus, calcium, folic acid, homocysteine level, 15-hydroxyvitamin D level
Monthly	P	Iron level and check all other laboratory indices that were previously found to be deficient until they are at an adequate level

*R = reasonable; P = pragmatic

TABLE 9-3 Recommendations for Weight Management and Monitoring

Weight Management	R/P*	Monitoring
Timing of pregnancy after surgery	P	No less than 12 months or until stable
Body mass index (BMI)	P	Measure at beginning of pregnancy
Weight gain	R	Individualize based on BMI: BMI 25–29.9: 15–25 pounds BMI > 30: 11–20 pounds
Weight monitoring	R	Every prenatal visit
Weight loss	P	Not recommended
*R = Reasonable; P = pragmatic		

that the individual who overeats or binge eats may be overeating in response to depression, which in turn results in weight gain (Kalarchian et al., 2007).

A controversial theory that is currently unproven suggests that bariatric surgery may enable a patient to lose weight, only to then have the patient transfer her food addiction to some other harmful addiction. Kalarchian et al. (2007) have also speculated that substance abuse and weight problems may have a shared diathesis. These researchers propose that eating behaviors increase when substance abuse is minimal and that risk of substance abuse behaviors may increase when eating behaviors are decreased. There may also be an increased risk of suicide among patients following bariatric surgery (Anderson, 2007). Retrospective studies have shown as much as a 58% increase in the rate of suicide among patients who are post bariatric surgery compared to individuals who are obese and did not have weight-loss surgery (Adams et al., 2007). Given this possibility, it is vitally important for the psychological assessment to include questions related to suicidal ideation in any patient evidencing symptoms of depression.

The clinician has a role in assessing the mental health status and needs of all women who present for gynecologic care. The familiarity between women and their clinician can provide a trusting atmosphere for mental health assessments. The clinician may be the first health professional a woman reaches out to when she has mental health problems.

Mental health assessments may take various forms: having the woman answer a questionnaire focused on mental health status; direct questions during the history and physical examination; and observation of the woman's affect, mood, and appearance during the visit. If a woman who is post bariatric surgery has a past history of depression or other mental health diagnosis, careful attention to her mental health needs should be given, especially after the first postsurgical year has passed. Studies suggest that women who are post bariatric surgery may relapse as a result of the psychosocial improvements that occurred in the first 6 to 18 postoperative months (Sarwer et al., 2005).Weight gain or lack of adherence to prescribed post-bariatric health regimens may indicate depression or other mood disorder. If the gynecologic patient is suspected to have psychosocial issues, the clinician should refer her to a mental health specialist.

Positive mental health benefits after bariatric surgery include improvement in body image. Less pain and fatigue associated with weight loss may also improve quality of life. Many women also report increased marital satisfaction and improved sexual functioning after successful weight loss surgery (Sarwer et al., 2005).

Conclusion

Bariatric surgery is an increasingly popular and viable weight-loss method for the woman with severe obesity. Clinicians who serve women in a general or gynecology practice need to be aware of the types of weight-loss surgery available, nutrient deficiencies that commonly occur after such surgery, and side effects that women may experience post bariatric surgery. Clinicians must also pay careful attention to the psychosocial needs of women who have undergone weight-loss surgery.

References

Adams, T. D., Gress, R. E., Smith, S. C., Halverson, R. C., Simper, S. C., Rosamond, W. D., ... Hunt, S. C. (2007). Long-term mortality after gastric bypass surgery. *New England Journal of Medicine, 357*, 753–761.

Anderson, P. (2007). *Higher-than-expected suicide rate following bariatric surgery.* Retrieved from http://www.medscape.com/viewarticle/564718

Anderson, C., Anderson, C. B., Fletcher, L., Mitchell, J. E., Thuras, P., & Crow, S. J. (2001). Weight loss and gender: An examination of physician attitudes. *Obesity Research, 9*(4), 257–263.

Barth, M. M., & Jenson, C. E. (2006). Postoperative nursing care of gastric bypass patients. *American Journal of Critical Care, 15*(4), 378–387.

Boan, J. (2005, April). Post-op management for bariatric surgery. *Clinical Advisor*, 30–35.

Campbell, C. D., Ganesh, J., & Ficicioglu, C. (2005). Two newborns with nutritional vitamin B_{12} deficiency: Challenges in newborn screening for vitamin B_{12} deficiency. *Haematologica, 90*, ECR45.

Centers for Disease Control and Prevention (CDC). (2006). *Overweight and obesity: trends among adults.* Retrieved, from http://usa.gov

Dao, T., Kuhn, J., Ehmer, D., Fisher, T., & McCarty, T. (2006). Pregnancy outcomes after bariatric surgery. *American Journal of Surgery, 192*(6), 762–766.

Deitel, M. (1998). Pregnancy after bariatric surgery. *Obesity Surgery, 8*, 1–4. Retrieved from http://clos.net

Drury, C. A. A. (2002). Exploring the association between body weight, stigma of obesity, and health care avoidance. *Journal of the American Academy of Nurse Practitioners, 14*(12), 554–561.

Firment, L., & Morrison, S. (2006). The skinny on weight-loss surgery. *American Association of Occupational Health Nurses Journal, 54*(9), 405–410.

Fujioka, K. (2005). Follow-up of nutritional and metabolic problems after bariatric surgery. *Diabetes Care, 28*(2), 481–484.

Graham, J. E. (2007). *Guidelines for prenatal care for post-bariatric women: An integrative review* (Unpublished doctoral dissertation). Oakland University, Rochester, MI.

Grange, D. K., & Finlay, J. L. (1994). Nutritional vitamin B_{12} deficiency in a breastfed infant following maternal gastric bypass. *Pediatric Hematology Oncology, 11*, 311–318.

Harvard Mental Health Letter. (2008, January). Retrieved from http://psychcentral.com/news/2007/12/20/bariatric-mental-health-needs/1687.html

Jacques, J. (2005). Nutritional implications of weight loss surgery. *Nutrition & the M.D., 31*(11), 1–5.

Kalarchian, M. A., Marcus, M. D., Levine, M. D., Courcoulas, A. P., Pilkonis, P. A., Ringham, R. M., . . . Rofey, D. L. (2007). Psychiatric disorders among bariatric surgery candidates: Relationship to obesity and functional health status. *American Journal of Psychiatry, 164*, 328–334.

Landsberger, E. J., & Gurewitsch, E. D. (2007). Reproductive implications of bariatric surgery: Pre- and postoperative considerations for extremely obese women of childbearing age. *Current Diabetes Report, 7*(4), 281–288.

McCook, J. G., Reame, N. E., & Thatcher, S. S. (2005). Health related quality of life issues in women with polycystic ovarian syndrome. *Journal of Obstetric, Gynecologic, and Neonatal Nursing, 34*(1), 12–20.

Merhi, Z. O. (2007). Challenging oral contraception after weight loss by bariatric surgery. *Gynecology Obstetric Investigation, 64*, 100–102.

Nelson, S. M., & Fleming, R. F. (2006). The preconceptual contraception paradigm: Obesity and infertility. *Human Reproduction.* Retrieved from http://humcontent/abstract/del1473v1rep.oxfordjournals.org/cgi

Norman, R. J., Noakes, M., Wu, R., Davies, M. J., Moran, L., & Wang, J. X. (2004). Improving reproductive performance in overweight/obese women with effective weight management. *Human Reproduction Update, 10*(3), 267–280.

Patel, J. A., Colella, J. J., Esaka, E., Patel, N. A., & Thomas, R. L. (2007). Improvement in infertility and pregnancy outcomes after weight loss surgery. *Medical Clinics of North America, 91*(3), 515–528.

Raymond, R. H. (2005). Hormonal status, fertility, and pregnancy before and after bariatric surgery. *Critical Care Nursing Quarterly, 28*(3), 263–268.

Roehrig, H. R., Xanthakos, S. S., Sweeney, J., Zeller, M. H., & Inge, T. H. (2007). Pregnancy after gastric bypass surgery in adolescents. *Obesity Surgery, 17*, 873–877.

Sarwer, D. B., Wadden, T. A., & Fabricatore, A. N. (2005). Psychosocial and behavioral aspects of bariatric surgery. *Obesity Research, 13*(4), 639–648.

Shuster, M., & Vasquez, N. A. (2005). Nutritional concerns related to Roux-en-Y gastric bypass. *Critical Care Nursing Quarterly, 28*(3), 227–260.

Smith, B. L. (2005). Bariatric surgery: It's no easy fix. *RN, 6*(6), 58–63.

Stetler, C. B., Morsi, D., Rucki, S., Broughton, S., Corrigan, B., Fitzgerald, J., . . . Sheridan, E. A. (1998). Utilization-focused integrative reviews in a nursing service. *Applied Nursing Research, 11*(4), 195–206.

Virij, A., & Murr, M. M. (2006). Caring for patients after bariatric surgery. *American Family Physician, 73*(8), 1–9.

Weiss, H. G., Nehoda, H., Labeck, B., Hourmont, K., Marth, C., & Aigner, F. (2001). Pregnancies after adjustable gastric banding. *Obesity Surgery, 11*, 303–306.

Zhao, Y., & Encinosa, W. (2007, January). *Bariatric surgery utilization and outcomes in 1998 and 2004* (Statistical brief #23). Retrieved from http://www.hcup-us.ahrq.gov/reports/statbriefs/sb23.pdf

CHAPTER 10

Gynecologic Health Care for Sexual and Gender Minorities

Linda A. Bernhard

Health is experienced in the context of each individual's life. "A feminist understanding of women's health conceptualizes the experience of health not as the experiences of a woman's body but rather as inseparable from the everyday experiences of an embodied life" (McDonald, McIntyre, & Anderson, 2003, p. 705). Health—and specifically gynecologic health—is experienced biologically, psychosocially, sexually, and spiritually. This is true for all women, including women of all sexual orientations and gender identities. This chapter considers the special gynecologic healthcare needs of lesbians, bisexual women, and transgender (LBT) individuals. These groups are increasingly being referred to collectively as sexual and gender minorities (SGMs). Both designations will be used in this chapter.

Definitions and Terminology

There are no official definitions for lesbian, bisexuality, or transgender. Indeed, definitions and labels are constantly evolving and highly complex. However, three components—identity, behavior, and attraction or desire—have come to be used to define sexual orientation for research and educational purposes (Solarz, 1999). Sexual identity refers to one's self-label as heterosexual, homosexual/lesbian, bisexual, or something else. Sexual behavior refers to one's sexual partners, as well as the sexual activities in which one engages. Attraction or desire refers to whom one desires sexually or about whom one fantasizes, and may be described as sexual preference. Any individual may have real or fantasized partners who are women, men, or both.

Traditionally, lesbians were defined by their sexual behavior: having sex with women meant that one was a lesbian. Similarly, having sex with both women and men meant that one was bisexual. Bisexual people respond erotically to both sexes, either serially or simultaneously.

However, when people claim their own identities, sexual identity and sexual behavior may not be congruent. Bisexuals may have partners of only one sex, or lesbians may have partners of both sexes. In addition, the terminology that SGMs use for themselves and their communities is specific to each individual.

Gender is a construct that includes psychological, social, and cultural factors, and is typically used to describe people as male or female. Biologic or natal *sex* is usually assigned at birth based on anatomy. *Gender identity* refers to one's self-label related to gender, regardless of biologic sex. Some people may choose a gender identity that is consistent with their biologic sex. Others choose a gender identity that is the opposite of their biologic sex. Still others choose a gender identity that is completely independent of sex; that is, they may consider themselves to be both female and male genders, transgender, or no gender.

Transgender is a broad construct that includes a wide variety of persons who have gender identities or behaviors that are not usually associated with their natal sex. Some transgender individuals have been called transsexuals, or people who feel that they *are* the other sex. The term "transsexual" is disappearing from use in favor of the more commonly used term "transgender." Transgender people with a natal sex of female who prefer a male gender identity can be referred to as FTM (female to male), transmen, or simply men. Similarly, transgender people with a natal sex of male who prefer a female gender identity can be referred to as MTF (male to female), transwomen, or simply women.

Sexual and gender identities are fluid and changing, and do not necessarily have anything to do with whom people choose for their sexual partners. For example, some women may claim to be heterosexual yet also have casual sex with women. Transgendered people may not have a sexual identity themselves but prefer partners of a particular sexual identity. People may vary in their sexual or gender identities at different times in their lives, in different places, or with different people.

All SGM people, including gay men, share the experience of being stigmatized by society and made to feel different for how and whom they love. It is the experience of stigma that brings them together for social support (Johnson, Mimiaga, & Bradford, 2008). Symbols of a shared culture, such as the rainbow flag and Pride marches, are reflections of how people who identify as SGMs support one another.

In every other way, SGM individuals are diverse. They can differ from one another in terms of race, ethnicity, class, age, religion, geographic location, citizenship, and ability status. Indeed, SGM people are found within every subgroup in society. Even so, it is impossible to know the actual number of SGM individuals in the United States, partly because of the difficulty in defining them, and partly because many are afraid to disclose their identity for fear of discrimination or other personal harm that will happen to them if they do. Thus, even though these groups may share some health needs and concerns, unique concerns arise within each group.

Homophobia and Heterosexism

Homophobia is an individual's irrational fear or hate of homosexual people. This may include bisexual or transgender persons, but sometimes the more distinct terms of *biphobia* or *transphobia*, respectively, are used. In health care, SGMs experience homophobia when clinicians and others think they are sick or immoral which may make them feel hassled, unwanted, or unsafe. Clinicians who are homophobic may avoid or refuse to care for LBT patients. In a recent example, two Christian infertility physicians refused to artificially inseminate a lesbian, citing their religious beliefs as grounds for refusal. The Supreme Court of California voted unanimously on August 18, 2008, that physicians in that state cannot discriminate against patients on the basis of the physicians' religious beliefs. In this case, the justices ruled that religion does not exempt physicians from following state law that imposes antidiscrimination obligations.

Heterosexism is the societal institutionalization of a dichotomy where one group of people—in this case, heterosexuals—are valued, and another group of people—in this case, SGMs—are devalued and oppressed. Heterosexism is the belief that heterosexuality is the best sexual orientation, and that all people should be heterosexual. In that way it is similar to other social dichotomies, such as racism or classism.

The experience of homophobia and heterosexism is also affected by other personal characteristics of an LBT individual, such as race, age, class, religion, and ability status. Of course, these characteristics cannot be divided; a person experiences all of them simultaneously. That is, an African American lesbian who is 80 years old and uses a wheelchair can experience racism, heterosexism, sexism, ageism, and ableism, all at the same time. She is an integrated human being, not just a lesbian or only an African American. Likewise, a white transgendered adolescent can experience heterosexism, transphobia, sexism, and ageism simultaneously.

Health Care for Sexual and Gender Minorities in a Societal Context

Social intolerance of homosexuality is still largely acceptable in the United States. Violence against SGMs is common. Consequently, SGM individuals live with a great deal of stress in a society that does not accept them. Stress comes either from *hiding* who one "really" is (i.e., being "in the closet"), so that she can avoid discrimination and loss, or from being "out" (of the closet) and thus risking discrimination and hate crimes because others know that she *is* a sexual or gender minority person. In many places, it is still legal to discriminate against homosexuals, so the threat associated with SGM identification is real. Even though laws are slowly changing, same-sex couples in nearly all states lack the legal rights of marriage and can experience discrimination in child custody situations, as well as in employment and housing.

"Coming out" is a developmental process that includes identifying and accepting oneself for who one is, and then identifying oneself as that to others. It is usually a gradual process, often accompanied by significant stress, because the person is afraid of what will happen and what kinds of changes one might experience if and when one does come out. Thus LBT individuals may be out in some aspects of their life and not in others. For example, one may be out to family and close friends, but not out at work. Coming out can occur at any time in a person's life. In addition, coming out is a never-ending process, because whenever an LBT person meets a new person (such as a healthcare clinician), one must choose whether to be out or not.

Coming out has multiple issues for transgender people. First, they recognize their gender identity; then, they choose to live it. This can be a long process, called *transitioning*. For MTF or FTM individuals, it will mean a complete change of identity, because living as the desired gender is a prerequisite for receiving hormones and gender assignment surgeries (World Professional Association for Transgender Health, 2001). When a transgendered person has fully transitioned and is identified exclusively as desired, the person may have great fear about being discovered as the person they no longer are.

An important part of the coming out process is becoming involved in lesbian, gay, bisexual, and transgender (LGBT) culture and community. Similar to other cultural groups, SGMs experience a sense of security in being with persons like themselves. With regard to health care, LGBT individuals have found security by developing health clinics and support groups for themselves outside the mainstream healthcare system. Many of these clinics were originally established in association with LGBT community centers or organizations.

Results of one study showed that lesbians were significantly more likely than heterosexual women to use complementary and alternative medicine (CAM) services (Matthews, Hughes, Osterman, & Kodl, 2005). In another study about lesbians' healthcare preferences, participants expressed interest in clinicians who incorporate integrative health into their care (Seaver, Freund, Wright, Tjia, & Frayne, 2008).

Health Care for Sexual and Gender Minorities in an Institutional Context

Institutions of health care include outpatient facilities as well as hospitals. Health care for LBT individuals and same-sex couples in healthcare institutions often is limited by institutional policies that define family in traditional ways, such as the nuclear family or blood relatives, or by staff who enforce outdated policies that prevent LBT individuals from being recognized as partners or family members. When these policies are implemented, LBT individuals may be denied access to information, participation in treatment decisions, or visitation.

One way that some LBT individuals protect themselves from such situations is by obtaining a durable power of attorney for health care. This document allows one person to appoint some other person, such as a lesbian partner, to make healthcare decisions for her, when she is unable to do so for herself. It serves as the proof of the patient's intentions for future health care and can provide access to institutions and clinicians for the designee.

Same-sex couples may also seek legal guardianship for their children or for partners who become disabled. In some states, individuals may legally adopt another person, regardless of age, and LBT individuals may use such adoptions as a way to maintain a legal relationship for health care and other purposes, such as inheritance.

In 2006, the Human Rights Campaign (HRC) Foundation and the Gay and Lesbian Medical Association (GLMA) began a process to promote a nationwide standard to decrease discrimination and promote quality care for LGBT patients. Hospitals voluntarily completed a survey about their policies related to nondiscrimination of patients, visitation and decision-making rights of partners, staff diversity training, and nondiscrimination employment practices. HRC and GLMA used the results to develop the Healthcare Equality Index (HEI), which rates healthcare facilities based on their policies and practices for LGBT patients. The HEI also includes recommendations to assist institutions to better meet the standards. The survey is distributed annually to hospitals and other healthcare institutions. The goal is for the HEI to become the gold standard for policies to ensure equal care and treatment for LGBT patients (HRC & GLMA, 2008).

Development of a Research Base for Lesbian, Bisexual, and Transgender Health

Although there is a paucity of evidence on LBT health, research within this arena is increasing. More is known about lesbian health than bisexual and transgender health, but lesbian health care has become a topic of significant discussion and research only since the 1980s. The first major study to identify lesbian health and mental health needs and concerns was the National Lesbian Health Survey (Bradford & Ryan, 1987). This national survey of 1900 self-identified lesbians is now considered a classic study. It was the first attempt to ask lesbians throughout the United States to describe their own healthcare needs, and it became a model that other researchers used to describe lesbian health needs locally, regionally, and nationally.

In 1997, the Institute of Medicine (IOM) created a committee to study lesbian health. Its landmark report, *Lesbian Health: Current Assessment and Directions for the Future* (Solarz, 1999), represents full recognition of the importance of lesbians and their health as worthy of attention and study. The eight recommendations developed as part of the IOM report were broad, including multiple topics for research, funding for research, conferences, and other mechanisms for dissemination of information about lesbian health.

As mentioned earlier, bisexual and transgender health research has lagged behind research about lesbian health. Studies conducted in this area remain very limited, and have focused primarily on sexually transmitted infections (STIs) and HIV. Recognizing the need to address the healthcare needs of all SGMs, the GLMA, along with other SGM activists and organizations across the United States, created the National Coalition for LGBT Health in 2000. The Coalition's purpose is to improve the health of LGBT persons by focusing on research, policy, education, and training. The Coalition has held healthcare summits, and it sponsors National LGBT Health Awareness Week in March on an annual basis.

Barriers to Health Care for Sexual and Gender Minorities

Barriers to quality health care for SGMs result from the homophobia and heterosexism in society, which all too often prevents equal access to health for all persons. SGMs experience many internal and external barriers to obtaining quality health care. Internal barriers—those that individuals themselves hold—may include reluctance to disclose their sexual or gender identity and distrust of medical institutions. However, clinicians cannot give complete care if they do not have complete information about their patients. If LBT individuals perceive that clinicians are gay positive, and if clinicians ask about sexual orientation, many LBT patients will disclose this information (Steele, Tinmouth, & Lu, 2006). Nonetheless, many LBT patients remain reluctant to disclose their identity to clinicians because they are afraid of homophobic responses, being humiliated, being mistreated, and having judgments made about them if they do so.

Three types of disclosure are possible: planned, passive, and unplanned (Bernhard, 2001). Planned disclosure occurs when an individual decides consciously to come out to the clinician. This is the safest form of disclosure for the LBT individual because she is in control, and can also plan actions, based on possible reactions to coming out. Results of research suggest that higher education is associated with more disclosure to healthcare clinicians, and disclosure to clinicians is associated with greater utilization of health care (Bergeron & Senn, 2003).

Passive disclosure occurs when the LBT individual does not specifically tell the clinician about being a sexual or gender minority, but assumes that the clinician knows, often because of appearance. However, the LBT individual does nothing to affirm or deny what she thinks the clinician knows. Unplanned disclosure occurs when an LBT individual had explicitly planned *not* to come out to a clinician, but something occurs during the interaction that causes her to think that she must disclose her status. For example, the triggering event could be an unnecessary procedure that she does not want. This is a very unsafe situation for the LBT individual because she did not consider options for how to deal with an unpleasant situation that developed.

External barriers to quality health care for SGMs are those within the healthcare system and among healthcare clinicians. The most significant of these barriers is the assumption by clinicians that all of their patients are heterosexual. In gynecology offices, this perspective is made obvious when clinicians assume that all women who come to them are seeking contraception. Although some LBT women may need contraception, many do not.

The heterosexual assumption is also made when there are no representations of SGMs in healthcare settings. Positive representations could include pictures or posters of same-sex couples, with or without children, as well as health information materials directed toward SGMs. It is also seen in intake materials that include a space for "husband," rather than spouse, partner, or significant other(s).

A key barrier to quality health care related to the heterosexual assumption is when clinicians lack knowledge about LBT individuals and their health. The education of clinicians is remarkably limited in the inclusion of topics related to health needs and concerns of SGMs. Although research on LBT health is still limited, evidence is increasing and clinicians must be as aware of the growing body of knowledge about SGM health, just as they stay up-to-date regarding health advances in other areas.

Another barrier to health care for LBT individuals concerns health insurance. As women, lesbians may not have health insurance because they work in jobs that do not provide insurance; this is not different from the situation faced by some heterosexual women. The difference is that many of those heterosexual women have health insurance from their husbands' employment. In a large national probability sample, women in same-sex relationships were significantly less likely than women in opposite-sex relationships to have health insurance, to have seen a clinician in the past year, and to have a regular source of health care (Heck, Sell, & Gorin, 2006). Although domestic partner benefits are increasingly being provided by employers, they are not available to many who could use them. Domestic partner benefits also reflect coverage for children, and same-sex parents may have difficulty obtaining coverage for their children if they are not the biologic or adoptive parent.

Even if transgendered individuals have health insurance, the medications many want and need most are hormones, which insurance often excludes. In addition, while many transgendered people do not choose to have surgical procedures in the process of transitioning, insurance usually excludes surgeries or any procedures related to changing sex or gender (Rachlin, Green, & Lombardi, 2008).

Eating Disorders

Societal norms for beauty and attractiveness require women to be extremely thin and fit to be happy and valued in society. Driven by this societal imperative, some women may develop eating disorders, such as binging and purging or highly restrictive diets, in an effort to attain or maintain thinness. Lesbians are often presumed—erroneously—to have less body dissatisfaction, dieting, and disordered eating behaviors than heterosexual women because lesbians are more able to resist societal norms.

The most current research suggests that the prevalence of eating disorders does not differ between lesbian and bisexual women and heterosexual women (Feldman & Meyer, 2007). In Feldman and Meyer's study, there were no significant differences in the prevalence of eating disorders between white, African American, and Latino lesbians; bisexuals; and gay men, although African Americans and Latinos had a higher prevalence.

Studies consistently demonstrate that lesbians, and in some cases bisexual women, have higher body weight (Boehmer, Bowen, & Bauer, 2007; Bowen, Balsam, & Ender, 2008; Valanis et al., 2000) and/or body mass index (BMI) than heterosexual women (Mays, Yancey, Cochran, Weber, & Fielding, 2002; Moore & Keel, 2003), including their own heterosexual sisters (Roberts, Dibble, Nussey, & Casey, 2003). Bisexual women seem to have fewer concerns about their weight when they are with a female partner than when they are with a male partner (Bowen, Balsam, Diergaarde, Russo, & Escamilla, 2006). Race has been shown to be an independent predictor of higher BMI in lesbians and bisexual women, with African American women having higher BMI (Yancey, Cochran, Corliss, & Mays, 2003). Although heterosexual women may prefer a lower body weight, lesbians who did not have partners had lower BMI than lesbians living with partners in one study (Yancey et al., 2003), suggesting that single lesbians may be similar to single heterosexual women who are dating.

Having a more positive lesbian identity (Joshua, 2003) and participating more frequently in lesbian social activities (Heffernan, 1999) have been considered buffers that may help lesbians avoid viewing themselves negatively. However, results of another study suggest that a lesbian identity may not serve as a buffer for a positive body image because the messages from the dominant culture about body image are so strongly internalized (Kelly, 2007). In addition, feminist identity and activities do not appear to serve as buffers against negative self-image (Guille & Chrisler, 1999; Heffernan, 1999).

Sexually Transmitted Infections and Bacterial Vaginosis Among Sexual and Gender Minorities

When caring for women with STIs, sexual behavior—rather than identity—is the most important concern. In one study, 13% of women who had only female sexual partners reported a history of STIs, and 15% of women who identified as lesbian reported having an STI (Bauer & Welles, 2001). Sexual partners and sexual behaviors, including risky practices such as not using condoms or other barriers during sexual activity, are what determine individuals' risk for contracting and transmitting STIs. Bisexual women are at very high risk for STIs because they often have large numbers of partners and engage in risky behaviors (Champion, Wilford, & Piper, 2005).

Although both lesbians and clinicians long thought that lesbians were at extremely low risk for development of STIs and vaginal infections, that myth has been debunked in recent decades. Research has demonstrated that human papillomavirus (HPV) (Marrazzo, 2000; Marrazzo, Koutsky, Kiviat, Kuypers, & Stine, 2001), bacterial vaginosis (BV) (Berger et al., 1995; Marazzo et al., 2002), and herpes simplex virus (HSV) 1 and 2 (Marrazzo, Stine, & Wald, 2003) all can be sexually transmitted from woman to woman. In addition, case reports suggest that trichomoniasis (Kellock & O'Mahony, 1996) and syphilis (Campos-Outcalt & Hurwitz, 2002) are sexually transmissible between women.

The myth that lesbians are at very low risk for STIs has been perpetuated based on the belief that lesbians do not have sex with men. In fact, research demonstrates consistently that most lesbians have had sex with men at some time in their lives, and many continue to have sex with men (Bauer & Welles, 2001; Diamant, Schuster, McGuigan, & Lever, 1999). Thus some lesbians and bisexual women may acquire STIs from male sexual partners and then transmit those infections to female sexual partners. In a study that compared lesbians, bisexual, and heterosexual women, all three groups reported behaviors—including sex with men who have sex with men, sex with male injection drug users, and sex while high on drugs—that placed them at increased risk for STIs (Koh, Gómez, Shade, & Rowley, 2005).

The prevalence of STIs in lesbians and women who have sex with women (WSW), which may include bisexual and transgender women, is not well known. Nevertheless, reports clearly demonstrate that STIs occur in these populations and should be diagnosed and treated. In a study of a population of WSW who reside in Minnesota, the highest self-reported incidence of STIs was genital warts (8%). Trichomoniasis and chlamydia were reported by 6%, genital herpes by 5%, and gonorrhea by 2% (Bauer & Welles, 2001). These rates are higher than those found in another study of WSW in the Seattle area, where the rates of diagnosed STIs in WSW were 2% for trichomoniasis and 1% for chlamydia (Marrazzo, Koutsky, & Handsfield, 2001). In addition, the reported prevalence of syphilis was 0.7% and that of vulvovaginal candidiasis was 15%.

Marrazzo, Koutsky, Kiviat, et al. (2001) found that in WSW the prevalence of HPV when tested by polymerase chain reaction was 13%. The seroprevalence of HSV in lesbians was 46% for HSV-1 and 8% for HSV-2; however, only 6% of the participants in this study self-reported genital herpes (Marrazzo et al., 2003).

Human immunodeficiency virus (HIV) has been identified in case studies of lesbians and women who report sex only with women (Kwakwa & Ghobrial, 2003). Similar to the situation with other STIs, lesbians themselves and clinicians often assume that lesbians are immune to HIV. Indeed, studies show that many lesbians think they are at low risk (Fishman & Anderson, 2003) or no risk (Montcalm & Myer, 2000) for contracting HIV, and the U.S. Centers for Disease Control and Prevention (CDC) continues to report that there are no confirmed cases of female-to-female transmission of HIV in the United States (CDC, 2006). Transmen (biologic females, living as men, who partner with women) also do not view themselves as at risk for HIV (Rachlin et al., 2008).

Recently, more lesbians—particularly if they have had multiple partners, and especially if those partners were male—have begun to be tested for HIV, because they believe that they *are* at risk (Dolan & Davis, 2008). Other reasons that women give for being tested include a health professional suggested testing, starting a new relationship, or being incarcerated.

Nearly 3% of all reported cases of HIV infection in women in the United States have occurred among women who reported having sex with women. However, in more than 60% of the reported cases of HIV in women, it is unknown whether the women had sex with women (CDC, 2006). A total of 534 cases of HIV infection in women who reported having sex only with women had been identified through 2004; however, 91% of those women also had another risk factor for acquisition of HIV. In the transmission hierarchy developed by the CDC, each individual is allowed only one exposure category, and categories are arranged hierarchically. However, multiple factors may account for transmission, and female-to-female transmission (which is not a category) may have occurred prior to, or concomitant with, heterosexual transmission or injection drug use.

Although HIV can be transmitted between women, this route of transmission appears to be rare. Presumably for this reason, HIV infection in transmen is also very uncommon. The prevalence in studies conducted between 1990 and 2003 was found to be in the range of 0 to 3% (Herbst et al., 2008).

Transmission of HIV from man to woman and from woman to man (called heterosexual contact by the CDC) is, of course, very likely. Heterosexual contact, which includes most bisexual women, was the source of 80% of the newly diagnosed cases of HIV in women in 2005 (CDC, 2008). Women of color are the most likely to be infected in this way.

Transgender women (MTF) have extremely high rates of HIV infection (Crosby & Pitts, 2007; Rachlin et al., 2008). In studies conducted between 1990 and 2003, the prevalence in this group was 28% (Herbst et al., 2008). One explanation for this high rate is that sex work is a cultural norm for transwomen, particularly when they are beginning the transition to female (Sausa, Keatley, & Operario, 2007). In a qualitative study of transwomen in San Francisco, respondents reported that sex work opens doors to other transwomen, providing social support. It also makes them feel independent by providing an income (Sausa et al., 2007). Transwomen need money to purchase hormones, and they often make more money if they have sex without condoms. To get through these experiences, they often use drugs and may share needles (Crosby & Pitts, 2007). All of these behaviors increase their risk for acquiring HIV, as well as other STIs.

Bacterial vaginosis is the most common cause of vaginitis, although its cause is unknown (Marrazzo, 2008). Although BV is not considered an STI, research has demonstrated both that BV is more prevalent in lesbians and other WSW than it is in heterosexual women, and that BV can be sexually transmitted between women (Evans, Scally, Wellard, & Wilson, 2008; Marrazzo, 2008). Concordance between partners for both the presence and the absence of BV ranges from 81% (Berger et al., 1995) to 95% of female couples (Marrazzo et al., 2002). However, couples with concordant BV apparently do not participate in different sexual activities than those who are discordant or do not have BV. No significant association between receptive oral sex and BV (a sexual practice not unique to WSW) was found in the first study to systematically examine that association (Evans et al., 2008). Nonetheless, why lesbians and WSW have an increased risk for BV is unknown.

A study by Bailey, Benato, Owen, and Kavanagh (2008) demonstrated that vulvovaginal candidiasis (VVC) also may be sexually transmissible between women. In a clinic sample of 708 women who completed a questionnaire about sexual practices and partners and demographics, and who had a complete genitourinary examination with cultures, the prevalence of VVC in WSW was found to be 18%; this group included both symptomatic and asymptomatic women. In the multivariate model, the only significant variable associated with a diagnosis of VVC was having two or more female partners in the past year.

Risky sexual behaviors in which LBT individuals may engage include unprotected oral, anal, or vaginal sex with female or male partners whose HIV status is positive or unknown; sex during menses; sharing sex toys; and sadomasochistic activities that result in a break in the skin. Low-income LBT individuals, especially if they are women of color or addicted to drugs, may also perform sex work for money or drugs, which increases their risk for STIs even more (Arend, 2003). Other risky behaviors that could result in HIV transmission because of transfer of blood are sharing razors, and brushing or flossing teeth prior to having sex (Fishman & Anderson, 2003).

Clinicians should counsel their patients about ways to prevent the spread of STIs and encourage them to be tested, especially for HIV. Women should know their own and their partners' HIV status, and use barriers consistently and correctly. Dental dams can be used as a barrier for oral sex, although many women find them too small or difficult to use. Clinicians can suggest using clear plastic wrap instead.

Polycystic Ovary Syndrome

Polycystic ovary syndrome (PCOS) may be more common in lesbians and FTM than in other women. This condition is characterized by polycystic ovaries, frequent anovulation resulting in oligomenorrhea or amenorrhea, and hyperandrogenism. PCOS is also associated with obesity. It is of concern because of the potential complications associated with it, including insulin resistance, dyslipidemia, and the metabolic syndrome (see Chapter 26).

Research has demonstrated that lesbians are significantly more likely than heterosexual women to have PCOS (Agrawal et al., 2004) and that transgender FTM individuals have a high prevalence of PCOS (Baba et al., 2007). A later study, however, did not find a significant difference in the prevalence of PCOS between FTM and controls, although FTM were more likely to have hyperandrogenism (Mueller et al., 2008).

Gynecologic Cancers and Lesbians

Most women are afraid of cancer, and LBT women are no different in this respect. When lesbians were asked to rank the health issues of greatest concern to them, breast cancer was rated number one, with cervical and ovarian cancers in the top ten (White & Dull, 1998). Like other women, including women who have a family history of breast cancer, lesbians overestimate their risk for breast cancer (McTiernan et al., 2001). However, WSW are also less likely than heterosexual women to be screened for cancer (Kerker, Mostashari, & Thorpe, 2006). Inadequate screening may increase the likelihood of later diagnosis of cancer, and greater morbidity and mortality.

Most of what will be discussed in this section concerns breast cancer, and most of the research has been conducted with lesbians. Some of the studies cited here included bisexual women, but virtually no research has been conducted with transgender people. In addition, there is a lack of information on most other gynecologic cancers in all LBT people.

Cancer Risk

In 1992, work by Suzanne Haynes at the National Cancer Institute caused a media furor, resulting in an ensuing uproar among lesbians, when it was reported that lesbians had a one in three risk of developing breast cancer, compared to the one in eight or nine risk for the general population of women. Haynes's analysis—not empiric research—was based on evidence suggesting that lesbians are less likely to have children, more likely to delay childbirth until after age 30, more likely to drink alcohol, and more likely to be overweight than heterosexual women. These risk factors have been associated with breast cancer, although certainly none of them is unique to lesbians.

As yet, no prospective empiric studies have definitively determined whether lesbians are at higher risk for breast cancer. Lesbians participating in the Women's Health Initiative (Valanis et al., 2000) did have higher self-reports of breast cancer (7%) compared to heterosexuals (5%), but bisexuals had the highest prevalence in that study (8%). In another case-control study of young women (ages 21 to 45 years) with and without breast cancer, the relative risk of women classified as lesbian in three different ways was higher than the relative risk of nonlesbians (Kavanaugh-Lynch, White, Daling, & Bowen, 2002). Risk factors that explained the difference were parity, breastfeeding, BMI, and use of alcohol.

When researchers used the Gail Model for risk assessment, they found lesbians had a significantly higher 5-year predicted risk and lifetime risk than their own heterosexual sisters (Dibble, Roberts, & Nussey, 2004) and other heterosexual women (Brandenburg, Matthews, Johnson, & Hughes, 2007). However, the results of these studies do not place lesbians in the high-risk category, which the Gail Model was developed to identify. Current research suggests that lesbians may be at somewhat higher risk for developing breast cancer than heterosexual women, but there is no evidence to indicate that it is the threefold higher risk that Haynes suggested in 1992.

Although men can develop breast cancer, it is rare in men. Even in the developing field of men's health, breast cancer is rarely discussed. Transwomen are biologic males, and it is estimated that their risk for breast cancer remains similar to that of other men, even though they may be taking estrogen. Many transmen have had mastectomies with or without plastic surgery to create a more masculine chest structure.

Lesbians do have different risk factors for some cancers than heterosexual women. Results of a retrospective study of risk factors for ovarian cancer revealed some differences between lesbian and heterosexual women (Dibble, Roberts, Robertson, & Paul, 2002). Not surprisingly, lesbians had lower parity and less use of oral contraceptives compared to heterosexual women. Both higher numbers of pregnancies and longer use of oral contraceptives are believed to protect against ovarian cancer. Lesbians had higher BMI than heterosexual women, but heterosexual women had higher rates of smoking; both of these issues are additional risk factors for ovarian cancer.

Cancer Screening

Regardless of whether lesbians are truly at higher risk for some types of cancers than other women, all women should have access to cancer screening. Clark, Bonacore, Wright, Armstong, and Rakowski (2003) conducted focus groups with legally unmarried women (which theoretically could include heterosexual, bisexual, lesbian, and transgender women) to discuss barriers to screening for breast, cervical, and colon cancer. Barriers included the cost of screening, lack of insurance, and pain (mostly associated with colon cancer), but the most important barrier was lack of acknowledgment and validation of women in the context of their lives. The women in the study indicated they were distressed with intake forms that did not allow them to identify emotional support persons. They also reported feeling devalued in offices that focused on reproductive health. Women who partner with women specifically reported being discriminated against if they disclosed their sexual orientation. Finally, women in the study reported delaying or avoiding screening due to feeling blamed or guilty about the size and shape of their bodies. Although these feelings were somewhat more frequent in women who were overweight or had large breasts, they were not unique to that group of participants (Clark et al., 2003). Lesbians older than age 50 years may avoid cancer screening specifically because they fear being identified as lesbian and/or because of the hostility that they expect to receive from clinicians based on their experiences with health care in the past (Dibble & Roberts, 2003).

There is no clear evidence that lesbians and other WSW participate in mammography screening more or less frequently than other women. Some studies show that lesbians are equally as likely as heterosexual women to have mammograms (Brandenburg et al., 2007; Valanis et al., 2000). Others indicate that lesbians are either significantly more likely than heterosexual women (Aaron et al., 2001) or less likely than heterosexual women to have mammograms (Kerker et al., 2006).

Research is less equivocal when it comes to Pap tests: Lesbians are less likely than heterosexual women to have regular Pap tests (Aaron et al., 2001; Mays et al., 2002; Powers, Bowen, & White, 2001). Mays et al. found that African American and Hispanic lesbians (but not Asian American lesbians) were significantly less likely to have had Pap tests within two years than African American and Hispanic heterosexual women. Using the transtheoretical model in a large Web-based survey of women, McGonigle (2003) found that lesbians were less likely to be in the maintenance stage of change than either bisexual or heterosexual women. Maintenance was defined as cervical screening on a regular basis. Lesbians who are younger than age 35 years and lesbians who are less educated were also less likely than other women to have regular Pap tests (Diamant, Schuster, & Lever, 2000). WSW were less likely than other women to have had Pap tests, but women whose behavior and identity were concordant (i.e., WSW who identified as lesbian) were more likely to have had Pap tests than women whose behavior and identity were discordant (i.e., WSW who identified as heterosexual) (Kerker et al., 2006).

One important reason why some lesbians have not had Pap tests is that clinicians have told them they did not need one because they were not having sex with men (Marrazzo, Koutsky, Kiviat, et al., 2001). Not surprisingly, women who have not had sex with men are less likely to have regular Pap screening (Marrazzo, Koutsky, Kiviat, et al., 2001). Unfortunately, older lesbians in the Women's Health Initiative who reported never having had sex with men had higher self-reports of cervical cancer than lesbians who reported having had sex with men (Valanis et al., 2000).

Cancer Diagnosis and Treatment

Lesbians have many similarities to heterosexual women concerning their responses to newly diagnosed breast cancer (Fobair et al., 2001). Fobair and colleagues compared the responses of lesbian and heterosexual women with breast cancer who had completed surgical treatment. Although there were no differences between the groups in terms of emotional distress, expression of feelings, and sexual satisfaction, lesbians were significantly less fatalistic, and more likely to express anger and use active coping than were heterosexuals. Lesbians had fewer body image problems and were more able to show their bodies to others.

Boehmer, Linde, and Freund (2005) studied coping and adjustment an average of 4 years after a breast cancer diagnosis in women who were members of a sexual minority group—lesbians, bisexual women, and women who partner with women. Overall, these researchers identified low levels of emotional distress among these women. Lesbians and bisexual women used significantly less cognitive avoidance coping than women who partner with women.

Fobair et al. (2001) found that lesbians with breast cancer received significantly more social support from their partners and friends, whereas heterosexual women received significantly more support from relatives. Boehmer, Freund, and Linde (2005) found that 77% of the sexual minority women in their study had a support person, and 79% of them were partners. Sexual minority women who had an identified support person perceived themselves as having more support than women who did not have an identified support person, even though the actual sizes of their support networks did not differ. In addition, the women and their partners did not differ in their levels of distress. Based on these findings, the researchers concluded that the emotional well-being of sexual minority women is dependent on their support person (Boehmer et al.).

Lesbians have been found to be significantly less satisfied with their physicians' care and inclusion of their partners in treatment discussions compared to heterosexual women (Fobair et al., 2001). Perhaps this difference arises because lesbians have often chosen not to disclose their sexual identity. Boehmer and Case (2004) found that 72% of the sexual minority women in their study actively disclosed their identity to their physicians; none of the physicians explicitly asked the women about their identity status. Disclosure resulted in a patient–clinician interaction that was unique to their sexual minority status, including respect for their partners and a more comprehensive approach to cancer care (Boehmer & Case, 2006).

Lesbians apparently do not receive different treatments for breast cancer than heterosexual women (Dibble & Roberts, 2002). The only difference between lesbians and heterosexual women concerning treatment for breast cancer identified by Dibble and Roberts was that lesbians experienced more side effects from chemotherapy compared to heterosexual women.

In the first study of its kind, Boehmer, Linde, and Freund (2007) investigated sexual minority women's decisions about breast reconstruction following mastectomy for breast cancer. Of the 15 women in the sample, eight elected reconstruction and seven decided against reconstruction. Both groups considered the same issues with regard to their decision making: breast size, self-image, and values rooted in their sexual minority identity status. Women who chose reconstruction experienced some problems and had some regrets, while women who did not choose reconstruction adjusted well. Women and their partners had similar levels of satisfaction, regardless of choice.

Interventions for Lesbians and Cancer

The legally unmarried women in the study by Clark and colleagues (2003) also made suggestions to clinicians for increasing the likelihood of their participation in cancer screening. Most importantly, they wanted a trusting relationship with a clinician whom they felt knew them and cared about them as whole persons. They wanted to make their own, informed decisions about health care and to have those decisions be respected by the clinician. And as a practical matter, they wanted to be able to schedule appointments for screening several months in advance and/or have multiple examinations scheduled on the same day.

Dibble and Roberts (2003) provided an intervention to women in senior centers for LGBT persons to enhance cancer screening for older lesbians. The intervention (a 1-hour didactic presentation by a lesbian clinician, followed by a 15-minute question-and-answer period) had a positive impact, based on a 6-month follow-up, with lesbians seeking mammography and pelvic examinations. Nevertheless, there was a very high (20%) refusal rate because these women were afraid of exposure and perceived lack of anonymity, even with a lesbian presenter and in a place known to them.

A 12-week Supportive-Expressive group therapy intervention for lesbians with breast cancer resulted in a significant increase in mood and family relations and a decrease in stress for the lesbians who participated in the program (Fobair et al., 2002). No changes in body image or sexuality were noted. These lesbians did report significantly less instrumental (helpful assistance) and informational (provision of knowledge) social support following the intervention, but that finding could reflect the fact that they no longer needed assistance or information.

Providing Culturally Sensitive Care

SGMs will feel most comfortable and safe in healthcare environments when they think that their sexuality or gender is *not* an issue and will not be the primary part of them being treated. To make that happen, clinicians must educate themselves about SGMs and their health needs and concerns, and create environments that are welcoming, nonthreatening, and normalized to SGMs. All staff should have sensitivity and/or diversity training related to LBGT issues.

A national training project for clinicians, *Removing the Barriers*, has been developed by the Mautner Project, a national health organization for lesbians, based in Washington, D.C., in collaboration with the CDC. This program is designed to improve clinicians' skills in working with lesbians and WSW and to enhance healthcare environments so that health care for lesbians is improved (Scout, Bradford, & Fields, 2001). The Mautner Project will partner with sites in any community across the United States. Clinicians can contact The Mautner Project (202-332-5536 or www.mautnerproject.org) to determine whether there is an opportunity available in their local communities to participate in the training and, if there is not, to initiate such a project.

Being educated includes having knowledge about both the provision and the content of care. To educate themselves about the content of health care for LBT women, clinicians should read current research and other literature about LBT health or attend conferences, such as the annual conference of the GLMA. They should also be willing to search for information, rather than simply dismiss questions that SGM patients might ask. They can talk with SGM individuals in their communities who are out and willing to assist with educating clinicians who want to learn; they can also work with local community LGBT agencies. Clinicians should be familiar with resources such as *Guidelines for Care of Lesbian, Gay, Bisexual, and Transgender Patients* (GLMA, 2006); *Bisexual Health: An Introduction and Model Practices for HIV/STI Prevention Programming* (Miller, André, Ebin, & Bessonova, 2007); and *Standards of*

Care for Gender Identity Disorders (World Professional Association for Transgender Health, 2001), as well as the CDC website on Lesbian, Gay, Bisexual, and Transgender Health (www .cdc.gov/lgbthealth).

Regarding the provision of care, clinicians must use good communication skills. Specifically, clinicians should use gender-neutral language, avoiding the heterosexual assumption. All personnel in healthcare settings should ask how a patient chooses to be identified and the preferred name and pronoun (some transgender people use the genderless pronouns *sie* and *hir*) regardless of the name or gender on insurance documents. Clinicians should also ask about important relationships, including who the patient defines as family and partner(s). When a family member or partner is present with the patient, clinicians should include them in discussion and care.

Clinicians should use a nonthreatening, nonjudgmental approach, and work specifically to build trust and make SGM patients feel at ease, comfortable, and safe. The clinician is responsible for setting the tone for the clinician–patient encounter. If the clinician is relaxed, it will help the patient to relax.

Clinicians should encourage disclosure of sexual or gender minority status when it is relevant to the presenting need. They may also disclose their own identity status, especially if they are LBT themselves and are able to come out. At the same time, clinicians should also explain to the patient whether and how the information obtained will be documented in the medical record. To avoid LBT patients believing that their sexuality is what is being treated, clinicians should always consider the full range of physical and psychosocial health problems for which LBT individuals may be seeking care, and explain why they are asking the questions they ask.

To make the healthcare environment welcoming and acceptable to SGMs, clinicians should consider the physical environment. Having images of all types of families, health information designed for bisexuals or transgendered people, and lesbian magazines, in the waiting area makes SGM individuals feel like they are welcome. Transmen, in particular, have reported feeling invisible in a gynecology waiting room (Hussey, 2006).

SGMs will also feel accepted when intake forms are inclusive of them. Reception staff must also be fully trained to be sensitive to the special needs of SGM patients, and to maintain their confidentiality and protect their privacy. Finally, clinicians should be aware of community resources and referrals, such as groups for lesbians with cancer, bisexual coming out, or transgender support, as well as mainstream referrals that are culturally sensitive to SGMs. If clinicians are seeking SGM patients, they should advertise in both LGBT-specific media and mainstream media.

Comfort in the examination room is also important for SGM patients. For those who have come for care when they may not have been in a healthcare environment for a long time (or ever) since coming out as LBT, the examination room can be particularly threatening. Examinations should be based on anatomy and organs present, not on the perceived gender of a patient. Pelvic examinations can be both physically and emotionally painful for butch women and transgender individuals. Encouraging the patient to have a support person present will be very useful.

Many SGMs avoid seeking health care because of bad experiences they have had in the past, or because they have heard about others' bad experiences. In a small community, such as the LBT community, people talk freely about both bad and good clinicians and institutions. When the community finds a "good" clinician with a positive attitude toward SGMs, others will go to that clinician. Moreover, SGMs tend to be loyal to clinicians who treat them with respect (Labig & Peterson, 2006).

Health Care for Special Groups

Youth and Adolescents

Youth and adolescents are less likely to identify themselves as lesbian or gay, regardless of their sexual behaviors (Austin, Conron, Patel, & Freedner, 2007; D'Augelli, 2004). Many find it difficult to choose a word that describes themselves, or they prefer the terms *queer* or *gender-queer*. Some younger people think that choosing an identity is too permanent, so they may prefer to define themselves as "mostly heterosexual" or "mostly homosexual." In a study of women college students, a group of "mostly straight" women were identified who were distinctly different from heterosexual, lesbian, or bisexual women (Thompson & Morgan, 2008).

Adolescents want to be like their friends, and coming out as LBT sets them apart in many ways. Self-identification as lesbian or gay is typically the last step in the process of coming out (D'Augelli, 2004). In addition, greater sexual experimentation among youth allows them to try various sexual behaviors without having to give themselves an identity label. Thus clinicians should not presume that girls for whom they provide care—even if they report being heterosexual—are not having sex with girls. Although clinicians should not make the assumption of heterosexuality with women of any age, this point may be even truer with youth.

LBT youth and adolescents typically engage in activities that put them at high risk for STIs, including HIV, pregnancy, and cervical cancer. Although LBT girls are no more likely than heterosexual girls to report ever having had sex with men, they have a higher current frequency of intercourse, and they are more likely to become pregnant (Saewyc, 2006). They are also less likely than heterosexual adolescents to use contraception, but when they do use contraception, they use effective methods.

The high rate of pregnancy among LBT adolescents is of concern; however, the explanations for it are unclear. It may be that the high frequency of sexual activity combined with the low rates of contraception produce this high rate of pregnancy. Perhaps the difference arises because LBT adolescents also have high rates of sexual abuse, homelessness, and prostitution or survival sex. And, finally, it may be that pregnancy is a deliberate goal of the adolescents (Saewyc, 2006).

In addition to unprotected sex, lesbian youth are likely to have body piercings or tattoos. Piercings of the tongue, abdomen, or genitalia (most commonly the clitoral hood or labia) can place youth at risk for bacterial infections and other STIs, especially during the initial healing period, with transfer of body fluids (Peterkin & Risdon, 2003). Full healing may take 6 to 8 weeks.

Smoking cigarettes is an important risk factor for the development of cervical cancer. Research shows that lesbian and bisexual girls are significantly more likely than heterosexual girls to use tobacco (Austin et al., 2004). Lesbian and bisexual girls, ages 12 to 17, are far more likely to report having smoked cigarettes in the previous week, month, and year, and to report that most or all of their friends smoke as well. Lesbian and bisexual women college students are also more likely to smoke than heterosexual women students (Ridner, Frost, & LaJoie, 2006). Even so, having only a high school education or less predicts smoking behavior (Hughes, Johnson, & Matthews, 2008). Clinicians should encourage all adolescents not to begin smoking and to assist those who have started smoking to stop.

Transgender youth are particularly concerned about safety issues and becoming victims of violence if they disclose their transgender status or if it is disclosed by others (Grossman & D'Augelli, 2006). While some transgender youth have parents who know and support them, others have been rejected by their families and peers. Consequently, they also fear rejection from clinicians. If transgender youth are younger than the age of 18, they may worry about obtaining hormones without parental consent (Corliss, Belzer, Forbes, & Wilson, 2007). In addition, these youth often cannot obtain employment because of discrimination based on their gender status, so they may engage in sex work to make enough money to buy the hormones they need.

When asked about the characteristics of clinicians and healthcare sites that would help them to trust a clinician or site, sexual minority youth in Philadelphia, ages 14 to 23, indicated that they wanted clinicians who maintain confidentiality, demonstrate respect and honesty, and are well educated (Ginsburg et al., 2002). Transgender youth want healthcare clinicians who are knowledgeable about their specific needs (Corliss et al., 2007).

Clinicians should be good listeners, nonjudgmental, and sensitive to LGBT issues. That is, they should not assume that LGBT youth have HIV or engage in risky sexual behaviors, and they should be understanding of same-sex partners' needs. Helpful clinicians are supportive, caring, trustworthy, nonjudgmental, and accessible (Corliss et al., 2007).

Concerning healthcare sites, the most important criterion, according to these youth, was that the place should be clean (Ginsburg et al., 2002). They also wanted a diverse staff, including diversity of race, gender, and sexual orientation. They hoped to see LGBT posters or magazines, making the place inviting, although those who were less out wanted LGBT health information available in private places, which could include individual examining rooms or restrooms.

Older Sexual and Gender Minorities

Older people, but especially older women, often experience age (and sex) discrimination. Older SGM individuals can also experience heterosexism. Many lesbian and bisexual women who are older (60 years and older) today lived their lives deeply in the closet, trying hard not to be identified as lesbian or bisexual, or specifically trying to "blend in" with other people in their communities (Jones & Nystrom, 2002). Some of these women are still afraid of being identified as lesbian. In the Women's Health Initiative, only 0.6% of older women identified themselves as lesbian and 0.8% identified as bisexual; however, 2.8% did not answer the question, and those women may very well be lesbians or bisexual women who were afraid of being "outed" (Valanis et al., 2000).

Some older lesbian and bisexual women were married to men and have children and grandchildren. Others do not have biologic children, but have children that they consider "theirs" (Claes & Moore, 2000). These older women have created networks of significant others who are their "chosen family." Clinicians need to be aware of the possibility of inter-generational relationships that are important to these women.

Older SGM individuals have similar concerns as other older people (e.g., housing, finances, illness, wanting to maintain control over their own lives), but their concerns for aging also include the impact of death of a partner, family, and friends that may or may not be recognized by society (Jones & Nystrom, 2002). Some lesbians will experience widowhood, although widowhood is not typically acknowledged for lesbians, except by their most immediate friends or family. The unpredictability of support to lesbian widows from family, friends, and clinicians can be stressful in itself. In a recent study, lesbian widows reported that positive support helped them to achieve more positive bereavement outcomes, including better quality of life and ability to move through their grief. Negative support resulted in hurt feelings, more difficulty with bereavement, and less resolution of grief (Bent & Magilvy, 2006). The lack of social acceptance or acknowledgment of their loss can make the experience even more painful, and may increase lesbians' risk for depression or other mental health problems.

Most older people fear institutionalization and losing their independence. For SGM people, these worries may be aggravated by fears about discrimination because of their sexual or gender minority status. Having advance directives completed can be one way to address some of those fears. In a recent study comparing heterosexual people with LGBT people, similar proportions of both groups believed that LGBT people were discriminated against in long-term care facilities, but significantly more heterosexual than LGBT people believed that LGBT people had equal access to social and healthcare services (Jackson, Johnson, & Roberts, 2008). Nonetheless, the majority of LGBT people in the study who believed that LGBT people are discriminated against in long-term care also speculated that they themselves would not hide their sexual or gender minority status if they had to go into a long-term care facility.

LGBT retirement communities are beginning to appear across the United States. Many LBGT people would prefer to live in such a center, believing that it would be a remedy for the discrimination that they perceive to exist in mainstream facilities.

Sexual and Gender Minorities with Disabilities

All women with disabilities face barriers to health care. For SGM women with disabilities, however, their disability is just one more factor that makes health care difficult. Disabilities may range from blindness or deafness to mobility problems to mental health problems, and vary depending on whether the disability is visible or invisible and whether it is lifelong or acquired. Consequently, SGMs with disabilities are an extremely heterogeneous group. The prevalence of disabilities may be higher among SGMs than in the general population. In a recent study, lesbians and bisexual women reported more major physical disabilities and functionally limiting disabilities than heterosexual women. They were also more likely to report receiving disability income (Cochran & Mays, 2007).

SGM women with disabilities share issues of disability with heterosexual women (e.g., the myth that women who are disabled are not sexually active) at the same time that they share healthcare issues with other SGMs (e.g., fear of disclosure to clinicians). Consequently, lesbians with disabilities may feel even more unsafe in gynecologic offices than other lesbians (O'Toole, 1996). It is incumbent upon clinicians to provide the same quality of care for SGMs with disabilities as they offer to all women.

Conclusion

SGM individuals are a diverse group of people who have health and gynecologic healthcare needs like all women, but who also have unique needs because of their SGM status. This chapter described some of these unique issues, as well as areas of similarities between SGMs and other women. Much more needs to be understood about the health of and care for these populations, and the research base is growing. Clinicians must strive to provide culturally sensitive care to their SGM patients.

References

Aaron, D. J., Markovic, N., Danielson, M. E., Honnold, J. A., Janosky, J. E., & Schmidt, N. J. (2001). Behavioral risk factors for disease and preventive health practices among lesbians. *American Journal of Public Health, 91*, 972–875.

Agrawal, R., Sharma, S., Bekir, J., Conway, G., Bailey, J., Balen, A. H., & Prelevic, G. (2004). Prevalence of polycystic ovaries and polycystic ovary syndrome in lesbian women compared with heterosexual women. *Fertility and Sterility, 82*(5), 1352–1357.

Arend, E. D. (2003). The politics of invisibility: HIV-positive women who have sex with women and their struggle for support. *Journal of the Association of Nurses in AIDS Care, 14*(6), 37–47.

Austin, S. B., Conron, K. J., Patel, A., & Freedner, N. (2007). Making sense of sexual orientation measures: Findings from a cognitive processing study with adolescents on health survey questions. *Journal of LBGT Health Research, 3*(1), 55–65.

Austin, S. B., Ziyadeh, N., Fisher, L. B., Kahn, J. A., Colditz, G. A., & Frazier, A. L. (2004). Sexual orientation and tobacco use in a cohort study of US adolescent girls and boys. *Archives of Pediatrics & Adolescent Medicine, 158*, 317–322

Baba, T., Endo, T., Honnma, H., Kitajima, Y., Hayashi, T., Ikeda, H., . . . Saito, T. (2007). Association between polycystic ovary syndrome and female-to-male transsexuality. *Human Reproduction, 22*(4), 1011–1016.

Bailey, J. V., Benato, R., Owne, C., & Kavanagh, J. (2008). Vulvovaginal candidiasis in women who have sex with women. *Sexually Transmitted Diseases, 35*(6), 533–536.

Bauer, G. R., & Welles, S. L. (2001). Beyond assumptions of negligible risk: Sexually transmitted diseases and women who have sex with women. *American Journal of Public Health, 91*, 1282–1286.

Bent, K. N., & Magilvy, J. K. (2006). When a partner dies: Lesbian widows. *Issues in Mental Health Nursing, 27*, 447–459.

Berger, B. J., Kolton, S., Zenilman, J. M., Cummings, M. C., Feldman, J., & McCormack, W. M. (1995). Bacterial vaginosis in lesbians: A sexually transmitted disease. *Clinical Infectious Diseases, 21*, 1402–1405.

Bergeron, S., & Senn, C. Y. (2003). Health care utilization in a sample of Canadian lesbian women: Predictors of risk and resilience. *Women & Health, 37*(3), 19–35.

Bernhard, L. A. (2001). Lesbian health and health care. *Annual Review of Nursing Research, 19*, 145–177.

Boehmer, U., Bowen, D., & Bauer, G. R. (2007). Overweight and obesity in sexual-minority women: Evidence from population-based data. *American Journal of Public Health, 97*(6), 1134–1140.

Boehmer, U., & Case, P. (2004). Physicians don't ask, sometimes patients tell: Disclosure of sexual orientation among women with breast cancer. *Cancer, 101*, 1882–1889.

Boehmer, U., & Case, P. (2006). Sexual minority women's interactions with breast cancer providers. *Women and Health, 44*(2), 41–58.

Boehmer, U., Freund, K. M., & Linde, R. (2005). Support providers of sexual minority women with breast cancer: Who they are and how they impact the breast cancer experience. *Journal of Psychosomatic Research, 59*, 307–314.

Boehmer, U., Linde, R., & Freund, K. M. (2005). Sexual minority women's coping and psychological adjustment after a diagnosis of breast cancer. *Journal of Women's Health, 14*(3), 214–224.

Boehmer, U., Linde, R., & Freund, K. M. (2007). Breast reconstruction following mastectomy for breast cancer: The decisions of sexual minority women. *Plastic and Reconstructive Surgery, 119*(2), 464–472.

Bowen, D. J., Balsam, K. F., Diergaarde, B., Russo, M., & Escamilla, G. M. (2006). Healthy eating, exercise, and weight: Impressions of sexual minority women. *Women & Health, 44*(1), 79–93.

Bowen, D. J., Balsam, K. F., & Ender, S. R. (2008). A review of obesity issues in sexual minority women. *Obesity, 16*(2), 221–227.

Bradford, J., & Ryan, C. (1987). *The National Lesbian Health Care Survey*. Washington, DC: National Lesbian and Gay Health Foundation.

Brandenburg, D. L., Matthews, A. K., Johnson, T. P., & Hughes, T. L. (2007). Breast cancer risk and screening: A comparison of lesbian and heterosexual women. *Women and Health, 45*(4), 109–130.

Campos-Outcalt, D., & Hurwitz, S. (2002). Female-to-female transmission of syphilis: A case report. *Sexually Transmitted Diseases, 29*, 119.

Centers for Disease Control and Prevention (CDC). (2006, June). *HIV/AIDS Among Women Who Have Sex with Women*. Fact sheet. Retrieved from http://www.cdc.gov/hiv/topics/women/resources/factsheets/wsw.htm

Centers for Disease Control and Prevention (CDC). (2008, August). *HIV/AIDS Among Women*. Fact sheet. Retrieved from http://www.cdc.gov/hiv/topics/women/resources/factsheets/women.htm

Champion, J. D., Wilford, K., & Piper, J. M. (2005). Risk and protective behaviours of bisexual minority women: A qualitative analysis. *International Nursing Review, 52*, 115–122.

Claes, J. A., & Moore, W. (2000). Issues confronting lesbian and gay elders: The challenge for health and human services providers. *Journal of Health and Human Services Administration, 23*(2), 181–202.

Clark, M. A., Bonacore, L., Wright, S. J., Armstrong, G., & Rakowski, W. (2003). The cancer screening project for women: Experiences of women who partner with women and women who partner with men. *Women & Health, 38*(2), 19–33.

Cochran, S. D., & Mays, V. M. (2007). Physical health complaints among lesbians, gay men, and bisexual and homosexually experienced heterosexual individuals: Results from the California Quality of Life Survey. *American Journal of Public Health, 97*(11), 2048–2055.

Corliss, H. L., Belzer, M., Forbes, C., & Wilson, E. C. (2007). An evaluation of service utilization among male to female transgender youth: Qualitative study of a clinic-based sample. *Journal of LGBT Health Research, 3*(2), 49–61.

Crosby, R. A., & Pitts, N. L. (2007). Caught between different worlds: How transgendered women may be "forced" into risky sex. *Journal of Sex Research, 44*(1), 43–48.

D'Augelli, A. R. (2004). High tobacco use among lesbian, gay, and bisexual youth. *Archives of Pediatrics & Adolescent Medicine, 158*, 309–310.

Diamant, A. L., Schuster, M. A., & Lever, J. (2000). Receipt of preventive health care services by lesbians. *American Journal of Preventive Medicine, 19*, 141–148.

Diamant, A. L., Schuster, M. A., McGuigan, K., & Lever, J. (1999). Lesbians' sexual history with men: Implications for taking a sexual history. *Archives of Internal Medicine, 159*, 2730–2736.

Dibble, S. L., & Roberts, S. A. (2002). A comparison of breast cancer diagnosis and treatment between lesbian and heterosexual women. *Journal of the Gay and Lesbian Medical Association, 6*, 9–17.

Dibble, S. L., & Roberts, S. A. (2003). Improving cancer screening among lesbians over 50: Results of a pilot study. *Oncology Nursing Forum, 30,* E71–E79.

Dibble, S. L., Roberts, S. A., & Nussey, B. (2004). Comparing breast cancer risk between lesbians and their heterosexual sisters. *Women's Health Issues, 14,* 60–68.

Dibble, S. L., Roberts, S. A., Robertson, P. A., & Paul, S. M. (2002). Risk factors for ovarian cancer: Lesbian and heterosexual women. *Oncology Nursing Forum, 29,* 29.

Dolan, K. A., & Davis, P. W. (2008). HIV testing among lesbian women: Social contexts and subjective meanings. *Journal of Homosexuality, 54*(3), 307–324.

Evans, A. I., Scally, A. J., Wellard, S. J., & Wilson, J. D. (2008). Prevalence of bacterial vaginosis in lesbians and heterosexual women in a community setting. *Sexually Transmitted Infections, 83,* 470–475.

Feldman, M. B., & Meyer, I. H. (2007). Eating disorders in diverse lesbian, gay, and bisexual populations. *International Journal of Eating Disorders, 40*(3), 218–226.

Fishman, S. J., & Anderson, E. H. (2003). Perception of HIV and safer sexual behaviors among lesbians. *Journal of the Association of Nurses in AIDS Care, 14*(6), 48–55.

Fobair, P., Koopman, C., Dimiceli, S., O'Hanlan, K., Butler, L. D., Classen, C.,... Spiegel, D. (2002). Psychosocial intervention for lesbians with primary breast cancer. *Psycho-Oncology, 11,* 427–438.

Fobair P., O'Hanlan, K., Koopman, C., Classen, C., Dimiceli, S., Drooker, N.,... Spiegel, D. (2001). Comparison of lesbian and heterosexual women's response to newly diagnosed breast cancer. *Psycho-Oncology, 10,* 40–51.

Gay and Lesbian Medical Association (GLMA). (2006). *Guidelines for care of lesbian, gay, bisexual, and transgender patients.* San Francisco: Author. Retrieved from http://www.glma.org

Ginsburg, K. R., Winn, R. J., Rudy, B. J., Crawford, J., Zhao, H., & Schwarz, D. F. (2002). How to reach sexual minority youth in the health care setting: The teens offer guidance. *Journal of Adolescent Health, 31,* 407–416.

Grossman, A. H., & D'Augelli, A. R. (2006). Transgender youth: Invisible and vulnerable. *Journal of Homosexuality, 51*(1), 111–128.

Guille, C., & Chrisler, J. C. (1999). Does feminism serve a protective function against eating disorders. *Journal of Lesbian Studies, 3*(4), 141–148.

Heck, J. E., Sell, R. L., & Gorin, S. S. (2006). Health care access among individuals involved in same-sex relationships. *American Journal of Public Health, 96*(6), 1111–1118.

Heffernan, K. (1999). Lesbians and the internalization of societal standards of weight and appearance. *Journal of Lesbian Studies, 3*(4), 121–127.

Herbst, J. H., Jacobs, E. D., Finlayson, T. J., McKleroy, V. S., Nemann, M. S., Crepaz, N., & HIV/AIDS Prevention Research Synthesis Team. (2008). Estimating HIV prevalence and risk behaviors of transgender persons in the United States: A systematic review. *AIDS Behavior, 12,* 1–17.

Hughes, T. L., Johnson, T. P., & Matthews, A. K. (2008). Sexual orientation and smoking: Results from a multisite women's health study. *Substance Use and Misuse, 43*(8–9), 1218–1239.

Human Rights Campaign Foundation (HRC) & Gay and Lesbian Medical Association (GLMA). (2008). *Healthcare equality index.* Washington, DC/San Francisco: Authors. Retrieved from http://www.hrc.org/hei

Hussey, W. (2006). Slivers of the journey: The use of photovoice and storytelling to examine female to male transsexuals' experience of health care access. *Journal of Homosexuality, 51*(1), 129–158.

Jackson, N. C., Johnson, M. J., & Roberts, R. (2008). The potential impact of discrimination fears of older gays, lesbians, bisexuals and transgender individuals living in small- to moderate-sized cities on long-term health care. *Journal of Homosexuality, 54*(3), 325–339.

Johnson, C. F., Mimiaga, M. J., & Bradford, J. (2008). Health care issues among lesbian, gay, bisexual, transgender and intersex (LGBTI) populations in the United States: Introduction. *Journal of Homosexuality, 54*(3), 213–224.

Jones, T. C., & Nystrom, N. M. (2002). Looking back, looking forward: Addressing the lives of lesbians 55 and older. *Journal of Women & Aging, 14*(3/4), 59–76.

Joshua, M. D. (2003). A model of the development of disordered eating among lesbians. *Dissertation Abstracts International, 63*(09), 4375.

Kavanaugh-Lynch, M. H. E., White, E., Daling, J. R., & Bowen, D. J. (2002). Correlates of lesbian sexual orientation and the risk of breast cancer. *Journal of the Gay and Lesbian Medical Association, 6,* 91–95.

Kellock, D. J., & O'Mahoney, C. P. (1996). Sexually acquired metronidazole-resistant trichomoniasis in a lesbian couple. *Genitourinary Medicine, 72,* 60–61.

Kelly, L. (2007). Lesbian body image perceptions: The context of body silence. *Qualitative Health Research, 17*(7), 873–883.

Kerker, B. D., Mostashari, F., & Thorpe, L. (2006). Health care access and utilization among women who have sex with women: Sexual behavior and identity. *Journal of Urban Health, 83*(5), 970–979.

Koh, A. S., Gómez, C. A., Shade, S., & Rowley, E. (2005). Sexual risk factors among self-identified lesbians, bisexual women, and heterosexual women accessing primary care settings. *Sexually Transmitted Diseases, 32*(9), 563–569.

Kwakwa, H. A., & Ghobrial, M. W. (2003). Female-to-female transmission of human immunodeficiency virus. *Clinical Infectious Diseases, 36*, e40–e41.

Labig, C. E., Jr., & Peterson, T. O. (2006). Sexual minorities and selection of a primary care physician in a Midwestern U.S. city. *Journal of Homosexuality, 51*(3), 1–5.

Marrazzo, J. M. (2000). Genital human papillomavirus infection in women who have sex with women: A concern for patients and providers. *AIDS Patient Care and STDs, 14*, 447–451.

Marrazzo, J. M. (2008). Elusive aetiology of bacterial vaginosis: Do lesbians have a clue? *Sexually Transmitted Infections, 83*, 424–425.

Marrazzo, J. M., Koutsky, L. A., Eschenbach, D. A., Agnew, K., Stine, K., & Hillier, S. L. (2002). Characterization of vaginal flora and bacterial vaginosis in women who have sex with women. *Journal of Infectious Diseases, 185*, 1307–1313.

Marrazzo, J. M., Koutsky, L. A., & Handsfield, H. H. (2001). Characteristics of female sexually transmitted disease clinic clients who report same-sex behavior. *International Journal of STD & AIDS, 12*, 41–46.

Marrazzo, J. M., Koutsky, L. A., Kiviat, N. B., Kuypers, J. M., & Stine, K. (2001). Papanicolaou test screening and prevalence of genital human papillomavirus among women who have sex with women. *American Journal of Public Health, 91*, 947–952.

Marrazzo, J. M., Stine, K., & Wald, A. (2003). Prevalence and risk factors for infection with herpes simplex virus type-1 and -2 among lesbians. *Sexually Transmitted Diseases, 30*, 890–895.

Matthews, A. K., Hughes, T. L., Osterman, G. P., & Kodl, M. M. (2005). Complementary medicine practices in a community-based sample of lesbian and heterosexual women. *Health Care for Women International, 26*, 430–447.

Mays, V. M., Yancey, A. K., Cochran, S. D., Weber, M., & Fielding, J. E. (2002). Heterogeneity of health disparities among African American, Hispanic, and Asian American women: Unrecognized influences of sexual orientation. *American Journal of Public Health, 92*, 632–639.

McDonald, C., McIntyre, M., & Anderson, B. (2003). The view from somewhere: Locating lesbian experience in women's health. *Health Care for Women International, 24*, 697–711.

McGonigle, T. H. (2003). *Surveying for sexuality in cyberspace: Sexual orientation and stage of change for cervical cancer screening* (Unpublished doctoral dissertation). Ohio State University, Columbus, OH.

McTiernan, A., Kuniyuki, A., Yasui, Y., Bowen, D., Burke, W., Culver, J. B., ... Durfy, S. (2001). Comparisons of two breast cancer risk estimates in women with a family history of breast cancer. *Cancer Epidemiology, Biomarkers & Prevention, 10*, 333–338.

Miller, M., André, A., Ebin, J., & Bessonova, L. (2007). *Bisexual health: An introduction and model practices for HIV/STI prevention programming.* New York: National Gay and Lesbian Task Force Policy Institute, Fenway Institute at Fenway Community Health, & BiNet USA.

Montcalm, D. M., & Myer, L. L. (2000). Lesbian immunity from HIV/AIDS: Fact or fiction? *Journal of Lesbian Studies, 4*, 131–147.

Moore, F., & Keel, P. K. (2003). Influence of sexual orientation and age on disordered eating attitudes and behaviors in women. *International Journal of Eating Disorders, 34*, 370–374.

Mueller, A., Gooren, L. J., Naton-Schötz, S., Cupisti, S., Beckmann, M. W., & Dittrich, R. (2008). Prevalence of polycystic ovary syndrome and hyperandrogenemia in female-to-male transsexuals. *Journal of Clinical Endocrinology and Metabolism, 93*(4), 1408–1411.

O'Toole, C. J. (1996). Disabled lesbians: Challenging monocultural constructs. In D. M. Krotoski, M. A. Nosek, & M. A. Turk (Eds.), *Women with physical disabilities: Achieving and maintaining health and well-being* (pp. 135–151). Baltimore: Paul H. Brooks.

Peterkin, A., & Risdon, C. (2003). *Caring for lesbian and gay people: A clinical guide.* Buffalo, NY: University of Toronto Press.

Powers, D., Bowen, D. J., & White, J. (2001). The influence of sexual orientation on health behaviors in women. *Journal of Prevention & Intervention in the Community, 22*(2), 43–60.

Rachlin, K., Green, J., & Lombardi, E. (2008). Utilization of health care among female-to-male transgender individuals in the United States. *Journal of Homosexuality, 54*(3), 243–258.

Ridner, S. L., Frost, K., & LaJoie, A. S. (2006). Health information and risk behaviors among lesbian, gay, and bisexual college students. *Journal of the American Academy of Nurse Practitioners, 18,* 374–378.

Roberts, S. A., Dibble, S. L., Nussey, B., & Casey, K. (2003). Cardiovascular disease risk in lesbian women. *Women's Health Issues, 13,* 167–174.

Saewyc, E. M. (2006). Pregnancy among lesbian, gay, and bisexual adolescents: Influences of stigma, sexual abuse, and sexual orientation. In A. M. Omoto & H. S. Kurtzman (Eds.), *Sexual orientation and mental health* (pp. 95–116). Washington, DC: American Psychological Association.

Sausa, L. A., Keatley, J., & Operario, D. (2007). Perceived risks and benefits of sex work among transgender women of color in San Francisco. *Archives of Sexual Behavior, 36,* 768–777.

Scout, J., Bradford, J., & Fields, C. (2001). Removing the barriers: Improving practitioners' skills in providing health care to lesbians and women who partner with women. *American Journal of Public Health, 91,* 989–990.

Seaver, M. R., Freund, K. M., Wright, L. M., Tjia, J., & Frayne, S. M. (2008). Healthcare preferences among lesbians: A focus group analysis. *Journal of Women's Health, 17*(2), 215–225.

Solarz, A. L. (Ed.). (1999). *Lesbian health: Current assessment and directions for the future.* Washington, DC: National Academy Press.

Steele, L. S., Tinmouth, J. M., & Lu, A. (2006). Regular health care use by lesbians: A path analysis of predictive factors. *Family Practice, 23,* 631–636.

Thompson, E. M., & Morgan, E. M. (2008). "Mostly straight" young women: Variations in sexual behavior and identity development. *Developmental Psychology, 44*(1), 15–21.

Valanis, B. G., Bowen, D. J., Bassford, T., Whitlock, E., Charney, P., & Carter, R. A. (2000). Sexual orientation and health: Comparisons in the Women's Health Initiative sample. *Archives of Family Medicine, 9,* 843–853.

White, J. C., & Dull, V. T. (1998). Room for improvement: Communication between lesbians and primary care providers. *Journal of Lesbian Studies, 2*(1), 95–110.

World Professional Association for Transgender Health. (2001). *Standards of care for gender identity disorders.* Retrieved from http://wpath.org/Documents2/socv6.pdf

Yancey, A. K., Cochran, S. D., Corliss, H. L., & Mays, V. M. (2003). Correlates of overweight and obesity among lesbian and bisexual women. *Preventive Medicine, 36,* 676–683.

11

Sexuality

Catherine Ingram Fogel

Despite the unalterable fact that women are sexual beings, it is difficult for many women and their clinicians to view sexual health as an essential component of health care or to discuss sexual concerns. Yet sexuality is an organic, normal, physical, and emotional function that is inextricably woven into the fabric of human life (Northrup, 1998). All women have a right to intimate and sexual lives and relationships that are voluntary, wanted, pleasurable, and noncoercive (World Health Organization [WHO], 2006). Women often ask questions and express concerns to their clinicians about their sexuality and sexual activity; and they expect nonjudgmental, open, and direct communication regarding sexual matters, sexual information, counseling, or therapy from those clinicians. Clinicians providing sexual health care need to understand the adverse impact that illnesses and their treatments can have on sexuality and sexual functioning. Additionally, an awareness of the detrimental impact of violence and coercive sexual experiences on sexual enjoyment is essential. All women are entitled to education regarding their health, including the provision of sexual information and resources, and to counseling to improve or sustain current sexual relationships or to solve a particular problem.

This chapter seeks to develop a solid knowledge base about sexuality for use in clinical practice from which sexual concerns may be addressed. It focuses on sexual desire, women's views of themselves and presentations to society, sexual response, and factors that influence sexual response, function, and dysfunction. Additionally, strategies for assessment are discussed as a foundation for management of female sexual dysfunction, which is addressed in Chapter 17.

Female Sexuality

Female sexuality is defined as the integrated, unique expression of self that includes the physiologic and psychologic processes inherent in sexual development. Included in sexual development are a view and presentation of oneself as a female, sexual desire, sexual response, and sexual orientation (Fogel, 2003). The complex process known as sexuality is coordinated by the neurologic, vascular, muscular, and endocrine systems (Baram & Basson, 2007). It encompasses a woman's values, attitudes, behaviors, physical appearance, beliefs, emotions, personality, and social and cultural orientations. Further, sexuality is a fundamental component of every woman's life and an important aspect of her health throughout her life. A woman's ability to express herself sexually lasts from birth to death. Indeed, there are few women for whom sex has not been important at some time in their lives.

Sexual expression is influenced by ethical, cultural, moral, and spiritual factors and is expressed differently at different times—alone, with one partner, or with many partners. In addition, no two women will express their sexuality in exactly the same way. Women express their identities and their need for emotional and physical closeness with others, in part, through their sexual relationships. When expressed positively, sexuality can bring much pleasure; however, sexuality also has the potential to cause great pain. A woman's sexuality is not limited by age, attractiveness, partner availability or participation, or sexual orientation.

Components of Sexuality

The unique human quality that is sexuality has several dimensions, including sexual desire, presentation of self as a sexual being, sexual orientation, and sexual lifestyles and relationships. Sexuality combines sex—that is, one's anatomic characteristics as male or female—with gender—that is, one's view and presentation of self as a man or a woman. Sexuality is more than just sexual intercourse; it involves a wide range of behaviors including fantasy, self-stimulation, noncoital pleasuring, erotic stimuli other than touch, communication about needs and desires, and the ability to define what is wanted and pleasurable in a relationship (Fogel & Woods, 2008). While acknowledging the influence of biology on sexuality, sexuality is also a social construct based on prescribed arrangements and sexual scripts that provide guidelines for appropriate sexual behaviors (Amaro, Navarro, Conron, & Raj, 2002).

Sexual desire, or interest in sexual experience, can occur spontaneously in women but usually is triggered by cues, such as romantic feelings toward a partner (McCall & Meston, 2006). The amount of sexual desire experienced varies from woman to woman, differs across a woman's life, and can be suppressed or repressed by many different factors. Kaplan (1979) considered sexual desire to be the innate urge for sexual activity, which is produced by the activation of a specific system in the brain and experienced as a specific sensation that motivates an individual to seek or respond to sexual experience. Although Kaplan defined sexual desire as a physical need, similar to hunger, a more accurate representation also includes recognition of women's needs for intimacy as a strong influence on sexual desire (Basson,

2000). Additional factors in the development of sexual desire include experiencing feelings of pleasure, enjoyment, dissatisfaction, or pain during sexual activity. Sexual desire can also develop from an interest in sexual activity, a preferred frequency of activity, and a gender preference for a sexual partner (Fogel, 2003). These scripts vary by gender, from culture to culture, and by cultural subgroups. In addition, an individual's expression of these scripts may vary due to cultural prescriptions and their personal situations (Amaro et al., 2002).

A view of self as a female and presentation of self as a sexual being begin to form in early childhood and evolve throughout a woman's life as life circumstances shape her identity. A woman's view of herself as female includes her gender identity, or the personal, private conviction that each person has about being feminine (sense of self as a woman); her sense of having characteristics customarily defined as feminine, masculine, or both (gender role); and body image (mental picture of one's body and its relationship to the environment) (Fogel, 2003). While gender identity can be influenced by one's biologic or anatomic sex, it is not necessarily consistent with biologic sex (Alexander, LaRosa, Bader, & Garfield, 2007).

Presentation of self as a woman (gender role behaviors) includes all those behaviors that women use to indicate to society that they are women, including dress, hairstyle, speech patterns, and walk. Gender role behaviors reflect a woman's internalization of societal and cultural stereotypes and expectations of what a woman's behavior should be (Alexander et al., 2007). Moreover, gender role prescriptions and expectations shape sexual expression. Beliefs about women and men and assumptions regarding appropriate behaviors for both affect sexual behavior, communication patterns, and expectations of sexual relationships.

Sexual orientation is the erotic or romantic attraction or preference for sharing sexual expression with persons of a specific gender. It also refers to the preference an individual develops for a partner, or the preference for the gender of the person with whom one has an emotional and physical attraction, and with whom one wishes to share sexual intimacy. Sexual preferences span a continuum ranging from total orientation to the same sex, to bisexuality, to total orientation to the other sex. Sexual orientation may be determined before birth, although orientation can also be influenced by social factors and personal experiences. It is important to understand that one's sexual practices may not necessarily indicate sexual orientation.

Sexual lifestyles and relationships provide the pattern and context for one's sexuality. While many options exist for women today, not all are equally accepted by society (Bernhard, 1995). The most frequently acknowledged pattern for women is heterosexual, marital monogamy, which is assumed to be the most desirable status by the majority of societies. In contrast, women who engage in serial heterosexual monogamy have an established pattern of conducting one monogamous relationship followed by another, similar relationship. Women who choose a pattern of nonmonogamous heterosexual marriage participate in sexual activity with other individuals or couples while married. Still other women elect to have sexual relations with one or more concurrent male partners without marriage (heterosexual coupling without marriage).

A woman is considered to be bisexual when her sexual and affectional preferences are directed toward individuals of either sex. Bisexual women may be married, have partners of both sexes simultaneously or serially, or have lesbian relationships as well as previous sexual relationships with men.

Women who partner with a woman (lesbians) direct their sexual and affectional preferences toward women. Lesbians may be coupled or single with one or many partners.

The celibate lifestyle involves the conscious choice to abstain from sexual activity. Women may view this choice positively as a means of giving one's time and energy and total attention to other activities. Alternatively, celibacy may be involuntary, as when women are between relationships.

Sexual Health

Defining sexual health is difficult. Indeed, for many people, it is not something that is considered until its absence is noticed. While experts do not agree on a definition of sexual health (Edwards & Coleman, 2004), the 1975 WHO definition provides a beginning point: "Sexual health is the integration of the somatic, emotional, intellectual, and social aspects of sexual being, in ways that are positively enriching and that enhance personality, communication, and love" (WHO Regional Office for Europe, 2001, p. 7). Essential elements of this definition include the capacity to enjoy and control sexual and reproductive behavior in accordance with a social and personal ethic; freedom from shame, fear, guilt, and misconceptions that inhibit sexual response and harm sexual relationships; and freedom from disease, illness, organic disorders, and deficiencies that interfere with sexual functioning. Essential to sexual health is an acceptance of one's gender identity, body image, sexual identity, and sexual orientation. Also important is the ability to comfortably communicate one's sexual feelings, needs, and desires. Thus sexual health may be considered those factors that enable women to enjoy and control their sexual and reproductive lives, including a physical and emotional state of well-being, and the quality of sexual and other close relationships.

Definitions of sexual health and sexual practices may contain value-laden terms that are susceptible to different interpretations. In many cases, cultural norms dictate what is acceptable or normal behavior. Before clinicians can provide sexual health care, they must be aware of how they define normal and abnormal sexual practices. Because it is not always easy to distinguish between aberrant and merely unconventional practices, clinicians should consider the questions found in **Box 11-1** to identify the attitudes and beliefs they hold regarding sexual practices.

Sexual Response in Women

Sexual response involves both capacity—that is, what a woman is capable of experiencing—and activity—that is, what she actually experiences. Emotion and physiology are interwoven within a woman's sexual response cycle.

Traditionally the Masters and Johnson (1966) model of sexual response, as adapted by Kaplan (1979), has been used to explain sexual response in both men and women. Although Masters and Johnson began the modern movement toward an understanding of the sexual

BOX 11-1 *Assessing a Sexual Behavior*

The following questions can be used when considering whether or not a particular behavior or practice is abnormal:

- What does the behavior mean to the woman?
- Does the behavior enrich or impoverish the sexual life of the woman and those with whom she shares sexual relations?
- Is the behavior tolerable to society?
- Is the behavior between two consenting adults?
- Does the behavior cause physical or psychological harm to the woman or her partner?
- Does the behavior involve coercion?

Source: MacLaren, 1995.

response cycle, their description focused solely on physiologic responses to stimuli. They identified two principal physiologic responses to sexual stimulation: vasocongestion and muscle tension. These responses are represented differently throughout the phases of the woman's sexual response cycle. Later authorities incorporated both biologic and psychological components (American Psychiatric Association, 1994; Kaplan).

The focus on genital responses and customary indicators of desire, such as sexual fantasies and the need for self-stimulation, does have some drawbacks, however. In particular, it ignores important components of women's sexual satisfaction, including intimacy, trust, and comfort with vulnerability, communication, respect, affection, and pleasure associated with sensual touching (Basson, 2000; Basson et al., 2004; Tiefer, 1991). Basson suggests that women's sexual response more commonly arises from needs for intimacy rather than a desire for physical sexual arousal, and that women's sense of sexual arousal arises only minimally from an awareness of genital congestion and other physiologic changes.

The traditional female sexual response cycle as described by Masters and Johnson and Kaplan, when modified to include the element of consent (Chalker, 1994), consists of four sequential phases: desire, excitement, orgasm, and resolution. The desire phase consists of sexual fantasy, thoughts, and awareness that sexual stimulation is wanted without physiologic changes. Vasocongestion, muscle tension, and other physiologic changes build, peak and release, then resolve during the excitement, orgasm, and resolution phases, respectively. During this cycle, progression occurs from a subjective sense of anticipation and pleasure to release and finally to relaxation.

While this model is useful for understanding male sexual response and dysfunction, it does not account for four fundamental aspects of women's healthy sexual functioning (Basson, 2000). First, women have a lower biologic urge to be sexual for the release of sexual tension than men. Second, women's motivations for sexual experiences are related to rewards that are not sexual in nature, and that occur in addition to and may be more relevant than their biologic urges. Although these rewards are not irrelevant to men, they may often be less of a motivating force. Men may experience their desire independent of context; thus desire may be more accurately labeled *drive* in this circumstance. Third, women's sexual arousal is a subjective mental excitement that may or may not be associated with an awareness of genital vasocongestion and other physical nongenital arousal symptoms. In fact, genital awareness may or may not be an erotic stimulus for women. Finally, women may or may not experience orgasmic release of sexual tension. When orgasmic release does occur, it can happen in a variety of ways, even in the same woman (Basson).

Basson (2000) suggests that while the Masters and Johnson model, as modified by Kaplan, may represent the beginning of a new understanding of sexual relationships for women, it is not truly representative of women's long-term sexual relationships, and that a different model would be more appropriate (**Figure 11-1**). Women move from a sexually neutral state to seeking sexual stimuli when they sense either an opportunity to be sexual or a partner's need, or when they have an awareness of one or more of the potential benefits of sexual activity. Sexual desire may be experienced as a craving for sexual sensations for their own sake, a desire to experience physical and subjective arousal, or possibly a release of sexual tension. In this model, sexual desire is a response rather than a spontaneous event. Although a woman may experience spontaneous desire in the form of sexual dreams, thoughts, or fantasies, she is more likely to be at a baseline neutral state at the onset of a partner experience (Basson, 2000).

Many sexually functional and satisfied women do not experience spontaneous sexual desire (Basson et al., 2004). Rather, sexual arousal and responsive sexual desire may occur simultaneously after the decision to experience sexual stimulation. The choice to engage in

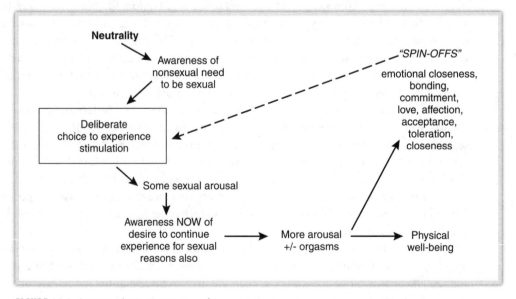

FIGURE 11-1 A woman's sex response cycle.

Source: Copyright © 2000 from *The female sexual response: A different model* by Rosemary Basson. Reproduced by permission of Taylor & Francis, Inc., http://www.taylorandfrancis.com.

sexual activity in such a case is initially based on needs other than a desire for physical sexual response and release. Likewise, women may experience physical well-being without orgasms and subsequent release. Emotional closeness with its attendant commitment, bonding, tolerance of imperfections in a relationship, and the appreciation of a partner's satisfaction are valued emotional rewards for women and will act as motivators to activate the next sexual cycle. Further, these rewards may be sufficient by themselves, or they may be accompanied by physical sexual hunger. Although a woman may be motivated to be sexual by experiencing increased intimacy, she also needs a pleasant physical experience for the motivation to continue over time.

Developmental Factors Influencing Sexuality

Adolescence

Adolescence, which is generally defined as the ages from 12 to 19 years, is a period of rapid physical change. It is also a time of potentially stressful psychosocial demands, including a time of awareness and change in sexual feelings. The development of adolescent sexuality focuses on five aspects:

- Physical changes of puberty and their relationship to self-esteem and body image
- Learning about normal bodily functions and sensual and sexual responses and needs
- Developing one's sense of self as a woman (gender identity) and comfort with one's sexual orientation
- Learning about sexual and romantic relationships
- Developing a personal sexual value system (Masters, Johnson, & Kolodney, 1995)

Sexuality is often defined through activities such as dating. During this time, adolescent females select companions, test ideas regarding themselves, and eventually experience sexual pleasure.

As adolescents develop a capacity for sexual intimacy, sexual curiosity and experimentation are common. In the United States, the likelihood of adolescents having ever had sexual intercourse increases steadily with age from 32.8% of ninth graders to 64.6% of twelfth graders (Eaton et al., 2008). Among U.S. adolescents in the twelfth grade, 20.1% of females and 23.3% of males report having had intercourse with four or more sexual partners (Eaton et al.). But not all such activity is welcome: 14.3% of 18- to 19-year-olds and 19.1% of 20- to 24-year-olds report having been forced to have intercourse or had a first intercourse that was nonvoluntary (Gavin et al., 2009). Oral sex is common among adolescents aged 15 to 19, with 54% of females and 55% of males in this age group having had oral sex (Lindberg, Jones, & Santelli, 2008). Adolescents often face peer pressure to be sexually active. An additional motivation for sexual activity for girls may be a desire for sexual intimacy rather than a wish for the physical act of intercourse.

Early Adulthood and Midlife

In early adulthood (ages 20 to 40 years), women achieve maturity in a sexual role and in the relationship tasks started in adolescence, including developing intimacy with another individual and development of long-term commitment to a sexual relationship. Important career and personal decisions are made and increasing responsibilities assumed; balancing relationships, career, and children is often a concern. Women face choices regarding sexual lifestyles and often experience several before settling into one. During these years, a woman continues to develop her personal sexual value system and must learn to be tolerant of others' sexual values. At some point during a woman's 20s and 30s, she faces decisions about childbearing. Throughout these years, frequency of sexual activity typically decreases (Fogel, 2003).

In midlife (40 to 60 years of age), women's sexuality is as varied as are women. Some women report that sex is very good, possibly the best ever. Others report that sex is not the driving force it once was, or that sex is less exciting and gratifying. The physiologic changes associated with menopause can affect sexual desire, expression, and functioning (North American Menopause Society [NAMS], 2007). Fluctuating levels of estrogen and related vasomotor instability can result in sleep disturbances associated with hot flashes; the resulting fatigue can adversely affect sexual desire. In the years immediately before and after menopause, some women may report a loss of sexual desire associated with decreased vaginal lubrication, vaginal dryness, dyspareunia, painful spasms of the vaginal muscles, loss of clitoral sensations, fewer orgasms, or decreased depth of orgasm (Bachmann & Leiblum, 2004; Northrup, 2001). In contrast, other women may report increased sexual desire, increased clitoral sensitivity, increased responsiveness, and an increase in orgasms (Northrup). For some women, a decreased concern of becoming pregnant may increase sexual desire and lessen inhibitions.

Older Adulthood

During older adulthood (after age 65), women continue to be sexual and enjoy sexual activity. Although sexual frequency and intensity may decline, sexual enjoyment sometimes increases with age (Alexander et al., 2007). The need for excitement, pleasure, and intimacy does not fade with aging. A critical issue for older women's sexual expression and activity is availability of a partner. Another important factor is which forms of intimacy a woman and her partner find acceptable, because many older women are interested in sexual activity that is not intercourse oriented (Baram & Basson, 2007).

Satisfaction with one's sexual function is also influenced by self-evaluation within the context of personal desires and expectations. Personal expectations are often based on cultural and social factors as well as past sexual experiences. The prevailing cultural view of older women as asexual beings can negatively affect sexual expression and activity, and often becomes a self-fulfilling prophecy. Further, the current cultural emphasis on youth, beauty, and thinness also contributes to societal expectations about asexuality in older women.

The physiologic changes associated with aging (decreased estrogen supply, decreased tissue elasticity, thinning of vaginal tissues) can cause irritation or discomfort with penetration and contribute to lessened desire and activity. In addition, the vascular changes that occur in arousal and the intensity of muscular contractions with orgasm may diminish moderately during and after menopause (NAMS, 2007). Loss of fatty tissue in the labia and mons pubis may result in tenderness and easily damaged tissue or abrasions, which may also decrease sexual libido and functioning. Orgasms may decrease in intensity and, in some women, become painful. Breast size also decreases and the breasts may sag. While these changes may alter a woman's sexual view of herself, they do not affect her ability to respond sexually. Rather, body changes may require that a woman and her partners alter how they engage in sexual activity. With aging, sexual practices may include the use of a water-soluble lubricant, increased foreplay for arousal, different sexual positions, and planning intercourse for times when energy levels are highest.

Childbearing

Sexuality is a concern for many women and their partners during pregnancy and postpartum as they experience the changes associated with childbearing. At the same time, these changes offer an opportunity to discuss sexuality and provide education for a couple's changing needs (Allen & Fountain, 2007). Women may experience changes in sexuality, including levels of libido and frequency of sexual activity, with each trimester of pregnancy. During the first trimester, desire and functioning may be inhibited by nausea and vomiting, breast tenderness, fatigue, and anxiety about the pregnancy. In the second trimester, women often express heightened desire as they feel better, although some may be inhibited by their increasing weight and bodily changes. Women may experience diminished sexual desire and activity during the third trimester associated with physical discomfort related to increasing size, especially when they are near term. Fears about the effect of intercourse on pregnancy maintenance and harming the fetus may decrease sexual interest or pleasure at any time during pregnancy. A woman's partner may also experience decreased interest in sexual activity as his view of her shifts from partner to mother. Both partners may experience reticence associated with the presence of a third person (the fetus) in their relationship (Fogel, 2003).

During the postpartum period, women frequently report lessened sexual desire and decreased sexual activity (Hicks, Goodall, Quattrone, & Lydon-Rochelle, 2004). Sleep loss, exhaustion, and physical discomforts, including dyspareunia, are common among women in the postpartum period (Declercq, Sakala, Corry, & Applebaum, 2008) and may contribute to decreased desire and activity. Early postpartum physical symptoms, such as lochia and increased vaginal discharge, are often not conducive to sexual desire or activity. Once the initial vaginal discharge has subsided, women may notice marked vaginal dryness associated with decreased levels of estrogen and progesterone. Although vaginal dryness is more common among women who are breastfeeding, it can occur in any postpartum woman and may require some form of lubrication to prevent dyspareunia (Palmer & Likis, 2003).

Finally, motherhood allows little privacy and little rest—both of which are necessary for sexual pleasure.

Infertility

Struggles with infertility and repeated attempts to conceive can have a negative effect on sexual desire, arousal, orgasm, and satisfaction (Nelson, Shindel, Naughton, Ohebshalom, & Mulhall, 2008). Fertility and virility seem to be inextricably linked in our society. A diagnosis of infertility may negatively affect a woman's sense of sexuality, her self-image, and even her marriage. For women who desire pregnancy, stress and the need to time intercourse may interfere with pleasure and communication, as couples no longer have sex for pleasure, but rather only for procreation. Years of attempting to conceive and bear a child may make spontaneous sex less likely to occur. Sexuality is an important source of communication and growth in the development of a couple's relationship. When the desired end result of sexual activity is reproduction, sex can become mechanical or demanding. Women may initiate sexual activity around the time of ovulation even if they are experiencing low or decreased desire. For their part, because they are reacting to a feeling of threat or perhaps resent the call for "sex on demand," men may experience reactive impotence, or the inability to perform sexually, especially around the time of ovulation.

Sociocultural Influences

Women's sexuality exists within the context of cultural expectations, individual experiences, and biologic potential. Social influences on sexuality first begin within the family. Through socialization of the individual, a family conveys its own, as well as society's, sexual attitudes and behaviors, and may contribute to later sexual dysfunction. Restrictive family upbringing or a belief that expressions of intimacy or sexuality are shameful or taboo may contribute to a woman's inability to express herself sexually.

Religion also influences sexual attitudes, beliefs, and values, and can exert a strong influence throughout a person's life. Religious proscriptions can contribute to sexual concerns or problems. For example, a view that sexual intercourse is acceptable only for procreation may raise concerns when pleasurable sensations are felt. Accepting or rejecting premarital sex, allowing or limiting contraception to prevent pregnancy, beliefs about monogamy for men and women, and condoning or rejecting homosexuality are examples of religious influences in a woman's life.

Society and culture are inextricably interwoven with sexuality and influence it as much as physiology and psychology. Society defines what sexual behavior is, defines the norms for that behavior, and guides the behavior of the individuals in a given culture. In part, women form their ideas of what is sexually appropriate and desirable from years of cultural scripting. These scripts are frequently different for men and women and can be the basis for many of the issues women experience in sexual relationships. The notions that men who are sexually aggressive are "macho" or "studs" and that sexually aggressive women are "whores" and "easy" are examples of such cultural beliefs. In addition, current sex role stereotypes prescribe that men initiate sexual activity and that women exercise control.

Sexual myths are common in every culture and society, are a source of sexual misinformation, and can be related to many sexual problems. Often they interfere with women reaching full sexual potential and establishing fulfilling sexual relationships. Many sexual myths exist today (Fogel, 2003; Smith, 1997). Examples include the ideas that women's needs are secondary to men's, that large amounts of sexual stimulation are needed to arouse a woman, and that when a woman says "no" she doesn't mean it. Other sexual myths are specific to elderly women, such as statements that older women are not interested in or capable of sexual expression, or that older women are physically unattractive and sexually undesirable.

A specific behavior may be defined as desirable by one cultural group and evil by another. Different views often exist regarding premarital, extramarital, and marital sex; appropriate sexual positions; accepted foreplay activities; and duration of coitus. Certainly cultural practices that physically alter sexual response, such as female circumcision (see Chapter 6), will affect sexuality.

Health-Related Influences

A number of health-related factors, including illness, surgery, disability, medications, and substance abuse, can influence sexuality and sexual performance. Illness may affect sexuality in a number of ways, and a variety of medical conditions can cause sexual dysfunction in women (**Box 11-2**). Chronic illness, with its associated fatigue, pain, and stress, affects sexual desire and arousal more often than it affects orgasm. Many medications can alter sexual functioning and cause sexual dysfunction, including anorgasmia and inadequate lubrication (**Box 11-3**). The degree of impairment is often dose related.

All cancers can affect sexuality and intimacy (Hordern, 2008). The accompanying changes in body image and self-concept may have a profound influence on sexuality (Rogers & Kristjanson, 2002). For example, in our society, where breasts are often viewed as sexual,

---

BOX 11-2 *Medical Conditions Associated with Altered Sexual Functioning in Women*

Adrenal disease	Hypertension
Arthritis	Malnutrition
Cancers	Neurologic disorders, such as multiple sclerosis
Cerebrovascular accident	and spinal cord injury
Chronic obstructive pulmonary disease	Oopherectomy
Coronary artery disease	Overactive bladder
Depression	Renal failure
Diabetes	Thyroid disorders
Hyperprolactinemia	Urinary incontinence

Sources: Adapted from Basson & Schultz, 2007; Clayton, 2007; EngenderHealth, 2004.

BOX 11-3 *Medications Adversely Affecting Sexual Functioning*

Antiandrogens	Diuretics
Cyproterone acetate	Spironolactone
Flutamide	Thiazides
Gonadotropin-releasing hormone (GnRH)	Estrogen
agonists	Narcotics
Anticonvulsants	Psychotropics
Antihistamines	Antidepressants
Antihypertensives	Antipsychotics
Alpha blockers	Benzodiazepines
Beta blockers	Mood stabilizers

Sources: Adpated from Baram & Basson, 2007; Basson & Schultz, 2007.

---

a woman with breast cancer may have sexuality concerns. Greater sexuality problems may be experienced by women who dislike their breasts, have a negative self-image, have been sexually abused, lack a support system, or are uncomfortable discussing personal or sexual concerns (Bernhard, 1995). Treatment of gynecologic cancer can affect sexual health as well. For example, radiation therapy can cause vaginal pain and dryness, and oophorectomy causes surgical menopause. The side effects of treatment, such as fatigue, nausea, and vomiting, can also adversely influence sexual functioning (Bodurka & Sun, 2006). Results of studies on the effect of a hysterectomy on sexuality vary, but most women report that experience improved sexual function after hysterectomy (Mokate, Wright, & Mander, 2006).

Disability can affect a woman's sexuality in various ways. Women who are disabled are often viewed as asexual by clinicians and the public alike (Cesario, 2002), and often are not encouraged to express their sexual feelings or to be sexually active. Clinicians often lack sufficient knowledge to provide women with disabilities with adequate information about sexuality (Schopp, Sanford, Hagglund, Gay, & Coatney, 2002). The specific physical effects of a given disability on sexual activity differ according to the condition and its severity. For example, women with spinal cord injuries commonly report autonomic dysreflexia (Schopp et al., 2002).

Sexually transmitted infections (STIs), including infection with the human immunodeficiency virus (HIV), are transmitted within the context of an interpersonal relationship and have the potential to affect a woman's sexuality and sexual functioning. Women who have been diagnosed with an STI often experience depression, low self-esteem, guilt, lack of trust, and anger (Fogel, 2003). The adoption of safer sex practices necessitates altered sexual practices. Sexual risk-reduction practices may require individuals to give up behavior that has been enjoyable, gratifying, highly reinforced, and often of long duration, and replace it with alternatives that are almost always less gratifying, more awkward, or inconvenient, and more difficult than current behaviors (Kelly & Kalichman, 1995). Women may decide to avoid the risk of contracting STIs by being celibate, by decreasing the number of their partners or avoiding certain partners, and by changing or avoiding specific sexual activities that increase risk. The risk of sexual coercion may be great for women in power-imbalanced relationships with men who resist using condoms. Sex roles and sexual double standards may hinder a woman's ability to ask for safer sex practices and contribute to a man's resistance toward implementing these practices.

Chemical dependency can have an adverse effect on sexual functioning and sexuality. Sexual dysfunction, especially sexual desire disorders, can occur with the use of substances such as alcohol, amphetamines, cocaine, opioids, sedatives, and tranquilizers (Zerbe, 1999). Women who use illicit substances may also trade sex for drugs and money.

Relationship and Partner Factors

Women are more likely than men to associate sex with love and commitment, and a woman's subjective perception of sexual pleasure is influenced by her perception of her relationship with her partner. Women have reported that their most pleasurable sexual feelings arose in response to intercourse with a partner, although their most profound physical responses occurred through masturbation (Darling, Davidson, & Jennings, 1991). Relationship discord may precipitate sexual dysfunction—so much so that many sex therapists believe that sexual dysfunction is a symptom of underlying relationship dysfunction. Open communication of one's sexual preferences, feelings, and desires is essential for sexual satisfaction. One or both partners may experience difficulty after disclosure of sexual activity outside the relationship. Sexual communication difficulties can be exacerbated by distrust, feelings of betrayal, and fear of disease. Sexual dysfunction in one partner may precipitate dysfunction in the other partner. For example, erectile difficulty in the male is often accompanied by lack of vaginal lubrication, orgasmic difficulties, and impaired desire disorders in the female.

Loss of one's partner can adversely affect sexuality. Many women define their identity through their relationships, such that loss of a partner may create a loss of sense of self. Further, the typical image of a widow is that of a grieving woman whose sexual life has ended. Factors that may be related to a woman's sexuality after loss of a partner are her extramarital sexual experiences, age, and sexual satisfaction in the marriage (Bernhard, 1995). Remarriage is correlated with age; the older a woman is when she loses a partner, the less likely she is to remarry.

Sexual Assessment

To provide satisfactory sexual health care, clinicians must be comfortable with their own sexuality, aware of their own biases, and have a sincere desire to assist their patients. When sexual health care is provided, it is essential that clinicians not make assumptions regarding a woman's sexual attitudes, values, feelings, or behavior. Additionally, clinicians need to know how various health problems, diseases, and their treatment affect sexual functioning and sexuality. Sexual health assessment includes a physiologic, psychologic, and sociocultural evaluation that entails obtaining a history, conducting a physical examination, and performing laboratory tests.

History

The sexual history is the most important aspect of the assessment process in relation to sexuality. Yet clinicians are often reluctant to ask about their patients' sexual histories or lifestyles (Warner, Rowe, & Whipple, 1999). Factors contributing to clinicians not obtaining adequate information about a woman's sexuality include not seeing the woman's sexual history as relevant to her health problem, inadequate training, embarrassment, and fear of offending.

Clinicians should take responsibility for introducing topics of sexual health problems. As with any interview, it is important to establish a positive tone before beginning. Rapport needs to be developed and sufficient time for building trust needs to be allowed before soliciting information that the woman may consider highly personal or intimate. Choose a quiet, private place where the woman can be comfortable and where interruptions can be minimized. Have the woman remain dressed and sit at eye level with her. Such measures foster a sense of acceptance and respect for the woman and reduce her possible feelings of intimidation. Do not allow anyone other than the woman to be present during this portion of the history to facilitate a candid, open discussion. Women should be assured that all information obtained during an oral history is confidential, although chart documentation is not. Further, any information that is obtained from a form completed by the woman also may not be confidential. It is not necessary to collect all the information at the same time, and a sexual history can be collected over several visits, especially when the woman is very anxious.

It is essential for clinicians to continually monitor their own responses for negative or uncomfortable feelings because these reactions are easily conveyed to patients. Usually more information is obtained if you begin with open-ended questions and allow the woman to tell her story in the way she is most comfortable. Women should be told why questions are being asked. Limits can be set if women offer excessive or irrelevant information. Women should be redirected if information becomes tangential, and encouragement should be provided if progress is slow.

It is best to begin with less threatening material, such as the woman's obstetric history or childhood sexual education, and move to more sensitive topics such as her current sexual practices. A general guide is to begin with questions about an individual's sexual education history (e.g., How did you learn about sex?), proceed to personal attitudes and beliefs about sexuality, and finally assess actual sexual behaviors.

Avoid using excessive medical terminology during an interview; both the clinician and the woman need to know the meaning of terms used. Euphemisms such as "slept with" should not be used. Only one question should be asked at a time, and the woman should be given enough time to answer. Statistical questions such as "How many times a week do you have sexual intercourse?" are not helpful because normal practices vary extensively among individuals. Rather than asking about a particular sexual experience, which people tend to deny, it is better to ask how many times the experience has occurred. This technique suggests that the experience is normal. Techniques such as universalizing or prefacing questions by comments such as "Many people …" or "Other women I have talked with have said …" may make a woman feel more comfortable when answering sensitive questions.

A sexual history can be incorporated into a total health history, or it can be more formal and inclusive. A number of formats are available for use, and the reader is referred to references that cover various approaches (Baram & Basson, 2007; Fogel, 2003; Frank, Mistretta, & Will, 2008; MacLauren, 1995). In most cases, sexual concerns or problems can be uncovered by asking a few questions (**Box 11-4**). While the specific form of sexual history to be used will vary depending on the woman, it is essential to include questions about her body image, concerns relating to sexual functioning, changes that have occurred in sexual function in the past six months or since the last visit, degree of satisfaction with sex life, and health conditions, medications, or treatments that affect sexual function. Women can also be asked to describe their present relationship and to rate this relationship with respect to communication, affection, sexual needs met, and sexual communication. If the woman is in more than one relationship, inquire about each relationship. A complete gynecologic history (see Chapter 6) is relevant and should also be obtained. Detailed assessment of risk for STIs can be found in Chapter 21.

Physical Examination and Diagnostic Studies

When it is indicated by history, reason for seeking care, treatment goals, or need for referral, a physical examination may be performed. While there are no studies specific to sexual assessment, often the history and physical examination may suggest that a specific laboratory test should be performed. Physical examination and diagnostic studies to be considered in the evaluation of sexual concerns can be found in Chapter 17.

BOX 11-4 *Questions Included in a Sexual History*

- Are you sexually active? Alternate questions include Are you sexually involved? and Are you having sexual relations?
- Are you having any sexual difficulties or problems at this time? Do you have any pain?
- Has any (illness, pregnancy, surgery) interfered with your being a partner? Has any (illness, surgery, medication, treatment) changed how you feel about yourself as a woman? Has any (disease, surgery, medication, treatment) altered your ability to function sexually?
- Is sex pleasurable for you (desire)? Are you having difficulty with lubrication during sex (arousal)? Are you able to have an orgasm/climax (orgasm)? Do you have any pain or discomfort during sexual activity (pain)?
- Are you satisfied with your sexual activity? Is it satisfactory? Are you happy with it?
- Do you have any sexual problems or questions?
- Do you limit physical contact with your partner because you are afraid it will lead to sex?
- Do you become irritated when your sexual partner initiates sex?
- Do you feel that having sex is an imposition?

Conclusion

Sexuality begins with conception and develops throughout a woman's life. Sexual problems are among the most common of human concerns and will be experienced by most people, if only briefly, at some point in their lives. It is essential for clinicians caring for women to have a working knowledge of sexual functioning and to provide a nonjudgmental, supportive approach so that women are comfortable in discussing issues related to sexuality. Clinicians can promote healthy sexual functioning by fostering communication, providing accurate information and counseling, and, when needed, making appropriate referrals to other health professionals.

References

Alexander, L. L., LaRosa, J. H., Bader, H., & Garfield, S. (2007). *New dimensions in women's health* (4th ed.). Sudbury, MA: Jones and Bartlett.

Allen, L., & Fountain, L. (2007). Addressing sexuality and pregnancy in childbirth education classes. *Journal of Perinatal Education, 16*, 32–36.

Amaro, H., Navarro, A. M., Conron, K. J., & Raj, A. (2002). Cultural influences on women's sexual health. In G. M. Wingood & R. J. DiClemente (Eds.), *Handbook of women's sexual and reproductive health* (pp. 71–92). New York: Kluwer Academic/Plenum.

American Psychiatric Association. (1994). *Diagnostic and statistical manual of mental disorders* (4th ed.). Washington, DC: Author.

Bachmann, G. A., & Leiblum, S. R. (2004). The impact of hormones on menopausal sexuality: A literature review. *Menopause: The Journal of the North American Menopause Society, 11*(1), 120–130.

Baram, D. A., & Basson, R. (2007). Sexuality, sexual dysfunction, and sexual assault. In J. S. Berek (Ed.), *Berek and Novak's gynecology* (14th ed., pp. 313–349). Philadelphia: Lippincott Williams & Wilkins.

Basson, R. (2000). The female sexual response: A different model. *Journal of Sex & Marital Therapy, 26*, 51–65.

Basson, R., Leiblum, S., Brotto, L., Derogatis, L., Fourcroy, J., Fugl-Meyer, K., ... Schultz, W. W. (2004). Revised definitions of women's sexual dysfunction. *Journal of Sexual Medicine, 1*, 40–48.

Basson, R., & Schultz, W. W. (2007). Sexual sequelae of general medical disorders. *Lancet, 369*, 409–424.

Bernhard, L. (1995). Sexuality in women's lives. In C. I. Fogel & N. F. Woods (Eds.), *Women's health care* (pp. 475–495). Thousand Oaks, CA: Sage.

Bodurka, D. C., & Sun, C. C. (2006). Sexual function after gynecologic cancer. *Obstetrics & Gynecology Clinics of North America, 33*, 621–630.

Cesario, S. K. (2002). Spinal cord injuries: Nurses can help affected women and their families achieve pregnancy, birth. *Association of Women's Health, Obstetric, and Neonatal Nurses Lifelines, 6*, 224–232.

Chalker, R. (1994). Updating the model of female sexuality. *Sexuality Information and Education Council of the United States, 22*, 1–6.

Clayton, A. H. (2007). Epidemiology and neurobiology of female sexual dysfunction. *Journal of Sexual Medicine, 4*(suppl 4), 260–268.

Darling, C. A., Davidson, J. K., & Jennings, D. A. (1991). The female sexual response revisited: Understanding the multiorgasmic experiences in women. *Archives of Sexual Behavior, 20*, 535.

Declercq, E. R., Sakala, C., Corry, M. P., & Applebaum, S. (2008). *New mothers speak out: National survey results highlight women's postpartum experiences.* New York: Childbirth Connection.

Eaton, D. K., Kann, L., Kinchen, S., Shanklin, S., Ross, J., Hawkins, J., ... Wechsler, H. (2008). Youth risk behavior surveillance—United States, 2007. *MMWR Surveillance Summaries, 57*(SS04), 1–131.

Edwards, W. M., & Coleman, E. (2004). Defining sexual health: A descriptive overview. *Archives of Sexual Behavior, 33*, 189–195.

EngenderHealth. (2004). Sexuality and sexual health: Online minicourse. Retrieved November 9, 2004, from http://www.engenderhealth.org/res/onc/sexuality/index.html

Fogel, C. I. (2003). Women and sexuality. In E. Q. Youngkin & M. S. Davis (Eds.), *Women's health: A primary* care clinical guide (3rd ed., pp. 109–129). Upper Saddle River, NJ: Pearson Prentice Hall.

Fogel, C. I., & Woods, N. F. (2008). Women's sexuality. In C. I. Fogel & N. F. Woods (Eds.), *Women's health care in advanced practice nursing* (pp. 295–312). New York: Springer.

Frank, J. E., Mistretta, P., & Will, J. (2008). Diagnosis and treatment of female sexual dysfunction. *American Family Physician, 77*, 635–642.

Gavin, L., MacKay, A. P., Brown, K., Harrier, S., Ventura, S. J., & Kann, L. (2009). Sexual and reproductive health of persons aged 10–24 years—United States, 2002–2007. *MMWR Surveillance Summaries, 58*(SS06), 1–58.

Hicks, T. L., Goodall, S. F., Quattrone, E. M., & Lydon-Rochelle, M. T. (2004). Postpartum sexual functioning and method of delivery: Summary of the evidence. *Journal of Midwifery & Women's Health, 49*, 430–436.

Hordern, A. (2008). Intimacy and sexuality after cancer: A critical review of the literature. *Cancer Nursing, 31*, E9–E17.

Kaplan, H. (1979). *Disorders of sexual desire and other new concepts and techniques in sex therapy*. New York: Brunner/Mazel.

Kelly, J. A., & Kalichman, S. C. (1995). Increased attention to human sexuality can improve HIV-AIDS prevention efforts: Key research issues and directions. *Journal of Consulting and Clinical Psychology, 63*(6), 907–918.

Lindberg, L. D., Jones, R., & Santelli, J. S. (2008). Noncoital sexual activities among adolescents. *Journal of Adolescent Health, 43*, 231–238.

MacLaren, A. (1995). Comprehensive sexual assessment. *Journal of Nurse-Midwifery, 40*(2), 104–119.

Masters, W., & Johnson, V. (1966). *The human sexual response cycle*. Boston: Little, Brown.

Masters, W. H., Johnson, V. E., & Kolodney, R. C. (1995). *Human sexuality* (5th ed.). New York: Harper-Collins.

McCall, K., & Meston, C. (2006). Cues resulting in desire for sexual activity in women. *Journal of Sexual Medicine, 3*, 838–852.

Mokate, R., Wright, C., & Mander, T. (2006). Hysterectomy and sexual function. *Journal of the British Menopause Society, 12*, 153–157.

Nelson, C. J., Shindel, A. W., Naughton, C. K., Ohebshalom, M., & Mulhall, J. P. (2008). Prevalence and predictors of sexual problems, relationship stress, and depression in female partners of infertile couples. *Journal of Sexual Medicine, 5*, 1907–1914.

North American Menopause Society (NAMS). (2007). *Menopause practice: A clinician's guide* (3rd ed.). Cleveland, OH: Author.

Northrup, C. (1998). *Women's bodies, women's wisdom*. New York: Bantam Books.

Northrup, C. (2001). *The wisdom of menopause*. New York: Bantam Books.

Palmer, A. R., & Likis, F. E. (2003). Lactational atrophic vaginitis. *Journal of Midwifery & Women's Health, 48*, 282–284.

Rogers, M., & Kristjanson, L. J. (2002). The impact on sexual functioning of chemotherapy-induced menopause in women with breast cancer. *Cancer Nursing, 25*(1), 57–65.

Schopp, L. H., Sanford, T. C., Hagglund, K. J., Gay, J. W., & Coatney, M. A. (2002). Removing service barriers for women with physical disabilities: Promoting accessibility in the gynecologic care setting. *Journal of Midwifery & Women's Health, 47*, 74–79.

Smith, R. P. (1997). *Gynecology in primary care*. Baltimore: Williams & Wilkins.

Tiefer, L. (1991). Historical, scientific, clinical, and feminist criticisms of "the human sexual response cycle." *Annual Review of Sex Research, 2*, 1–23.

Warner, P. H., Rowe, T., & Whipple, B. (1999). Shedding light on the sexual history. *American Journal of Nursing, 99*(6), 34–40.

World Health Organization (WHO). (2006). *Defining sexual health: Report of a technical consultation on sexual health, 28–31 January 2002, Geneva*. Geneva, Switzerland: Author.

World Health Organization (WHO) Regional Office for Europe. (2001). *WHO regional strategy on sexual and reproductive health*. Copenhagen, Denmark: Author.

Zerbe, K. J. (1999). *Women's mental health in primary care*. Philadelphia: Saunders.

12

Contraception

Patricia Aikins Murphy
Katherine Morgan
Frances E. Likis

Contraceptive management is often a challenging undertaking, but providing family planning services offers clinicians the opportunity to empower people by helping them to make choices that can truly alter their life courses. More than 62 million women of reproductive age reside in the United States. Seven in 10 of these women, or about 43 million women, are sexually active and do not want to become pregnant (Alan Guttmacher Institute, 2010). The average woman in the United States desires two children and, therefore, must use contraception for approximately three decades of her life. Sixty-three percent of U.S. women of reproductive age who practice contraception use reversible methods (Alan Guttmacher Institute). Among women experiencing an unintended pregnancy, 46% had not used a contraceptive method during the month they became pregnant. The majority of women who were using some contraceptive method at the time of an unintended pregnancy report inconsistent or incorrect use (Jones, Darroch, & Henshaw, 2002).

When it comes to contraception, the challenge lies in helping each woman choose the method that best meets her needs and providing education so that she can use the chosen method correctly and consistently. Unfortunately, there is no perfect contraceptive method—one that requires no effort, never fails, has no side effects, is easily affordable, and reverses immediately. The good news is that more contraceptive options are available now than ever before.

Contraceptive users today want more than efficacy from a method. They desire a method that is safe, convenient, and cost-effective, and that has few side effects. How a method affects a woman's life—from side effects such as daily spotting to the need to remember to do something every day—may be a major determinant in consistency of use. In addition, knowledge about the noncontraceptive health benefits of some methods is increasing; this background enables women to make contraceptive choices that can have positive implications for their health. Most therapeutic uses of contraception are not approved by the U.S. Food and Drug Administration (FDA), although many are supported by evidence gathered through research studies. Clinicians frequently prescribe medications for conditions other than those for which they have FDA approval, and this off-label use is within the scope of prescriptive authority when sound rationale and evidence are used (FDA, 2009).

Contraceptive counseling should never be guided by a clinician's biases about what is best for a particular patient. Rather, the best method for any woman is the one that she wants and is motivated to use. Clinicians should present all of the choices that are reasonable (i.e., those that are acceptable in light of the individual history) and assist each woman to find her own best option. Clinicians should rely only on evidence-based contraindications to avoid unnecessarily restricting contraceptive options when determining whether the patient's history makes a particular method acceptable. The U.S. *Medical Eligibility Criteria for Contraceptive Use* (Centers for Disease Control and Prevention [CDC], 2010), which are adapted from the World Health Organization's (WHO) *Medical Eligibility Criteria for Contraceptive Use* (2009), are helpful in determining whether a woman is a candidate for a particular method (see Appendix 12-A for these guidelines). A thorough knowledge of the contraceptive methods available is imperative for providing contraceptive counseling that leads to a fully informed choice. Women usually use contraception in the context of a relationship, so their partners may need education as well. A woman may at times need supportive counseling to negotiate contraceptive issues within her relationship.

This chapter provides an overview of the various methods of contraception. Data on efficacy and effectiveness, safety and side effects, noncontraceptive benefits, and the advantages and disadvantages of each method are presented. A full discussion of contraceptive counseling and management is beyond the scope of this chapter, but interested readers are referred to the bibliography at the end of the chapter, which suggests resources for further research.

Contraceptive Efficacy and Effectiveness

The effectiveness of contraceptive methods is described in several ways. *Efficacy*, sometimes referred to as "method failure" or "perfect use" failure rates, is how well a method works inherently. Efficacy describes the likelihood that an unintended pregnancy will occur even when the method is used consistently and exactly as prescribed. In most research studies, pregnancies that result from inconsistent use or incorrect use are not included in "method failure" rates. *Effectiveness*, also termed "user failure" or "typical use" failure rates, is how well a method works in actual practice. Effectiveness describes all unintended pregnancies that occur if a method is not used properly, such as in the case of inconsistent or incorrect use. The terms "efficacy" and "effectiveness" are often used interchangeably when discussing contraception (Grimes, 2009; Trussell, 2007).

Not all contraceptive failures qualify as "user failures." Indeed, all contraceptive methods have inherent failure rates. Unintended pregnancies may occur even with highly effective methods such as sterilization (**Table 12-1**). Methods that are highly dependent on user

TABLE 12-1 Percentage of Women Experiencing an Unintended Pregnancy During the First Year of Typical Use and the First Year of Perfect Use of Contraception and the Percentage Continuing Use at the End of the First Year, United States

Method	% of Women Experiencing an Unintended Pregnancy Within the First Year of Use		% of Women Continuing Use at One Year[3]
	Typical Use[1]	Perfect Use[2]	
No method[4]	85	85	—
Spermicides[5]	29	18	42
Withdrawal	27	4	43
Fertility awareness–based methods	25	—	51
Standard days method[6]	—	5	—
Two-day method[6]	—	4	—
Ovulation method[6]	—	3	—
Sponge			
Parous women	32	20	46
Nulliparous women	16	9	57
Diaphragm[7]	16	6	57
Condom[8]			
Female (Reality)	21	5	49
Male	15	2	53
Combined pill and progestin-only pill	8	0.3	68
Evra patch	8	0.3	68
NuvaRing	8	0.3	68
Depo-Provera	3	0.3	56
IUD			
ParaGard (copper T)	0.8	0.6	78
Mirena (LNG-IUS)	0.2	0.2	80
Implanon	0.05	0.05	84
Female sterilization	0.5	0.5	100
Male sterilization	0.15	0.10	100

(continues)

TABLE 12-1 Percentage of Women Experiencing an Unintended Pregnancy During the First Year of Typical Use and the First Year of Perfect Use of Contraception and the Percentage Continuing Use at the End of the First Year, United States   *(Continued)*

Emergency contraceptive pills: Treatment initiated within 72 hours after unprotected intercourse reduces the risk of pregnancy by at least 75%.[9]

Lactational amenorrhea method (LAM): LAM is a highly effective, *temporary* method of contraception.[10]

---

[1] Among *typical* couples who initiate use of a method (not necessarily for the first time), the percentage who experience an accidental pregnancy during the first year if they do not stop use for any other reason. Estimates of the probability of pregnancy during the first year of typical use for spermicides, withdrawal, periodic abstinence, the diaphragm, the male condom, the pill, and Depo-Provera are taken from the 1995 National Survey of Family Growth corrected for underreporting of abortion; see the text for the derivation of estimates for the other methods.

[2] Among couples who initiate use of a method (not necessarily for the first time) and who use it *perfectly* (both consistently and correctly), the percentage who experience an accidental pregnancy during the first year if they do not stop use for any other reason. See the text for the derivation of the estimate for each method.

[3] Among couples attempting to avoid pregnancy, the percentage who continue to use a method for 1 year.

[4] The percentages becoming pregnant in columns (2) and (3) are based on data from populations where contraception is not used and from women who cease using contraception in order to become pregnant. Among such populations, about 89% become pregnant within 1 year. This estimate was lowered slightly (to 85%) to represent the percentage who would become pregnant within 1 year among women now relying on reversible methods of contraception if they abandoned contraception altogether.

[5] Foams, creams, gels, vaginal suppositories, and vaginal film.

[6] The ovulation and two-day methods are based on evaluation of cervical mucus. The standard days method avoids intercourse on cycle days 8 through 19.

[7] With spermicidal cream or jelly.

[8] Without spermicides.

[9] The treatment schedule is one dose within 120 hours after unprotected intercourse, and a second dose 12 hours after the first dose. Both doses of Plan B can be taken at the same time. Plan B (1 dose is 1 white pill) is the only dedicated product specifically marketed for emergency contraception. The U. S. Food and Drug Administration has in addition declared the following 22 brands of oral contraceptives to be safe and effective for emergency contraception: Ogestrel or Ovral (1 dose is 2 white pills), Levlen or Nordette (1 dose is 4 light-orange pills), Cryselle, Levora, Low-Ogestrel, Lo/Ovral or Quasence (1 dose is 4 white pills), Tri-Levlen or Triphasil (1 dose is 4 yellow pills), Jolessa, Portia, Seasonale or Trivora (1 dose is 4 pink pills), Seasonique (1 dose is 4 light-blue-green pills), Empresse (1 dose is 4 orange pills), Alesse, Lessina or Levlite (1 dose is 5 pink pills), Aviane (1 dose is 5 orange pills), and Lutera (1 dose is 5 white pills).

[10] However, to maintain effective protection against pregnancy, another method of contraception must be used as soon as menstruation resumes, the frequency or duration of breastfeeds is reduced, bottle feeds are introduced, or the baby reaches 6 months of age.

Source: Reprinted with permission from Trussell, J. (2007). Contraceptive efficacy. In R. A. Hatcher, J. Trussell, A. L. Nelson, W. Cates, F. H. Stewart, & D. Kowal (Eds.), *Contraceptive technology* (19th ed.). New York: Ardent Media.

---

consistency may have higher failure rates, but not all unintended pregnancies occur as a result of user errors. Clinicians should avoid implying that unintended pregnancies are the user's fault.

In addition to inherent method efficacy and using a method consistently and correctly, several other factors affect contraceptive failure rates. Most failures are concentrated in early usage: More fertile women will have earlier failures, and women who use contraception incorrectly or inconsistently will get pregnant sooner. In addition, older women are less fecund (able to get pregnant) than younger woman; thus any method used by younger women will have a higher failure rate than when the same method is used by older women. Other factors contributing to contraceptive success include the fertility of the male partner, the motivation to avoid pregnancy (as opposed to simply wanting to space pregnancies), relationship status, and frequency of sexual intercourse (Trussell, 2007).

Nonhormonal Methods

The nonhormonal contraceptive methods can be grouped into three general categories:

- Physiologic methods: abstinence, coitus interruptus, lactational amenorrhea method (breastfeeding), and fertility awareness–based (FAB) methods
- Barrier methods: male condoms, vaginal barrier methods, and spermicides
- Sterilization: male and female

One additional contraceptive method that does not contain hormones—the copper intrauterine device (IUD)—is covered in the section on intrauterine contraception. The reversible nonhormonal contraceptive options (physiologic and barrier methods) generally require motivated users, and most of these methods necessitate taking action with every act of sexual intercourse. In general, their efficacy is less than that of hormonal methods, but these options do not have systemic side effects. In addition, many barrier methods do not require involvement of a clinician. Nonhormonal methods may also be chosen because they fit within the woman's cultural beliefs. The irreversible contraceptive options, male and female sterilization, are the only permanent forms of contraception and require certainty that future childbearing is not desired.

Physiologic Methods

Abstinence

Abstaining from penile–vaginal intercourse is the only certain way to avoid pregnancy. Abstinence is most often practiced in conjunction with FAB methods or prior to becoming sexually active. Although abstinence is generally promoted as the method of choice for adolescents, counseling should include all contraceptive options.

Efficacy and Effectiveness Abstinence is 100% effective at preventing pregnancy.

Safety and Side Effects There are no contraindications to or side effects from using abstinence.

Noncontraceptive Benefits There are no noncontraceptive benefits of abstinence.

Advantages and Disadvantages Abstinence is readily available and completely effective. Abstinence prevents sexually transmitted infections (STIs), including infection with the human immunodeficiency virus (HIV) via penile–vaginal transmission, but users must be cautioned to avoid other sexual practices (e.g., oral sex and anal sex) that put them at risk for STIs (see Chapter 21). The major disadvantage of abstinence is that it is unrealistic for most couples in long-term relationships to use abstinence exclusively for an extended period of time.

Coitus Interruptus

Coitus interruptus, also known as withdrawal, is the removal of the penis from the vagina prior to ejaculation. Coitus interruptus prevents pregnancy by keeping sperm from entering the vagina. While only 2.5% of women in the United States using contraception employ coitus interruptus as their primary method, 5.4% of women in the 2002 National Survey of Family Growth report having used withdrawal during the month of their interview and 56% at some time in their lives (Chandra, Martinez, Mosher, Abma, & Jones, 2005).

Efficacy and Effectiveness The theoretical efficacy of coitus interruptus is high, but significant typical-use failure rates have been reported (Table 12-1). However, findings from the 2002 National Survey of Family Growth indicate that the typical-use failure rate of withdrawal is 18%, which is almost the same as the 17% rate for the male condom (Kost, Singh, Vaughan, Trussell, & Bankole, 2008). Studies have also refuted the long-held belief that pre-ejaculatory fluid contains sperm, which could cause pregnancy even if withdrawal was used correctly (Jones, Fennell, Higgins, & Blanchard, 2009; Zukerman, Weiss, & Orvieto, 2003).

Safety and Side Effects There are no contraindications to or side effects from using coitus interruptus.

Noncontraceptive Benefits There are no noncontraceptive benefits of coitus interruptus.

Advantages and Disadvantages Coitus interruptus is readily available, requires no supplies or cost, and is user controlled. Couples can use coitus interruptus intermittently when other methods are unavailable. Disadvantages include the need to use this method with every act of intercourse, and the need to exert the self-discipline and control necessary to stop intercourse. Coitus interruptus does not prevent STI transmission because penile–vaginal contact occurs, and HIV and other STIs can be present in pre-ejaculatory fluid. Women who use coitus interruptus should be educated about emergency contraception as a backup method.

Lactational Amenorrhea Method

Infant suckling during breastfeeding increases maternal prolactin levels, which in turn inhibits ovulation; this is the physiologic basis of the lactational amenorrhea method (LAM) of contraception. Three conditions must be met for LAM to be effective: (1) exclusive or near exclusive breastfeeding, (2) amenorrhea, and (3) infant is younger than 6 months old (Kennedy & Trussell, 2007). Breastfeeding education and support are beneficial for women using LAM.

Efficacy and Effectiveness Breastfeeding is an extremely effective method of contraception if the conditions for use are met (Table 12-1). Failures typically occur when breastfeeding is nonexclusive or after the infant is 6 months old. In these instances, the likelihood of ovulation increases and the woman may be unaware of her return to fertility.

Safety and Side Effects There are no contraindications to LAM, but breastfeeding is not recommended for women who are HIV positive in countries such as the United States where infant formula is accessible, or for women who are taking medications that could be harmful to the infant. The only side effects of LAM are those associated with breastfeeding, such as sore nipples and mastitis.

Noncontraceptive Benefits Women who breastfeed their infants have decreased risk of ovarian, endometrial, and breast cancers (Collaborative Group on Hormonal Factors in Breast Cancer, 2002; Newcomb & Trentham-Dietz, 2000; Whittemore, 1994). Breastfeeding also has numerous benefits for infant health.

Advantages and Disadvantages LAM is readily available, free, and can be used immediately postpartum. The disadvantages of LAM are that it is available only to women who are breastfeeding, its duration of use is limited, and women may have difficulty sustaining the patterns of breastfeeding required to maintain contraceptive effectiveness. In addition, LAM does not provide protection from STIs/HIV.

Fertility Awareness–Based Methods

FAB methods involve determining when a woman is most fertile during each month and using either abstinence or barrier contraception during that time to prevent pregnancy. The "fertile window" or time when intercourse is most likely to result in pregnancy comprises the five days before plus the day of ovulation (Wilcox, Weinberg, & Baird, 1995). FAB methods are also referred to as natural family planning and the rhythm method. Among women in the United States who use contraception, 1% use FAB methods (Chandra et al., 2005).

The fertile window can be identified with calendar methods or by using signs and symptoms of ovulation. Calendar methods require counting the days in the menstrual cycle. The calendar rhythm method entails the woman recording the length of 6 to 12 menstrual cycles and determining the longest and shortest cycles. She then uses that information to identify the first (days in shortest cycle minus 18) and last (days in longest cycle minus 11) fertile day each month. Calculations must be updated with each cycle (Jennings & Arévalo, 2007). This method requires careful calculations that can be confusing; thus the standard days method (SDM) was developed as a simpler calendar method. Women using the SDM are advised to use abstinence or a barrier contraceptive on days 8 to 19 of the menstrual cycle. A color-coded set of beads called CycleBeads can be used in conjunction with the SDM to help women keep track of their fertile window (http://www.cyclebeads.com). The SDM is recommended for women whose cycles are 26 to 32 days in length (Arévalo, Jennings, & Sinai, 2002).

The postovulation method is another variation on the calendar method. With this method, the woman subtracts 14 days from her average cycle length to predict the day of ovulation. Abstinence or a barrier method is used during the first half of the cycle until the fourth morning after the predicted day of ovulation. This method requires the longest period of abstinence or use of additional contraception.

Signs and symptoms of ovulation include a rise in the basal body temperature (BBT) and changes in cervical mucus. The BBT increases at the time of ovulation and remains elevated for the rest of the cycle. Using BBT charting in conjunction with the postovulation observations is beneficial, but predicting the fertile period with BBT is difficult because ovulation has already occurred once the rise in temperature is observed.

The Billings ovulation method uses assessment of cervical mucus to determine the fertile window. Women check daily for the increased, clear, stretchy, slippery cervical secretions associated with ovulation. The fertile time lasts from the day when ovulatory cervical secretions are first observed until four days after they are last observed (Billings, 2001).

The two-day method is a simplified version of the ovulation method. The woman checks daily for cervical secretions and is considered fertile any day that she has cervical secretions present or had them present the day before (Arévalo, Jennings, Nikula, & Sinai, 2004).

The symptothermal method involves observing multiple indicators of the fertile window; the most common combination is assessment of cervical mucus and daily BBT charting. The cervical secretions can be used to identify the beginning of the fertile window, and the BBT can be used to detect the end. Some women using the symptothermal method also assess cervical position and signs of ovulation (e.g., mittelschmerz). Home ovulation tests originally used for women with infertility (e.g., Clearblue Easy Fertility Monitor) can be used in conjunction with the calendar, ovulation, or symptothermal methods to improve their effectiveness (Fehring, 2005).

The detailed information required for patient education about FAB methods is beyond the scope of this chapter. Readers are referred to the websites listed in **Box 12-1** for further information, including training courses for clinicians.

Efficacy and Effectiveness The theoretical efficacy of FAB methods varies according to the specific technique used (Table 12-1). The typical-use failure rate reflects the difficulty of using these methods correctly and consistently.

BOX 12-1 *Websites for Fertility Awareness–Based Methods Information*

Institute for Natural Family Planning: www.marquette.edu/nursing/natural-family-planning
Institute for Reproductive Health: www.irh.org

Safety and Side Effects   There are no health concerns with the use of FAB methods, but certain circumstances or conditions complicate their use. These factors include the postpartum period, breastfeeding, having an abortion immediately before their use, recent menarche or perimenopause when cycles may be irregular, medications that alter the regularity of cycles or fertility signs, vaginal discharge, irregular vaginal bleeding, and conditions associated with elevated body temperature (CDC, 2010). There are no side effects of FAB methods.

Noncontraceptive Benefits   The principles of FAB methods can also be used to conceive when couples decide they want children.

Advantages and Disadvantages   Patients may have to pay for FAB methods training or supplies (e.g., basal body thermometer, CycleBeads), but there is no ongoing cost unless a barrier contraceptive is used during the fertile window. These methods are user controlled and may be the only acceptable form of contraception for some religions and cultures. Disadvantages include the need for detailed education, ongoing attention to identifying the fertile window, and abstaining from intercourse or using an additional contraceptive method several days each month. FAB methods do not protect either partner from STIs, and users should be educated about emergency contraception.

Barrier Methods

The use of physical and chemical barriers for contraception is as old as history. In ancient times, women used vaginal suppositories of crocodile dung, wool, seaweed, or crushed root, often mixed with honey and herbs. Other methods included sea sponges moistened with lemon or vinegar. Condoms made of linen or animal intestines were also commonly used (Tone, 2001). With the development of technology for vulcanized rubber in the mid-1800s, manufacture of condoms and "womb veils" (the term used for devices such as diaphragms and caps) increased dramatically. By the 1870s, women in the United States could purchase these devices from mail-order companies, pharmacies, dry-goods stores, and rubber vendors. Until the development of hormonal and intrauterine contraception in the latter half of the 1900s, these were the only methods other than FAB methods that were available to couples desiring to control their fertility (Tone).

All barrier methods are coitus dependent. They must be applied at the time of intercourse, before any penile penetration, and ideally before any genital contact to avoid disruption in sex play. This requirement may be a problem for some couples due to the need to plan ahead, or for others who find application disruptive. Couples can be taught to make application or insertion of the barrier method part of their sex play. The coitus-dependent nature of barrier methods may be an advantage for couples who have infrequent intercourse.

Although these methods are less effective in preventing pregnancy than contemporary hormonal or intrauterine methods, interest in barrier contraception is on the rise again. This trend partly reflects the hormone-free aspects of barrier methods, but largely indicates recognition of their potential role as dual protection against pregnancy and STIs, including

HIV. The cervix is the point of entry for many sexually transmitted pathogens. Protecting the cervix via chemical or physical barriers is an expanding area of research in the prevention of STIs. Finally, barrier contraceptives can be used by most people because contraindications to the use of these methods are rare (CDC, 2010).

Male Condoms

The male condom is a thin sheath that is placed over the erect penis. It serves as a barrier to pregnancy by trapping seminal fluid and sperm and offers protection against STIs. In fact, early descriptions of condom use in the 1500s emphasized the condom's role in protection from syphilis and other diseases (Tone, 2001).

Latex condoms were first introduced in the mid-1800s. With few exceptions, the design has changed little since then. They are manufactured and packaged with a rolled rim, designed to be applied to the tip of the penis and then rolled down over the erect penis. It is important to note that there is a right side and a wrong side when the condom is rolled up; applying the condom with the wrong side out will prevent it from being placed properly, and potentially contaminate the outside of the condom with seminal fluid. Minor design changes over the years to this rolled-rim construction have included enlarged tips to contain ejaculated fluid (**Figure 12-1**), as well as variety in colors, sizes, flavors, and textured surfaces that are purported to enhance sexual pleasure. Some condoms add lubricants as well, including spermicidal lubricants.

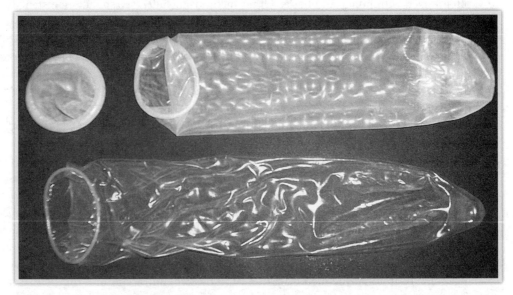

FIGURE 12-1 Male condoms: rolled rim condom as packaged; unrolled condoms with rounded and extended tips.

Nonlatex condoms were developed in response to several concerns about latex condoms. These condoms are made of polyurethane or a latex-like material called styrene ethylene butylene styrene (SEBS). Nonlatex condoms are odorless, colorless, and nonallergenic. They transmit body heat better, and have a looser fit, theoretically allowing more sensitivity. They can be used with any lubricant, and do not usually deteriorate with the use of oil-based lubricants or under adverse storage conditions. Many users prefer the nonlatex condoms over latex (Gallo, Grimes, Lopez, & Schulz, 2006), and these preferences may translate into more consistent use of condoms. Consistent use and consumer familiarity with and education about the product may reduce the higher rates of breakage and slippage that have been reported in studies.

Efficacy and Effectiveness When used correctly and consistently, latex condoms are an effective form of contraception (Gallo et al., 2006) (Table 12-1). Condom failures are commonly related to breakage of the condom, or slippage during intercourse or while removing the condom. In general, pregnancy rates for nonlatex condoms are slightly higher than the corresponding rates for latex condoms, but within the range considered acceptable for barrier methods. However, nonlatex condoms have higher reported rates of breakage and slippage than latex condoms (Gallo et al.). It is unclear whether this difference is related to the product, or to a lack of familiarity with the product.

Safety and Side Effects Latex condoms should not be used by persons with known latex allergies. Some women report genital irritation and discomfort from the use of condoms. This issue may be related either to the condom or to concomitant lubricant use. Some condoms are lubricated with a spermicide (nonoxynol-9), which may produce genital irritation in some women (see the section on spermicides). One study of a polyurethane condom evaluated genital irritation in both men and women. Although no differences were observed among the men in each group, the female partners in the polyurethane group had significantly less genital pain, pruritus, and vaginal pain than their counterparts in the latex condom group (Steiner, Dominik, Rountree, & Dorflinger, 2003).

Noncontraceptive Benefits Condoms are routinely recommended for their noncontraceptive benefit of protection from STIs. Consistent use of latex condoms in sexually active HIV-serodiscordant couples can result in an 80% reduction in the incidence of HIV infection (Weller & Davis-Beaty, 2002). Condoms also offer statistically significant protection against gonorrhea, chlamydia, herpes simplex virus (HSV) type 2, and syphilis, and they may protect women from trichomoniasis (Holmes, Levine, & Weaver, 2004). While condoms do not appear to offer protection against human papillomavirus (HPV) infection, their use is associated with higher rates of cervical intraepithelial neoplasia regression and cervical HPV infection clearance (Holmes et al.).

Advantages and Disadvantages Condoms have the advantage of being widely available on an over-the-counter basis, without the need for clinician visit or prescription. The nonlatex condoms tend to be more expensive than their latex counterparts. The effectiveness of condoms is coitus dependent. (**Box 12-2**). Correct use is critical to prevent breakage, slippage, and resultant unintended pregnancy. A potential disadvantage of using condoms as a contraceptive method is that they are male controlled. Women who are in relationships where they cannot negotiate condom use with their partners need a method they can control.

Spermicides

Spermicides are chemical barriers that are used either alone or in conjunction with a physical barrier (such as a condom, diaphragm, or sponge) to prevent pregnancy. In earlier centuries, douching with chemical substances, insertion of cocoa butter or gelatin suppositories, and foaming tablets made of sodium bicarbonate with boric acid or quinine were popular, albeit not very effective, methods of contraception (Tone, 2001).

All spermicides currently marketed in the United States contain nonoxynol-9 (N-9). This product may be formulated as a gel, cream, foam, suppository, foaming tablet, or film, and is generally provided in 50 to 150 milligram (mg) dosages. Other spermicidal compounds are available in other countries, such as octoxynol-9, benzalkonium chloride, and menfegol. Fewer than 2% of women report using N-9 formulations as their sole method of contraception (Bensyl, Iuliano, Carter, Santelli, & Gilbert, 2005).

Efficacy and Effectiveness Studies comparing N-9 in various formulations (vaginal contraceptive film, foaming tablets, suppositories, and gels), each used without condoms or other physical barriers, showed typical-use pregnancy rates over 6 months that ranged from 10% to 15% to a high of 28% (Raymond, Chen, & Luoto, 2004; Raymond & Dominik, 1999) (Table 12-1). These rates are higher than those for other barrier contraceptives. Formulations containing at least 100 mg of N-9 were associated with lower unintended pregnancy rates.

BOX 12-2 *Advantages and Disadvantages of Barrier Methods*

Advantages:
- Nonhormonal
- Do not require daily action
- Some are available without prescription.
- Some offer protection against STIs

Disadvantages:
- Require planning
- Require application at the time of intercourse and may be interruptive
- Breakage or slippage of barrier methods at time of intercourse may increase risk of unintended pregnancy.

Note: All women relying on barrier or coitus-dependent methods should be aware of emergency contraception and be offered an advance prescription.

Although the effectiveness of spermicides used as a sole agent is less than that of other contraceptive methods, spermicide use is certainly more effective than using no method at all.

Safety and Side Effects N-9 is a surfactant, and surfactants can disrupt cell membranes. By extension, many believed that the surfactant in this product would also act against pathogenic organisms and protect the user against gonorrhea, chlamydia, herpes, and syphilis. Studies from the late 1980s suggested that N-9 could inactivate HIV and other STIs (Louv, Austin, Alexander, Stagno, & Cheeks, 1988; Malkovsky, Newell, & Dalgleish, 1988; Polsky et al., 1988).

More recently, studies have shown that N-9 is an irritant to both animal and human tissue. Frequent use is associated with increased reports of vaginal irritation. As an irritant, N-9 has the potential to disrupt or damage epithelial tissue in both the vagina and the rectum. The risk of this disruption increases with frequency of use and dose (Wilkinson, Tholandi, Ramjee, & Rutherford, 2002). Because intact tissue is the first defense against infection, N-9 could, therefore, potentially increase the risk of transmission of infection by causing microabrasions in the epithelium. In addition, strong evidence indicates that N-9 does not reduce STIs among sex workers or women attending STI clinics (Wilkinson et al., 2002); in fact, it may even increase the risk of HIV acquisition in high-risk women (Van Damme et al., 2002).

Current recommendations for the use of N-9–based spermicides are as follows:

- N-9 should not be used for purposes of STI protection.
- N-9 should not be used by women who engage in multiple daily acts of intercourse.
- N-9 should not be used by women at high risk for HIV acquisition.
- N-9 should not be used rectally.

For women at low risk of HIV acquisition, however, N-9 products remain a valid contraceptive option (WHO, 2001). In fact, N-9 is intended to be used with other female cervicovaginal barriers.

The likelihood of women who use N-9 for contraception developing specific genitourinary symptoms after 6 to 7 months of use is 13% to 17% for a yeast infection, 8% to 12% for bacterial vaginosis, 19% to 27% for vulvovaginal irritation, and 11% to 15% for urinary tract symptoms (but only 3% to 6% for culture-proven urinary tract infection). The likelihood of irritation and other genitourinary symptoms in the male partner ranges from 6% to 14% after 6 to 7 months of use. In the studies that produced these findings, there was no comparison group to indicate whether these rates are higher, lower, or the same as the rates in the general population of sexually active women using contraception (Raymond et al., 2004). However, the reported rates are high enough to warrant counseling women to report symptoms so that they can be evaluated, diagnosed, and properly treated.

Noncontraceptive Benefits Despite concerns about the potential for cervicovaginal epithelial disruption with N-9–based spermicides, the appeal of vaginally applied chemical barriers remains high. This attraction stems largely from their potential to provide dual protection—they are both spermicidal and microbicidal. Woman-controlled, vaginally applied, lubricating microbicides offer great potential for protection against STIs, including HIV. Microbicide development and clinical trials are ongoing.

Advantages and Disadvantages Spermicides containing N-9 are widely available as over-the-counter products and do not require a prescription or clinician visit. Thus they are readily accessible to women who need personally controlled, discreet, low-cost contraception. The effectiveness of spermicides is coitus dependent (Box 12-2). Disadvantages include the low contraceptive effectiveness and the potential for symptoms of cervicovaginal irritation. As noted earlier, women who engage in multiple daily acts of intercourse or who are at high risk for STIs/HIV should avoid use of spermicides containing N-9.

Diaphragms

The traditional diaphragm has a long history as a contraceptive device (Tone, 2001). Currently fewer than 1% of women in the United States using contraception use the diaphragm (Chandra et al., 2005). Nevertheless, this device is well recognized as a woman-controlled method that provides not only contraceptive protection, but also potential protection against some STIs.

Efficacy and Effectiveness The contraceptive efficacy of the diaphragm is similar to that of the male condom (Table 12-1). Traditional diaphragms are designed to be used in conjunction with a spermicide. The only study comparing differences in the contraceptive effectiveness of a diaphragm depending on whether spermicide is used was underpowered and, therefore, could not reach firm conclusions (Bounds, Guillebaud, Dominik, & Dalberth, 1995). During sexual excitement the upper part of the vagina expands; thus diaphragms and other devices that might be in contact with the vaginal walls during fitting may no longer provide a complete physical barrier to sperm migration during intercourse. Theoretically, an additional and important function of the diaphragm would be to maintain spermicide in contact with the cervical os, thereby ensuring that sperm are trapped by the chemical barrier.

Safety and Side Effects The spermicide side effects discussed earlier in this chapter may also be experienced by diaphragm users. The only diaphragm available in the United States as of this writing is made of silicone and can be used by women with latex allergies. Irritation or even abrasions of the vaginal mucosa have been noted in women with improperly sized diaphragms or with prolonged retention of the diaphragm in the vagina. Although no clear association with toxic shock syndrome has been demonstrated, diaphragms and other contraceptive barrier devices should not be left in the vagina for more than 24 hours, and their use during menses is discouraged.

Urinary tract infections are more common in diaphragm users than among women using hormonal contraceptives. Two factors may explain this phenomenon. The first is mechanical: The rim of the diaphragm may exert pressure against the urethra, which might be perceived as frequency or dysuria, or incomplete bladder emptying, and may lead to infection. The second reason is that the spermicides used with the diaphragm can alter normal vaginal flora and may increase the likelihood of *E. coli* bacteriuria.

Noncontraceptive Benefits The diaphragm has possible value in protecting the cervix from infection, but data demonstrating a protective effect are not currently available.

Advantages and Disadvantages Diaphragms are user-controlled, nonhormonal contraceptive methods that are needed only at the time of intercourse (Box 12-2). The devices come in multiple sizes, varying in diameter (**Figure 12-2**). They must be fit by a clinician and require a prescription to purchase. Thus diaphragms have a higher initiation cost than condoms, but can be used for years with proper care. The only additional cost is the spermicide that must be used with the diaphragm. Diaphragms are washable and reusable. Proper use is important. Users should be counseled on the timing of insertion and removal, use of spermicide, appropriate care of the device, and need for periodic reevaluation of the size.

Cervical Caps

Cervical caps are cuplike devices that cover the cervix. Smaller than diaphragms or vaginal barriers, they maintain their position over the cervix by suction, adhering to the cervix, or via a design that uses vaginal walls for support. Caps have long been popular in Europe, where several types of latex caps and a disposable silicone cap are available. The FemCap is the only cervical cap device available in the United States.

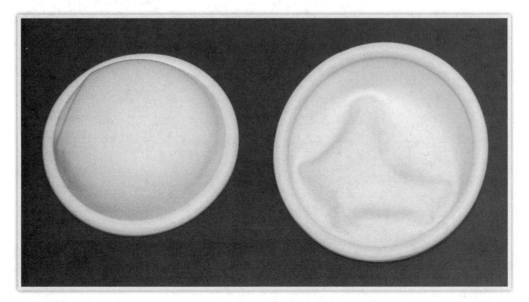

FIGURE 12-2 Diaphragms.

The FemCap is made of silicone and has a design like an inverted sailor's cap (**Figure 12-3**). The dome covers the cervix, and the longer side of the brim fits into the back of the vagina. Three sizes are available, and selection is determined by obstetric history. The Fem-Cap can be worn for as long as 48 hours, but, as with all vaginal devices, should not be used during menses. The device is designed to be used with a thin layer of spermicide around the outer brim.

Efficacy and Effectiveness The FemCap was not as effective in preventing pregnancy as the traditional diaphragm in clinical studies; the extrapolated annual failure rates slightly exceed 20% (Gallo, Grimes, & Schulz, 2002). Some design issues were felt to contribute to the failure rates in the research studies, however (Mauck, Callahan, Weiner, & Dominik, 1999); these problems were corrected via a subsequent design of the cap, and the device that was approved by the FDA is the modified design. Cervical caps may be less effective in women who have had children than in those who have not.

Safety and Side Effects In a randomized trial comparing FemCap to the traditional diaphragm, FemCap users had significantly fewer urinary tract infections (7.5%) than those in the diaphragm group (12.4%). In this same study, there were no differences in vaginitis, irritation, dysmenorrhea, or Pap test changes between the groups (Mauck et al., 1999).

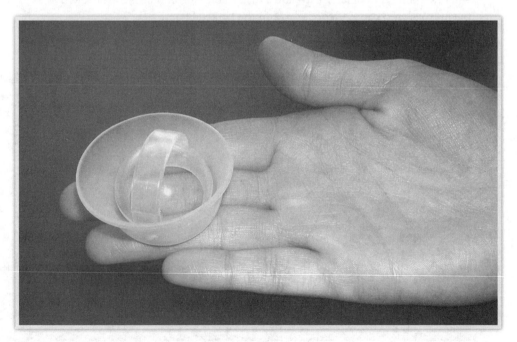

FIGURE 12-3 The FemCap.
Source: Courtesy of the Cervical Barrier Advancement Society.

Noncontraceptive Benefits As with all barrier methods, protection of the cervix by the cervical cap may offer some noncontraceptive benefit in the prevention of STIs, especially those that are acquired via the cervix.

Advantages and Disadvantages Cervical caps are coitus dependent (Box 12-2), and may be appropriate for women who do not want or cannot use hormonal contraception. The latex-free FemCap is appropriate for women who have, or whose partners have, latex allergies. Insertion and removal of cervical caps may be complex for some women; these women will need additional teaching and counseling to use this contraceptive method consistently and correctly. In a comparative study, more insertion and removal problems were noted with FemCap than with the traditional diaphragm. Approximately 10% to 15% of potential research participants could not be fit with the FemCap, or were unable to insert or remove it (Mauck et al., 1999).

Caps require an initial cost for fitting and purchase, but should last for approximately 2 years with proper care. Ongoing costs include the purchase of spermicides. The FemCap is available only with a prescription. These cervical caps are available through Planned Parenthood affiliates, individual clinicians, or clinics, or may be ordered directly from the manufacturer. The FemCap website (http://www.femcap.com) provides detailed information about obtaining this device.

Vaginal Sponge

The Today sponge is a single-use, soft, absorbent, polyurethane device that contains approximately 1000 mg of nonoxynol-9 spermicide; when moistened, the sponge gradually releases 125 to 150 mg of spermicide over 24 hours of use (**Figure 12-4**). Its primary contraceptive effectiveness derives from the gradual release of spermicide; it also provides a physical barrier to the cervix and absorbs semen. The vaginal sponge can be used for multiple episodes of coitus over 24 hours without inserting more spermicide.

Efficacy and Effectiveness Pregnancy rates are somewhat higher among women who use contraceptive sponges than among women who use diaphragms (Kuyoh, Toroitich-Ruto,

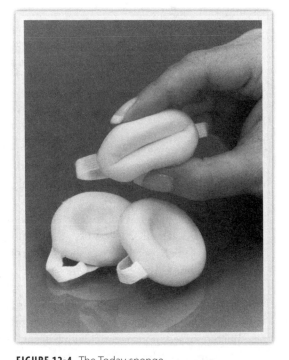

FIGURE 12-4 The Today sponge.

Source: Courtesy of Allendale Pharmaceuticals, Inc. (http://www.allendalepharm.com).

Grimes, Schulz, & Gallo, 2003). As with the cervical cap, the higher rates occur among women who have had children, as opposed to women who have never given birth (McIntyre & Higgins, 1986) (Table 12-1).

Safety and Side Effects Women who use the vaginal sponge tend to discontinue use of their method at higher rates than women who use the diaphragm; more than 40% of the women who use both methods stopped using them in research studies. Allergic-type reactions, such as dermatitis, erythema, irritation, and vaginal itching, were more common with the sponge, although they occurred in only 4% of users (Kuyoh, et al., 2003). Four cases of toxic shock syndrome among users of the sponge were reported in 1983. These were associated with recent childbirth, use of the method for more than 24 hours, and/ or difficult removal with fragmentation of the sponge. Given the number of sponges sold during that time, experts estimated that the risk of toxic shock syndrome was extremely low: approximately 10 cases per year per 100,000 women using sponges ("Leads from the *MMWR*," 1984).

Noncontraceptive Benefits The vaginal sponge may offer some noncontraceptive benefit in the prevention of STIs by physical protection of the cervix. This is a theoretical advantage; actual protection from STIs has not been demonstrated.

Advantages and Disadvantages The sponge shares the advantages and disadvantages of other nonhormonal barrier, coitus-dependent methods (Box 12-2). It does not require a clinician visit or fitting and is available on an over-the-counter basis. Its single-use application may prove more expensive over time than methods that can be reused.

Female Condom

The female condom was developed as an alternative to male condoms, to give women a nonprescription barrier contraceptive method that they could control, and also use to reduce their exposure to STIs. It has been available in the United States since 1993 (Hoffman, Mantell, Exner, & Stein, 2004). The original female condom, FC1 (Reality), was made of polyurethane. In 2009, a second-generation model made of nitrile, known as FC2, was approved by the FDA. The FC2 is less expensive and quieter than the FC1.

The female condom is a sheath approximately 6.5 inches long that has a flexible ring at both ends (**Figure 12-5**). The smaller ring, at the closed end of the sheath, is inserted high in the vagina. The larger ring rests outside the vagina against the vulva and acts as a guide during penetration. This ring also maintains the sheath covering the full length of the vagina, and prevents it from "bunching up" inside the vagina. The sheath is coated with a silicone-based, nonspermicidal lubricant, and women can use additional lubricant as well. The female condom should not be used simultaneously with a male condom, as the risk of breakage increases.

Efficacy and Effectiveness The effectiveness of the female condom in preventing pregnancy is in the same range as that of other barrier methods (Table 12-1).

Safety and Side Effects Female condoms are made of polyurethane and so do not present problems for people with latex allergies.

Noncontraceptive Benefits Laboratory studies demonstrate that polyurethane can block transmission of smaller viruses such as herpes virus and HIV. Studies suggest that the female condom is at least as effective as male condoms in preventing STIs (Hoffman et al., 2004).

Advantages and Disadvantages The female condom is a nonhormonal, female-controlled method that is available as an over-the-counter product. The results of a randomized crossover

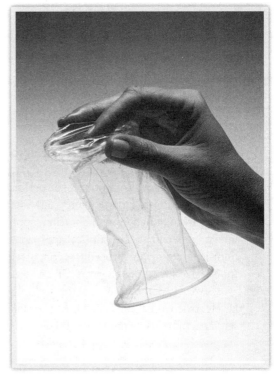

FIGURE 12-5 A female condom.
Source: © Photodisc

trial suggested that most users prefer the male condom to the female condom (Kulczycki, Kim, Duerr, Jamieson, & Macaluso, 2004). The population in this study, however, may not be representative of women who desire female-controlled barrier methods and protection from STIs.

Some women find the female condom difficult to insert, although this problem decreases with proper education. Although it is a female-controlled method, male partner cooperation may still be necessary for consistent use; the partner's lack of acceptance is often cited as a reason for discontinuation. Female condoms can be used only once, so this method can be costly over time.

Sterilization

Sterilization is one of the most prevalent contraceptive methods in the United States. Among U.S. women aged 15 to 44, 17% use female sterilization and 6% use male sterilization as their contraceptive method. The percentage of women using female sterilization increases with age from 2.2% of women aged 20 to 24 to 34.7% of those aged 40 to 44. The same is true for vasectomy, which is used by 0.5% of women aged 20 to 24 and 12.7% of those aged 40 to 44 (Chandra et al., 2005). Approximately 700,000 tubal sterilizations and 500,000 vasectomies are performed annually in the United States (American College of Obstetricians and Gyne-cologists, 2003).

Sterilization is considered a permanent procedure. People choose sterilization when they are sure they want no more children. Thus the person's age and his or her number of living children are important determining factors when considering sterilization.

Female Sterilization

Female sterilization involves permanently blocking the fallopian tubes, which prevents sperm from ascending the reproductive tract and thereby meeting and fertilizing an egg released from the ovary. Female sterilization can be performed postpartum, post abortion, or as an "interval" procedure unrelated to pregnancy. Few sterilization procedures in the United States are performed in conjunction with abortion; approximately half are done postpartum, and half are interval procedures. The surgical approaches most commonly employed include laparoscopy, mini-laparotomy, and procedures concurrent with a cesarean birth. Newer approaches include transcervical methods (Bartz & Greenberg, 2008).

A variety of methods exist for occluding the fallopian tubes, including unipolar or bipolar electrocoagulation; mechanical occlusion using clips, rings, or bands; and ligation or salpingectomy, using one of several techniques. Procedures other than transcervical methods are generally effective immediately (Bartz & Greenberg, 2008).

There are currently two FDA-approved transcervical sterilization methods, Essure and Adiana, both of which are performed via hysteroscopy and can be done in an office setting. Essure involves placement of micro-inserts of metal and fibers into the fallopian tubes. Adiana uses tubal endocoagulation followed by implantation of a silicone matrix within the treated area. After these procedures, tissue grows into the insert or matrix, effectively blocking the tubes. A hysterosalpingogram (HSG) must be performed 3 months after either procedure to confirm tubal occlusion, and women must use reliable contraception until sterilization effectiveness is confirmed with HSG (Smith, 2009).

Efficacy and Effectiveness Tubal sterilization is a highly effective contraceptive method (Table 12-1). Although its overall failure rate is low, failures do occur and are more frequent in women who are younger at the time of sterilization. Failure rates are similar to those of other highly effective, long-term contraceptive methods such as implants and intrauterine contraception. In an extensive study of surgical sterilization efficacy, postpartum partial salpingectomy and unipolar coagulation were the most effective sterilization methods. The method with the highest failure was laparoscopic spring clip application (Peterson et al., 1996). The effectiveness of Essure is at least as high as, if not greater than, that of surgical sterilization methods. Long-term data for Adiana are not yet available, but initial trial participants had a 1.1% failure rate at 1 year and a 1.8% at 2 years after placement (Smith, 2009). Many experts recommend timing an interval procedure during the follicular phase of the menstrual cycle and using a highly sensitive pregnancy test prior to surgery to reduce the risk of luteal-phase pregnancies that are conceived but not recognized before sterilization is performed.

Safety and Side Effects Sterilization is a very effective method of contraception, but when pregnancy does occur after tubal sterilization, the risk of ectopic pregnancy is high. In the largest study of sterilization, one-third of all poststerilization pregnancies were ectopic (Peterson et al., 1997). Other risks are related to the surgical procedures used, and include infection, hemorrhage, anesthesia complications, and surgical trauma or injury. The likelihood of these complications is very low, occurring in fewer than 1% of all procedures. The transcervical sterilization methods avoid the risks of abdominal incisions and anesthesia.

A "post-tubal syndrome" has been described, which typically includes increased dysmenorrhea and abnormalities in the menstrual cycle. Most authorities believe such symptoms are more likely related to discontinuing hormonal contraceptives, or simply getting older and entering the perimenopause. There is no consistent evidence of a true post-tubal syndrome within the first 2 years after the procedure (Peterson et al., 2000).

Noncontraceptive Benefits There is a decreased risk of ovarian cancer following tubal sterilization. In addition, studies have shown a lower risk of pelvic inflammatory disease (PID) among women who have been sterilized when compared to women who have not (Bartz & Greenberg, 2008). The reasons for this effect are not entirely clear but could be related to mechanical blockage of an ascending spread of pathologic organisms.

Advantages and Disadvantages Tubal sterilization is a highly effective permanent method of contraception, well suited to women who have completed their families. The surgical procedures are expensive, however, and insurance coverage for them varies. Additional barriers to access include requirements for a waiting period after signing consent and minimum age requirements. Studies in the United States suggest that women who have been sterilized are less likely to return for annual checkups or to use other preventive health services such as Pap tests. They are also less likely to use condoms for prevention of STIs. Counseling for women contemplating or undergoing sterilization should focus on the continued need for preventive health services (Winkler et al., 1999).

The younger the woman is at the time of her sterilization, the more likely she is during subsequent years to express regret about having the procedure. Younger women are also more likely to inquire about or seek a reversal of the procedure than older women (Hillis, Marchbanks, Tylor, & Peterson, 1999).

Male Sterilization

Male sterilization, or vasectomy, cuts or blocks both the right and the left vas deferens, which are the small tubes that carry sperm from the testes to become part of the seminal fluid. Sperm account for only 5% of the semen that is produced by the prostate and other glands; thus there is only a minimal decrease in the amount of seminal fluid following male sterilization. Vasectomies have no effect on sex drive, male hormone production, or sexual function.

Two types of vasectomy procedures are currently in use, and both can be performed in an outpatient setting. The conventional vasectomy requires one midline or two lateral incisions in the scrotum. The vas is lifted out through the incision and occluded using one of a variety of methods such as ligation, cautery, excision of a segment of the vas, and/or application of clips. The opening is then sutured. With the "no-scalpel" method, the skin of the scrotum is pierced and the vas exposed and blocked through an opening so small it does not require stitches (Pollack, Thomas, & Barone, 2007).

Vasectomy is not immediately effective. Sperm are continually produced and transported through the male reproductive tract, so some sperm will continue to be present distal to the site of the vasectomy. Generally it takes between 15 and 20 ejaculations to clear all sperm from the reproductive tract and be assured of contraception. The current recommendation is for men to wait 3 months, rather than a specific number of ejaculations, before relying on vasectomy (WHO, 2004). Men are usually advised to have a follow-up visit and examination of ejaculate to ensure the absence of sperm before they stop using other contraceptive methods.

Efficacy and Effectiveness The first-year failure rate for vasectomy is estimated to be very low, but good research on this topic is lacking. Recent attempts to systematically review and summarize studies of vasectomy have led to the conclusion that most studies are of poor quality and better research is needed. Vasectomy failure rates are similar to those for female sterilization (Pollack et al., 2007) (Table 12-1).

Safety and Side Effects Most men will experience some degree of postoperative discomfort; infection and scrotal hematoma occur on rare occasions. Some men experience chronic testicular pain after vasectomy, but only a small percentage (3% or fewer) report pain that negatively affects their life or causes them to regret having had the procedure (Pollack et al., 2007). Antisperm antibodies are more common among men who have had vasectomies than the general population, although there is no evidence that any adverse health consequences are associated with this condition. Vasectomy does not increase the risk of prostate cancer (Pollack et al.).

Noncontraceptive Benefits No benefits other than contraception have been demonstrated to date for vasectomy.

Advantages and Disadvantages Vasectomy is a simple procedure that is less complicated and less costly than female sterilization for couples wishing permanent contraception. As is true with tubal sterilization, regret may occur with certain unanticipated life changes. Reversal has a better chance of success when performed within 10 years of vasectomy; pregnancy rates decrease as the interval between vasectomy and reversal increases (Pollack et al., 2007). Men need to be counseled that vasectomy does not prevent STIs.

Hormonal Methods

The FDA approval of combined oral contraceptives (COCs) in 1960 marked a revolutionary change in reproductive rights and responsibilities for women around the world. For the first time, women had access to a nearly 100% effective form of contraception that did not require the participation of the male partner and was independent of the act of coitus. COCs (or "the Pill") are some of the best-studied and most widely used medications available today; they remain the most popular form of reversible contraception in the United States (Alan Guttmacher Institute, 2010).

Two types of hormonal contraceptives are available: those that contain progestin (progestin-only), and those that contain progestin and estrogen (combined). Progestin, the synthetic version of the endogenous hormone progesterone, is highly effective alone as a contraceptive, but may cause irregular bleeding. The addition of estrogen to progestin in combined methods results in more predictable bleeding patterns due to stabilization of the endometrium. Estrogen as a single agent for contraception requires doses that may cause unacceptable risks of serious side effects, such as thromboembolic events and endometrial hyperplasia. The synergistic activity of estrogen and progestin makes it possible to combine these hormones in lower doses to produce successful contraception than would be possible using either hormone alone (Wallach & Grimes, 2000).

The combined contraceptive methods include COCs, the patch, and the vaginal ring. The progestin methods include progestin-only pills, the depot medroxyprogesterone acetate injection, and the subdermal implant. Each method is described in this section. An additional contraceptive method that contains progestin, the LNG-IUS, is discussed later in this chapter in the section on intrauterine contraception.

Both progestin and estrogen inhibit the hypothalamic–pituitary–ovarian axis and subsequent steroidogenesis. Progestins have several contraceptive effects, including preventing the luteinizing hormone (LH) surge and thereby inhibiting ovulation; thickening the cervical mucus, which inhibits sperm penetration and transport; changing the motility of the fallopian tubes so that transport of sperm or ova is impaired; and causing the endometrium to become atrophic, although it is unknown whether these changes are sufficient to prevent implantation in the rare event that fertilization occurs. Estrogen suppresses the production of follicle-stimulating hormone (FSH), thereby preventing the selection and emergence of a dominant follicle. The primary mechanism of action of all hormonal contraceptive methods, with the exception of progestin-only pills (POPs) and the LNG-IUS, is preventing ovulation. Other contraceptive effects of progestin represent secondary mechanisms to prevent pregnancy should ovulation occur. POPs and the LNG-IUS do not consistently inhibit ovulation, and their primary mechanism of action is thickening the cervical mucus.

None of the hormonal methods provide STI/HIV protection. For this reason, it is important to stress the concomitant use of barrier methods in women who are at risk of exposure to STIs.

Combined Hormonal Methods

Early formulations of COCs contained unnecessarily high doses of hormones, consisting of 80 to 100 micrograms (mcg) of either ethinyl estradiol or mestranol and 1 to 5 mg of progestins. Since the 1970s, the trend has been to develop lower-dose formulations that are equally effective, safer, and have a better side-effect profile. In addition to improving COC formulations, alternative delivery systems for combined contraception have been developed that allow women to avoid a daily dosing schedule. These newer methods, which include the combined contraceptive patch and vaginal ring, allow the circulating doses of estrogen and progestin to be lowered even further. This section begins by providing information about COCs, which is then followed by a discussion of the patch and the vaginal ring.

Combined Oral Contraceptives

Since the milestone introduction of COCs in the United States in 1960, many formulations of COCs have been developed. Each is unique while on patent, but today more generic formulations are available than patented options, so the same formulation may have several names. COCs are classified as monophasic or multiphasic (biphasic or triphasic), depending on whether the dosage of hormones is constant or varies. There is no evidence that either monophasic or multiphasic formulations are a superior choice.

Most of the COCs available today contain 20 to 35 mcg of ethinyl estradiol, although a few COCs contain 50 mcg of ethinyl estradiol or mestranol, the methyl ether of ethinyl estradiol. Approximately 30% of mestranol is lost as it is converted to ethinyl estradiol; thus a 50-mcg mestranol pill is bioequivalent to a 35-mcg ethinyl estradiol pill.

COCs also contain one of several different progestins. The progestins are often referred to as belonging to the first, second, or third generation, although this is actually an inappropriate categorization. With the exception of drospirenone, all progestins in COCs available in the United States are derived from 19-nortestosterone. These derivatives can be classified into two categories: (1) the estranes, or chemical derivatives of norethindrone (norethindrone, norethindrone acetate, and ethynodiol diacetate), and (2) the gonanes, or chemical derivatives of norgestrel (norgestrel, its active isomer levonorgestrel, desogestrel, and norgestimate). Members of these categories differ in terms of both their bioavailability and their half-life. Caution should be exercised when comparing the potency or purported androgenicity of the various type of progestin by category. Rather, formulations should be judged on the clinical response of the patient.

Drospirenone, the only non-testosterone-derived progestin, is an analogue of the diuretic spironolactone. Drospirenone has a mild potassium-sparing diuretic effect, necessitating that potassium levels be checked during the first cycle in women using angiotensin-converting enzyme (ACE) inhibitors, chronic daily nonsteroidal anti-inflammatory drugs (NSAIDs), angiotensin-II receptor antagonists, potassium-sparing diuretics, heparin, and aldosterone antagonists (Bayer HealthCare Pharmaceuticals, 2010). Women with conditions that predispose them to hyperkalemia should not use COCs containing drospirenone.

The initial choice of a particular COC should be made with the goal of providing the woman with safe, effective contraception. All low-dose (less than 50 mcg) COCs meet this requirement, so it is reasonable to provide a woman with whatever formulation is most cost-effective, or whatever pill she requests by name.

Instructions contained in the pill package insert include options for a Sunday start, a first day start, and a day 5 start. All of these options are based on the principle that as long as

COCs are begun within the first 5 days of the menses, there is contraceptive protection in the first cycle. The Sunday start has been the traditional approach in the United States, because the appearance of COC packages often reflects that regimen, and the withdrawal bleed does not usually occur on the weekend, which couples may find preferable. The advantage of the first day start is that no backup contraceptive method is required in the first cycle. Women are advised to use additional contraception, such as condoms, with the other start regimens for the first 7 days.

A new approach is to utilize a "quick start" by beginning the pill regardless of where the woman is in her menstrual cycle, if pregnancy is excluded and with additional contraception for the first 7 days. Instructions are given to take a pregnancy test in 2 to 3 weeks if unprotected sex occurred during the cycle. This practice has been shown to increase continuation rates for this contraceptive method and is not associated with an increased incidence of adverse bleeding patterns (Westhoff et al., 2002; Westhoff, Morroni, Kerns, & Murphy, 2003).

According to the traditional cyclic schedule, women take 21 days of active COCs followed by 7 days of inactive pills or no pills. Some newer regimens have a shorter hormone-free interval of 4 or 5 days. During the hormone-free interval, bleeding from the withdrawal of estrogen and progestin occurs. This is technically a withdrawal bleed, rather than menses, and is based primarily on convention rather than on science. Extended (omitting the hormone-free interval for two or more cycles) and continuous (omitting the hormone-free interval indefinitely) COC regimens are becoming increasingly popular, both for medical indications and convenience. Monophasic pills are generally preferred for this use.

Efficacy and Effectiveness COCs require the woman's daily adherence to the dosing schedule, which can be compromised by many factors, resulting in a gap between efficacy and effectiveness (Table 12-1). Based on worldwide data related to pill use, it appears that more than 2 million women become pregnant unintentionally each year due to incorrect pill use (Zlidar, 2000). Common reasons for COC failure include not starting a new pack on time, missing pills, "taking a break" from the pill, and discontinuing the pill in response to normal side effects. The counseling and education provided by the clinician are critical to the ultimate success of the woman in avoiding unwanted pregnancy.

The most important pills to take in each cycle are the first and last active COCs, which ensure that the hormone-free interval does not exceed 7 days. During the hormone-free interval, pituitary stimulation of the ovary by FSH is likely to resume and follicular development may begin in many women (Elomaa et al., 1998; Killick, Bancroft, Oelbaum, Morris, & Elstein, 1990). Immature follicles stimulated during the hormone-free phase generally regress once the hormonal pills are resumed, and 7 consecutive days of pill use have been shown to be sufficient in suppressing any follicular function (Letterie & Chow, 1992). Hormone-free intervals of less than 7 days may become the standard recommendation in the future. Patient instructions must stress the importance of starting a new pack on time and not taking more than 7 days off of the active pills. If a woman does extend the hormone-free interval beyond 7 days, she should be instructed to abstain from intercourse or use additional contraception until 7 consecutive pills have been taken.

Missing pills is almost universal among women who choose the pill for contraception. Missing a random pill now and then is unlikely to lead to a method failure. Unfortunately, this fact may lead to complacency regarding the importance of daily adherence to the schedule, as women come to believe that inconsistent pill use is adequate. The probability of pill failure increases with repeated missed pills, however. This issue is complicated by the fact that instructions for women who miss a pill can be confusing. Simplified instructions include a "7-day rule": If the first pill in the pack is missed, or if two or more pills in a row are missed in the cycle, the woman should abstain or use barrier methods for 7 days. If only one pill is missed, the next pill should be taken as soon as possible, but no backup is required. In the case where a woman has missed three or more consecutive pills, and if a withdrawal bleed has begun, she may discard the old pill pack and begin a new cycle. Again, she should not have more than 7 days of inactive pills or pill-free days.

Many women incorrectly believe that temporarily discontinuing or "taking a break from" COCs is beneficial. It is important to convey to patients that the hormones found in the pill do not accumulate in the body, and that the occurrence of a withdrawal bleed indicates that the endometrium is responding to the absence of hormones. There are no differences in the long-term fertility of women who use the pill intermittently and those who use the pill for many years. Among women who take a break, however, the rate of unintended pregnancy increases 25% (Guillebaud, 2000).

As many as one-third of women in the United States who begin taking oral contraceptives discontinue their use before the end of 1 year stating they are dissatisfied with using pills because of the side effects (Table 12-1). A misunderstanding about the management of side effects may compound this dissatisfaction. Clear information about the side effects commonly encountered during the first three cycles of pill use should be given. Whenever a woman begins a new COC, she should be advised to contact the clinician prior to discontinuing the pills if she experiences unwanted side effects. This way, a different pill may be substituted without interrupting effective contraception. Many references are available to assist the clinician in fine-tuning COC formulations to each woman's needs (see the bibliography at the end of this chapter).

A number of medications can modify the effectiveness of COCs. Pharmacologic mechanisms that alter medication metabolism include induction of liver enzymes, alterations in sex hormone-binding globulin (SHBG), and medications that impact the first-pass effect in the gut. Medications that can reduce the effectiveness of COCs include antiretroviral therapy, rifampin, rifabutin, and some anticonvulsants (e.g., lamotrigine, carbamazepine, phenytoin, barbiturates, primidone, topiramate, and oxcarbazepine) (CDC, 2010). Some research indicates that the over-the-counter herbal supplement St. John's wort may also interfere with the effectiveness of COCs (Nelson, 2007). Broad-spectrum antibiotics have been blamed for COC failures, although pharmacologic evidence to support this contention is lacking (CDC, 2010). Given the prevalence of antibiotic use, any pill failures are more likely to be coincidence or to be associated with missed pills. Women who are concerned about reduced COC efficacy while on antibiotics can shorten or eliminate the placebo pills in the pill pack, or use an additional contraceptive, but it is not necessary to routinely recommend these precautions.

Safety and Side Effects COCs are one of the most extensively studied medications available and are known to be extremely safe for healthy women. Many of the side effects are bothersome but not dangerous; however, serious complications are possible and are the basis of contraindications to COC use. These contraindications may be related to the direct effects of the hormonal ingredient, as in breast cancer, or they may result from hormonal effects on other systems, as in thromboembolism. The U.S. *Medical Eligibility Criteria for Contraceptive Use* (CDC, 2010; see Appendix 12-A) provide an evidence-based guide to the contraindications to COC use. One must always weigh the risks of pregnancy in relation to the risks associated with contraceptive use.

All COCs increase the risk of venous thromboembolism (VTE). The risk appears to be related to the dose of estrogen and is greatest for women with known clotting disorders, such as factor V Leiden, or a family history of thrombosis. The various progestin components may contribute to the risk of VTE to a differing degree; however, the difference between pills is small, and the studies showing their relative risks have been subject to methodological errors (Fritz & Speroff, 2011). COCs containing less than 50 mcg of estrogen do not appear to increase the risk of arterial thrombosis (myocardial infarction or stroke) in healthy, nonsmoking women, including women older than 40 years. COCs may increase blood pressure in some women through an increase in plasma angiotensin. Because hypertension is a cofactor in the development of cardiovascular disease, blood pressure should be monitored in COC users.

Metabolic effects of COCs include development of benign hepatocellular adenomas, although this side effect is very rare with the low-dose pills. There does not appear to be an association between these benign tumors and the development of liver cancer. Low-dose COCs appear to create negligible changes in insulin levels or glucose levels and have no effect on the development of diabetes. There is no difference in weight gain in pill users versus nonusers in large studies; however, a few women may experience an anabolic response to COCs, though they are able to lose weight once the oral contraceptive is discontinued (Fritz & Speroff, 2011).

History of COC use, regardless of duration, does not affect breast cancer risk. Current COC users experience an increased risk of breast cancer cases; however, this risk is small, and may represent a detection bias, as pill users are more likely to receive regular screening (Fritz & Speroff, 2011). Some studies have noted an increase in the incidence of cervical cancer in COC users. It is difficult to determine whether this finding reflects a true increase or a result of the fact that women who use COCs have more sexual partners, HPV infections, and Pap tests, the latter of which causes detection bias (Fritz & Speroff).

Mood changes and changes in libido have been noted among pill users and may respond to a change in the pill formulation. Depression, although rare, may justify the use of alternative methods of contraception. Other side effects specific to estrogen include nausea, cervical ectopy and leukorrhea, telangiectasis, chloasma (darkening of sun-exposed skin), growth of breast tissue (ductal tissue or fat deposition), increase in the cholesterol content within the bile (which can lead to gallstones), benign hepatocellular adenomas, and changes in the clotting cascade. Effects specific to the androgenic impact of progestins include increased appetite and subsequent weight gain, mood changes and depression, fatigue, complexion changes, changes in carbohydrate metabolism, increased low-density lipoprotein (LDL) and decreased high-density lipoprotein (HDL) cholesterol, decreased libido, and pruritus. Effects that can be either estrogen or progestin related include headaches, hypertension, and breast tenderness. Many of the side effects that women associate with COCs occur either during the 7 hormone-free days or appear to be associated with the demise of follicles recruited during the hormone-free interval (Sulak, Scow, Preece, Riggs, & Kuehl, 2000). In turn, a trial of extended use as described previously may improve the symptoms that women experience at predictable times in their pill cycles.

Noncontraceptive Benefits The noncontraceptive benefits of COCs are numerous and underappreciated (American College of Obstetricians and Gynecologists, 2010). Some evidence indicates that the relative risk of ovarian cancer is decreased by 20% for each 5 years of COC use. This reduction in risk persists more than 30 years after pills are discontinued, although the extent of risk reduction diminishes somewhat with time (Collaborative Group on Epidemiological Studies of Ovarian Cancer, 2008). Likewise, COC use reduces the risk of endometrial cancer by approximately 50%. This risk lessens with increasing duration of use and persists for as long as 20 years after the COCs are stopped (Cibula et al., 2010).Women on COCs also experience lower rates of PID requiring hospitalization, fewer ectopic pregnancies, and a lower incidence of endometriosis (Nelson, 2007). These conditions are the most common causes of infertility; thus the pill helps preserve fertility, not by conservation of ovulation, but rather through prevention of causes of subfertility. Other well-documented noncontraceptive benefits of the pill include menstrual-related effects (discussed in the next paragraph), improvement in acne and hirsutism, and reduced incidence of benign breast conditions (Nelson). Older studies demonstrated reduced risk of developing functional ovarian cysts while on COCs, but this effect is less profound with the lower doses of hormones in currently used COCs. Limited evidence suggests that COCs may also improve bone density, reduce the risk of uterine fibroids, and decrease sickle cell crises (American College of Obstetricians and Gynecologists; Nelson).

In addition to being effective contraception, COCs have many other therapeutic uses. COCs regulate menstrual cycles and are useful in the management of abnormal bleeding patterns. While taking COCs, women experience lighter "periods" (withdrawal bleeds) that may treat or improve anemia. COCs can also be an effective treatment for mittelschmerz, dysmenorrhea, endometriosis, premenstrual symptoms, and the vasomotor symptoms of perimenopause (American College of Obstetricians and Gynecologists, 2010; Nelson, 2007). Women who experience catamenial conditions—those that rise and fall in synchronicity with the menstrual cycle, such as menstrual migraines—may also find improvement with COCs. Decreasing the number of withdrawal bleeding episodes per year may further diminish these problems.

Advantages and Disadvantages COC use is unrelated to coitus. Most women in the United States are familiar with the instructions for COC use, and this method is widely available in pharmacies and clinics. Confidence in the product is high due to the fact it has been on the market for more than 50 years and has been continually researched. Additionally, more than 30 different formulations of the pill are available, allowing for individualization based on response to the products.

The obvious disadvantage of COCs is the need for daily pill taking. The ongoing cost of the method can be problematic as well. Particularly for young women, lack of privacy may also be an issue. Finally, some women experience side effects with COCs that they are unable to tolerate.

Combined Contraceptive Patch and Vaginal Ring

The contraceptive patch (Ortho Evra) and vaginal ring (NuvaRing) share many similarities with COCs, yet have some distinct differences. The patch and ring utilize delivery systems that allow for simpler dosing than daily pill taking. Both methods avoid the first-pass metabolism of COCs, allowing for lower-dose administration and potentially avoiding interactions with other medications.

The patch releases 20 mcg/day of ethinyl estradiol and 150 mcg/day of the progestin norelgestromin, the active metabolite of norgestimate. These active ingredients are rapidly absorbed and reach therapeutic serum concentrations within 24 to 48 hours (Nanda, 2007). The thin, beige patch, which is approximately the size of a matchbook (**Figure 12-6**), is applied by the woman and worn for 1 week at a time. The patch is changed weekly on the same day of the week for 3 weeks,

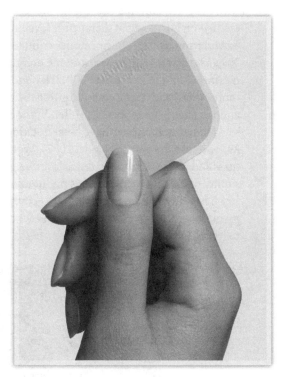

FIGURE 12-6 Combined contraceptive patch (Ortho Evra).

Source: Reprinted with permission from Ortho McNeil Pharmaceuticals.

and then no patch is worn for 1 week to allow for a withdrawal bleed. As with COCs, no more than 7 days should pass between removal of the last patch and the beginning of the next patch cycle. The patch can be worn on the buttocks, upper arm, abdomen, and anywhere on the upper torso except the breasts (Nanda, 2007).

The vaginal ring is colorless and flexible, with an outer diameter of about 2 inches (**Figure 12-7**). It releases 15 mcg/day of ethinyl estradiol and 120 mcg/day of the progestin etonogestrel, the active metabolite of desogestrel (Nanda, 2007). The active ingredients of the ring rapidly diffuse across the mucous membrane of the vagina and reach a steady state in the serum. The ring is left in place in the vagina for 21 days and then removed for 1 week allowing for a withdrawal bleed. The ring provides a steady delivery of hormones, which allows for a very low serum concentration—approximately half of the serum concentration found with a 35-mcg COC (Nanda, 2007).

Efficacy and Effectiveness The patch and the vaginal ring have the same theoretical efficacy and typical-use failure rates as COCs (Table 12–1). There is less opportunity for user error with the patch and ring as these methods need not be remembered daily. Each patch continues to emit hormones at therapeutic levels for at least 9 days (Abrams, Skee, Natarajan, Wong, & Anderson, 2002). The hormones emitted by the ring also remain at therapeutic levels after 3 weeks; therefore, there is also some margin of error if women forget to change the products on time (Mulders & Dieben, 2001). Extended (omitting the patch/ring-free week for two or more cycles) and continuous (omitting the patch/ring-free week indefinitely) use of the patch and ring has been reported (Miller, Verhoeven, & Hout, 2005; Stewart et al., 2005).

Higher failure rates have been documented in women weighing more than 198 lb (90 kg) who use the patch (Nanda, 2007). Women who weigh more than 198 lb or have a body mass index (BMI) categorized as overweight or obese should be cautioned about the possibility of increased failure rates but not denied the methods.

The patch is effective only if it is completely attached to the skin; even partial detachment necessitates replacement. The exact placement of the ring in the vagina is not critical to its efficacy.

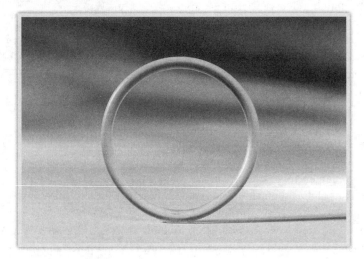

FIGURE 12-7 Combined contraceptive ring (NuvaRing).

Source: Reprinted with permission from Organon USA, Inc. NuvaRing is a registered trademark of N.V. Organon.

Safety and Side Effects The U.S. *Medical Eligibility Criteria for Contraceptive Use* (CDC, 2010) are currently the same for COCs, the patch, and the ring except for in women who have undergone malabsorptive bariatric surgery procedures (see Appendix 12-A and Chapter 9). It is theoretically possible that the nonoral delivery systems may result in different safety and side-effect profiles, but to date no evidence has been published to support this hypothesis. Clinicians are cautioned to not presume the patch and ring are "safer" than COCs. A woman who is not a candidate for COCs should not be given the patch or ring either.

The patch has been associated with heightened concern about an increased risk of VTE (deep vein thromboses and pulmonary emboli). In 2005, a warning was added to the label of the patch that includes the following statement:

> The pharmacokinetic (PK) profile for the ORTHO EVRA patch is different from the PK profile for oral contraceptives in that it has higher steady state concentrations and lower peak concentrations. AUC and average concentration at steady state for ethinyl estradiol (EE) are approximately 60% higher in women using ORTHO EVRA compared with women using an oral contraceptive containing EE 35 mcg. In contrast, peak concentrations for EE are approximately 25% lower in women using ORTHO EVRA. Inter-subject variability results in increased exposure to EE in some women using either ORTHO EVRA or oral contraceptives. However, inter-subject variability in women using ORTHO EVRA is higher. It is not known whether there are changes in the risk of serious adverse events based on the differences in pharmacokinetic profiles of EE in women using ORTHO EVRA compared with women using oral contraceptives containing 35 mcg of EE. Increased estrogen exposure may increase the risk of adverse events, including venous thromboembolism. (Ortho-McNeil-Janssen-Pharmaceuticals, 2010)

Studies have produced conflicting results on this topic, with one showing a higher risk of VTE with the patch compared to COCs (Cole, Norman, Doherty, & Walker, 2007), and another showing a similar risk for VTE with the patch and COCs (Jick, Kaye, Russmann, & Jick, 2006). While hormone levels with the patch are typically higher than those with COCs, the clinical implications of these pharmacokinetic findings are unclear and do not necessarily indicate any increased risk of serious side effects (Nanda, 2007).

In general, the side effects of the patch and the vaginal ring are very similar to those of COCs, such as breakthrough bleeding and nausea. In addition, the patch and ring have some unique side effects related to their delivery systems. In studies of the patch, approximately 20% of participating women experienced some skin irritation at the site of application, but less than 3% discontinued use for this reason (Audet et al., 2001). The ring may be felt during intercourse; however, this is not commonly cited as a reason for discontinuation. There is no increase in vaginitis or cervical cytologic changes with the vaginal ring (Veres, Miller, & Burington, 2004).

Noncontraceptive Benefits It is theoretically plausible that the noncontraceptive benefits of COCs may be realized with the patch and ring as well, because these methods affect the hypothalamic–pituitary–ovarian axis in the same way as COCs; however, epidemiologic studies to support this theory are lacking. Caution must be exercised in attributing the same long-term benefits of COCs to the patch and ring in the absence of published evidence of this effect.

Advantages and Disadvantages The intrinsic advantage of the patch and ring is the absence of daily dosing, which may lead to greater effectiveness. A specific advantage of the vaginal ring is the absence of visible evidence of its use, which may appeal to some women, particularly adolescents, who want to keep their contraceptive use private. The patch may appeal to women who are not comfortable with vaginal placement, but desire a nondaily method of contraception.

One current disadvantage of the patch and ring is that only one formulation of each method is available. The development of a variety of products may allow for individual variations in response to hormones, and patch color choices may appeal to some women as well. These methods are also associated with ongoing costs. A final disadvantage of the patch and the ring is that both methods still contain large amounts of active ingredients upon their disposal. The presence of these chemicals has prompted environmental concerns about the effect of high doses of estrogen and progestin seeping into the water supply. In the future, a recommendation may be issued to place the used devices into a biohazard waste container instead of landfills.

Progestin Hormonal Methods

Progestin contraceptives are used continuously; there is no hormone-free week as with combined methods. Progestin contraceptive methods are generally considered safer for women who are unable to take estrogen. In spite of this belief, the product labeling for some progestin-only products mimics the labeling for products containing estrogen. The U.S. *Medical Eligibility Criteria for Contraceptive Use* (CDC, 2010; see Appendix 12-A) are useful for determining appropriate candidates for progestin-only contraception. Progestin contraceptives do not provide the same cycle control as methods with estrogen.

Progestin-Only Pills

The POPs or "mini-pills" available in the United States contain 0.35 mg of norethindrone. Each pill contains active ingredients; there is no hormone-free week as with COCs. POPs must be taken not only daily, but also at the same time each day.

Efficacy and Effectiveness POPs do not suppress ovulation as reliably as COCs; thus they rely primarily on the contraceptive effect of thickened cervical mucus. In a woman who ovulates while taking the progestin-only pill, taking the pill as few as 3 hours late may allow the cervical mucus to return to its fertile spinnbarkeit state and render the contraceptive effect temporarily void. When POPs are used in combination with lactation, the two are nearly 100% effective.

Safety and Side Effects Contraindications to POP use can be found in Appendix 12-A. Irregular bleeding and spotting are the side effects most commonly associated with POPs. Other side effects include headache, nausea, breast tenderness, depression, and benign ovarian cysts (Raymond, 2007b). Decreased effectiveness of POPs is possible when these agents are used in combination with rifampin or rifabutin (CDC, 2010).

Noncontraceptive Benefits Similar to other hormonal methods, there is a reduction in menorrhagia and dysmenorrhea with POPs (Raymond, 2007b). Other possible noncontraceptive benefits include a decrease in premenstrual symptoms and a decrease in upper reproductive tract infections due to the thickened cervical mucus. The reductions in ovarian and endometrial cancer rates seen with COCs have not been reported with POPs.

Advantages and Disadvantages Each package of POPs contains one type of pill (versus two or more in a package of COCs), so there may be less confusion about which pill is to be taken. POPs are a safe method for many women who cannot take estrogen for medical reasons. Similarly, women who are sensitive to even low-estrogen pills, as manifested by nausea, breast tenderness, or hypertension, but who still want an oral contraceptive, may do well on POPs. POPs are preferable to COCs for lactating women because they do not cause adverse effects on the volume or quality of breastmilk (Raymond, 2007b). The contraceptive effect ends immediately upon discontinuation of POPs.

Disadvantages of POPs, other than the side effects previously mentioned, include the need for careful adherence to the dosing schedule. Utilizing an alarm or watch that beeps daily at the same time may enhance compliance.

Progestin Injection

The depot medroxyprogesterone acetate (DMPA) injection (Depo-Provera) has been approved for contraception since 1995, although the clinical trials were conducted in the 1960s and 1970s and the medication was used for the treatment of endometriosis and as an off-label contraceptive prior to FDA approval. DMPA is given as either a 150-mg intramuscular injection or a 104-mg subcutaneous injection that can be self-administered. Either injection is given every 12 weeks. DMPA is a synthetic progestogen in the pregnane family, but it is different than the estrane and gonane progestins found in oral contraceptives. When given at 12-week intervals, DMPA is a powerful inhibitor of the hypothalamic–pituitary axis at the level of the hypothalamus (Schwallie & Assenzo, 1973). Ovulatory suppression often lasts longer than 12 weeks, but because in a minority of women the contraceptive effect expires, all women are instructed to return for repeat doses at 12-week intervals.

Ideally, the first DMPA injection should be given during the first 5 days of the menses or at 6 weeks postpartum prior to the resumption of intercourse, and it can be provided immediately post abortion. If these circumstances are not practical, it is reasonable to provide the injection once pregnancy has been ruled out. In this case, the woman should be advised to take a highly sensitive pregnancy test 2 to 3 weeks after the first injection, as amenorrhea may be interpreted as a normal effect of the method. If DMPA is given in early pregnancy, it does not appear to stimulate fetal anomalies or miscarriage (it was previously used to prevent miscarriage); nevertheless, it is important to detect pregnancy as soon as possible to facilitate entry to prenatal care or abortion care. Women given DMPA "off cycle" (outside the previously mentioned ideal parameters for initiation of the method) should be instructed to use a barrier method for the first 7 days while the serum levels are reaching adequate concentrations. The same instructions apply to women who are late for their injections. If she has engaged in unprotected intercourse in the previous 5 days, a woman should be offered emergency contraception as well.

Efficacy and Effectiveness   The failure rates for DMPA are listed in Table 12-1. The difference between theoretical efficacy and typical use probably reflect the pattern of patients not returning on time for subsequent injections.

Safety and Side Effects   Like POPs, DMPA is safer than combination products overall and can be used by women who are not candidates for estrogen contraceptives. Refer to Appendix 12-A for a complete list of contraindications and precautions regarding DMPA use.

In 2004, the following warning was added to the DMPA label:

> Women who use Depo-Provera Contraceptive Injection may lose significant bone mineral density. Bone loss is greater with increasing duration of use and may not be completely reversible. It is unknown if use of Depo-Provera Contraceptive Injection during adolescence or early adulthood, a critical period of bone accretion, will reduce peak bone mass and increase the risk for osteoporotic fracture in later life. Depo-Provera Contraceptive Injection should not be used as a long-term birth control method (i.e., longer than 2 years) unless other birth control methods are considered inadequate. (Pfizer, 2010)

While bone mineral density (BMD) does decrease during DMPA use, a systematic review of the literature determined that this decline in BMD reverses after DMPA discontinuation (Kaunitz, Arias, & McClung, 2008). This pattern is similar to the BMD changes seen in women who breastfeed. Changes in BMD are an intermediate outcome, but the truly important clinical outcome is fracture risk. Studies examining fracture risk in low-risk women who previously used DMPA are not yet available (American College of Obstetricians and Gynecologists, 2008; Kaunitz et al., 2008). The American College of Obstetricians and Gynecologists does not recommend restricting DMPA initiation or continuation based on concerns about BMD. Likewise, use of DMPA is not considered an indication for BMD screening or medications to prevent osteoporosis, such as estrogen, bisphosphonates, or selective estrogen receptor modulators (American College of Obstetricians and Gynecologists; Kaunitz et al.). All women, regardless of contraceptive method, should be counseled about osteoporosis prevention, including adequate intake of calcium and vitamin D via diet and/or supplements.

As with all progestin-only methods, side effects associated with DMPA include changes in bleeding patterns, with breakthrough bleeding and spotting occurring in the majority of women in the first 6 months of use. After 12 months of use, approximately 40% to 50% of women will have become amenorrheic, with this rate increasing to 80% after 5 years of use (Goldberg & Grimes, 2007). With appropriate counseling, many women see amenorrhea as a benefit of DMPA.

Weight gain with DMPA is common but does not occur in all women (Goldberg & Grimes, 2007). With obesity and its attendant health risks at epidemic proportions, counseling about healthy weight management is essential for all women, with close attention being paid to this issue in women using DMPA. Other side effects reported in a small minority of women on DMPA include depression, headache, decreased libido, and nervousness (Goldberg & Grimes).

Noncontraceptive Benefits Noncontraceptive benefits of DMPA include a reduction in the number of seizures in women with epilepsy and seizure disorders (Goldberg & Grimes, 2007). DMPA is not affected by the anticonvulsant medications, making it ideal for the patient with seizure disorders who does not want to become pregnant (CDC, 2010). DMPA is also associated with a reduction in sickle cell crises in patients with sickle cell disease (Goldberg & Grimes). DMPA is not affected by any medications except aminoglutethimide, which is used to treat Cushing's disease.

As is the case with all hormonal contraceptive options, women have less menorrhagia and less dysmenorrhea with DMPA. Ectopic pregnancy, PID, and endometriosis are all common causes of infertility. Because of the high degree of ovulatory suppression, ectopic pregnancies are decreased when compared to women using no contraception. PID may also be decreased, as with other hormonal methods, and DMPA is also a successful treatment for endometriosis. Altogether, DMPA may have the effect of preserving fertility by avoiding these conditions.

Another unique benefit of DMPA is that it is private, which has contributed to the appeal of this method among the adolescent population.

Advantages and Disadvantages Advantages of DMPA include its high degree of efficacy and long-term nature and its noninterference with coitus. For women who want to keep their contraceptive choice private, there is no visible evidence of their use of DMPA. DMPA can be used during lactation without compromise of the breastmilk quality or quantity. Women 35 years of age and older who smoke are able to use DMPA even during the later reproductive years, a time when prevention of pregnancy can be as critical as for the younger woman. DMPA has long been used in patients with mental disabilities to achieve amenorrhea in women who cannot manage their menses.

The long-term nature of DMPA may also be considered a disadvantage, as the contraceptive effect may not cease immediately upon discontinuation. In fact, the median time to conception following the supposed end of the DMPA effects is 10 months, with a range of 4 to 31 months (Pfizer, 2010). DMPA requires intramuscular injections be provided by a trained healthcare professional, which requires that the patient make regular visits for injections. The subcutaneous formulation might improve continuation of contraception among women who find it difficult to get to a clinician's office. However, there remains the possibility of allergic reaction to either the progestin or the vehicle used for injection, or vagal reactions to the injection itself. Like all hormonal methods, DMPA does not provide any protection from STIs.

Progestin Implant

The subdermal progestin implant is among the most effective methods of contraception, and the American College of Obstetricians and Gynecologists (2009) recommends that this long-acting reversible contraceptive be offered as a first-line method and its use encouraged among most women as a contraceptive option. The single-rod etonogestrel implant (Implanon) is 40 mm long and 2 mm in diameter and contains 68 mg of etonogestrel that is released slowly over 3 years (**Figure 12-8**). Etonogestrel is the active metabolite of desogestrel. As with its predecessors (Norplant and Norplant-2), training of clinicians is needed to ensure appropriate placement and skilled removal. Removal of the new implant is reported to be easier than was the case with the previously used multiple-rod systems for several reasons: It is a single rod, it is slightly larger in size than the multiple-rod systems, and it is made of ethylene vinyl acetate, which is less flexible than the silastic used to make older rods. The implant should be inserted during the first 7 days of the menses, postpartum, or post abortion, to avoid pregnancy in the first cycle. Fertility returns rapidly after removal of the implant, with 1-year pregnancy rates similar to those of women discontinuing barrier methods (Glasier, 2002).

Efficacy and Effectiveness The failure rates for the implant are listed in Table 12-1. This high rate of efficacy is related to the intrinsic efficacy of the product and the fact that once inserted, there is no room for user error.

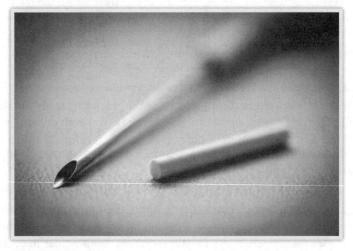

FIGURE 12-8 Single-rod etonogestrel implant (Implanon).
Source: © GARO/PHANIE/Photo Researchers, Inc.

Safety and Side Effects Based on worldwide data, the implant appears to be as safe as other progestin-only methods and is associated with similar side effects, such as irregular bleeding and amenorrhea (Booranabunyat & Taneepanichskul, 2004). Irregular bleeding is the most common reason for discontinuation (Glasier, 2002). Low-dose subdermal contraception has a history of association with the development of benign follicular cysts that rarely require intervention, but can be a cause for anxiety among women when encountered. Other side effects of the method include bruising and irritation at the insertion site and possible weight increase (Raymond, 2007a).

Noncontraceptive Benefits The implant can decrease dysmenorrhea and endometriosis symptoms (Raymond, 2007a).

Advantages and Disadvantages Advantages of the subdermal implant include the presence of highly effective contraception following a single insertion procedure. The contraceptive effect is immediately reversible upon removal of the device. The implant is discreet but palpable, providing reassurance to the woman that it is in place and has not migrated.

Disadvantages of subdermal contraception include the relative recency of its market introduction as well as a corresponding shortage of research on its use in the United States. However, if the Norplant experience proves educational, it is likely that the method will be well received among appropriately counseled women who are cared for by trained clinicians who are skilled in insertion and removal techniques. The high initial cost and a need for clinician insertion and removal may be barriers to use of the implant for some women.

Intrauterine Contraception

The use of medical devices placed in the uterus to prevent pregnancy dates back to the early 1900s. Although the infection risk with early devices was high, design improvements led to a variety of intrauterine devices (IUDs) becoming available in the 1960s and 1970s (Tone, 2001). Popular devices were generally made of inert plastic, with single filament threads that protruded through the cervix into the vagina.

The one memorable exception to this design was the Dalkon Shield, which was introduced in 1970. This device quickly became associated with a high risk of pelvic infection. It had a multifilament tail enclosed in a sheath; when the strings were cut, the protective sheath was compromised and bacteria could ascend into the uterus inside the sheath (Nelson, 2000). Although other IUDs did not have the same design flaw, the adverse publicity and lawsuits associated with the Dalkon Shield tainted all IUDs, and use of the device fell out of favor by the late 1970s.

Recent developments in design and scientific review of the risks and benefits associated with intrauterine contraception have led to a revival of interest in this contraceptive method. Recognizing that IUDs represent a long-acting reversible contraceptive in the top tier of efficacy, the American College of Obstetricians and Gynecologists (2009) recommends intrauterine contraception be offered as a first-line method and its use encouraged among most women as an option.

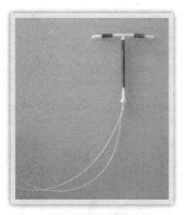

FIGURE 12-9 Copper T380A
intrauterine device (ParaGard).

Source: Reprinted with permission
from FEI Women's Health.

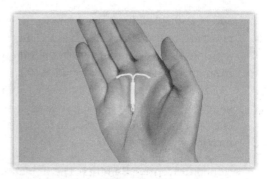

FIGURE 12-10 Levonorgestrel intrauterine system
(Mirena).

Source: Reprinted with permission from Berlex.

Two intrauterine contraceptives are available in the United States, though others are used in other countries. The copper IUD (T380A, ParaGard) is a T-shaped device of polyethylene with copper wire wound around the stem and arms (**Figure 12-9**). A monofilament polyethylene thread is attached to a ball on the end of the stem. The copper adds spermicidal and other effects that allow the device to be smaller than a plain plastic device. The primary contraceptive effect is provided by the reaction to having a foreign body in the reproductive tract: a sterile inflammatory response that is spermicidal (Alvarez et al., 1988). The LNG-IUS (Mirena) is also T-shaped, but contains no copper. Instead, it features a reservoir that releases levonorgestrel at a rate of 20 mcg per day (**Figure 12-10**). The local delivery of progestin produces thickening of the cervical mucus and an endometrial reaction, in addition to the foreign body (Jonsson, Landgren, & Eneroth, 1991). The LNG-IUS also has a monofilament thread. Both devices are effective; the major difference between them is that the copper IUD may stay in place for at least 10 years, while the LNG-IUS may stay in place for at least 5 years.

The copper IUD may be inserted at any time during the menstrual cycle when pregnancy can be ruled out. The LNG-IUS is inserted within 7 days of the onset of menses. Many clinicians perform insertion of either device during menses to be certain the woman is not pregnant. Postabortion, postplacental (within 10 minutes after expulsion of the placenta), and immediate postpartum (within the first week after childbirth and preferably within the first 48 hours) insertion may also be performed. The procedures for copper IUD and LNG-IUS insertion differ and are beyond the scope of this chapter. The manufacturers provide insertion training for clinicians and can be contacted via their websites (http://www.paragard.com and http://www.mirena-us.com).

Effectiveness and Efficacy Intrauterine contraception is extremely effective (Table 12-1). Nevertheless, both the copper IUD and the LNG-IUS can be spontaneously expelled from the uterus. While expulsion may be associated with cramping or bleeding, it may be unnoticed. Women should be taught to check periodically for the strings to ensure the device is still placed properly. There is little room for user error with intrauterine contraception, other than not checking the strings and thus not recognizing an expulsion.

Safety and Side Effects Despite the negative experience associated with the Dalkon Shield, contemporary intrauterine contraceptives with monofilament threads are very safe for most women (see Appendix 12-A). There is no evidence that they increase the risk of PID or infertility. A temporary increase in infection rates during the first weeks after insertion has been noted, which is probably related to the insertion process or preexisting infection prior to insertion (Grimes, 2000, 2007). Use of an IUD does not increase the rate of ectopic pregnancy. When an IUD user becomes pregnant, the pregnancy is more likely to be ectopic, but because the chance of pregnancy itself is so rare, the actual rate of ectopic pregnancy is very low. Perforation of the uterus during insertion is a rare but possible risk.

The most common side effects associated with the copper IUD are bleeding and dysmenorrhea. Menstrual blood loss increases with copper IUDs, as can the length of the menses. NSAIDs can be used to treat excessive bleeding (Grimes, 2007).

Irregular bleeding is common with the LNG-IUS. Initially, intermenstrual bleeding may occur. As the duration of use increases, there is a reduction in menstrual flow and often amenorrhea develops. Counseling prior to insertion of the device may help reduce anxiety about the irregular bleeding. Women should be counseled that the bleeding does not represent hormonal fluctuations, but rather the shedding of the endometrial lining as an atrophic state is achieved. Other side effects linked to the LNG-IUS include lower abdominal pain, complexion changes, back pain, breast tenderness, headaches, mood changes, and nausea, although all of these effects decline with time, and they are noted in only a minority of patients. In general, few hormonal side effects are observed with this low dose of progestin. As with other progestin-only methods, benign follicular cysts are common, occurring in 8% to 12% of IUD users. Most cysts resolve spontaneously (Pakarinen, Suvisaari, Luukkainen, & Lahteenmaki, 1997).

Noncontraceptive Benefits Menstrual flow is reduced by as much as 90% with use of the LNG-IUS (Grimes, 2007), and the device is FDA approved to treat heavy menstrual bleeding. The LNG-IUS can be used to treat idiopathic menorrhagia as well as heavy menstrual bleeding associated with perimenopause, uterine fibroids, and adenomyosis (American College of Obstetricians and Gynecologists, 2010). The LNG-IUS may also be useful in the treatment of endometrial hyperplasia, endometriosis, and dysmenorrhea (American College of Obstetricians and Gynecologists). The progestin in the device is sufficient to protect the endometrium as a component of hormone therapy. The LNG-IUS can be inserted in the late reproductive years and then left in place through the transition to menopause.

Another emerging noncontraceptive benefit is that the cervical mucus barrier and atrophic endometrium created by the LNG-IUS may actually protect the user from PID (Li, Lee, & Pun, 2004). Studies show the risk of PID to be equal in IUD users and nonusers and related to the risk of STIs rather than IUD use (Otero-Flores, Guerrero-Carreno, & Vasquez-Estrada,

2003). In addition, some evidence suggests that the copper IUD and LNG-IUS are associated with a reduced risk of endometrial cancer (Grimes, 2007).

Advantages and Disadvantages Intrauterine contraception has the advantage of providing long-term contraception that is not coitus dependent and does not require adjustments to daily activities (such as remembering to take a pill every day). Contemporary intrauterine contraception options have effectiveness rates that are comparable to those of sterilization. Unlike permanent sterilization, intrauterine contraception offers the added advantage of being rapidly reversible, making this method ideal for young women who desire long-term contraception. IUDs are also discreet and private methods. Copper devices are hormone free. The reduced bleeding with the LNG-IUS can lead to substantial savings in the cost of sanitary products.

There can be a high upfront cost for intrauterine contraception. The copper IUD and LNG-IUS cost several hundred dollars, and a visit to a skilled clinician is needed for their insertion. Many clinicians also require a pre-insertion visit to test for infections, and a post-insertion visit after the first menses to ensure the device has not been expelled. However, these are long-term contraceptives with no additional costs; thus they are among the least expensive methods over time.

Emergency Contraception

Emergency contraception entails the use of contraceptive methods after intercourse to prevent pregnancy. Four emergency contraceptive methods are available in the United States: levonorgestrel emergency contraceptive pills (ECPs), combined ECPs, ulipristal acetate, and the copper IUD. Emergency contraception works by preventing or delaying ovulation, preventing fertilization, and/or preventing implantation. Emergency contraception does not cause an abortion, has no effect on an established pregnancy, and does not offer any protection from STIs or HIV. Access to emergency contraception has the potential to reduce the incidence of unintended pregnancy, which would have a tremendous positive impact on the lives of women, men, and their families by reducing the need for abortion and minimizing the social costs associated with unplanned pregnancy and childbearing (see Chapter 18).

Levonorgestrel ECPs contain either a 1.5-mg single dose (Plan B One-Step) or two doses of 0.75 mg taken 12 hours apart (Next Choice and Plan B, although the latter product is being phased out and is no longer available in all pharmacies). Women can take both doses in the two-dose products (Next Choice and Plan B) as a single dose. Although the instructions for the levonorgestrel ECP products state the pills must be taken within 72 hours after unprotected intercourse, they are actually effective as long as 120 hours after unprotected intercourse. However, taking the pills as soon as possible is ideal because effectiveness declines with time (Zieman et al., 2010). Levonorgestrel ECPs are available over the counter to women and men age 17 and older; women 16 and younger need a prescription to obtain them.

Combined ECPs must contain at least 100 mcg of ethinyl estradiol and 0.50 mg of levonorgestrel per dose. A dedicated combined ECP product is not available in the United

States, but numerous COCs can be used as combined ECPs (see Table 12-1, footnote 9). COCs containing norgestrel are preferable to those with norethindrone, as failure rates are slightly higher with norethindrone (Zieman et al., 2010). Combined ECPs should be started as soon as possible, and within 120 hours, after unprotected intercourse. Two doses are taken 12 hours apart. The second dose can be taken outside the 120-hour window, but as with the levonorgestrel ECPs, the effectiveness declines the later the combined ECPs are started (Zieman et al.).

Ulipristal acetate (ella) is a selective progesterone receptor modulator that was approved by the FDA in 2010. For use as an ECP, a single 30-mg dose is taken within 120 hours of unprotected intercourse. The effectiveness of ulipristal acetate does not decline within the 120-hour window as is the case for levonorgestrel and combined ECPs (Fine et al., 2010). Ulipristal acetate is available only by prescription.

The copper IUD can be inserted as long as 5 days after unprotected intercourse. This method is rarely utilized as emergency contraception in the United States; however, recent evidence suggests many women might choose the copper IUD if it is offered as an emergency contraception option. In a study in which 57 women in Utah requesting emergency contraception were allowed to choose between levonorgestrel ECPs and the copper IUD without charge for either method, 40% chose the copper IUD (Turok et al., 2010).

Efficacy and Effectiveness The percentage of women who become pregnant after using emergency contraception ranges from 0.4% (early start, less than 12 hours after unprotected intercourse) to 2.7% (late start, 1 to 3 days after unprotected intercourse) with levonorgestrel ECPs, ranges from 0.5% (early start) to 4.2% with combined ECPs, and is 0.1% with the copper IUD (Zieman et al., 2010). In a meta-analysis of two studies comparing ulipristal acetate and levonorgestrel ECPs, ulipristal acetate halved the risk of becoming pregnant compared with levonorgestrel ECPs when administered within 120 hours after unprotected intercourse (Glasier et al., 2010).

Safety and Side Effects Levonorgestrel ECPs, combined ECPs, and ulipristal acetate should not be given to women with a known or suspected pregnancy; there are no other contraindications to their use. The usual contraindications and precautions for ongoing COC and POP use do not apply to ECPs (CDC, 2010). The usual contraindications and precautions to copper IUD use apply when using this method for emergency contraception (see Appendix 12-A).

Combined ECPs frequently cause nausea and vomiting, which can be reduced by giving an antiemetic, such as promethazine, prior to treatment. Spotting, changes in next menses, headache, breast tenderness, and mood changes can also occur. These same side effects are sometimes noted with levonorgestrel ECPs but are much less frequent and less severe with this option (Zieman et al., 2010). Headache, dysmenorrhea, nausea, and abdominal pain are the most frequently observed side effects with ulipristal acetate (Fine et al., 2010; Glasier et al., 2010). The copper IUD can cause the side effects discussed in the section on intrauterine contraception.

Advantages and Disadvantages Emergency contraception is the only contraceptive method that can be used after intercourse. It cannot be used as an ongoing method of contraception, however, and it provides no STI/HIV protection. Access to emergency contraception remains limited because only one method—levonorgestrel ECPs—is available without prescription, and even then is available only to women 17 and older. Clinicians can increase access to emergency contraception by providing advance prescriptions to women 16 and younger for levonorgestrel ECPs and all patients of reproductive age for ulipristal acetate. Studies have shown that having ECPs at home increases the likelihood that they will be used when needed and does not promote sexual risk taking (Glasier & Baird, 1998; Raine, Harper, Leon, & Darney, 2000). Providing emergency contraception prescriptions over the phone as needed is another way to increase access.

References

Abrams, L. S., Skee, D. M., Natarajan, J., Wong, F. A., & Anderson, G. D. (2002). Pharmacokinetics of a contraceptive patch (Evra/Ortho Evra) containing norelgestromin and ethinyloestradiol at four application sites. *British Journal of Clinical Pharmacology, 53*, 141–146.

Alan Guttmacher Institute. (2010). *Facts on contraceptive use*. Retrieved from http://www.guttmacher.org/pubs/fb_contr_use.html

Alvarez, F., Brache, V., Fernandez, E., Guerrero, B., Guiloff, E., Hess, R.,…Zacharias, S. (1988). New insights on the mode of action of intrauterine contraceptive devices in women. *Fertility and Sterility, 49*(5), 768–773.

American College of Obstetricians and Gynecologists. (2003). Benefits and risks of sterilization (Practice Bulletin No. 46). *Obstetrics and Gynecology, 102*, 647–658.

American College of Obstetricians and Gynecologists. (2008). Depot medroxyprogesterone acetate and bone effects (Committee Opinion No. 415). *Obstetrics and Gynecology, 112*, 727–730.

American College of Obstetricians and Gynecologists. (2009). Increasing use of contraceptive implants and intrauterine devices to reduce unintended pregnancy (Committee Opinion No. 450). *Obstetrics and Gynecology, 115*, 206–218.

American College of Obstetricians and Gynecologists. (2010). Noncontraceptive uses of hormonal contraceptives (Practice Bulletin No. 110). *Obstetrics and Gynecology, 115*, 206–218.

Arévalo, M., Jennings, V., Nikula, M., & Sinai, I. (2004). Efficacy of the new two-day method of family planning. *Fertility and Sterility, 82*, 885–892.

Arévalo, M., Jennings, V., & Sinai, I. (2002). Efficacy of a new method of family planning: The Standard Days Method. *Contraception, 65*, 333–338.

Audet, M. C., Moreau, M., Koltun, W. D., Waldbaum, A. S., Shangold, G., Fisher, A. C., & Creasy, G. W. (2001). Evaluation of contraceptive efficacy and cycle control of a transdermal contraceptive patch versus an oral contraceptive: A randomized controlled trial. *Journal of the American Medical Association, 285*, 2347–2354.

Bartz, D., & Greenberg, J. A. (2008). Sterilization in the United States. *Reviews in Obstetrics and Gynecology, 1*, 23–32.

Bayer HealthCare Pharmaceuticals. (2010). *Yasmin physician labeling*. Retrieved from http://berlex.bayerhealthcare.com/html/products/pi/fhc/Yasmin_PI.pdf?WT.mc_id=www.berlex.com

Bensyl, D. M., Iuliano, A. D., Carter, M., Santelli, J., & Gilbert, B. C. (2005). Contraceptive use—United States and territories, Behavioral Risk Factor Surveillance system, 2002. *MMWR Surveillance Summaries, 54*(SS06), 1–72.

Billings, E. L. (2001). *Teaching the Billlings Ovulation Method* (3rd ed.). Retrieved from http://www.woomb.org/bom/lit/teach/teach.pdf

Booranabunyat, S., & Taneepanichskul, S. (2004). Implanon use in Thai women above the age of 35 years. *Contraception, 69*, 489–491.

Bounds, W., Guillebaud, J., Dominik, R., & Dalberth, B. T. (1995). The diaphragm with and without spermicide: A randomized, comparative efficacy trial. *Journal of Reproductive Medicine, 40*, 764–774.

Centers for Disease Control and Prevention (CDC).

(2010). U.S. medical eligibility criteria for contraceptive use, 2010: Adapted from the World Health Organization medical eligibility criteria for contraceptive use (4th ed.). *Morbidity and Mortality Weekly Report, 59*, 1–86.

Chandra, A., Martinez, G. M., Mosher, W. D., Abma, J. C., & Jones, J. (2005). Fertility, family planning, and reproductive health of U.S. women: Data from the 2002 National Survey of Family Growth. *Vital Health Statistics, 23*, 1–160.

Cibula, D., Gompel, A., Mueck, A. O., La Vecchia, C., Hannaford, P. C., Skouby, S. O.,...Dusek, L. (2010). Hormonal contraception and risk of cancer. *Human Reproduction Update, 16*, 631–650.

Cole, J. A., Norman, H., Doherty, M., & Walker, A. M. (2007). Venous thromboembolism, myocardial infarction, and stroke among transdermal contraceptive system users. *Obstetrics and Gynecology, 109*, 339–346.

Collaborative Group on Epidemiological Studies of Ovarian Cancer. (2008). Ovarian cancer and oral contraceptives: Collaborative reanalysis of data from 45 epidemiological studies including 23 257 women with ovarian cancer and 87 303 controls. *Lancet, 371*, 303–314.

Collaborative Group on Hormonal Factors in Breast Cancer. (2002). Breast cancer and breastfeeding: Collaborative reanalysis of individual data from 47 epidemiological studies in 30 countries, including 50 302 women with breast cancer and 96 973 women without the disease. *Lancet, 360*, 187–195.

Elomaa, K., Rolland, R., Brosens, I., Moorrees, M., Deprest, J., Tuominen, J., & Lähteenmäki, P. (1998). Omitting the first oral contraceptive pills of the cycle does not automatically lead to ovulation. *American Journal of Obstetrics and Gynecology, 179*, 41–46.

Fehring, R. J. (2005). New low and high tech calendar methods of family planning. *Journal of Midwifery and Women's Health, 50*, 31–38.

Fine, P., Mathé, H., Ginde, S., Cullins, V., Morfesis, J., & Gainer, E. (2010). Ulipristal acetate taken 48–120 hours after intercourse for emergency contraception. *Obstetrics and Gynecology, 115*, 257–263.

Food and Drug Administration (FDA). (2009). *"Off-label" and investigational use of marketed drugs, biologics and medical devices*. Retrieved from http://www.fda.gov/ScienceResearch/SpecialTopics/RunningClinicalTrials/GuidancesInformationSheetsandNotices/ucm116355.htm

Fritz, M. A., & Speroff, L. (2011). *Clinical gynecologic endocrinology and infertility* (8th ed.). Baltimore: Lippincott Williams & Wilkins.

Gallo, M. R., Grimes, D. A., Lopez, L. M., & Schulz, K. F. (2006). Nonlatex versus latex male condoms for contraception. *Cochrane Database of Systematic Reviews, 1*, CD003550.

Gallo, M. F., Grimes, D. A., & Schulz, K. F. (2002). Cervical cap versus diaphragm for contraception. *Cochrane Database of Systematic Reviews, 4*, CD003551.

Glasier, A. (2002). Implantable contraceptives for women: Effectiveness, discontinuation rates, return of fertility, and outcome of pregnancies. *Contraception, 65*, 29–37.

Glasier, A., & Baird, D. (1998). The effects of self-administering emergency contraception. *New England Journal of Medicine, 339*, 1–4.

Glasier, A. F., Cameron, S. T., Fine, P. M., Logan, S. J., Casale, W., Van Horn, J.,...Gainer, E. (2010). Ulipristal acetate versus levonorgestrel for emergency contraception: A randomised non-inferiority trial and meta-analysis. *Lancet, 375*, 555–562.

Goldberg, A. B., & Grimes, D. A. (2007). Injectable contraceptives. In R. A. Hatcher, J. Trussell, A. L. Nelson, W. Cates, F. Stewart, & D. Kowal (Eds.), *Contraceptive technology* (19th ed., pp. 157–179). New York: Ardent Media.

Grimes, D. A. (2000). Intrauterine device and upper-genital-tract infection. *Lancet, 356*, 1013–1019.

Grimes, D. A. (2007). Intrauterine devices (IUDs). In R. A. Hatcher, J. Trussell, A. L. Nelson, W. Cates, F. Stewart, & D. Kowal (Eds.), *Contraceptive technology* (19th ed., pp. 117–143). New York: Ardent Media.

Grimes, D. A. (2009). Forgettable contraception. *Contraception, 80*, 497–499.

Guillebaud, J. (2000). *Contraception today: A pocketbook for general practitioners* (4th ed.). London: Martin Dunitz.

Hillis, S. D., Marchbanks, P. A., Tylor, L. R., & Peterson, H. B. (1999). Poststerilization regret: Findings from the United States Collaborative Review of Sterilization. *Obstetrics and Gynecology, 93*, 889–895.

Hoffman, S., Mantell, J., Exner, T., & Stein, Z. (2004). The future of the female condom. *Perspectives on Sexual and Reproductive Health, 36*, 120–126.

Holmes, K. K., Levine, R., & Weaver, M. (2004). Effectiveness of condoms in preventing sexually transmitted infections. *Bulletin of the World Health Organization, 82*, 454–461.

Jennings, V. H., & Arévalo, M. (2007). Fertility awareness–based methods. In R. A. Hatcher, J. Trussell, A. L. Nelson, W. Cates, F. Stewart, & D. Kowal (Eds.), *Contraceptive technology* (19th ed., pp. 343–360). New York: Ardent Media.

Jick, S. S., Kaye, J. A., Russmann, S., & Jick, H. (2006). Risk of nonfatal venous thromboembolism in women using a contraceptive transdermal patch and oral contraceptives containing norgestimate and 35 microg of ethinyl estradiol. *Contraception, 73*, 223–228.

Jones, R. K., Darroch, J. E., & Henshaw, S. K. (2002). Contraceptive use among U.S. women having abortions in 2000–2001. *Perspectives on Sexual and Reproductive Health, 34*, 294–303.

Jones, R. K., Fennell, J., Higgins, J. A., & Blanchard, K. (2009). Better than nothing or savvy risk-reduction practice? The importance of withdrawal. *Contraception, 79*, 407–410.

Jonsson, B., Landgren, B. M., & Eneroth, P. (1991). Effects of various IUDs on the composition of cervical mucus. *Contraception, 43*, 447–458.

Kaunitz, A. M., Arias, R., & McClung, M. (2008). Bone density recovery after depot medroxyprogesterone acetate injectable contraception use. *Contraception, 77*, 67–76.

Kennedy, K. I., & Trussell, J. (2007). Postpartum contraception and lactation. In R. A. Hatcher, J. Trussell, A. L. Nelson, W. Cates, F. Stewart, & D. Kowal (Eds.), *Contraceptive technology* (19th ed., pp. 403–431). New York: Ardent Media.

Killick, S. R., Bancroft, K., Oelbaum, S., Morris, J., & Elstein, M. (1990). Extending the duration of the pill-free interval during combined oral contraception. *Advances in Contraception, 6*, 33–40.

Kost, K., Singh, S., Vaughan, B., Trussell, J., & Bankole, A. (2008). Estimates of contraceptive failure from the 2002 Survey of National Family Growth. *Contraception, 77*, 10–21.

Kulczycki, A., Kim, D. J., Duerr, A., Jamieson, D. J., & Macaluso, M. (2004). The acceptability of the female and male condom: A randomized crossover trial. *Perspectives on Sexual and Reproductive Health, 36*, 114–119.

Kuyoh, M. A., Toroitich-Ruto, C., Grimes, D. A., Schulz, K. F., & Gallo, M. F. (2003). Sponge versus diaphragm for contraception: A Cochrane review. *Contraception, 67*, 15–18.

Leads from the *MMWR*: Toxic-shock syndrome and the vaginal contraceptive sponge. (1984). *Journal of the American Medical Association, 251*, 1015–1016.

Letterie, G. S., & Chow, G. E. (1992). Effect of "missed" pills on oral contraceptive effectiveness. *Obstetrics and Gynecology, 79*, 979–982.

Li, C. F., Lee, S. S., & Pun, T. C. (2004). A pilot study on the acceptability of levonorgestrel-releasing intrauterine device by young, single, nulliparous Chinese females following surgical abortion. *Contraception, 69*, 247–250.

Louv, W. C., Austin, H., Alexander, W. J., Stagno, S., & Cheeks, J. (1988). A clinical trial of nonoxynol-9 for preventing gonococcal and chlamydial infections. *Journal of Infectious Disease, 158*, 518–523.

Malkovsky, M., Newell, A., & Dalgleish, A. G. (1988). Inactivation of HIV by nonoxynol-9. *Lancet, 1*(8586), 645.

Mauck, C., Callahan, M., Weiner, D. H., & Dominik, R. (1999). A comparative study of the safety and efficacy of FemCap, a new vaginal barrier contraceptive, and the Ortho All-Flex diaphragm. The FemCap Investigators' Group. *Contraception, 60*, 71–80.

McIntyre, S. L., & Higgins, J. E. (1986). Parity and use-effectiveness with the contraceptive sponge. *American Journal of Obstetrics and Gynecology, 155*, 796–801.

Miller, L., Verhoeven, C. H., & Hout, J. (2005). Extended regimens of the contraceptive vaginal ring: A randomized trial. *Obstetrics and Gynecology, 106*, 473–482.

Mulders, T. M., & Dieben, T. O. (2001). Use of the novel combined contraceptive vaginal ring NuvaRing for ovulation inhibition. *Fertility and Sterility, 75*, 865–870.

Nanda, K. L. (2007). Contraceptive patch and vaginal contraceptive ring. In R. A. Hatcher, J. Trussell, A. L. Nelson, W. Cates, F. Stewart, & D. Kowal (Eds.), *Contraceptive technology* (19th ed., pp. 271–295). New York: Ardent Media.

Nelson, A. L. (2000). The intrauterine contraceptive device. *Obstetrics and Gynecology Clinics of North America, 27*, 723–740.

Nelson, A. L. (2007). Combined oral contraceptives. In R. A. Hatcher, J. Trussell, A. L. Nelson, W. Cates, F. Stewart, & D. Kowal (Eds.), *Contraceptive technology* (19th ed., pp. 193–270). New York: Ardent Media.

Newcomb, P. A., & Trentham-Dietz, A. (2000). Breast feeding practices in relation to endometrial cancer risk, USA. *Cancer Causes & Control, 11*, 663–667.

Ortho-McNeil-Janssen-Pharmaceuticals. (2010). *Ortho Evra prescribing information.* Retrieved from http://www.orthoevra.com/sites/default/files/assets/Ortho EvraPI_0.pdf

Otero-Flores, J. B., Guerrero-Carreno, F. J., & Vazquez-Estrada, L. A. (2003). A comparative randomized study of three different IUDs in nulliparous Mexican women. *Contraception, 67*, 273–276.

Pakarinen, P. I., Suvisaari, J., Luukkainen, T., & Lahteenmaki, P. (1997). Intracervical and fundal administration of levonorgestrel for contraception: Endometrial thickness, patterns of bleeding, and persisting ovarian follicles. *Fertility and Sterility, 68*, 59–64.

Peterson, H. B., Jeng, G., Folger, S. G., Hillis, S. A., Marchbanks, P. A., & Wilcox, L. S. (2000). The risk of menstrual abnormalities after tubal sterilization. U.S. Collaborative Review of Sterilization Working Group. *New England Journal of Medicine, 343*, 1681–1687.

Peterson, H. B., Xia, Z., Hughes, J. M., Wilcox, L. S., Tylor, L. R., & Trussell, J. (1996). The risk of pregnancy after tubal sterilization: Findings from the U.S. Collaborative Review of Sterilization. *American Journal of Obstetrics and Gynecology, 174*, 1161–1168.

Peterson, H. B., Xia, Z., Hughes, J. M., Wilcox, L. S., Tylor, L. R., & Trussell, J. (1997). The risk of ectopic pregnancy after tubal sterilization. U.S. Collaborative Review of Sterilization Working Group. *New England Journal of Medicine, 336*, 762–767.

Pfizer. (2010). *Depo-Provera full prescribing information.* Retrieved from http://www.pfizer.com/files/products/uspi_depo_provera_contraceptive.pdf

Pollack, A. E., Thomas, L. J., & Barone, M. A. (2007). Female and male sterilization. In R. A. Hatcher, J. Trussell, A. L. Nelson, W. Cates, F. Stewart, & D. Kowal (Eds.), *Contraceptive technology* (19th ed., pp. 361–401). New York: Ardent Media.

Polsky, B., Baron, P. A., Gold, J. W., Smith, J. L., Jensen, R. H., & Armstrong, D. (1988). In vitro inactivation of HIV-1 by contraceptive sponge containing nonoxynol-9. *Lancet, 1*(8600), 1456.

Raine, T., Harper, C., Leon, K., & Darney, P. (2000). Emergency contraception: Advance provision in a young, high-risk clinic population. *Obstetrics and Gynecology, 96*, 1–7.

Raymond, E. G. (2007a). Contraceptive implants. In R. A. Hatcher, J. Trussell, A. L. Nelson, W. Cates, F. Stewart, & D. Kowal (Eds.), *Contraceptive technology* (19th ed., pp. 145–156). New York: Ardent Media.

Raymond, E. G. (2007b). Progestin-only pills. In R. A. Hatcher, J. Trussell, A. L. Nelson, W. Cates, F. Stewart, & D. Kowal (Eds.), *Contraceptive technology* (19th ed., pp. 181–191). New York: Ardent Media.

Raymond, E. G., Chen, P. L., & Luoto, J. (2004). Contraceptive effectiveness and safety of five nonoxynol-9 spermicides: A randomized trial. *Obstetrics and Gynecology, 103*, 430–439.

Raymond, E., & Dominik, R. (1999). Contraceptive effectiveness of two spermicides: A randomized trial. *Obstetrics and Gynecology, 93*, 896–903.

Schwallie, P. C., & Assenzo, J. R. (1973). Contraceptive use: Efficacy study utilizing medroxyprogesterone acetate administered as an intramuscular injection once every 90 days. *Fertility and Sterility, 24*, 331–339.

Smith, R. D. (2009). Contemporary hysteroscopic methods for female sterilization [Electronic publication ahead of print]. *International Journal of Gynecology & Obstetrics.* doi: 10.1016/j.ijgo.2009.07.026

Steiner, M. J., Dominik, R., Rountree, R. W., & Dorflinger, L. (2003). Contraceptive effectiveness of a polyurethane condom and a latex condom: A randomized controlled trial. *Obstetrics and Gynecology, 101*, 539–547.

Stewart, F. H., Kaunitz, A. M., Laguardia, K. D., Karvois, D. L., Fisher, A. C., & Friedman, A. J. (2005). Extended use of transdermal norelgestromin/ethinyl estradiol: A randomized trial. *Obstetrics and Gynecology, 105*, 1389–1396.

Sulak, P. J., Scow, R. D., Preece, C., Riggs, M. W., & Kuehl, T. J. (2000). Hormone withdrawal symptoms in oral contraceptive users. *Obstetrics and Gynecology, 95*, 261–266.

Tone, A. (2001). *Devices and desires: A history of contraceptives in America.* New York: Hill & Wong.

Trussell, J. (2007). Choosing a contraceptive: Efficacy, safety, and personal considerations. In R. A. Hatcher, J. Trussell, A. L. Nelson, W. Cates, F. Stewart, & D. Kowal (Eds.), *Contraceptive technology* (19th ed., pp. 19–47). New York: Ardent Media.

Turok, D. K., Gurtcheff, S. E., Handley, E., Simonsen, S. E., Sok, C., & Murphy, P. (2010). A pilot study of the copper T380A IUD and oral levonorgestrel for emergency contraception. *Contraception, 82*, 520–5252.

Van Damme, L., Ramjee, G., Alary, M., Vuylsteke, B., Chandeying, V., Rees, H.,…Laga, M. (2002). Effectiveness of COL-1492, a nonoxynol-9 vaginal gel, on HIV-1 transmission in female sex workers: A randomised controlled trial. *Lancet, 360*, 971–977.

Veres, S., Miller, L., & Burington, B. (2004). A comparison between the vaginal ring and oral contraceptives. *Obstetrics and Gynecology, 104*, 555–563.

Wallach, M., & Grimes, D. A. (Eds.). (2000). *Modern oral contraception.* Totowa, NJ: Emron.

Weller, S. C., & Davis-Beaty, K. (2002). Condom effectiveness in reducing heterosexual HIV transmission. *Cochrane Database of Systematic Reviews, 1,* CD003255.

Westhoff, C., Kerns, J., Morroni, C., Cushman, L. F., Tiezzi, T., & Murphy, P. A. (2002). Quick Start: A novel oral contraceptive initiation method. *Contraception, 66,* 141–145.

Westhoff, C., Morroni, C., Kerns, J., & Murphy, P. A. (2003). Bleeding patterns after immediate versus conventional oral contraceptive initiation: A randomized controlled trial. *Fertility and Sterility, 79,* 322–329.

Whittemore, A. S. (1994). Characteristics relating to ovarian cancer risk: Implications for prevention and detection. *Gynecologic Oncology, 55*(Pt. 2), S15–S19.

Wilcox, A. J., Weinberg, C. R., & Baird, D. D. (1995). Timing of sexual intercourse in relation to ovulation. *New England Journal of Medicine, 333,* 1517–1521.

Wilkinson, D., Tholandi, M., Ramjee, G., & Rutherford, G. W. (2002). Nonoxynol-9 spermicide for prevention of vaginally acquired HIV and other sexually transmitted infections: Systematic review and meta-analysis of randomised controlled trials including more than 5000 women. *Lancet Infectious Diseases, 2,* 613–617.

Winkler, H. A., Anderson, P. S., Fields, A. L., Runowicz, C. D., De Victoria, C., & Goldberg, G. L. (1999). Compliance with Papanicolaou smear screening following tubal ligation in women with cervical cancer. *Journal of Women's Health, 8,* 103–107.

World Health Organization (WHO). (2001). *WHO/CONRAD technical consultation on nonoxynol-9: Summary report.* Retrieved from http://www.who.int/reproductivehealth/publications/rtis/RHR_03_8/en

World Health Organization (WHO). (2004). *Selected practice recommendations for contraceptive use* (2nd ed.). Geneva, Switzerland: Author. Retrieved October 11, 2009, from http://www.who.int/reproductivehealth/publications/family_planning/9241562846index/en/index.html

World Health Organization (WHO). (2009). *Medical eligibility criteria for contraceptive use* (4th ed.). Retrieved February 12, 2011, from http://whqlibdoc.who.int/publications/2010/9789241563888_eng.pdf

Zieman, M., Hatcher, R. A., Cwiak, C., Darney, P. D., Creinen, M. D., & Stosur, H. R. (2010). *Managing contraception: 2010–2012.* Atlanta, GA: Bridging the Gap Communications.

Zlidar, V. M. (2000). Helping women use the pill (Series A, No. 10). *Population Reports, 28*(2).

Zukerman, Z., Weiss, D. B., & Orvieto, R. (2003). Does preejaculatory penile secretion originating from Cowper's gland contain sperm? *Journal of Assisted Reproduction and Genetics, 20,* 157–159.

Bibliography

Dickey, R. P. (2010). *Managing contraceptive pill patients* (14th ed.). Dallas, TX: EMIS Medical.

Fritz, M. A., & Speroff, L. (2011). *Clinical gynecologic endocrinology and infertility* (8th ed.). Baltimore: Lippincott Williams & Wilkins.

Hatcher, R. A., Trussell, J., Nelson, A. L., Cates, W., Stewart, F. H., & Kowal, D. (Eds.). (2007). *Contraceptive technology* (19th ed.). New York: Ardent Media.

Office of Population Research and the Association of Reproductive Health Professionals. (2011). *The emergency contraception web site.* Retrieved from www.not-2-late.com

Speroff, L., & Darney, P. D. (2010). *A clinical guide for contraception* (5th ed.). Baltimore: Lippincott Williams & Wilkins.

Zieman, M., Hatcher, R. A., Cwiak, C., Darney, P. D., Creinen, M. D., & Stosur, H. R. (2010). *Managing contraception: 2010–2012.* Atlanta, GA: Bridging the Gap Communications.

12-A

Selected Medical Eligibility Criteria for Contraceptive Use

The U.S. *Medical Eligibility Criteria for Contraceptive Use* (CDC, 2010) is a comprehensive, evidence-based guide for determining whether women have relative or absolute contraindications to contraceptive methods. The *Medical Eligibility Criteria* uses the following four classification categories of whether a person can use or should not use a method:

- *Category 1*—A condition for which there is no restriction for the use of the contraceptive method
- *Category 2*—A condition where the advantages of using the method generally outweigh the theoretical or proven risks
- *Category 3*—A condition where the theoretical or proven risks usually outweigh the advantages of using the method
- *Category 4*—A condition that represents an unacceptable health risk if the contraceptive method is used

The following table is a summary of selected criteria for contraceptive use. The table is a quick reference and not inclusive of the full guidelines. Readers are referred to the complete Medical Eligibility Criteria (available online, see citation at the end of the appendix) for clarifications of category classification, complete references, and conditions and contraceptive methods that are not included in this table. Abbreviations for the methods in the table are as follows:

- *COC/P/R*—Low-dose (≤ 35 mcg ethinyl estradiol) combined oral contraceptives, patch, and vaginal ring
- *POP*—Progestin-only pills
- *DMPA*—Depot medroxyprogesterone acetate injection
- *Implants*—Levonorgestrel/etonogestrel implants
- *Cu-IUD*—Copper intrauterine device
- *LNG-IUD*—Levonorgestrel intrauterine device

When there is a differentiation between criteria for initiation and continuation of a method, these are noted with the abbreviations "I" and "C" next to the category number.

Condition	COC/P/R	POP	DMPA	Implants	Cu-IUD	LNG-IUD
Personal Characteristics and Reproductive History						
Pregnancy					4	4
Age	Menarche to <40 = 1 ≥40 = 2	Menarche to <18 = 1 18–45 = 1 >45 = 1	Menarche to <18 = 2 18–45 = 1 >45 = 2	Menarche to <18 = 1 18–45 = 1 >45 = 1	Menarche to <20 = 2 ≥20 = 1	Menarche to <20 = 2 ≥20 = 1
Parity a) Nulliparous b) Parous	1 1	1 1	1 1	1 1	2 1	2 1
Breastfeeding a) < 21 days	4	2	2	2		
b) 21 to < 30 days i) With other risk factors for venous thromboembolism (VTE) (such as age ≥ 35 years, previous VTE, thrombophilia, immobility, transfusion at birth, body mass index [BMI] ≥ 30 kg/m², postpartum hemorrhage, post–cesarean birth, preeclampsia, or smoking)	3–4	2	2	2		
ii) Without other risk factors for VTE	3	2	2	2		
c) 30–42 days i) With other risk factors for VTE (such as age ≥ 35 years, previous VTE, thrombophilia, immobility, transfusion at birth, BMI ≥ 30 kg/m², postpartum hemorrhage, postcesarean birth, preeclampsia, or smoking)	3–4	1	1	1		
ii) Without other risk factors for VTE	2	1	1	1		
d) > 42 days	2	1	1	1		

Condition	COC/P/R	POP	DMPA	Implants	Cu-IUD	LNG-IUD
Postpartum (in nonbreastfeeding women)						
a) < 21 days	4			1		
b) 21–42 days						
i) With other risk factors for VTE (such as age ≥ 35 years, previous VTE, thrombophilia, immobility, transfusion at birth, BMI ≥ 30 kg/m², postpartum hemorrhage, post–cesarean birth, preeclampsia, or smoking)	3–4			1		
ii) Without other risk factors for VTE	2	1	1	1		
c) > 42 days	1	1	1	1		
Postpartum (in breastfeeding women)						
a) < 21 days	3	1	1	1		
b) ≥ 21 days	1	1	1	1		
Postpartum (breastfeeding or nonbreastfeeding women, including post–cesarean section)						
a) < 10 minutes after delivery of the placenta					1	2
b) 10 minutes after delivery of the placenta to < 4 weeks					2	2
c) ≥ 4 weeks					1	1
d) Puerperal sepsis					4	4
Postabortion						
a) First trimester	1	1	1	1	1	1
b) Second trimester	1	1	1	1	2	2
c) Immediate postseptic abortion	1	1	1	1	4	4
Past ectopic pregnancy	1	2	1	1	1	1
History of pelvic surgery	1	1	1	1	1	1
Smoking						
a) Age < 35	2	1	1	1	1	1
b) Age ≥ 35						
i) < 15 cigarettes/day	3	1	1	1	1	1
ii) ≥ 15 cigarettes/day	4	1	1	1	1	1

(continues)

275

Condition	COC/P/R	POP	DMPA	Implants	Cu-IUD	LNG-IUD
Obesity						
a) ≥ 30 kg/m² BMI	2	1	1	1	1	1
b) Menarche to < 18 years and ≥ 30 kg/m² BMI	2	1	2	1	1	1
History of bariatric surgery						
a) Restrictive procedures: decrease storage capacity of the stomach	1	1	1	1	1	1
b) Malabsorptive procedures: decrease absorption of nutrients and calories by shortening the functional length of the small intestine	COCs = 3 P/R = 1	3	1	1	1	1
Cardiovascular Disease						
Multiple risk factors for arterial cardiovascular disease (such as older age, smoking, diabetes, and hypertension)	3/4	2	3	2	1	2
Hypertension						
a) Adequately controlled hypertension	3	1	2	1	1	1
b) Elevated blood pressure levels (properly take measurements)						
i) Systolic 140–159 mm HG or diastolic 90–99 mm HG	3	1	2	1	1	1
ii) Systolic > 160 mm HG or diastolic ≥ 100 mm HG	4	2	3	2	1	2
c) Vascular disease	4	2	3	2	1	2
History of high blood pressure during pregnancy (where current blood pressure is measurable and normal)	2	1	1	1	1	1
Deep venous thrombosis (DVT)/pulmonary embolism (PE)						

Condition	COC/P/R	POP	DMPA	Implants	Cu-IUD	LNG-IUD
a) History of DVT/PE, not on anticoagulant therapy						
i) Higher risk for recurrent DVT/PE (≥ 1 risk factor)	4	2	2	2	1	2
ii) Lower risk for recurrent DVT/PE (no risk factors)	3	2	2	2	1	2
b) Acute DVT/PE	4	2	2	2	2	2
c) DVT/PE and established anticoagulant therapy for at least 3 mos						
i) Higher risk for recurrent DVT/PE (≥ 1 risk factor)	4	2	2	2	2	2
ii) Lower risk for recurrent DVT/PE (no risk factors)	3	2	2	2	2	2
d) Family history (first-degree relatives)	2	1	1	1	1	1
e) Major surgery						
i) With prolonged immobilization	4	2	2	2	1	2
ii) Without prolonged immobilization	2	1	1	1	1	1
f) Minor surgery without immobilization	1	1	1	1	1	1
Known thrombogenic mutations (e.g. factor V Leiden; prothrombin mutation; protein S, protein C, and antithrombin deficiencies)	4	2	2	2	1	2
Superficial venous thrombosis						
a) Varicose veins	1	1	1	1	1	1
b) Superficial thrombophlebitis	2	1	1	1	1	1
Current and history of ischemic heart disease	4	I2/C3	3	I2/C3	1	I2/C3
Stroke (history of cerebrovascular accident)	4	I2/C3	3	I2/C3	1	2
Known hyperlipidemias (screening is NOT necessary for safe use of contraceptive methods)	2/3	2	2	2	1	2
Valvular heart disease						
a) Uncomplicated	2	1	1	1	1	1
b) Complicated (pulmonary hypertension, risk for atrial fibrillation, history of subacute bacterial endocarditis)	4	1	1	1	1	1

(continues)

Condition	COC/P/R	POP	DMPA	Implants	Cu-IUD	LNG-IUD
Peripartum cardiomyopathy						
a) Normal or mildly impaired cardiac function						
i) < 6 mos	4	1	1	1	2	2
ii) ≥ 6 mos	3	1	1	1	2	2
b) Moderately or severely impaired cardiac function	4	2	2	2	2	2
Rheumatic Diseases						
Systemic lupus erythematosus (SLE)						
a) Positive (or unknown) antiphospholipid antibodies	4	3	I3/C3	3	I1/C1	3
b) Severe thrombocytopenia	2	2	I3/C2	2	I3/C2	2
c) Immunosuppressive treatment	2	2	I2/C2	2	I2/C1	2
d) None of the above	2	2	I2/C2	2	I1/C1	2
Rheumatoid arthritis						
a) On immunosuppressive therapy	2	1	2/3	1	I2/C1	I2/C1
b) Not on immunosuppressive therapy	2	1	2	1	1	1
Neurologic Conditions						
Headaches						
a) Nonmigrainous (mild or severe)	I1/C2	I1/C1	I1/C1	I1/C1	1	I1/C1
b) Migraine						
i) Without aura						
Age < 35	I2/C3	I1/C2	I2/C2	I2/C2	1	I2/C2
Age ≥ 35	I3/C4	I1/C2	I2/C2	I2/C2	1	I2/C2
ii) With aura (at any age)	I4/C4	I2/C3	I2/C3	I2/C3	1	I2/C3
Epilepsy	1	1	1	1	1	1
Depressive Disorders						
Depressive disorders	1	1	1	1	1	1

Condition	COC/P/R	POP	DMPA	Implants	Cu-IUD	LNG-IUD
Reproductive Tract Infections and Disorders						
Vaginal bleeding patterns						
a) Irregular pattern without heavy bleeding	1	2	2	2	1	I1/C1
b) Heavy or prolonged bleeding (includes regular and irregular patterns)	1	2	2	2	2	I1/C2
Unexplained vaginal bleeding (suspicious for serious conditions)						
Before evaluation	2	2	3	3	I4/C2	I4/C2
Endometriosis	1	1	1	1	2	1
Benign ovarian tumors (including cysts)	1	1	1	1	1	1
Severe dysmenorrhea	1	1	1	1	2	1
Gestational trophoblast disease						
a) Decreasing or undetectable β-hCG	1	1	1	1	3	3
b) Persistently elevated β-hCG levels or malignant disease	1	1	1	1	4	4
Cervical ectropion	1	1	1	1	1	1
Cervical intraepithelial neoplasia (CIN)	2	1	2	2	1	2
Cervical cancer (awaiting treatment)	2	1	2	2	I4/C2	I4/C2
Breast disease						
a) Undiagnosed mass	2	2	2	2	1	2
b) Benign breast disease	1	1	1	1	1	1
c) Family history of cancer	1	1	1	1	1	1
d) Breast cancer						
i) Current	4	4	4	4	1	4
ii) Past and no evidence of current disease for 5 years	3	3	3	3	1	3

(continues)

Condition	COC/P/R	POP	DMPA	Implants	Cu-IUD	LNG-IUD
Endometrial hyperplasia	1	1	1	1	1	1
Endometrial cancer	1	1	1	1	I4/C2	I4/C2
Ovarian cancer	1	1	1	1	1	1
Uterine fibroids	1	1	1	1	2	2
Anatomical abnormalities a) That distort the uterine cavity b) That do not distort the uterine cavity					4 2	4 2

Pelvic inflammatory disease (PID)
a) Past PID (assuming no current risk factors of STIs)
  i) With subsequent pregnancy
  ii) Without subsequent pregnancy
b) Current PID
	1
	1
	1
		1
		1
		1
			1
			1
			1
				1
				1
				1
					I1/C1
					I2/C2
					I4/C2
						I1/C1
						I2/C2
						I4/C2

STIs a) Current purulent cervicitis or chlamydial infection or gonorrhea	1	1	1	1	I4/C2	I4/C2
b) Other STIs (excluding HIV and hepatitis)	1	1	1	1	I2/C2	I2/C2
c) Vaginitis (including *Trichomonas vaginalis* and bacterial vaginosis)	1	1	1	1	I2/C2	I2/C2
d) Increased risk of STIs	1	1	1	1	I2-3/C2	I2-3/C2
HIV/AIDS						
High risk for HIV	1	1	1	1	I2/C2	I2/C2
HIV infection	1	1	1	1	I2/C2	I2/C2
AIDS Clinically well on ARV therapy (see *antiretroviral therapy* below)	1	1	1	1	I3/C2 I2/C2	I3/C2 I2/C2

Condition	COC/P/R	POP	DMPA	Implants	Cu-IUD	LNG-IUD
Other Infections						
Schistosomiasis						
a) Uncomplicated	1	1	1	1	1	1
b) Fibrosis of the liver (if severe, see *cirrhosis*)	1	1	1	1	1	1
Tuberculosis						
a) Non-pelvic	1	1	1	1	I1/C1	I1/C1
b) Pelvic	1	1	1	1	I4/C3	I4/C3
Malaria	1	1	1	1	1	1
Endocrine Conditions						
Diabetes						
a) History of gestational disease	1	1	1	1	1	1
b) Nonvascular disease						
i) Noninsulin-dependent	2	2	2	2	1	2
ii) Insulin-dependent	2	2	2	2	1	2
c) Nephropathy/retinopathy/ neuropathy	3/4	2	3	2	1	2
d) Other vascular disease or diabetes of > 20 years' duration	3/4	2	3	2	1	2
Thyroid disorders						
a) Simple goiter	1	1	1	1	1	1
b) Hyperthyroid	1	1	1	1	1	1
c) Hypothyroid	1	1	1	1	1	1
Gastrointestinal Conditions						
Inflammatory bowel disease (IBD) (ulcerative colitis, Crohn disease)	2/3	2	2	1	1	1
Gallbladder disease						
a) Symptomatic						
i) Treated by cholecystectomy	2	2	2	2	1	2
ii) Medically treated	3	2	2	2	1	2
iii) Current	3	2	2	2	1	2
b) Asymptomatic	2	2	2	2	1	2

(continues)

Condition	COC/P/R	POP	DMPA	Implants	Cu-IUD	LNG-IUD
History of cholestasis						
a) Pregnancy-related	2	1	1	1	1	1
b) Past COC-related	3	2	2	2	1	2
Viral hepatitis						
a) Acute or flare	I3-4/C2	1	1	1	1	1
b) Carrier	I1/C1	1	1	1	1	1
c) Chronic	I1/C1	1	1	1	1	1
Cirrhosis						
a) Mild (compensated)	1	1	1	1	1	1
b) Severe (decompensated)	4	3	3	3	1	3
Liver tumors						
a) Benign						
i) Focal nodular hyperplasia	2	2	2	2	1	2
ii) Hepatocellular adenoma	4	3	3	3	1	3
b) Malignant (hepatoma)	4	3	3	3	1	3
Anemias						
Thalassemia	1	1	1	1	2	1
Sickle cell disease	2	1	1	1	2	1
Iron-deficiency anemia	1	1	1	1	2	1
Solid Organ Transplantation						
a) Complicated: graft failure (acute or chronic), rejection, cardiac allograft vasculopathy	4	2	2	2	I3/C2	I3/C2
b) Uncomplicated	2	2	2	2	I2/C2	I2/C2

Condition	COC/P/R	POP	DMPA	Implants	Cu-IUD	LNG-IUD
Drug Interactions						
Antiretroviral (ARV) therapy						
a) Nucleoside reverse transcriptase inhibitors (NRTIs)	1	1	1	1	I2-3/C2	I2-3/C2
b) Nonnucleoside reverse transcriptase inhibitors (NNRTIs)	2	2	1	2	I2-3/C2	I2-3/C2
c) Ritonavir-boosted protease inhibitors	3	3	1	2	I2-3/C2	I2-3/C2
Anticonvulsant therapy						
a) Certain anticonvulsants (phenytoin, carbamazepine, barbiturates, primidone, topiramate, oxcarbazepine)	3	3	1	2	1	1
b) Lamotrigine	3	1	1	1	1	1
Antimicrobial therapy						
a) Broad-spectrum antibiotics	1	1	1	1	1	1
b) Antifungals	1	1	1	1	1	1
c) Antiparasitics	1	1	1	1	1	1
d) Rifampicin or rifabutin therapy	3	3	1	2	1	1

Source: Adapted from Centers for Disease Control and Prevention. (2010). U.S. medical eligibility criteria for contraceptive use, 2010: Adapted from the World Health Organization medical eligibility criteria for contraceptive use, 4th edition. _Morbidity and Mortality Weekly Report, 59,_ 1–86. Retrieved from http://www.cdc.gov/reproductivehealth/unintendedpregnancy/USMEC.htm

12-B

Primary* Mechanisms of Action of Contraceptive Methods

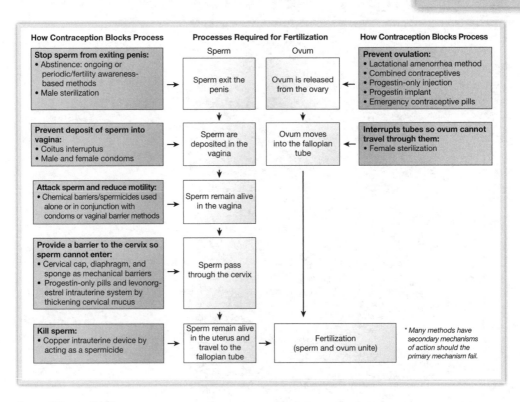

How Contraception Blocks Process	Processes Required for Fertilization		How Contraception Blocks Process
	Sperm	Ovum	
Stop sperm from exiting penis: • Abstinence: ongoing or periodic/fertility awareness-based methods • Male sterilization	Sperm exit the penis	Ovum is released from the ovary	**Prevent ovulation:** • Lactational amenorrhea method • Combined contraceptives • Progestin-only injection • Progestin implant • Emergency contraceptive pills
Prevent deposit of sperm into vagina: • Coitus interruptus • Male and female condoms	Sperm are deposited in the vagina	Ovum moves into the fallopian tube	**Interrupts tubes so ovum cannot travel through them:** • Female sterilization
Attack sperm and reduce motility: • Chemical barriers/spermicides used alone or in conjunction with condoms or vaginal barrier methods	Sperm remain alive in the vagina		
Provide a barrier to the cervix so sperm cannot enter: • Cervical cap, diaphragm, and sponge as mechanical barriers • Progestin-only pills and levonorgestrel intrauterine system by thickening cervical mucus	Sperm pass through the cervix		
Kill sperm: • Copper intrauterine device by acting as a spermicide	Sperm remain alive in the uterus and travel to the fallopian tube	Fertilization (sperm and ovum unite)	*Many methods have secondary mechanisms of action should the primary mechanism fail.*

Source: © Frances E. Likis.

13

Menopause

Ivy M. Alexander
Linda C. Andrist

Menopause, which is often thought of as the closure of reproductive capability, has emerged as one of the predominant health issues for midlife women. A major reason that menopause is receiving so much attention is the increasing numbers of women reaching midlife, which encompasses the perimenopausal years (ages 35 to 50 years) to menopause (ages 50 to 60 years) (Davis & Huber, 2004; Fogel & Woods, 2008). The baby boom generation—that is, people born between 1945 and 1960—is the largest middle-aged cohort ever recorded. In 2004, women who reached age 65 had an average 20 years of life expectancy (Administration on Aging, 2008). Because the life span continues to increase, women will live one-third of their lives after menopause.

The emphasis on the end of reproduction ignores the myriad issues facing women at midlife. Midlife brings with it many changes, such as children leaving home, illness or death of parents, and career changes. Transitions that accompany midlife include adjusting to the idea of mortality, adapting to changes in family relationships, becoming more authentic, and assessing and appreciating one's life experiences (Sampselle, Harris, Harlow, & Sowers, 2002).

During midlife, women continue to grow and develop psychologically. Increasingly, menopause is being understood as another life stage with potential for growth and development. The challenges experienced during this transition may serve as the basis for personal reflection and growth (Busch, Barth-Olofsson, Rosenhagen, & Collins, 2003).

Many researchers have elucidated women's unique growth and development. For example, Gilligan (1982) found that relationships were a priority for women. Jordan and colleagues (1991) found that women develop in relationship with others, and development means increasing complexity, connection, and mutuality. Collins (1990) recognized the uniqueness of African American women's experience. The major premise in many of the published works is the importance of recognizing the variation in women's development based on culture, race, and socioeconomic variables.

To that end, Sampselle et al. (2002) conducted focus groups with 32 Caucasian and African American women who were in midlife to identify factors that enhanced their well-being, and to determine whether these factors differed between the two groups. These researchers found that Caucasian participants were concerned about menopause as a sign of aging and the loss of youthful appearance, whereas the African American women were welcoming of menopause as a normal event. All of the women identified childbearing and child launching as major stages in women's lives. The potential for further personal development was enhanced by fewer childcare demands, and women felt few feelings of loss.

Quinn (1991) developed a theoretical model, known as "Integrating a New Me," through a qualitative study with 12 women. Four processes that women experienced were identified:

- Tuning into me: The beginning of the awareness of entering perimenopause
- Facing a paradox of feelings: Both positive and negative feelings about situations such as getting older, reproduction, physical vulnerability, and uncertainty about the future
- Contrasting impressions: The processing of conflicting information, women developing their own symbolic meaning through integrating interactions with others, and their own self-appraisal
- Making adjustments: The changes and alterations that women make in response to their emotional, physical, and life changes in daily living

Arnold (2005) interviewed 23 women about the transition in moving from their 40s to their 50s. The women described these changes as "stepping out of the mold" of society's "rules" about how they should behave, and "letting go" of material things as well as previous expectations they had of themselves. "I feel competent and no longer have to prove my abilities" (p. 641). "Walking in balance" was a theme that women described as "characterizing self as peaceful, accepting, and in line with their interests and needs" (p. 642). They described themselves as "moving in new directions," finding a new zest for life and interests for creative self-expression. At this stage of their lives, they were "redefining relationships" with family and particularly female friends. Finally they expressed a freedom "to be" strong resourceful women.

Building on Sheehy's (1976, 1995) work, Wilmoth (1996) proposed a conceptual framework that includes disassembling, evaluating, and reassembling, as a means to find one's own truth. Disassembling entails taking apart our psychological lives and examining them from a new perspective. This phase includes a natural mourning process for lost youth, loss of procreative abilities, and lost opportunities, and is similar to Quinn's first process. The evaluation process that accompanies disassembling requires that women look into themselves to see who they are and whether they like themselves. Wilmoth argues that the context of each woman's experience depends on her lived experience and life situation—hence the variation in women's experiences. Reassembling incorporates a coming of age and a movement toward mastery.

Ballard, Kuh, and Wadsworth (2001) described the menopause transition as a status passage based on a longitudinal study, which includes five stages: (1) expectations of symptoms, (2) experience of symptoms and loss of control, (3) confirmation of the menopause, (4) regaining control, and (5) freedom from menstruation.

All of the aforementioned models include three major phases: assessment, adjusting to change, and acceptance. It is noteworthy that many researchers have found that menopause itself—that is, the cessation of menstruation—is just one event in the overall context of women's lives during midlife.

The Medicalization of Menopause: A Historical Perspective

Menopause is a remarkable example of the medicalization of women's bodies. The biomedical model of the twentieth century perpetuated menopause as a deficiency disease (MacPherson, 1981) or endocrinopathy (Utian, 1987). Science attempted to establish hormone therapy (HT; **Table 13-1**) as the panacea for prevention of diseases in old age, and pharmaceutical corporations aggressively marketed their products as representing "the fountain of youth."

In 1938, researchers in England produced the first synthetic estrogen, diethylstilbestrol, which was heralded as the cure for postmenopausal symptoms. Premarin, a medication

TABLE 13-1 Recommended Hormone Therapy Terminology*

Term	Abbreviation/Explanation
Estrogen therapy alone	ET
Estrogen-progestogen therapy	EPT
Hormone therapy	HT; encompassing term for ET/EPT
Continuous-combined daily estrogen-progestogen therapy	CC-EPT
Continuous-sequential estrogen-progestogen therapy (estrogen daily, progestogen added on a set sequence)	CS-EPT
Preparations of ET or EPT that have a systemic—not solely vaginal—effect	Systemic HT
Preparations of ET that have a predominantly vaginal—not systemic—effect	Local ET
Progestogen	Encompassing term for progesterone and progestin

*The North American Menopause Society (NAMS) has urged clinicians, researchers, and the media to standardize terminology, which it considers essential for ensuring accurate communication. Note that the word *replacement* has been deleted from the terms *hormone replacement therapy* and *estrogen replacement therapy*.

Source: Adapted from NAMS, 2010a.

introduced by Wyeth-Ayerst in 1942, was the first nonsynthetic estrogen produced from the urine of pregnant mares. Although this therapy was prescribed for many women, the use of HT did not increase significantly until the 1960s, particularly after the publication of *Feminine Forever* by gynecologist Robert Wilson (1966). The major message in this highly popular book—100,000 copies of which were sold in the first seven months after its publication—was that after menopause women would become eunuchs with withered breasts and begin a "living decay" (Wilson, p. 43). Estrogen use, which was then referred to as hormone replacement therapy (HRT), promised women the fountain of youth and was praised by Wilson as "one of the greatest biological revolutions in the history of civilization" (Wilson, p. 16). Interestingly, Wilson's work was funded by the pharmaceutical manufacturers Ayerst, Searle, and Upjohn.

Between the years 1967 and 1975, sales of Premarin (conjugated equine estrogens [CEE]) tripled. By the time its association with endometrial cancer became known, Premarin was the fifth most popular drug in the United States. In 1975, researchers began to link estrogen use with an increased incidence of endometrial cancer, and the sales of Premarin dropped dramatically. By 1979, the National Institute on Aging convened a consensus conference and agreed that "women using estrogens should take them only for the shortest possible time, in the lowest possible dose," because HT increases the risk for endometrial cancer (U.S. Department of Health, Education, and Welfare, 1979, p. 1). Additionally, the committee concluded that HT was effective only for hot flashes and vaginal dryness (National Women's Health Network, 2000). It is noteworthy that this is the same recommendation put forward by the North American Menopause Society (NAMS) in 2003.

During the 1980s, epidemiologic data demonstrated that the addition of a progestogen to estrogen therapy (ET) lowered the risk of endometrial cancer. Once again, HT increased in popularity. When researchers demonstrated that HT could decrease the risk of osteoporosis in the early 1980s (Weiss, Ure, Ballard, William, & Daling, 1980), the promotion of HT changed from an emphasis on symptom relief to prevention of disease in old age. By the late 1980s, several observational studies had shown that HT was protective against heart disease. Indeed, until the release of the findings of the Women's Health Initiative (WHI) in 2002, clinicians continued recommending HT to nearly all postmenopausal women for long-term prevention of heart disease. The U.S. Preventive Services Task Force (USPSTF) made the recommendation in the 1990s that all women should be counseled about and consider preventive HT (USPSTF, 1996). The USPSTF did not, however, offer a recommendation about whether women should actually take HT. Studies linking estrogen use and breast cancer were glossed over, and women were told that the risk of heart disease outweighed the risk of breast cancer. Studies were published linking the use of HT and reduced risk of Alzheimer's disease, memory loss, skin integrity, and colon cancer.

The WHI is the largest clinical trial ever to be conducted on health risks of postmenopausal women. As part of this study, nearly 17,000 women were randomized into HT or placebo groups between 1993 and 1998. The estrogen with progestogen arm of the study was halted in 2002, after a mean of 5.2 years of follow-up, because the health risks outweighed the benefits. These deleterious outcomes included increased risk of breast cancer, coronary events, stroke, and pulmonary embolism (Rossouw et al., 2002). In March 2004, the estrogen arm of the study was also stopped because researchers found an increased risk of stroke. The study group reported that estrogen did not appear to increase or decrease heart disease or breast cancer (Anderson et al., 2004; National Institutes of Health [NIH], 2004). Results from the WHI established that ET prevents osteoporosis-related hip fractures and protects the spine and small bones against the development of osteoporosis. While CEE preparations are still indicated for the prevention of postmenopausal osteoporosis, most experts recommend the use of nonestrogen medications for this purpose (Liu, 2004).

Some experts have pointed out the limitations of the WHI results, such as the age of participants. The mean age of women participating in the study was 63 years, which is significantly older than newly menopausal women. The study also used only one HT product, Prempro, which contains CEE and medroxyprogesterone acetate (MPA). Although findings from the WHI may apply to all HT products, additional clinical trials are needed to clarify the risks and benefits of other products. Finally, the WHI did not address quality of life issues for women with moderate to severe vasomotor symptoms related to menopause. In fact, these women were excluded from the study. For these reasons, it remains difficult to evaluate differences in HT response between women who initiate HT before the cessation of menses and those who begin later (Wysocki, Alexander, Schnare, Moore, & Freeman, 2003).

Women's use of postmenopausal HT declined shortly after the results of the WHI were published. Some resources reported that only 16% of women reinitiated HT, with women with diabetes, hyperlipidemia, or cardiovascular disease and those who were taking ET alone being more likely to restart HT (Newton et al., 2008). A meta-analysis of 30 clinical trials (26,708 women) and data from the Nurses' Health Study (121,700 women) demonstrated that the timing of initiating HT is an important factor, at least in terms of preventing heart disease. Women who started HT nearer to the menopause obtained a greater benefit from this therapy (Grodstein, Manson, & Stampfer, 2006; Salpeter, Walsh, Greyber, Ormiston, & Salpeter, 2004).

NAMS released position statements on the use of HT in menopausal women in 2004, 2007, 2008, and 2010 based on all of the studies subsequent to the WHI. The 2010 statement has specific recommendations:

- HT is not indicated for the sole purpose of preventing cardiovascular disease. Beginning HT in women aged 50 to 59 years or within 10 years of menopause to treat menopausal symptoms should not increase coronary heart disease risk. A growing body of evidence suggests that beginning HT at that time may decrease this risk.
- ET taken for fewer than 5 years seems to have little effect on the risk for breast cancer.
- HT is not recommended for prevention of cognitive aging or dementia.
- Although there have been no randomized clinical trials (RCTs) involving the lowest effective doses of ET and EPT, using the lowest dose that results in effectiveness should be the therapeutic goal for individual women.
- Duration of use must be individualized and based on the woman's profile and risk–benefit ratio.

- All women with an intact uterus should receive systemic progestogen with estrogen to decrease the risk of endometrial carcinoma (NAMS, 2010a).

The evolution of the use of HT for the prevention of disease has been challenged based on RCTs, and epidemiologic and observational data. The opening page of the NAMS's 2010 publication *Menopause Practice: A Clinician's Guide*, Fourth Edition, begins with these words: "Menopause is a normal, natural event ..." (NAMS, 2010b, p. 1.1). This shift from the 1980s view of menopause as pathologic, along with the increase in research on women's experiences of menopause, indicates a paradigm shift is occurring, which is effectively dismantling the concept of menopause as a disease. Nurse researchers, in particular, have demonstrated that menopause is a normal developmental stage in women's lives. Some women will need HT to increase their quality of life, but the practice is no longer standard treatment for all women during midlife.

Natural Menopause

Menopause is defined as the point in time in which there has been a cessation of menstruation for at least 12 consecutive months. Menopause occurs in response to normal physiologic changes in the hypothalamic–pituitary–ovarian axis (see Chapter 5 for a detailed description of the menstrual cycle). During the perimenopausal period, which spans approximately 2 to 8 years prior to the last menstrual period, and for the 12 months of amenorrhea preceding menopause, fewer ovarian follicles develop in each menstrual cycle. The follicles that do develop are less responsive to follicle-stimulating hormone (FSH), and the ovaries produce less estradiol, progesterone, and androgens. Thus the usual negative feedback effect from elevated estrogen and progesterone levels on hypothalamic production of gonadotropin-releasing hormone (GnRH) is lost, and the anterior pituitary production of FSH and leuteinizing hormone (LH) continues. Irregular menstrual cycles—characterized by longer or shorter cycles, heavier or lighter flow, periods of amenorrhea, and worsening or newly developing premenstrual symptoms—are common during this time. Eventually, ovarian follicle production stops, estrogen and progesterone levels remain low, FSH and LH levels remain high, and menstruation ceases. The postmenopausal period refers to the first 5 years or so following menopause when hormonal fluctuations often continue to occur (NAMS, 2010b; Soules et al., 2001; Utian, 1999a, 1999b, 2001).

A woman is born with approximately 1.2 million ovarian follicles. Throughout her life, some of these follicles are used during ovulation, but most are lost through atresia until menopause when about 1000 follicles remain.

Although it sounds like a smooth process, the perimenopausal transition is anything but smooth for most women. Hormone levels can fluctuate wildly from day to day, causing many of the symptoms associated with the perimenopause and menopause transition (**Table 13-2**). Hormone fluctuation is related to many factors including the reduced number of responsive ovarian follicles.

Contrary to popular belief, women continue to produce estrogen and androgens after menopause. Three types of estrogen of exist. Estradiol (E_2), which is the most potent of

TABLE 13-2 Symptoms Associated with Perimenopause and Menopause

Acne	Headache	Poor concentration
Arthralgia	Hirsutism/virilization	Recurrent cystitis
Asthenia	Hot flashes/flushes	Recurrent vaginitis
Decreased libido	Irregular menses/bleeding	Skin dryness/atrophy
Decreased vaginal lubrication	Irritability/mood disturbances	Sleep disturbances/insomnia
Depression	Mastalgia	Stress urinary incontinence*
Dizziness	Myalgia	Urinary frequency
Dry eyes	Nervousness/anxiety	Urinary urgency
Dry/thinning hair	Night sweats	Vaginal atrophy
Dyspareunia	Nocturia	Vaginal/vulvar burning
Dysuria	Odor	Vaginal/vulvar irritation
Fatigue	Palpitations	Vaginal/vulvar pruritis
Forgetfulness	Paresthesia	
Formication		

*Data are inconclusive.

Sources: Data from Alexander et al., 2003; Avis et al., 2001; Greendale, Lee, & Arriola, 1999; Jacobs Institute on Women's Health, 2003; McKinlay, 1996.

the three, is the main estrogen produced during the reproductive years; it is present in low amounts in the postmenopausal years following peripheral conversion of androstenedione. Estriol (E_3) is secreted by the placenta and synthesized from androgens produced by the fetus during pregnancy, and is present in nonpregnant women in small amounts as a by-product of estradiol and estrone. Estrone (E_1), the weakest estrogen, is the primary estrogen present in postmenopausal women, children, and men. In the postmenopausal period, estrone is produced by adipose conversion of androstenedione secreted by the adrenals (95%) and, to a lesser extent, the ovaries (5%), as well as by metabolism of estradiol.

Although the ovaries no longer produce functional follicles after menopause, the corticostromal and hilar cells of the stromal tissue are steroidogenic and produce significant levels of both androstenedione and testosterone for many years. Circulating levels of androstenedione in postmenopausal women are approximately half those of premenopausal women. Conversely, circulating levels of testosterone remain relatively constant in women who are either premenopausal or postmenopausal, partly due to the presence of high FSH and LH levels, which stimulate the ovarian stromal tissues to increase their testosterone production.

Natural menopause occurs for most women between the ages of 48 and 55 years. Fifty-one is the average age for women in the Western world (Soules et al., 2001; Utian, 1999b). The age at menopause is difficult to predict for an individual woman, but does correlate with the age when her mother or older sisters had menopause (Cramer, Xu, & Harlow, 1995; de

Bruin et al., 2001). A number of factors that may affect the age at menopause have been studied, such as parity, age at menarche, obesity, height, and oral contraceptive use (Bromberger et al., 1997; Cooper, Sandler, & Bohlig, 1999; Dvornyk et al., 2006; Gold et al., 2001; Santoro et al., 2007; Santoro et al., 2004; van Noord, Dubas, Dorland, Boersma, & te Velde, 1997). In contrast, studies of gene mutations and models to predict age for menopause have had limited success (Hefler et al., 2006; Huber et al., 2006). Smoking has consistently been found to have a relationship with age at menopause, and is associated with menopause occurring 1½ years earlier among smokers versus nonsmokers (Bromberger et al., 1997; Cooper et al.; Gold et al.; van Noord et al.). Menstrual cycle changes, including length of cycle, amount of bleeding, and 2- and 3-month periods of amenorrhea are associated with a shorter time to menopause (Garcia et al., 2005; Harlow et al., 2006). Cycle lengths less than 21 days have been associated with the early stages of the menopause transition (Van Voorhis, Santoro, Harlow, Crawford, & Randolph, 2008). A combination of symptoms—including irregular cycles, changed hormone levels, age, and smoking—was identified to be predictive in the Study of Women's Health Across the Nation (SWAN) (Santoro et al., 2007).

Ethnicity also may have an effect on age at menopause. A few studies have found that African American women experience menopause slightly earlier than other women, with an average age at menopause of 49.6 years and a median age of 49.3 or 50 years (Bromberger et al., 1997; Palmer, Rosenberg, Wise, Horton, & Adams-Campbell, 2003). However, no significant difference in age at menopause was identified in black versus white women (average age = 51.4 years for both groups) in the SWAN study (Gold et al., 2001). Interestingly, the SWAN study did identify statistically significant differences in average age at menopause among Hispanics (51.0 years) and Japanese Americans (51.8 years), as compared with Caucasians (51.4 years). Body size could also be a factor (Santoro et al., 2004), because women with higher body weights often have more adipose tissue, which stores androstenedione and converts it to estrogen (Fritz & Speroff, 2011).

A serum blood test for anti-Müllerian hormone (AMH) may be the preferred predictor in the future. Research has identified that AMH, which reflects the number of follicles, may be helpful in identifying when women older than the age of 30 can expect to be postmenopausal (van Disseldorp et al., 2008). More research is needed to determine exactly how this measure, which is currently used for infertility evaluations, might be applied for predicting menopause.

Menopause from Other Causes

Menopause can also occur due to several other causes (NAMS, 2010b; Utian, 1999a). Induced menopause occurs following either surgical excision of both ovaries (bilateral oophorectomy) or ovarian function ablation caused by medication, chemotherapy, or radiation. Although menstruation and fertility cease immediately following surgical menopause, both may persist for several months after ablative treatments are given. Premature menopause is menopause that occurs before the age of 40. It often follows the pattern of natural menopause, and results in the permanent loss of menstruation and fertility. Idiopathic ovarian insufficiency or premature ovarian failure (POF) also occurs in women younger than 40 years old; however, unlike premature menopause, POF is not always permanent and is often associated with other health problems, such as autoimmune and genetic disorders. Temporary menopause can occur at any age when normal ovarian function is lost and then resumes. This condition can be idiopathic, related to a disease entity, or induced by medications.

Women who experience induced or premature menopause have early loss of fertility and often experience more severe symptoms. They are at greater risk for developing cardiovascular disease (CVD) and osteoporosis (Gallagher, 2007; Lobo, 2007), and may also face significant health problems related to underlying disease processes.

Diagnosing Menopause

Menopause is actually a retrospective diagnosis because it is based on the clinical absence of menses for 12 consecutive months. Serial FSH testing that revealed levels sustained at less than 40 mIU/mL was used in the past to determine menopause status. However, because FSH levels can return to normal and estrogen levels can unexpectedly rise high enough to trigger the LH surge needed for ovulation, serum FSH testing is no longer recommended for determining perimenopausal or menopausal status (Bastian, Smith, & Nanda, 2003; NAMS, 2010a, 2010b). Similarly, perimenopause is most accurately identified based on a variety of factors, including age and symptoms such as hot flashes, irregular menses, and vaginal dryness. Due to the potential for unexpected ovulation, women who are perimenopausal need to continue to use a reliable form of birth control (see Chapter 12 for information about contraception). Perimenopausal women experience a high rate of unintended pregnancies with as many as 40% to 50% of pregnancies in these women reported as unintended (Finer & Henshaw, 2006; Sherman, Harvey, & Noell, 2005).

Differential Diagnoses

Other health problems can mimic the symptoms of menopause and must also be considered when a woman presents with perimenopausal and menopausal symptoms (NAMS, 2010b). These diagnoses may include diabetes, hypertension, arrhythmias, thyroid disorders (hypothyroid or hyperthyroid), anemia, depression, tumors, or carcinoma. A sample list of differential diagnoses is provided in **Table 13-3**. Medications, alcohol, or drug use can also cause many symptoms similar to perimenopause and menopause.

Each woman presenting with menopausal symptoms must be carefully evaluated with a thorough history, a physical examination, and selective laboratory testing (such as a complete blood count, fasting glucose, and serum thyroid-stimulating hormone level) to accurately identify the cause of her symptoms. Often a woman has several diagnoses to contend with at once, such as hypertension, diabetes, and menopause. Controlling her diabetes and hypertension may also reduce her menopausal symptoms enough so that they no longer are bothersome for her.

TABLE 13-3 Sample of Differential Diagnoses That Have Symptoms Similar to Perimenopause and Menopause

Diagnosis	Symptoms Similar to Perimenopause/Menopause
Anemia	Fatigue
	Cognitive changes
Anovulation	Amenorrhea
Pregnancy	Irregular bleeding
Arrhythmias	Fatigue
	Palpitations
Arthritis	Joint aches/pain
Depression	Fatigue
	Moodiness
	Anxiety
	Sleep disturbances, insomnia
Diabetes	Fatigue
	Hot flashes/heat intolerance
Hypertension	Headaches
Hyperthyroidism	Sleep disturbance, insomnia
	Nervousness, irritability
	Heat intolerance
Hypothyroidism	Fatigue
	Dry skin
	Cognitive problems
Infections (viral illnesses, HIV, influenza, fever, tuberculosis, sexually transmitted infections)	Vasomotor symptoms
	Dyspareunia
	Cystitis symptoms
	Vaginitis
Pregnancy	Menstrual changes
Spontaneous abortion	Menorrhagia
Uterine fibroids	
Uterine polyps	
Endometriosis	
Adenomyosis	
Ovarian cysts	
Ovarian tumors	

TABLE 13-3 Sample of Differential Diagnoses That Have Symptoms Similar to Perimenopause and Menopause *(Continued)*

Diagnosis	Symptoms Similar to Perimenopause/Menopause
Vulvar dystrophy	Vaginal atrophy
	Dyspareunia

Presentation and Variation of the Menopause Experience

The experience of menopause is unique and personal. Some women have severe symptoms that disrupt all aspects of their lives, whereas others find menopause to be almost a "non-event" and report no bothersome symptoms. Most symptoms that do occur are related to reduced levels of estrogen and progesterone. Two types of estrogen receptors have been identified (alpha and beta), which are located in the cognitive and vasomotor centers of the brain, eyes, skin, heart, vascular system, gastrointestinal tract, breast tissue, urogenital tract, and bone. Progesterone receptors have been identified in the hypothalamus, pituitary, and vasomotor areas of the brain, as well as in the heart, vascular tissues, lung, breast, pancreas, gynecologic organs, and bones. As hormone levels rise and fall, symptoms may develop. An individual woman's symptom experience may be related to her body size as adipose tissues store and convert androstenedione to estrogen (Fritz & Speroff, 2011). Additionally, women with greater abdominal adiposity are more likely to experience hot flashes than their slimmer counterparts (Thurston et al., 2008).

Both the type (Table 13-2) and severity of menopausal symptoms can vary. Symptoms usually begin in the perimenopausal period and may gradually increase in severity. Postmenopausal women typically experience more symptoms with greater severity than do perimenopausal women (Avis et al., 2001). The symptoms women report most frequently are vasomotor in nature, including hot flashes, or hot flushes, and sweats. Hot flashes are most frequent in the first 5 to 7 years following menopause but can last for many more years in some women (Kronenberg, 1990).

Hot flashes are experienced as an intense heat sensation and may or may not be followed by sweating, which can be profuse. They are characterized by a measurable increase in skin temperature and conductance that is followed by a decrease in core body temperature. Hot flushes are similar to hot flashes but include a flushing over the face and upper chest, most likely due to peripheral vascular dilatation. Vasomotor symptoms that occur during the night are termed night sweats. Hot flashes occur concurrently with a surge in LH levels. Although the relationship between LH secretion and body temperature change is not well understood, the same mechanisms that trigger the hypothalamic event that causes the temperature increase also stimulate GnRH secretion and cause LH elevation. Some women experience a prodrome prior to a hot flash. Many women feel cold following a hot flash owing to the reduction in core temperature; this effect is exacerbated if sweating is also present. Postmenopausal women are more sensitive to core temperature changes because their thermoneutral zone—the range of internally recognized normal core body temperature—narrows (Freedman & Blacker, 2002). Thus, when core temperature rises, they feel overly hot; conversely, when it falls, they feel overly chilled.

Sleep disruptions are also common among menopausal women. Some of these sleep changes are related to normal aging, such as reduced time in sleep stages three (early deep sleep) and four (deep sleep and relaxation), more periods of brief arousal, and an overall decreased need for sleep—an average of five to seven hours for adults (Blackman, 2000). Hot flashes and sweats can further interrupt sleep (Baker, Simpson, & Dawson, 1997; Kronenberg, 1990; NAMS, 2010b). Sleep loss, in turn, causes daytime fatigue and has been associated with irritability; emotional lability; stress; depression; headache; poor functioning at home, work, or school; and difficulty concentrating, reasoning, and remembering (NIH, 2007).

Urogenital changes leading to atrophy affect all women, may cause vaginal dryness and dyspareunia, and can predispose women to urinary incontinence. The risk of urinary incontinence increases with age, but this condition is never considered normal. (See Chapter 23 for additional information on urnary incontinence.) Lower estrogen levels are associated with urethral atrophy, which can increase the likelihood of developing incontinence further.

Many normal changes of aging can also affect sexual function in women, such as longer time to achieve vaginal lubrication and production of fewer vaginal secretions overall; reduced vaginal elasticity, pigment, rugation, and number of superficial epithelial cells, leading to increased petechiae and bleeding following minor trauma (including sexual activity); reduced lactobacilli populations, which increase pH and the risk of infection; and atrophy of adipose and collagen tissue in the vulva. Women may also experience lowered libido, lessened sexual activity, problems with their partner's sexual performance, or relationship problems that make them less interested in sex (Dennerstein, Dudley, & Burger, 2001). Whatever the causes of dyspareunia or sexual dysfunction may be, this subject is often difficult for women to broach with their clinicians. It is important for clinicians to ask women about sexual function and satisfaction, and remain open to the fact that sexual expression can take many forms (see Chapters 11 and 17).

Cultural or racial background may have an effect on menopausal symptoms. The SWAN study indicated that while Caucasian and Hispanic women reported the greatest number of psychosomatic symptoms, such as moodiness, headaches, and palpitations (Avis et al., 2001), the severity of vasomotor symptoms (hot flashes, sweats) was highest among African American women, followed by Hispanic, Caucasian, Chinese, and Japanese women (Gold et al., 2000). Vaginal dryness was more common among African American and Hispanic women, and Hispanic women were more likely to report urine leakage, forgetfulness, and heart pounding or racing than Caucasian women. However, Caucasian women were more likely to experience difficulty sleeping than women of other races (Gold et al.). In the WHI study, Hispanic women were more likely to have experienced urogenital symptoms such as dryness, irritation, discharge, and itching (Pastore, Carter, Hulka, & Wells, 2004). Additionally, some symptoms may be more bothersome for certain women. For example, African American women have described a high degree of discomfort attributable to vaginal and body odor, sleep changes and night sweats, weight gain, moodiness, "rage," and irritability

(Alexander et al., 2003). Asian women have reported more severe problems with joint pain and stiffness, especially in the neck, shoulders, and back (Gold et al.).

A woman's expectations for menopause may also affect her experience. Expectations can range from no expectations, to positive or negative expectations, to uncertainty (Woods & Mitchell, 2008). Similarly, a woman's response to menopause can affect her experience. Many women view menopause as a natural life transition and may not be interested in any treatment options besides lifestyle changes. Others see it as a disruption of their lives and a sign of aging that they want to minimize as much as possible. Many women identify menopause as a time for reflection and reevaluation of their lives and health (Alexander et al., 2003; Woods & Mitchell).

Midlife Health Issues

Health risks change for women at midlife, partly due to the changed hormonal milieu and partly due to other normal aging processes. In particular, women are at greater risk for developing heart disease, osteoporosis, and diabetes. Weight management is also a significant issue. See Chapter 8 for a full discussion of routine health screening for midlife women.

Overweight and Obesity

As women age, weight management often becomes a struggle. Although women tend to associate increased weight with menopause, it is not related specifically to hormonal changes but rather can be a natural part of aging. Women gain an average of 5 pounds at midlife (NAMS, 2010b). This increase is partly due to the decrease in muscle mass that occurs with age and slows down the rate at which calories are burned, and partly due to a decrease in activity that often accompanies midlife. Maintaining one's weight through midlife usually requires both a reduction in caloric intake and an increase in activity.

Not only does weight increase at midlife, but the distribution of body fat also changes. Adipose tissue tends to accumulate at the hips and thighs in younger women (the "pear" shaped body). As women age, adipose tissue is redistributed and begins to accumulate at the waist (the "apple" shaped body). Abdominal adiposity and weight gain at midlife are significant issues. This concern relates not only to the potentially negative body-image concerns for women, but also to the fact that both obesity—defined as a body mass index (BMI) greater than 30 kg/ m^2 and a waist circumference larger than 35 inches—are individually associated with a greater risk for developing insulin resistance that can lead to CVD and diabetes (American Diabetes Association [ADA], 2004a). In addition, obesity is associated with osteoarthritis, cholecystic disease, and urinary incontinence, as well as with cancers such as breast, endometrial, and colorectal (American Obesity Association, 2002; Centers for Disease Control and Prevention, 2011). Furthermore, having a BMI greater than 27 kg/m^2 was associated with a greater frequency of hot flashes, night sweats, and soreness or stiffness in the back, shoulders, and neck in the SWAN study (Gold et al., 2000).

Cardiovascular Disease

The number one cause of mortality for both women and men in the United States is CVD. Approximately 500,000 women die from CVD each year in the United States. This number is higher than that from the next seven causes of mortality in women combined and exceeds the CVD mortality rate in men (American Heart Association [AHA], 2002, 2004). Notably, heart disease disproportionately affects women of color. After the age of 50 years, more than 50% of all deaths among women are attributed to some type of CVD. CVD includes hypertension, valvular heart disease, coronary artery disease, or coronary heart disease (leading to angina or myocardial infarction), stroke, arrhythmias, congestive heart failure, and congenital heart defects.

Women are at a significantly increased risk for developing heart disease following menopause (AHA, 2004; NAMS, 2010a, 2010b). Some of this increased risk is due to changes in cholesterol levels that are found in postmenopausal women. Low-density lipoprotein (LDL) and very-low-density lipoprotein (VLDL) levels increase, and LDL oxidation is enhanced. Additionally, high-density lipoprotein (HDL) levels may decrease somewhat. However, the HDL changes are far less significant than the LDL changes. Other changes, such as the reduced elasticity in the vascular system and associated hypertension, may be related to decreased levels of estrogen and progesterone. Moreover, production of some precoagulation factors (e.g., fibrinogen, factor VII) and some fibrinolytic factors (e.g., plasminogen, antithrombin III) increase, and may interact with hormonal and vascular changes to further increase risk. General risk factors for CVD include cigarette smoking, a sedentary lifestyle, stress, obesity, preexisting hypertension, abnormal serum lipids, and diabetes mellitus. Women who experience premature menopause may have an even greater risk, especially if they smoke (Lobo, 2007; NAMS, 2010b).

Diabetes Mellitus

The likelihood of developing type 2 diabetes mellitus increases with age and disproportionately affects women of minority racial and ethnic groups, such as Native Americans, Hispanics or Latinas, African Americans, Asian Americans, and Pacific Islanders. General risk factors for developing diabetes include being overweight or obese (BMI of 25 or greater), having abdominal adiposity (waist circumference over 35 inches in women), a sedentary lifestyle, insulin resistance, a history of gestational diabetes or polycystic ovary syndrome, and a family history of diabetes. Hypertension and dyslipidemia also predispose an individual to developing diabetes. Individuals with impaired fasting glucose levels (100–125 mg/dL) or impaired glucose tolerance (2-hour post 75-gm glucose load of 140–199 mg/dL) are identified as having pre-diabetes, and 30% to 40% of them will develop type 2 diabetes within 5 years (ADA, 2004b; Mayer-Davis, D'Antonio, & Tudor-Locke, 2003). In addition to significantly increasing the risk for CVD and cerebrovascular disease, diabetes increases the risk for developing infections, foot ulcers, peripheral vascular disease, peripheral neuropathy, nephropathy, and retinopathy (ADA, 2004a; Franz, 2003). The American Association of

Clinical Endocrinologists (AACE, 2008) recommends aggressive treatment for both women and men with pre-diabetes (elevated fasting blood sugars in the 100–125 mg/dL range).

Managing diabetes is more difficult for women during perimenopause due to fluctuations in hormone concentrations. Insulin resistance increases with reduced levels of estrogen, causing higher serum glucose levels. Progesterone changes have a converse effect on glucose, causing lower levels due to the increase in insulin sensitivity that accompanies falling progesterone concentrations. After menopause, glucose levels tend to be lower because insulin sensitivity increases and insulin use becomes more efficient as estrogen and progesterone concentrations stabilize (Gaspar, Gotta, & van den Brule, 1995; Godsland, 1996; Porth & Kunert, 2002). At the same, other midlife changes, such as weight gain and slowed metabolism, affect glucose levels; thus numerous adjustments in medications and regimens are often necessary to maintain adequate glucose control.

Cancer

In 2011, the leading cause of mortality from cancer among women in the United States was estimated to be lung and bronchus cancer (26%), followed by breast (15%), and colon (9%) cancers (American Cancer Society [ACS], 2011). These same three types of cancer were expected to be the most often diagnosed forms among women in 2011 (ACS). Mortality from cancer has decreased overall among women, with the exception of lung cancer, for which mortality is leveling off.

The risk for developing cancer increases as women age. A woman's risk for developing breast cancer is approximately 1 out of 30 at the age of 50, then increases gradually to approximately 1 out of 9 for a woman who lives into her 80s. The lifetime risk for a woman to develop breast cancer is about 1 in 7 (ACS, 2011; National Cancer Institute, 2003, 2008). Chapter 8 provides cancer screening recommendations, and Chapter 16 offers further information on breast cancer.

Osteoporosis

Osteoporosis is a disorder of the skeletal system characterized by reduced bone strength that increases the risk for fracture (Hodgson & Watts, 2003). Bone strength incorporates factors of both bone density and bone quality. Bone density is the volume of bone, whereas bone quality refers to the rate of turnover, bone architecture, mineralization, and accumulated damage.

There are two types of osteoporosis: primary and secondary (Dawson-Hughes, Lindsay, et al., 2008). Secondary osteoporosis occurs in response to medication (e.g., corticosteroids, anticonvulsants, or methotrexate) or other disease processes (e.g., hyperthyroidism, chronic liver disease, or gastrointestinal diseases, such as malabsorption) that interfere with the normal process of bone formation and can affect women or men at any age. Primary osteoporosis is associated with aging and affects women much more significantly than men. Adults achieve peak bone mass in their late 20s to mid-30s, after which time the rates of bone resorption and formation become relatively stable. However, as women age, their bone resorption rate slowly begins to exceed that of bone formation, resulting in a slow decline of bone mass. Because of the loss of estrogen, the rate of bone loss in the first year after menopause is especially rapid, between 1% and 5%, but then slows to approximately 1% per year. In contrast, bone mass is lost in men at a rate of 0.2% to 0.5% per year. **Table 13-4** lists risk factors for osteoporosis. Screening recommendations can be found in Chapter 8.

The gold standard for diagnosing osteopenia or osteoporosis is bone mineral density (BMD) measurement by dual-energy x-ray absorptiometry (DEXA or DXA)—a technique that is used to evaluate central BMD at the spine and hip. Although DXA can also be used to evaluate the wrist BMD, central testing is much more predictive of overall BMD and fracture risk. Quantitative computed tomography (CT) scan can be used to perform spine measurements and is particularly useful for testing individuals with arthritis, as it is less likely to reflect osteocytes. BMD results are reported as *T*-scores and *Z*-scores. The *T*-score identifies the number of standard deviations the patient's BMD is above or below that for a young adult and a gender-matched norm. Osteopenia is present when the *T*-score is –1.0 to –2.5. Osteoporosis is present when the *T*-score is –2.5 or less. Severe or established osteoporosis is present when the *T*-score is –2.5 or less and fragility fractures are present. The *Z*-score provides a

TABLE 13-4 Risk Factors for Osteoporosis

Potentially Modifiable Risk Factors	Nonmodifiable Risk Factors
Body weight < 127 pounds	Advanced age
Body mass index < 22–24	Female gender
Amenorrhea (due to eating disorder or excessive exercise)	Race (Caucasian and Asian women at greatest risk, followed by Hispanic and African American women)
Nulliparity	
Low estrogen levels (e.g., menopause)	Personal history of fracture during adulthood
Lifestyle factors (e.g., cigarette smoking, excessive alcohol or caffeine intake, sedentary activity level, or inadequate calcium or vitamin D intake)	Family history of osteoporosis
	First-degree relative with a history of fracture
Medications (e.g., thyroid hormone, corticosteroids, anticonvulsants, aluminum-containing antacids, lithium, methotrexate, gonadotropin-releasing hormone, cholesteramine, heparin, warfarin)	
Chronic diseases (e.g., endocrine disorders, gastrointestinal disorders, connective tissue diseases, bone disorders, chronic liver disease, cystic fibrosis, seizure disorders, hematologic malignancies, prolonged immobility, eating disorders, chronic renal failure, or frailty)	

Sources: Data from Dawson-Hughes, Lindsay, et al., 2008; Hodgson & Watts, 2003.

comparison in BMD for the patient to an age-matched mean and is used for diagnosis only in children (Dawson-Hughes, Lindsay, et al., 2008).

Women with osteoporosis are at increased risk for fracture. Interestingly, fracture rates are even higher among women with osteopenia (Dawson-Hughes, Lindsay, et al., 2008). Although osteoporosis and osteopenia by themselves are painless and not functionally problematic, the risk for fractures puts a patient at significant risk. Following a hip fracture, there is a 10% to 20% increase in mortality. Among survivors, 30% to 40% sustain some degree of permanent disability and 24% to 50% never return to independent living (Dawson-Hughes, Tosteson, et al., 2008; Hodgson & Watts, 2003).

Prevention is a key factor in osteoporosis management. For perimenopausal and postmenopausal women, prevention strategies focus on the following considerations:

- Adequate intake of calcium
  - 1000 mg/day for premenopausal women and postmenopausal women on HT
  - 1200 mg/day for perimenopausal or premenopausal women older than 50 years
  - 1500 mg/day for postmenopausal women not taking HT and women older than 65 years
- Adequate intake of vitamin D (400–800 international units/day)
- Weight bearing and resistance exercise
- Fall prevention
- Avoiding tobacco
- Moderating alcohol intake (Dawson-Hughes, Tosteson, et al., 2008; Hodgson & Watts, 2003; NIH, 1994)

Exercise is site specific and needs to be continued to maintain bone strength. Medication management is recommended for women with T-scores of –2.5 or lower, and for those with hip or vertebral fractures (Dawson-Hughes, Lindsay, et al., 2008). For women with T-scores in the osteopenic range (–1.0 to –2.5), medication is recommended if they also have fractures or are at high risk for fracture (e.g., are immobilized, are taking glucocorticoids, are at high risk for falls).

For other women with T-scores in the osteopenic range, use of the World Health Organization's (WHO's) Fracture Risk Assessment Tool (FRAX) is recommended to identify those who would realize a cost-effective benefit from initiating medication therapy (Dawson-Hughes, Tosteson, et al., 2008; Tosteson et al., 2008; WHO, 2007). The FRAX tool is accessible online (http://www.shef.ac.uk/FRAX/) and is applicable for women who have not previously been treated with medications. Information is entered for 11 different risk factors plus the hip raw BMD value (in g/cm^2) to calculate the 10-year probability for a hip fracture and the 10-year probability for any type of major osteoporotic fracture. If the rates for hip fracture probability are greater than 3% or the rate for any major osteoporotic fracture is greater than 20%, medication therapy is recommended (Dawson-Hughes, Lindsay, et al., 2008).

The treatment decision must be weighed against the clinical presentation, with the clinician recognizing the limitations of FRAX. "The FRAX provides an estimated fracture risk in a given individual but does not identify the level of fracture risk at which treatment should be started ('intervention threshold')." (Lane & Silverman, 2008). Many of the variables entered are dichotomous ("yes/no") and do not capture the increased risk present with a higher level on a continuous variable scale (e.g., use of higher doses of corticosteroid increases risk for fracture). Additionally, the T-score used in the FRAX calculations is not the same as that obtained with DXA testing. A conversion program is available on the National Osteoporosis Foundation (NOF) website that can be downloaded to the clinician's computer for use, however. The converted T-score should then be entered into the FRAX program.

Repeat BMD testing for osteoporosis is recommended every 2 years after treatment is initiated, to monitor the effects of therapy (Dawson-Hughes, Lindsay, et al., 2008). **Table 13-5** summarizes the available pharmacologic treatment options for osteoporosis in postmenopausal women. Combination therapy, initiated by an osteoporosis specialist, is also possible; usually a bisphosphonate (alendronate or risedronate) is combined with another class (e.g., estrogen or raloxifene).

Thyroid Disease and Depression

Thyroid disease and depression are other health issues that must be considered at midlife. Thyroid disease affects women more than men, and its incidence increases with age (Baskin, 2002). Symptoms of hyperthyroidism or hypothyroidism can mimic perimenopause and menopause symptoms.

The risk of depression also increases during midlife both due to symptoms caused by hormonal fluctuations and midlife stresses such as financial concerns, employment issues, relationship problems, family changes, or health issues of self or family members (NAMS, 2010b). Depression rates are approximately three times as high in perimenopausal women as they are in premenopausal women (Cohen, 2004). These problems and other differential diagnoses (Table 13-3) must be considered when a woman presents with menopausal symptoms.

Lifestyle Approaches for Symptom Management

Several lifestyle alterations can be implemented to reduce menopausal symptoms. Some of these interventions also afford additional health benefits such as reducing risk for CVD or osteoporosis. Lifestyle management may encompass dietary changes, exercise, vitamins or supplements, vaginal lubricants and moisturizers, changes in clothing, smoking cessation, stress management techniques, sleep aids, and activities to enhance memory function.

Dietary Changes

Several dietary substances have been linked with more frequent or more severe hot flashes. They include sugar (especially refined), caffeine (including hot and cold beverages and other foods, such as chocolate, that contain caffeine), spicy foods, and alcohol (Alexander et al., 2003; NAMS, 2010b). Avoidance or moderate intake of these substances should be recommended.

TABLE 13-5 Pharmacologic Treatment Options for Osteoporosis in Postmenopausal Women*

Medication	FDA Approved For	Considerations
Alendronate (Fosamax)	• Prevention—5 mg orally daily or 35 mg orally weekly • Treatment—10 mg orally daily or 70 mg orally weekly (70-mg dose also available with cholecalciferol/vitamin D3 as Fosamax Plus D)	• Use with caution if the patient has upper gastrointestinal disease, owing to its clinical association with dysphagia, esophagitis, and ulceration • Take first thing in the morning on an empty stomach with an 8-oz glass of water, remain upright and take no other food or drink for at least 30 minutes • Take 2 hours before antacids/calcium
Risedronate (Actonel)	• Prevention—5 mg orally daily or 35 mg orally weekly • Treatment—5 mg orally daily, 35 mg orally weekly (35-mg dose is also available in a delayed release formulation as Atelvia or packaged with calcium carbonate as Actonel with Calcium), 75 mg orally 2 consecutive days each month, 150 mg orally once a month	• Same as alendronate
Ibandronate (Boniva)	• Prevention or treatment—150 mg orally once a month or 2.5 mg orally daily • Treatment—3 mg intravenously every 3 months	• Same as alendronate for tablets but must remain upright and take no other food or drink for at least 60 minutes • Intravenous injection is administered over a period of 15 to 30 seconds
Zoledronic acid (Reclast)	• Prevention—5 mg intravenously once every 2 years • Treatment—5 mg intravenously once a year	• Intravenous infusion is administered over a period of no less than 15 minutes
Calcitonin (Miacalcin, Fortical)	• Treatment—200 international units intranasal spray daily or 100 international units subcutaneous injection every other day	• Usually administered as nasal spray • Has an analgesic effect on osteoporotic fractures

TABLE 13-5 Pharmacologic Treatment Options for Osteoporosis in Postmenopausal Women* *(Continued)*

Medication	FDA Approved For	Considerations
Estrogen (i.e., Premarin, Ogen, Alora, Climara, Estrace, Menostar, Vivelle, Vivelle-Dot, Estraderm, Premphase,† Prempro,† femhrt,† Activella,† Prefest,† Climara Pro†)	• Prevention—Doses and routes vary‡	• Also effective in alleviating most symptoms of menopause • Comes in pills or patch
Raloxifene (Evista)	• Prevention or treatment—60 mg orally daily	• May cause hot flashes • Not recommended if the patient is taking ET or EPT
Teriparatide (Forteo)	• Treatment—20 mcg subcutaneously daily	• Reserved for use after failure of first-line agents
Denosumab (Prolia)	• Treatment—60 mg subcutaneously every 6 months	• Reserved for use after failure of first-line agents

*See prescribing reference for full information on doses, side effects, contraindications, and cautions.
†Also contain progestogens, which should be used in women with an intact uterus.
‡Lowest effective dose should be used. The FDA recommends considering nonestrogen osteoporotic agents when ET/EPT use is solely for the purpose of osteoporosis prevention.
Source: Data from NAMS, 2011a.

Increased water intake is also recommended because of the augmented insensible loss of fluids through sweating. Water intake, especially cold water, has been reported to help with reducing symptoms such as skin dryness, and it reduces the discomfort associated with hot flashes and sweating (Alexander et al., 2003; NAMS, 2004). The usual water intake of six to eight glasses per day should be recommended. However, for women who experience urinary incontinence, water consumption may need to be restricted for social occasions when there is no easy access to a bathroom, or limited to the morning for women who experience nocturia.

Exercise

Lower levels of physical activity have been linked with a higher frequency of menopausal symptoms, especially forgetfulness, difficulty sleeping, heart pounding or racing, and stiffness or soreness (Gold et al., 2000). Similarly, higher levels of physical activity have been associated with reduced severity of menopausal symptoms such as vasomotor symptoms, depression, and forgetfulness (Alexander, Ruff, & Udemezue, n.d.; NAMS, 2004, 2010b). In addition to mediating menopause symptoms, exercise reduces cardiovascular and osteoporosis risks, improves sleep, and assists with maintaining a healthy weight, relieving stress, reducing moodiness, and improving mental function.

Vitamins and Supplements

Several vitamins and supplements may be useful for minimizing menopausal symptoms and improving overall health. For example, calcium (1200–1500 mg/day) and vitamin D (400–800 international units/day) are needed for postmenopausal women to maintain bone strength (NIH, 1994).

Vitamin E in doses up to 800 international units/day has shown to produce either small improvements or no changes in hot flashes in clinical trials (Barton et al., 1998; Blatt, Weisbader, & Kupperman, 1953). A meta-analysis indicated that vitamin E did not provide a reduction in overall mortality, cerebrovascular accident, or cardiovascular death (Vivekananthan, Penn, Sapp, Hsu, & Topol, 2003). In the same meta-analysis, beta-carotene was shown to have a slightly increased risk for all-cause mortality. Vitamin E has, however, been linked with a reduced risk for developing Alzheimer's disease (Klatte, Scharre, Nagaraja, Davis, & Beversdorf, 2003; Onofrj et al., 2002; Thomas, Iacono, Bonanni, D'Andreamatteo, & Onofrj, 2001).

The B vitamins are known to reduce homocysteine levels; high levels of homocysteine are associated with cerebrovascular accident, CVD, Alzheimer's disease, and osteoporotic fracture. For reduction of homocysteine and to partly compensate for the lack of fruits and vegetables usually found in the U.S. diet, daily supplementation with a multivitamin containing the B vitamins (folate, B_6, and B_{12}) is recommended (Fairfield & Fletcher, 2002; Fletcher & Fairfield, 2002; McLean et al., 2004; van Meurs et al., 2004). Formulations that include iron should be avoided unless there is a documented need for iron supplementation, as excess iron can have negative effects on the cardiovascular system or liver over time.

Vaginal Lubricants and Moisturizers

Vaginal lubricants can be used to relieve vaginal dryness and dyspareunia caused by reduced vaginal secretions. Several nonhormonal water-based preparations are available as over-the-counter products (e.g., K-Y Personal Lubricant, Astroglide, Lubrin, Moist Again) and can be used for daily comfort for vaginal dryness and during sexual activity. Longer-acting vaginal moisturizers (e.g., Replens, K-Y Long-Lasting Vaginal Moisturizer) may be more appropriate for some women. The moisturizers replenish and maintain fluids in the vaginal epithelial cells and provide longer relief. Moisturizers may be particularly beneficial for women who experience daily discomfort and can reduce vaginitis by supporting a normal pH (Nachtigall, 1994).

Women must be cautioned against using any oil-based products, such as petroleum jelly (Vaseline), as these preparations can injure vaginal tissue and are not easily removed. Vitamin E oil, when applied topically to the vaginal walls, is an exception to this caution. It can provide relief for vaginal dryness without interfering with condom or diaphragm function, and it rarely irritates tissues. Other products that contain oils or fragrances should also be discouraged as they often cause vaginitis or irritation. Douching is not effective for moisturizing and will remove normal flora, thereby increasing the risk for infection (NAMS, 2010b; Willhite, 2001).

Clothing and Environment

Wearing layered clothes, breathable fabrics such as cotton or linen, or moisture-wicking fabrics, such as those worn by runners, is recommended to reduce discomfort with hot flashes and sweats (Alexander et al., 2004; NAMS, 2010b). Avoiding turtlenecks, fabrics that do not allow circulation or absorb sweat (e.g., polyester and silk), and extra layers (e.g., slips and full-length stockings) is also recommended. Keeping the room temperature cool, having an open window or using a fan to circulate air, and ingesting cold foods or beverages can reduce core body temperature and are also helpful in reducing the symptoms of menopause (NAMS, 2004, 2010b).

Smoking Cessation

Smoking is associated with increased morbidity and mortality, especially related to CVD and cancers; earlier age at menopause; increased rate of bone loss; and increased prevalence of all menopausal symptoms except vaginal dryness (Gold et al., 2000, 2001; NAMS, 2010b). Various smoking cessation programs are available, but the most successful program is ultimately the one that is of interest to a specific woman. She needs to be both interested in quitting and motivated to quit. Support from a clinician and use of medications or patches can significantly improve cessation rates (ACS, 2007).

Stress Management

Stress has been reported to increase menopause symptoms (Alexander et al., 2003). Additionally, stress is associated with poor sleep and can increase depression or moodiness. At midlife, women may face multiple stressors such as health changes for themselves or family members, financial concerns, loss of a parent, children leaving home, or relationship struggles with a partner, child, or parent.

Managing stress must be individualized, as each woman may find different tactics helpful. Some suggestions include regular exercise, meditation, relaxation techniques such as deep breathing, yoga, tai-chi, taking a bath, reading, having a massage, seeking support from friends, or activities related to spirituality or religion. Few studies have evaluated the effects of such techniques on menopausal symptoms; however, reports indicate that avoiding and effectively managing stress are associated with less intense and fewer hot flashes (Alexander et al., 2003). While studies have not shown that progressive muscle relaxation and biofeedback control produce any significant change in hot flashes, paced respiration has been linked with a significant reduction in hot flashes (Freedman & Woodward, 1992; Freedman, Woodward, Brown, Javaid, & Pandy, 1995; Irvin, Domar, Clark, Zuttermeister, & Freidman, 1996). Many women find that yoga breathing—a variation of paced respiration—can enhance relaxation and reduce hot flashes. Yoga breathing consists of a deep inhalation for the count of four, holding the breath for a count of seven, and slowly exhaling over a count of eight.

Sleep

Evaluating the cause of sleep disruptions is important for developing a plan of management. If sleep disruption is related to hot flashes or other menopausal symptoms, control of those symptoms will usually restore normal sleep patterns. Light blankets, cotton sleepwear or moisture-wicking pajamas, and a well-ventilated room are recommended for reducing nocturnal hot flashes. However, if sleep disruption is unrelated to hot flashes, a more generalized approach is needed.

Developing good sleep hygiene is especially important for perimenopausal and menopausal women. Sleep hygiene refers to actions that cue the mind that it is time for sleep and allow the part of the brain that controls the body during sleep to take over. Developing regular routines prior to bedtime, such as brushing the teeth or changing into sleepwear, and doing something relaxing, such as paced respirations, progressive relaxation, guided imagery, taking a warm bath, reading a relaxing book, or drinking a warm beverage without caffeine, can help cue the mind that it is time to sleep. Similarly, activities that tend to stimulate the mind should be avoided just before bed, such as watching television, reading a fast-paced or stimulating book, doing work, or exercise. The bedroom should be reserved for sleep and sexual activities. This is especially important for individuals who have difficulty falling asleep, as doing work or watching television in bed can have a stimulating effect. Establishing regular times for sleep and waking is also important for developing good sleep patterns, as this consistency will help in developing normal daily routines.

Lifestyle changes that can help restore sleep patterns include avoiding use of stimulants, such as caffeine, alcohol, or nicotine, and engaging in exercise. The effects of caffeine can last as long as 20 hours in some individuals, so total elimination is preferable (Landolt, Werth, Borbely, & Dijk, 1995). Although alcohol initially can have a sedative effect, it can cause interruptions in normal sleep patterns after falling asleep, including fragmented sleep and rebound awakening (Landolt, Rioth, Dijk, & Borbely, 1996). Similarly, nicotine can cause increased sleep latency and reduces overall sleep duration. Exercise can enhance sleep quality, reduce sleep latency, and increase the amount of time spent in deep sleep. However, timing for exercise is important, as engaging in exercise right before bedtime will increase sleep latency.

For those with short sleep duration, sleep-restriction therapy can be tried (Morin et al., 1999). First the current average duration of sleep is identified, along with a needed and consistent time for awakening. The woman is instructed to go to bed four hours prior to the determined time for wakening, and to get up at the predetermined wake time. She needs to stay awake except for the determined sleep time (no napping). After she is sleeping more than 95% of this time for several nights consistently, the time to go to bed is moved to one half hour earlier. This pattern is continued until the desired sleep time is achieved.

It is also important to educate women that they require less sleep as they age. Few postmenopausal women need 8 hours of sleep per night; rather, 6 to 7 hours is the norm.

Mental Function

A slow decline in mental function is expected with aging. However, some women experience bothersome cognitive changes that develop as menopausal symptoms occur. Poor mental functioning is often associated with lack of sleep or high levels of stress, but cognitive impairment can also be related to a myriad of medical problems. Thus the first step in evaluating mental function is to complete a comprehensive assessment to identify potential causes of the cognitive problems.

For women who are experiencing reduced cognitive function that is unrelated to other organic problems, several simple memory aids may be of use. Noting appointments and dates of importance in a calendar, or writing lists to use for completing tasks, work activities, or shopping can help reduce stress associated with forgetting these items. Participating in activities that keep the mind engaged, such as intellectually stimulating work, puzzles, or other activities, can also help to maintain cognitive function.

Pharmacologic Options for Menopause Symptom Management

NAMS (2010a, 2010b) recommends lifestyle changes alone or in combination with nonprescription remedies for women with mild vasomotor symptoms; however, prescription systemic hormone products remain the standard for women with moderate to severe symptoms. The U.S. Food and Drug Administration (FDA) defines moderate to severe hot flashes as 7 to 8 episodes per day or at least 60 episodes per week. It is important to note that hot flashes will eventually resolve over time without medication in most women.

The Cochrane Group conducted a meta-analysis of 21 randomized, double-blind, placebo-controlled clinical trials that enrolled 2511 women. The researchers reported that systemic ET/EPT reduced hot flash severity and frequency significantly more than placebos. Some antidepressant, antihypertensive, and anticonvulsant agents have also been shown to reduce vasomotor symptoms (NAMS, 2004, 2010b). **Table 13-6** lists currently available HT products. Note that in their review of efficacy of various preparations, the NAMS researchers concluded that there is no evidence to claim that one product is superior to another in terms of ability to yield symptom relief. **Table 13-7** lists nonhormonal prescription options and **Table 13-8** lists vaginal preparations.

There is no FDA-approved therapy for treating hot flashes in women who are at high risk for, or who have been diagnosed with, breast cancer. Nonhormonal agents may provide hot flash relief for women who have had breast cancer. Herbal alternatives to HT should be used with caution because they can have estrogen-like activity.

Therapy Considerations

Prior to prescribing HT, it is imperative that clinicians and their patients review any cautions or contraindications to hormone use (**Table 13-9**). The clinician must engage the patient in the decision-making process and weigh the risks, benefits, and scientific uncertainty with

TABLE 13-6 Hormone Therapy Options*

Type	Product Name	Active Ingredient	Dosage
Estrogens, oral	Cenestin	Conjugated estrogens	0.3 mg, 0.45 mg, 0.625 mg, 0.9 mg, or 1.25 mg once daily
	Enjuvia	Conjugated estrogens	0.3 mg, 0.45 mg, 0.625 mg, 0.9 mg, or 1.25 mg once daily
	Estrace	17β-estradiol	0.5 mg, 1 mg, or 2 mg once daily
	Femtrace	Estradiol acetate	0.45 mg, 0.9 mg, or 1.8 mg once daily
	Menest	Esterified estrogens	0.3 mg, 0.625 mg, 1.25 mg, or 2.5 mg once daily
	Ortho-Est	Estropipate	0.625 mg (0.75 estropipate, calculated as sodium estrone sulfate 0.625), 1.25 (1.5) mg, 2.5 (3) mg, or 5 (6) mg once daily
	Premarin	Conjugated equine estrogens (CEE)	0.3 mg, 0.45 mg, 0.625 mg, 0.9 mg, 1.25 mg once daily
Estrogens, transdermal and topical preparations	Esclim, Vivelle, Vivelle-Dot	17β-estradiol matrix patch	0.025 mg, 0.0375 mg, 0.05 mg, 0.075 mg, or 0.1 mg twice weekly
	Alora	17β-estradiol matrix patch	0.025 mg, 0.05 mg, 0.075 mg, or 0.1 mg twice weekly
	Climara	17β-estradiol matrix patch	0.025 mg, 0.0375 mg, 0.05 mg, 0.075 mg, or 0.1 mg once weekly
	Fempatch	17β-estradiol matrix patch	0.025 mg once weekly
	Menostar	17β-estradiol matrix patch	0.014 mg once weekly
	Estraderm	17β-estradiol reservoir patch	0.05 mg or 0.1 mg twice weekly
	EstroGel	17β-estradiol transdermal gel	0.035 mg once daily (1 metered pump of 1.25 gm of gel applied from wrist to shoulder)
	Elestrin	17β-estradiol transdermal gel	0.0125 mg or 0.0375 mg once daily (1–2 metered pumps of 0.87 gm of gel applied to the upper arm and shoulder)
	Divigel	17β-estradiol transdermal gel	0.003 mg, 0.009 mg, or 0.027 mg once daily (0.25-, 0.5- or 1-gm packet of gel applied to the upper thigh)
	Estrasorb Cream	17β-estradiol topical emulsion	0.05 mg once daily (two packets of 1.74 gm of emulsion each applied one to each upper leg)
	Evamist	17β-estradiol transdermal spray	1.53 mg, 3.06 mg, or 4.59 mg once daily (applied as 1–3 sprays to the forearm)

(continues)

309

TABLE 13-6 Hormone Therapy Options* *(Continued)*

Type	Product Name	Active Ingredient	Dosage
Progestogens, oral	Provera	Medroxyprogesterone acetate (MPA)	2.5 mg, 5 mg, or 10 mg continuously or on set cycle schedule
	Prometrium	Micronized progesterone	100 mg or 200 mg continuously or on set cycle schedule
	Micronor, Nor-QD	Norethindrone	0.35 mg continuously or on set cycle schedule
	Aygestin	Norethindrone acetate	5 mg continuously or on set cycle schedule
	Megace	Megestrol acetate	20 mg or 40 mg continuously or on set cycle schedule
Combination estrogen-progestogen products, oral	Premphase	CEE (14 tabs), then CEE + MPA (14 tabs)	0.625 mg E, then 0.625 mg E + 5 mg P once daily sequentially
	Prempro	CEE + MPA	0.3 mg E + 1.5 mg P once daily 0.45 mg E + 1.5 mg P once daily 0.625 mg E + 2.5 mg P once daily, or 0.625 mg E + 5 mg P once daily continuously
	Femhrt	Ethinyl estradiol + norethindrone acetate	2.5 mcg E + 5 mg P or 5 mcg E + 1 mg P once daily, continuously
	Angeliq	17β-estradiol + drospirenone	1 mg E + 0.5 mg P or 1 mg E + 1 mg P once daily, continuously
	Activella	17β-estradiol + norethindrone acetate	0.5 mg E + 0.1 mg P once daily
	Prefest	17β-estradiol (3 tabs) then 17β-estradiol + norgestimate (3 tabs)	1 mg E, then 1 mg E + 0.09 mg P, once daily sequentially
Combination estrogen-progestogen products, transdermal	Climara Pro	17β-estradiol + levonorgestrel	0.045 mg E + 0.015 mg P once weekly
	CombiPatch	17β-estradiol + norethindrone acetate	0.05 mg E + 0.14 mg P or 0.05 mg E + 0.25 mg P twice weekly

*See prescribing reference for full information on doses, side effects, contraindications, and cautions.

310

TABLE 13-7 Nonhormonal Pharmacologic Options for Vasomotor Symptoms*

Category	Drug	Dosage	Comments	Side Effects	Contraindications
Antidepressants	Venlafaxine (Effexor)	37.5–75 mg/day; up-titrate when starting therapy	Response is immediate	Nausea, vomiting, mouth dryness, decreased appetite	Concomitant use of MAO inhibitors; taper when discontinuing
	Fluoxetine (Prozac)	20 mg/day; uptitrate when starting therapy	Response is immediate	Asthenia, sweating, nausea, somnolence, anorgasmia, decreased libido	Concomitant use of MAO inhibitors or thioridazine; caution with warfarin; taper when discontinuing
	Paroxetine (Paxil)	12.5–25 mg/day; up-titrate when starting therapy	Response is immediate	See fluoxetine; weight gain, blurred vision	See fluoxetine; taper when discontinuing
Anticonvulsants	Gabapentin (Neurontin)	Initial dose 300 mg/day at bedtime, can increase to up to 300 mg three times per day at 3–4 day intervals		Somnolence, dizziness, ataxia, fatigue, weight gain	Avoid antacids within 2 hours of use; taper when discontinuing
Antihypertensives	Clonidine (Catapres)	0.05–0.1 mg twice daily	Available as a patch, less effective than antidepressants or gabapentin	Dry mouth, drowsiness, dizziness, weakness, constipation, rash, myalgia, urticaria, insomnia, nausea, agitation, orthostatic hypotension, impotence, arrhythmias	Taper when discontinuing
	Methyldopa (Aldomet) and belladonna, ergotamine, and phenobarbitol (Bellergal)		NAMS does not recommend due to limited efficacy data and potential for adverse effects		

*See prescribing reference for full information on doses, side effects, contraindications, and cautions.
Sources: Data from Grady, 2002; NAMS, 2010b.

TABLE 13-8 Vaginal and Intrauterine Hormone Products*

Type	Product Name	Active Ingredient	Dose
Estrogen			
Vaginal hormone creams	Estrace	17β-estradoil	2–4 gm daily for 1–4 weeks, then 1 gm daily 1–3 times per week for 1–3 weeks. Maintenance: 1 gm 1–3 times a week, cyclically (3 weeks on, 1 week off). Taper dosage or discontinue at 3–6 month intervals
	Premarin	Conjugated equine estrogens	0.5–2 g intravaginally daily cyclically (3 weeks on, 1 week off). Reevaluate periodically. Tapering is frequently appropriate but not specified in product information
Vaginal tablets	Vagifem	Estradiol hemihydrate	25 mcg once daily for two weeks then twice weekly
Ring	Estring	Micronized 17β-estradoil	7.5 mcg/24 hours, replace every 90 days
	Femring	Estradiol acetate	0.05 mg/day or 0.1 mg/day, replace every 3 months
Progestogen			
Gel	Crinone	Progesterone	4% gel–45 mg, 1 applicator every other day, give 6 doses; increase to 8% if no response
Intrauterine device	Mirena	Levonorgestrel	20 mcg daily, lasts for 5 years

*See prescribing reference for full information on doses, side effects, contraindications, and cautions.

Source: Data from NAMS, 2011b.

TABLE 13-9 Contraindications to HT and Adverse Effects

Absolute Contraindications to Estrogen Use	Adverse Effects of ET
Known or suspected cancer of the breast	Uterine bleeding
Known or suspected estrogen-dependent neoplasia	Breast tenderness
	Nausea
History of uterine or ovarian cancer	Abdominal bloating
History of coronary heart disease or stroke	Fluid retention in extremities
History of biliary tract disorder	Headache
Undiagnosed, abnormal genital bleeding	Dizziness
History of or active thrombophlebitis or thromboembolic disorders	Hair loss
Absolute Contraindications to Progestogen Use	**Adverse Effects of EPT**
Active thrombophlebitis or thromboembolic disorders	Mood changes
Liver dysfunction or disease	Possible increased uterine bleeding than if taking ET alone
Known or suspected cancer of the breast	
Undiagnosed abnormal vaginal bleeding	
Pregnancy	

each woman to individualize her treatment options. The risk of breast cancer increases after 3 to 5 years of EPT. As mentioned earlier, HT should not be used for protection against CVD, although some data indicate that beginning HT use in early menopause may have a cardioprotective effect. Recent data do not support decreased risk of dementia (NAMS, 2010a).

Women considering using HT should have the recommended screening tests for health promotion and disease prevention in addition to a complete history and physical examination (see Chapter 8 for screening recommendations). Special attention should be paid to any personal or family history of health problems that would contraindicate ET or EPT use. If the woman is considered an appropriate candidate for this therapy, the clinician explains the various protocols for administering HT: ET alone (for women without an intact uterus), EPT continuously or sequentially, or local ET.

HT Protocols and Formulations

Estrogen Therapy ET has been prescribed exclusively for women who have had a hysterectomy because the evidence reported in 1975 suggested that unopposed estrogen increases risk for endometrial hyperplasia and cancer. Side effects of ET are listed Table **13-10**.

Estrogen–Progestogen Therapy Combination estrogen and progestogen therapy can be taken either sequentially (CS-EPT) or continuously (CC-EPT). In the sequential regimen,

TABLE 13-10 Management of HT Side Effects

Side Effect	Strategy
Fluid retention	Decrease salt intake; maintain adequate water intake; exercise; recommend an herbal diuretic or mild prescription diuretic
Bloating	Change to low-dose transdermal estrogen; lower the progestogen dose to a level that still protects the uterus; change the progestogen or try micronized progesterone
Breast tenderness	Lower the estrogen dose; change the estrogen; decrease salt intake; change the progestogen; decrease caffeine and chocolate consumption
Headaches	Change to transdermal estrogen; lower the estrogen and/or progestogen dose; change to a CC-EPT regimen; ensure adequate water intake; decrease salt, caffeine, and alcohol use
Mood changes	Lower the progestogen dose; change to a CC-EPT regimen; ensure adequate water intake; restrict salt, caffeine, and alcohol consumption
Nausea	Take hormones with meals; change the estrogen; change to transdermal estrogen; lower the estrogen or progestogen dose

Source: Adapted with permission from North American Menopause Society. (2010). *Menopause core curriculum study guide* (4th ed.). Cleveland, OH: Author.

an estrogen is taken daily with the addition of a progestogen in a cyclic fashion, usually on days 1 to 12 of the month. One side effect often noted with this therapy is that most women will have a withdrawal bleed monthly. To avoid this consequence, the continuous regimen was developed in which the estrogen and progestogen are taken on a daily basis. Another option includes pulsed combination therapy, wherein the progestogen is taken for two days, followed by a day off, in a repeating pattern. The original idea was to reduce potential side effects from the progestogen; however, breakthrough bleeding is usually more problematic with this regimen. A less frequently used regimen is the cyclic regimen, where estrogen is taken daily for the first 21 days of the cycle and then progestogen is added for days 12 to 21. A withdrawal bleed usually occurs between days 22 and 28, during which neither estrogen nor progestogen is taken. However, menopausal symptoms usually rebound when the estrogen is not taken; therefore, few women opt for the cyclic regimen.

Estrogens A variety of estrogen compounds exist: estrogens that are bioidentical and transformed into human estrogens, such as 17-beta estradiol, estriol, and estrone; synthetic estrogen analogs, such as ethinyl estradiol; and nonhuman estrogens, such as CEE. CEE is the most widely used estrogen and has been the product used in the majority of clinical trials, including the WHI and HERS.

Estrogens differ in target tissue response and in dose equivalency. They can be administered either systemically or locally. Systemic preparations are available as oral tablets or transdermal patches. Local preparations are available as creams, tablets, or rings. The vaginal ring containing 0.5 mg or 0.1 mg/day of estradiol acetate over three months is the only local treatment that has proved effective in treating hot flashes (NAMS, 2010b). Local treatment with estrogen theoretically avoids systemic absorption; however, in a review of the studies on vaginal preparations, Crandall (2002) found that the ring has slightly more systemic absorption. Women who want to avoid systemic effects, such as breast cancer survivors, should probably use a different preparation until more evidence is available.

Progestogens Progestogens are hormones that possess progestational properties. The most commonly prescribed progestogen has been MPA, but others are being used with more regularity, such as micronized progesterone (which is bioidentical), norgestimate, and nore-thindrone acetate. Side effects of adding progestogens to estrogens are listed in Table 13-9.

Estrogen–Androgen Therapy Therapy combining androgens and estrogens has been theorized to improve loss of libido in postmenopausal women; however, there is not enough scientific evidence from randomized clinical trials to say with certainty that testosterone plus estrogen is more effective than estrogen alone. One older study of 40 women showed no significant differences in levels of self-reported sexual enjoyment and desire (Dow, Hart, & Forrest, 1982). Another crossover study from the same era compared estrogen alone, estrogen plus testosterone, testosterone, and placebo. These researchers found that women reported significantly improved levels of sexual desire, arousal, and fantasies while taking testosterone and estrogen plus testosterone (Sherwin, Gelfand, & Brender, 1985). Additional clinical trials are currently being conducted. Known side effects of androgens include alopecia, acne, deepening of the voice, and hirsutism. As of this writing, there are no androgen therapies approved by the FDA for use in women. See Chapter 17 for additional information on use of androgen preparations in women with decreased sexual desire.

Plan of Care and Patient Education

NAMS recommends initiating ET and EPT at lower than standard doses, such as 0.3 mg CEE, 0.25 to 0.5 mg 17-beta estradiol patch, or the equivalent. Studies have shown that these dosages provide adequate vasomotor relief, although the level of endometrial protection afforded by these regimens has not been evaluated in long-term clinical trials. Vasomotor symptoms usually begin to resolve in 2 to 6 weeks after initiating HT.

Patients should be offered anticipatory guidance about management of side effects, should they occur. Research evidence has absolved HT from contributing to weight gain; however, fluid retention may make women feel as if they are gaining weight. Table 13-10 lists possible side effects and strategies.

Patients should return for a follow-up visit with the clinician in 6 to 8 weeks to evaluate their progress; if the initial dose of ET/EPT does not provide adequate symptom relief, it can be increased or taken on a daily divided dose schedule. The decision to continue or discontinue HT should be revisited at least annually. Some women will have symptoms for a short time, such as a few months to a year. Others remain symptomatic for years and may need to continue HT as long as 5 years (Wysocki et al., 2003).

When the patient seeks to discontinue therapy, she should be advised there is about a 50% chance symptoms will recur. Rates of recurrence are similar whether HT is tapered or stopped abruptly; therefore, NAMS (2010a) makes no recommendation about how to discontinue therapy.

Complementary and Alternative Medicine Options for Menopause Symptom Management

The use of complementary and alternative medicine (CAM) is on the rise in the United States (Eisenberg et al., 1993; Eisenberg et al., 1998; Kessler et al., 2001), especially among women (Upchurch & Chyu, 2005). Visits to alternative providers now exceed visits to primary care clinicians, and most patients who use CAM do not report this usage to their primary care clinicians. Furthermore, women are the largest group of CAM users, and the use of CAM to manage menopause symptoms is growing (Bair et al., 2005; Brett & Keenan, 2007; Daley et al., 2006; Newton, Buist, Keenan, Anderson, & LaCroix, 2002). It is imperative for clinicians to ask patients about the use of CAM and to become knowledgeable about the CAM therapies that women are using.

Natural Versus Bioidentical Hormones

Many women seek "natural" hormones, believing that they are less likely to cause harmful side effects than manufactured hormones (Alexander, 2006). The term *natural* actually refers to any product with principal components that originate from plant, animal, or mineral sources. Thus this definition encompasses pharmaceutically manufactured hormones, which are also derived from animal, plant, or mineral substances. Natural hormones are not necessarily identical to the hormones produced by a woman's body.

Several hormones are available that are "bioidentical" to the hormones produced in women's bodies, however. Frequently women requesting "natural hormones" are actually seeking bioidentical formulations (Alexander, 2006). Bioidentical hormones are available through prescription from both usual and compounding pharmacies. Several forms of estrogen are available in bioidentical formulations such as estrone, estriol, and 17-beta estradiol. Bioidentical progesterone is also available in micronized form.

Many women prefer to get estrogens through compounding pharmacies. Two commonly available preparations that contain bioidentical estrogens are Bi-est and Tri-est. Bi-est contains 2 mg estriol (80%) and 0.5 mg estradiol (20%); Tri-est contains 2 mg estriol (80%), 0.25 mg estrone (10%), and 0.25 mg estradiol (10%). These products are advertised as containing 80% estriol, which is correct. However, they contain significant amounts of estradiol and, therefore, may require progesterone for endometrial protection (Gaudet, 2004). Estriol also can be compounded as a vaginal cream.

The FDA (2008) has recently taken action against compounding pharmacies to stop unwarranted and misleading claims in advertisements that their products are safer than the estrogen products produced by traditional pharmaceutical companies. In reality, all estrogens carry a similar safety and risk profile.

Herbals

Although many women seek relief of menopausal symptoms, especially hot flashes, from herbal preparations, few studies exist to offer information regarding their efficacy or safety. Because these products are generally identified as diet supplements, rather than as medications, they are not regulated by the FDA in the same way as prescription medications and other over-the-counter products. Federal regulations for these products do exist, but they are poorly enforced. This lax supervision raises questions regarding the purity, contents, and consistency from package to package or tablet to tablet. Various preparations of the same herbal product may contain dramatically different amounts of active ingredients (e.g., extract versus tincture), and many products consist of mixtures of many different herbs in a single preparation, making dosing difficult. Furthermore, little is known regarding the interactions between various herbal products and prescription medications or other herbal products.

Despite these concerns, herbal products are widely used for menopausal symptom relief. Several of them are commonly used in combination products or in Chinese herb mixtures. **Table 13-11** provides information about some of these preparations.

Isoflavones

Isoflavones are compounds derived from plants that have both estrogenic and nonestrogenic properties. They are present in foods, such as soy and red clover, as well as in commercial preparations. Isoflavones are often referred to as phytoestrogens because of their ability to bind weakly with estrogen receptors, especially the beta receptors, and have been extensively studied for reducing hot flashes. Several recent placebo-controlled trials show little or no statistically significant differences in hot flash reduction in treatment versus control groups (Lewis et al., 2006; Nikander et al., 2003; Penotti et al., 2003; Tice et al., 2003). Nelson and colleagues (2006) analyzed 17 studies evaluating the effectiveness of soy for menopause-related hot flashes; in the 11 soy extract trials considered, 4 showed some improvement or mixed results, while mixed results or no differences were found in 6 studies of red clover.

Despite these disappointing findings, soy is a healthy food that the FDA has allowed to be identified as reducing the risk of heart disease. There is no evidence that soy predisposes women to breast cancer, and it can be used by breast cancer survivors. Some data suggest that use of soy for 5 years or more could cause endometrial overgrowth (Unfer et al., 2004). Women who choose to add soy to their diets need to be educated to use the soy to replace something else, rather than adding extra calories through soy nuts, shakes, or cereals.

TABLE 13-11 Herbals Commonly Used for Menopausal Symptom Relief*

Product	Usual Dosage†	Purpose in Menopause	Comments
Black cohosh (*Cimicifuga racemosa*)	20 mg twice daily (proprietary standardized extract)	Vasomotor symptoms	Multiple products and formulations available
			Research evidence suggests beneficial effect on menopausal symptoms, benefit similar to estrogen for hot flash relief
			Safety for use > 6 months not established
			Product labels frequently recommend much higher doses
			Can potentiate antihypertensives
			Wide variations in product ingredients, extraction processes, and purity
			Side effects rare, usually intestinal upset, headache, dizziness, hypotension, or painful extremities; more common with higher doses
Chastetree berry (*Vitex agnus castus*)	Effective dose unknown, hard to find standardized extract	Menstrual irregularity	More popular in Europe than the United States; approved in Germany for premenstrual syndrome (PMS), mastalgia, and menopause symptoms
			Often found in combination products
			Research focuses on PMS symptoms, no data on relief of menopause symptoms
			Side effects rare, usually headache, intestinal upset
Dong quai (*Angelica sinensis*)	2 capsules two to three times per day; usually in combination products	Gynecologic conditions	Widely used in Asia
			Research found no benefit for menopause symptoms
			Often in Chinese herb combination products (*Chinese Materia Medica* advises against giving it alone)
			A "heating" herb, can cause a red face, hot flashes, sweating, irritability, or insomnia
			Contains coumarin derivatives, contraindicated in those taking warfarin
			Can cause photosensitivity, hypotension
Evening primrose oil (*Oenothera biennis*)	3–4 gm daily in divided doses	Hot flashes Mastalgia	Data show no benefit in treatment versus controls
			Potentiates risk for seizure if taken with seizure disorder, phenothiazines, and other medications that lower the seizure threshold
			Side effects include diarrhea and nausea

Herb	Dose	Indication	Comments
Ginkgo (Ginkgo biloba)	40–80 mg of standardized extract three times daily	Memory changes	Insufficient research on safety and efficacy Memory changes often related to sleep disturbances, menopausal sleep disturbances frequently related to vasomotor symptoms or other life stressors Side effects include gastrointestinal distress, hypotension; chronic use has been linked with subarachnoid hemorrhage, subdural hematoma, and increased bleeding times
Ginseng (Panax ginseng)	1–2 gm root daily in divided doses	General "tonic" Improved mood, fatigue	Heavily adulterated Research showed no benefit on menopausal symptoms; showed benefits on well-being, general health, and depression Can cause uterine bleeding, mastalgia Contraindicated with breast cancer, and with monoamine oxidase inhibitors, stimulants, or anticoagulants; may potentiate digoxin and others (multiple drug interactions) Side effects include rash, nervousness, insomnia, hypertension
Kava (Piper methysticum)	150–300 mg of root extract daily in divided doses	Irritability Insomnia	Banned in several countries due to hepatotoxicity, thus not recommended Contraindicated with depression Side effects include gastrointestinal discomfort, impaired reflexes and motor function, weight loss, hepatotoxicity, rash
Licorice root (Glycyrrhiza glabra)	5–15 mg of root equivalent daily in divided doses	Menopause-related symptoms	Found in many Chinese herb mixtures No data supporting relief of hot flashes High doses can lead to primary aldosteronism cardiac arrhythmias, cardiac arrest Contraindicated if hepatic or renal disease, diabetes, hypertension, arrhythmia, hypokalemia, hypertonis, pregnancy, or on diuretics
Passion flower (Passiflora incarnata)	3–10 grains daily in divided doses	Sedative	Research shows mixed results in sleep improvement Menopausal sleep disturbances frequently related to vasomotor symptoms or other life stressors

(continues)

TABLE 13-11 Herbals Commonly Used for Menopausal Symptom Relief* *(Continued)*

Product	Usual Dosage†	Purpose in Menopause	Comments
St. John's wort (*Hypericum perforatum*)	300 mg three times daily (standardized extract)	Vasomotor symptoms Irritability Depression	No data supporting vasomotor relief Research findings support use for depression, there are no clinical trials for menopause symptom treatment Often combined with black cohosh for menopause symptom treatment Interferes with metabolism of many medications that are metabolized in the liver (C 450) (e.g., estrogen, digoxin, theophylline), reduces international normalized ratio (INR) levels, not to be used concomitantly with antidepressants, monoamine oxidase inhibitors, or immunosuppressants Side effects include photosensitivity, rash, constipation, cramping, dry mouth, fatigue, dizziness, restlessness, insomnia
Valerian root (*Valeriana officinalis*)	300–600 mg aqueous extract 1/2–1 hour before bed (insomnia); 150–300 mg aqueous extract each morning and 300–400 mg each evening (anxiety)	Sedative Antianxiety	Used for insomnia in intermittent dosing, for anxiety with chronic dosing Research showed improvement in sleep and depression/mood scales Side effects include headache, uneasiness, excitability, arrhythmias, morning sedation, gastrointestinal upset, cardiac function disorders (with long-term use)
Wild yam (*Dioscorea villosa*)	Unknown	Menopausal symptoms	Products claim that creams are converted to progesterone; however, the human body cannot convert topical or ingested wild yam into progesterone Research showed no benefit on menopausal symptoms

*See prescribing reference for full information on doses, side effects, contraindications, and cautions.

†Dosages vary and differ according to form (e.g., tincture, liquid extract, drops, essential oil, standardized extract).

Sources: Decker & Myers, 2001; Gaudet, 2004; Low Dog, 2004; NAMS, 2010b.

Other classes of phytoestrogens include flavonoids, lignans, and coumestrans. These classes have much lower hormonal affinity and are generally not thought to be useful for menopausal symptom management. They are found in some foods and food products and carry some of the cardioprotective properties of isoflavones. Lignans are found in flaxseed oil, whole grains, and some fruits and vegetables. Flavonoids are found in oils, spices, wine, tea, and some vegetables. Coumestrans are found in alfalfa sprouts, red beans, split peas, spinach, and some species of clover; these phytoestrogens can interfere with bleeding profiles and may have interactions with warfarin.

Progesterone Creams

Several different progesterone creams are available over-the-counter. FDA regulations are not currently enforced for these products, again raising concerns about their purity and content. Progesterone creams include products such as PhytoGest, Pro-Gest, Endocreme, and Pro-Dermex, and the stated progesterone content varies from less than 2 mg to 700 mg. These creams can also be prescribed using compounding pharmacies.

Although some women taking systemic estrogens may want to use progesterone creams for endometrial protection to avoid systemic progesterone effects, there are no data that support the use of progesterone creams for endometrial protection. At least one randomized, controlled study identified improvement in vasomotor symptoms for women using transdermal progesterone cream as compared with controls (Leonetti, Longo, & Anasti, 1999). Topical progesterone creams may be a promising option if future research supports these findings.

Acupuncture

Research findings evaluating acupuncture for the relief of menopause-related hot flashes have been contradictory. One small study of 24 women identified no differences in subjects treated with electroacupuncture versus controls (Wyon, Lindgren, Lundberg, & Hammar, 1995). In contrast, a more recent study (N = 17) identified significant reductions in hot flashes and sleep disturbances in women treated over a six-week period with acupuncture at menopause symptom-specific sites as compared with controls who were treated with a general tonic acupuncture (Cohen, Rousseau, & Carey, 2003). Some other studies comparing effects of acupuncture to sham or placebo have demonstrated a reduction in severity, but not frequency, of hot flashes (Huang, Nir, Chen, Schnyer, & Manber, 2006; Nir, Huang, Schnyer, Chen, & Manber, 2007), while others showed no differences (Deng et al., 2007; Vincent et al., 2007). Acupuncture may prove to provide some benefit but further research is needed to clarify its usefulness.

Conclusion

Menopause is a marker in the lives of middle-aged women. While a normal developmental stage, it gives women the opportunity to evaluate their health and risks for diseases of aging, thereby instituting lifestyle changes that prevent disease and promote health. Although many women will transition through perimenopause to postmenopause without incident, many will also experience mild to severe vasomotor symptoms. Treatments for these problems can decrease symptoms and improve women's quality of life. As the numbers of postmenopausal women increase, clinicians are in a prime position to counsel their patients about healthy aging.

References

Administration on Aging. (2008). *A profile of older Americans: 2008*. Washington, DC: Author. Retrieved from http://www.aoa.gov/AoARoot/Aging_Statistics/Profile/2008/docs/2008profile.pdf

Alexander, I. M. (2006). Bioidentical hormones for menopause therapy: Separating the myths from the reality. *Women's Health Care: A Practical Journal for Nurse Practitioners, 5*(1), 7–17.

Alexander, I. M., Ruff, C., Rousseau, M. E., White, K., Motter, S., McKie, C., & Clark, P. (2003). Menopause symptoms and management strategies identified by black women [Abstract]. *Menopause, 10*(6), 601.

Alexander, I. M., Ruff, C., Rousseau, M. E., White, K., Motter, S., McKie, C., et al. (2004, April). *Experiences and perceptions of menopause and midlife health among black women*. Paper presented at the meeting of the Eastern Nursing Research Society 16th Annual Scientific Sessions, Quincy, MA.

Alexander, I. M., Ruff, C. C., & Udemezue, C. (n.d.). *Correlation between lifestyle behaviors and severity of menopausal symptoms in black women. [Unpublished data.]* P20 pilot study in the Yale-Howard Center for reducing health disparities through self- and family-management (Grant No. 1P20NR08349-01). Bethesda, MD: National Institute of Nursing Research.

American Association of Clinical Endocrinologists (AACE). (2008). *Diabetes experts recommend one-two punch for treating patients with pre-diabetes.* Retrieved from http://media.aace.com/article_display.cfm?article_id=4828

American Cancer Society (ACS). (2007). *Guide to quitting smoking.* Retrieved from http://www.cancer.org/docroot/PED/content/PED_10_13X_Guide_for_Quitting_Smoking.asp

American Cancer Society (ACS). (2011). *Cancer facts and figures 2011.* Atlanta, GA: Author. Retrieved from http://www.cancer.org/Research/CancerFacts Figures/CancerFactsFigures/cancer-facts-figures-2011

American Diabetes Association (ADA). (2004a). Position statement: Diagnosis and classification of diabetes mellitus. *Diabetes Care, 27*(suppl 1), S5–S10.

American Diabetes Association (ADA). (2004b). Position statement: Screening for type 2 diabetes. *Diabetes Care, 27*(suppl. 1), S11–S14.

American Heart Association (AHA). (2002). *Heart disease and stroke statistics: 2003 update.* Dallas, TX: Author.

American Heart Association (AHA). (2004). *Women and cardiovascular disease.* Retrieved from http://www.americanheart.org

American Obesity Association. (2002). *Obesity fact sheets* (Updated March 24, 2004). Retrieved from http://www.obesity.org

Anderson, G. L., Limacher, M., Assaf, A. R., Bassford, T., Beresford, S. A., Black, H.,... Wassertheil-Smoller, S. (2004). Effects of conjugated equine estrogen in postmenopausal women with hysterectomy: The Women's Health Initiative randomized controlled trial. *Journal of the American Medical Association, 291*(14), 1701–1712.

Arnold, E. (2005). A voice of their own: Women moving into their fifties. *Health Care for Women International, 26*(8), 630–651.

Avis, N. E., Stellato, R., Crawford, S., Bromberger, J., Ganz, P., Cain, V., & Kagawa-Singer, M. (2001). Is there a menopausal syndrome? Menopausal status and symptoms across racial/ethnic groups. *Social Science and Medicine, 52*(3), 345–356.

Bair, Y. A., Gold, E. B., Azari, R. A., Greendale, G., Sternfeld, B., Harkey, M. R., & Kravitz, R. L. (2005). Use of conventional and complementary health care during the transition to menopause: Longitudinal results from the Study of Women's Health Across the Nation (SWAN). *Menopause, 12*(1), 31–39.

Baker, A., Simpson, S., & Dawson, D. (1997). Sleep disruption and mood changes associated with menopause. *Journal of Psychosomatic Research, 43*(4), 359–369.

Ballard, K. D., Kuh, D. J., & Wadsworth, M. E. J. (2001). The role of the menopause in women's experiences of the "change of life." *Sociology of Health and Illness, 23*(4), 397–424.

Barton, D. L., Loprinzi, C. L., Quella, S. K., Sloan, J. A., Veeder, M. H., Egner, J. R., ... Novotny, P. (1998). Prospective evaluation of vitamin E for hot flashes in breast cancer survivors. *Journal of Clinical Oncology, 16*(2), 495–500.

Baskin, H. J. (2002). American Association of Clinical Endocrinologists' medical guidelines for clinical practice for the evaluation and treatment of hyperthyroidism and hypothyroidism. *Endocrine Practice, 8*(6), 457–469.

Bastian, L. A., Smith, C. M., & Nanda, K. (2003). Is this woman perimenopausal? *Journal of the American Medical Association, 289*(7), 895–902.

Blackman, M. R. (2000). Age-related alterations in sleep quality and neuroendocrine function: Interrelationships and implications. *Journal of the American Medical Association, 284*(7), 879–881.

Blatt, M. H. G., Weisbader, H., & Kupperman, H. S. (1953). Vitamin E and the climacteric syndrome. *Archives of Internal Medicine, 91,* 792–796.

Brett, K. M., & Keenan, N. L. (2007). Complementary and alternative medicine use among midlife women for reasons including menopause in the United States: 2002. *Menopause, 14*(2), 300–307.

Bromberger, J. T., Matthews, K. A., Kuller, L. H., Wing, R. R., Meilahn, E. N., & Plantinga, P. (1997). Prospective study of the determinants of age at menopause. *American Journal of Epidemiology, 145*(2), 124–133.

Busch, H., Barth-Olofsson, A. S., Rosenhagen, S., & Collins, A. (2003). Menopause transition and psychological development. *Menopause, 10*(2), 179–187.

Centers for Disease Control and Prevention. (2011). *Overweight and obesity.* (Updated October 11, 2011.) Retrieved from http://www.cdc.gov

Cohen, L. (2004, April). *Depression rates in perimenopausal and premenopausal women: A longitudinal study.* Paper presented at the meeting of the American Psychiatric Association, New York.

Cohen, S. M., Rousseau, M. E., & Carey, B. (2003). Can acupuncture ease the symptoms of menopause? *Holistic Nursing Practice, 17*(6), 295–299.

Collins, P. H. (1990). *Black feminist thought: Knowledge, consciousness, and the politics of empowerment.* Boston: Unwin Hyman.

Cooper, G. S., Sandler, D. P., & Bohlig, M. (1999). Active and passive smoking and the occurrence of natural menopause. *Epidemiology, 10*(6), 771–773.

Cramer, G., Xu, H., & Harlow, B. L. (1995). Family history as a predictor of early menopause. *Fertility and Sterility, 64,* 740–745.

Crandall, C. (2002). Vaginal estrogen preparations: A review of safety and efficacy for vaginal atrophy. *Journal of Women's Health, 11*(10), 857–877.

Daley, A., MacArthur, C., McManus, R., Stokes-Lampard, H., Wilson, S., Roalfe, A., & Mutrie, N. (2006). Factors associated with the use of complementary medicine and non-pharmacological interventions in symptomatic menopausal women. *Climacteric, 9*(5), 336–346.

Davis, R., & Huber, K. (2004). Class, ethnicity, age, physical status, and sexual orientation: Implications for health and healthcare. In M. Condon (Ed.), *Women's health* (pp. 21–40). Upper Saddle River, NJ: Prentice Hall.

Dawson-Hughes, B., Lindsay, R., Khosla, S., Melton, L. J., Tosteson, A. N., Favus, M., & Baim, S. (2008). *Clinician's guide to prevention and treatment of osteoporosis* (Vol. 2008). Washington, DC: National Osteoporosis Foundation.

Dawson-Hughes, B., Tosteson, A. N., Melton, L. J., 3rd, Baim, S., Favus, M. J., Khosla, S., & Lindsay, R. L. (2008). Implications of absolute fracture risk assessment for osteoporosis practice guidelines in the USA. *Osteoporosis International, 19*(4), 449–458.

de Bruin, J. P., Bovenhuis, H., van Noord, P. A. H., Pearson, P. L., van Arendonk, J. A. M., te Velde, E. R., ... Dorland, M. (2001). The role of genetic factors in age at natural menopause. *Human Reproduction, 16*(9), 2014–2018.

Decker, G. M., & Myers, J. (2001). Commonly used herbs: Implications for clinical practice [insert]. *Clinical Journal of Oncology Nursing, 5*(2), 13p.

Deng, G., Vickers, A., Yeung, S., D'Andrea, G. M., Xiao, H., Heerdt, A. S., ... Cassileth, B. (2007). Randomized, controlled trial of acupuncture for the treatment of hot flashes in breast cancer patients. *Journal of Clinical Oncology, 25*(35), 5584–5590.

Dennerstein, L., Dudley, E., & Burger, H. (2001). Are changes in sexual functioning during midlife due to aging or menopause? *Fertility & Sterility, 76*(3), 456–460.

Dow, M. G., Hart, D. M., & Forrest, C. A. (1982). Hormonal treatments of sexual unresponsiveness in postmenopausal women: A comparative study. *British Journal of Obstetrics and Gynaecology, 90*, 361–366.

Dvornyk, V., Long, J. R., Liu, P. Y., Zhao, L. J., Shen, H., Recker, R. R., & Deng, H. W. (2006). Predictive factors for age at menopause in Caucasian females. *Maturitas, 54*(1), 19–26.

Eisenberg, D. M., Davis, R. B., Ettner, S. L., Appel, S., Wilkey, S., Van Rompay, M., & Kessler, R. C. (1998). Trends in alternative medicine use in the United States, 1990–1997: Results of a follow-up national survey. *Journal of the American Medical Association, 280*(18), 1569–1575.

Eisenberg, D. M., Kessler, R. C., Foster, C., Norlock, F. E., Calkins, D. R., & Delbanco, T. L. (1993). Unconventional medicine in the United States: Prevalence, costs, and patterns of use. *New England Journal of Medicine, 328*(4), 246–252.

Fairfield, K. M., & Fletcher, R. H. (2002). Vitamins for chronic disease prevention in adults: Scientific review. *Journal of the American Medical Association, 287*(23), 3116–3126.

Finer, L. B., & Henshaw, S. K. (2006). Disparities in rates of unintended pregnancy in the United States, 1994 and 2001. *Perspectives on Sexual and Reproductive Health, 38*(2), 90–96.

Fletcher, R. H., & Fairfield, K. M. (2002). Vitamins for chronic disease prevention in adults: Clinical applications. *Journal of the American Medical Association, 287*(23), 3127–3129.

Fogel, C. I., & Woods, N. F. (Eds.). (2008). *Women's health care in advanced practice nursing.* New York: Springer.

Food and Drug Administration (FDA). (2008). *FDA takes action against compounded menopause hormone therapy drugs.* Retrieved from http://www.fda.gov/NewsEvents/Newsroom/PressAnnouncements/2008/ucm116832.htm

Franz, M. J. (Ed.). (2003). *A CORE curriculum for diabetes education: Diabetes and complications* (5th ed.). Chicago: American Association of Diabetes Educators.

Freedman, R. R., & Blacker, C. M. (2002). Estrogen raises the sweating threshold in postmenopausal women with hot flashes. *Fertility and Sterility, 77*(3), 487–490.

Freedman, R. R., & Woodward, S. (1992). Behavioral treatment of menopausal hot flashes: Evaluation by ambulatory monitoring. *American Journal of Obstetrics and Gynecology, 167*, 436–439.

Freedman, R. R., Woodward, S., Brown, B., Javaid, J. I., & Pandy, G. N. (1995). Biochemical and thermoregulatory effects of treatment for menopausal hot flashes. *Menopause, 2*, 211–218.

Fritz, M. A., & Speroff, L. (2011). *Clinical gynecologic endocrinology and infertility* (8th ed.). Baltimore: Lippincott Williams & Wilkins.

Gallagher, J. C. (2007). Effect of early menopause on bone mineral density and fractures. *Menopause, 14*(3 Pt 2), 567–571.

Garcia, C. R., Sammel, M. D., Freeman, E. W., Lin, H., Langan, E., Kapoor, S., & Nelson, D. B. (2005). Defining menopause status: Creation of a new definition to identify the early changes of the menopausal transition. *Menopause, 12*(2), 128–135.

Gaspar, U. J., Gotta, J. M., & van den Brule, F. A. (1995). Post menopausal changes of lipid and glucose metabolism: A review of the main aspects. *Maturitas, 21*, 171–178.

Gaudet, T. W. (2004). CAM approaches to menopause management: Overview of the options. *Menopause Management: Women's Health Through Midlife & Beyond, 13*(suppl 1), 48–50.

Gilligan, C. (1982). *In a different voice: Psychological theory and women's development.* Cambridge, MA: Harvard University Press.

Godsland, I. F. (1996). The influence of female sex steroids on glucose metabolism and insulin action. *Journal of Internal Medicine, 738*(suppl), 1–60.

Gold, E. B., Bromberger, J., Crawford, S., Samuels, S., Greendale, G. A., Harlow, S. D., & Skurnick, J. (2001). Factors associated with age at natural menopause in a multiethnic sample of midlife women. *American Journal of Epidemiology, 153*(9), 865–874.

Gold, E. B., Sternfeld, B., Kelsey, J. L., Brown, C., Mouton, C., Reame, N., … Stellato, R. (2000). Relation of demographic and lifestyle factors to symptoms in a multi-racial/ethnic population of women 40–55 years of age. *American Journal of Epidemiology, 152*(5), 463–473.

Grady, D. (2002). A 60-year-old woman trying to discontinue hormone replacement therapy. *Journal of the American Medical Association, 287*(16), 2130–2137.

Greendale, G. A., Lee, N. P., & Arriola, E. R. (1999). The menopause. *Lancet, 353*(9152), 571–580.

Grodstein, F., Manson, J. E., & Stampfer, M. J. (2006). Hormone therapy and coronary heart disease: The role of time since menopause and age at hormone initiation. *Journal of Women's Health (Larchmont), 15*(1), 35–44.

Harlow, S. D., Cain, K., Crawford, S., Dennerstein, L., Little, R., Mitchell, E. S.,…Yosef, M. (2006). Evaluation of four proposed bleeding criteria for the onset of late menopausal transition. *Journal of Clinical Endocrinology and Metabolism, 91*(9), 3432–3438.

Hefler, L. A., Grimm, C., Bentz, E. K., Reinthaller, A., Heinze, G., & Tempfer, C. B. (2006). A model for predicting age at menopause in white women. *Fertility and Sterility, 85*(2), 451–454.

Hodgson, S. F., & Watts, S. F. (2003). American Association of Clinical Endocrinologists medical guidelines for clinical practice for the prevention and treatment of postmenopausal osteoporosis: 2001 edition with selected updates for 2003. *Endocrine Practice, 9*(6), 544–564.

Huang, M. I., Nir, Y., Chen, B., Schnyer, R., & Manber, R. (2006). A randomized controlled pilot study of acupuncture for postmenopausal hot flashes: Effect on nocturnal hot flashes and sleep quality. *Fertility and Sterility, 86*(3), 700–710.

Huber, A., Grimm, C., Huber, J. C., Schneeberger, C., Leodolter, S., Reinthaller, A.,…Hefler, L. A. (2006). A common polymorphism within the steroid 5-alpha-reductase type 2 gene and timing of menopause in Caucasian women. *European Journal of Obstetrics, Gynecology, and Reproductive Biology, 125*(2), 221–225.

Irvin, J. H., Domar, A. D., Clark, C., Zuttermeister, P. C., & Freidman, R. (1996). The effects of relaxation response training on menopausal symptoms. *Journal of Psychosomatic Obstetrics and Gynaecology, 17*, 202–207.

Jacobs Institute on Women's Health. (2003). *Expert panel on menopause counseling.* Retrieved from http://www.jiwh.org/menodownload.htm

Jordan, J. V., Kaplan, A. G., Miller, J. B., Stiver, I. P., & Surrey, J. L. (1991). *Women's growth in connection.* New York: Guilford Press.

Kessler, R. C., Davis, R. B., Foster, D. F., Van Rompay, M. I., Walters, E. E., Wilkey, S. A., et al. (2001). Long-term trends in the use of complementary and alternative medical therapies in the United States. *Annals of Internal Medicine, 135*(4), 262–268.

Klatte, E. T., Scharre, D. W., Nagaraja, H. N., Davis, R. A., & Beversdorf, D. Q. (2003). Combination therapy of donepezil and vitamin E in Alzheimer disease. *Alzheimer Disease & Associated Disorders, 17*(2), 113–116.

Kronenberg, F. (1990). Hot flashes: Epidemiology and physiology. *Annals of the New York Academy of Sciences, 592*, 52–86, 123–133.

Landolt, H. P., Rioth, C., Dijk, D. J., & Borbely, A. A. (1996). Late-afternoon ethanol intake affects nocturnal sleep and the sleep EEG in middle-aged men. *Journal of Clinical Psychopharmacology, 16*, 428–436.

Landolt, H. P., Werth, E., Borbely, A. A., & Dijk, D. J. (1995). Caffeine intake (200 mg) in the morning affects human sleep and EEG spectra at night. *Brain Research, 675*, 67–74.

Lane, N., & Silverman, S. (2008). *Hotline: New NOF guidelines and the WHO Fracture Assessment Tool or FRAX.* Retrieved from http://www.rheumatology.org/publications/hotline/03_18_flax.asp

Leonetti, H. B., Longo, S., & Anasti, J. N. (1999). Transdermal progesterone cream for vasomotor symptoms and postmenopausal bone loss. *Obstetrics & Gynecology, 94*(2), 225–228.

Lewis, J. E., Nickell, L. A., Thompson, L. U., Szalai, J. P., Kiss, A., & Hilditch, J. R. (2006). A randomized controlled trial of the effect of dietary soy and flaxseed muffins on quality of life and hot flashes during menopause. *Menopause, 13*(4), 631–642.

Liu, J. (2004). Use of conjugated estrogens after the Women's Health Initiative. *The Female Patient, 29*, 8–13.

Lobo, R. A. (2007). Surgical menopause and cardiovascular risks. *Menopause, 14*(3 Pt 2), 562–566.

Low Dog, T. (2004). CAM approaches to menopause management: The role for botanicals in menopause. *Menopause Management: Women's Health Through Midlife & Beyond, 13*(suppl 1), 51–53.

MacPherson, K. I. (1981). Menopause as disease: The social construction of a metaphor. *Advances in Nursing Science, 3*, 95–113.

Mayer-Davis, E. J., D'Antonio, A., & Tudor-Locke, C. (2003). Lifestyle for diabetes prevention. In M. J. Franz (Ed.), *A core curriculum for diabetes education: Diabetes in the life cycle and research* (5th ed., pp. 1–30). Chicago: American Association of Diabetes Educators.

McKinlay, S. M. (1996). The normal menopause transition: An overview. *Maturitas, 23*(2), 137–145.

McLean, R. R., Jacques, P. F., Selhub, J., Tucker, K. L., Samelson, E. J., Broe, K. E.,…Kiel, D. P. (2004). Homocysteine as a predictive factor for hip fracture in older persons. *New England Journal of Medicine, 350*(20), 2042–2049.

Morin, C. M., Hauri, P. J., Espie, C. A., Speilman, A. J., Buysse, D. J., & Bootzin, R. R. (1999). Nonpharmacologic treatment of chronic insomnia: An American Academy of Sleep Medicine review. *Sleep, 22,* 1134–1156.

Nachtigall, L. E. (1994). Comparative study: Replens versus local estrogen in menopausal women. *Fertility & Sterility, 61,* 178–180.

National Cancer Institute (NCI). (2003). *Probability of developing or dying of cancer.* Retrieved from http://srab.cancer.gov/devcan

National Cancer Institute (NCI). (2008). *Cancer facts and figures, 2008.* Retrieved from http://www.cancer.org/downloads/STT/2008CAFFfinalsecured.pdf

National Institutes of Health (NIH). (1994). *Optimal calcium intake: NIH consensus statement.* Retrieved from http://text.nlm.nih.gov/nih/cdc/www/ 97txt .html

National Institutes of Health (NIH). (2004). NIH asks participants in Women's Health Initiative Estrogen-Alone Study to stop study pills, begin follow-up phase. Retrieved from http://www.nhlbi.nih.gov/new/press/04-03-02.htm

National Institutes of Health (NIH). (2007). National Center on Sleep Disorder Research and Office of Prevention, Education, and Control. Retrieved from www.nhlbi.nih.gov/health/prof/sleep/pslp_pat. htm

National Women's Health Network. (2000). *Taking hormones and women's health: Choices, risks, and benefits.* Washington, DC: Author.

Nelson, H. D., Vesco, K. K., Haney, E., Fu, R., Nedrow, A., Miller, J.,…Humphrey, L. (2006). Nonhormonal therapies for menopausal hot flashes: Systematic review and meta-analysis. *Journal of the American Medical Association, 295*(17), 2057–2071.

Newton, K. M., Buist, D. S., Keenan, N. L., Anderson, L. A., & LaCroix, A. Z. (2002). Use of alternative therapies for menopause symptoms: Results of a population-based survey. *Obstetrics and Gynecology, 100*(1), 18–25.

Newton, K. M., Buist, D. S., Yu, O., Hartsfield, C. L., Andrade, S. E., Wei, F.,…Chan, K. A. (2008). Hormone therapy initiation after the Women's Health Initiative. *Menopause, 15*(3), 487–493.

Nikander, E., Kilkkinen, A., Metsa-Heikkila, M., Adlercreutz, H., Pietinen, P., Tiitinen, A., & Ylikorkala, O. (2003). A randomized placebo-controlled crossover trial with phytoestrogens in treatment of menopause in breast cancer patients. *Obstetrics & Gynecology, 101*(6), 1213–1220.

Nir, Y., Huang, M. I., Schnyer, R., Chen, B., & Manber, R. (2007). Acupuncture for postmenopausal hot flashes. *Maturitas, 56*(4), 383–395.

North American Menopause Society (NAMS). (2003). Estrogen and progestogen use in peri- and postmenopausal women: September 2003 position statement of the North American Menopause Society. *Menopause, 10*(6), 497–506.

North American Menopause Society (NAMS). (2004). Treatment of menopause-associated vasomotor symptoms: Position statement of the North American Menopause Society. *Menopause, 11*(1), 11–33.

North American Menopause Society (NAMS). (2007). *Menopause practice: A clinician's guide* (3rd ed.). Cleveland, OH: Author.

North American Menopause Society (NAMS). (2008). Estrogen and progestogen use in postmenopausal women: July, 2008 position statement of the North American Menopause Society. *Menopause: The Journal of the North American Menopause Society, 15*(4), 584–603.

North American Menopause Society (NAMS). (2010a). Estrogen and progestogen use in postmenopausal women: 2010 position statement of the North American Menopause Society. *Menopause, 17*(2), 242–255.

North American Menopause Society (NAMS). (2010b). *Menopause practice: A clinician's guide* (4th ed.). Cleveland, OH: Author.

North American Menopause Society (NAMS). (2011a, September 30). *Government approved postmenopausal osteoporosis drugs in the United States and Canada.* Retrieved from http://www.menopause. org/otcharts.pdf

North American Menopause Society (NAMS). (2011b, October 25). *Hormone products for postmenopausal use in the United States and Canada.* Retrieved from http://www.menopause.org/htcharts.pdf

Onofrj, M., Thomas, A., Luciano, A. L., Iacono, D., Di Rollo, A., D'Andreamatteo, G., & Di Iorio, A.. (2002). Donepezil versus vitamin E in Alzheimer's disease: Part 2: Mild versus moderate–severe Alzheimer's disease. *Clinical Neuropharmacology, 25*(4), 207–215.

Palmer, J. R., Rosenberg, L., Wise, L. A., Horton, N. J., & Adams-Campbell, L. L. (2003). Onset of natural menopause in African American women. *American Journal of Public Health, 93*(2), 299–306.

Pastore, L. M., Carter, R. A., Hulka, B. S., & Wells, E. (2004). Self-reported urogenital symptoms in post-menopausal women: Women's Health Initiative. *Maturitas, 49*(4), 292–303.

Penotti, M., Fabio, E., Modena, A. B., Rinaldi, M., Omo-dei, U., & Vigano, P. (2003). Effect of soy-derived isoflavones on hot flushes, endometrial thickness, and the pulsatility index of the uterine and cerebral arteries. *Fertility & Sterility, 79*(5), 1112–1117.

Porth, C. M., & Kunert, M. P. (Eds.). (2002). *Pathophysiology concepts of altered health states* (6th ed.). Philadelphia: Lippincott Williams & Wilkins.

Quinn, A. A. (1991). A theoretical model of the perimenopausal process. *Journal of Nurse-Midwifery, 36*(1), 25–29.

Rossouw, J. E., Anderson, G. L., Prentice, R. L., LaCroix, A. Z., Jackson, R. D., Beresford, S. A. A.,…Ockene, J. (2002). Risks and benefits of estrogen plus progestin in healthy postmenopausal women: Principal results from the Women's Health Initiative Randomized Controlled Trial. *Journal of the American Medical Association, 288*(3), 321–333.

Salpeter, S. R., Walsh, J. M. E., Greyber, E., Ormiston, T. M., & Salpeter, E. E. (2004). Mortality associated with hormone replacement therapy in younger and older women. *Journal of General Internal Medicine, 19*(7), 791–804.

Sampselle, C. M., Harris, V. H., Harlow, S. D., & Sowers, M. (2002). Midlife development and menopause in African American and Caucasian women. *Health Care for Women International, 23*(4), 351–363.

Santoro, N., Brockwell, S., Johnston, J., Crawford, S. L., Gold, E. B., Harlow, S. D.,…Sutton-Tyrrell, K. (2007). Helping midlife women predict the onset of the final menses: SWAN, the Study of Women's Health Across the Nation. *Menopause, 14*(3 Pt 1), 415–424.

Santoro, N., Lasley, B., McConnell, D., Allsworth, J., Crawford, S., Gold, E. B.,…Weiss, G. (2004). Body size and ethnicity are associated with menstrual cycle alterations in women in the early menopausal transition: The Study of Women's Health Across the Nation (SWAN) Daily Hormone Study. *Journal of Clinical Endocrinology & Metabolism, 89*(6), 2622–2631.

Sheehy, G. (1976). *Passages: Predictable crises of adult life.* New York: Dutton.

Sheehy, G. (1995). *New passages: Mapping your life across time.* New York: Random House.

Sherman, C. A., Harvey, S. M., & Noell, J. (2005). "Are they still having sex?" STI's and unintended pregnancy among mid-life women. *Journal of Women and Aging, 17*(3), 41–55.

Sherwin, B. B., Gelfand, M. M., & Brender, W. (1985). Androgen enhances sexual motivation in females: A prospective crossover study of sex steroid administration in the surgical menopause. *Psychosomatic Medicine, 47*, 339–351.

Soules, M. R., Sherman, S., Parrott, E., Rebar, R., Santoro, N., Utian, W., & Woods, N. (2001). Executive summary: Stages of Reproductive Aging Workshop (STRAW). *Fertility & Sterility, 76*(5), 874–878.

Thomas, A., Iacono, D., Bonanni, L., D'Andreamatteo, G., & Onofrj, M. (2001). Donepezil, rivastigmine, and vitamin E in Alzheimer disease: A combined P300 event-related potentials/neuropsychologic evaluation over 6 months. *Clinical Neuropharmacology, 24*(1), 31–42.

Thurston, R. C., Sowers, M. R., Sutton-Tyrrell, K., Everson-Rose, S. A., Lewis, T. T., Edmundowicz, D., & Matthews, K. A. (2008). Abdominal adiposity and hot flashes among midlife women. *Menopause, 15*(3), 429–434.

Tice, J. A., Ettinger, B., Ensrud, K., Wallace, R., Blackwell, T., & Cummings, S. R. (2003). Phytoestrogen supplements for the treatment of hot flashes: The Isoflavone Clover Extract (ICE) Study: A randomized controlled trial. *Journal of the American Medical Association, 290*(2), 207–214.

Tosteson, A. N., Melton, L. J., 3rd, Dawson-Hughes, B., Baim, S., Favus, M. J., Khosla, S., & Lindsay, R. L. (2008). Cost-effective osteoporosis treatment thresholds: The United States perspective. *Osteoporosis International.* Retrieved from http://www.ncbi.nlm.nih.gov/entrez/query.fcgi?cmd=Retrieve&db=PubMed&dopt=Citation&list_uids=18292976

Unfer, V., Casini, M. L., Costabile, L., Mignosa, M., Gerli, S., & Di Renzo, G. C. (2004). Endometrial effects of long-term treatment with phytoestrogens: A randomized, double-blind, placebo-controlled study. *Fertility and Sterility, 82*(1), 145–148, quiz 265.

Upchurch, D. M., & Chyu, L. (2005). Use of complementary and alternative medicine among American women. *Women's Health Issues, 15*(1), 5–13.

U.S. Department of Health, Education, and Welfare, National Institute on Aging. (1979). *Summary of conclusions of the NIH Conference on Estrogen Use and Postmenopausal Women.* Washington, DC: Author.

U.S. Preventive Services Task Force (USPSTF). (1996). *Guide to preventive services*. Rockville, MD: Agency for Healthcare Research and Quality.

Utian, W. H. (1987). Overview on menopause. *American Journal of Obstetrics and Gynecology, 156*, 1280–1283.

Utian, W. (1999a). The International Menopause Society: Menopause-related terminology definitions. *Climacteric, 2*, 284–286.

Utian, W. H. (1999b). An historical perspective of natural and surgical menopause. *Menopause, 6*(2), 83–86.

Utian, W. H. (2001). Semantics, menopause-related terminology, and the STRAW reproductive aging staging system. *Menopause, 8*(6), 398–401.

van Disseldorp, J., Faddy, M. J., Themmen, A. P., de Jong, F. H., Peeters, P. H., van der Schouw, Y. T., & Broekmans, F. J. (2008). Relationship of serum anti-Müllerian hormone concentration to age of menopause. *Journal of Clinical Endocrinology and Metabolism, 93*(6), 2129–2134.

van Meurs, J. B. J., Dhonukshe-Rutten, R. A. M., Pluijm, S. M. F., van der Klift, M., de Jonge, R., Lindemans, J.,...Uitterlinden, A. G. (2004). Homocysteine levels and the risk of osteoporotic fracture. *New England Journal of Medicine, 350*(20), 2033–2041.

van Noord, P. A., Dubas, J. S., Dorland, M., Boersma, H., & te Velde, E. (1997). Age at natural menopause in a population-based screening cohort: The role of menarche, fecundity, and lifestyle factors. *Fertility & Sterility, 68*(1), 95–102.

Van Voorhis, B. J., Santoro, N., Harlow, S., Crawford, S. L., & Randolph, J. (2008). The relationship of bleeding patterns to daily reproductive hormones in women approaching menopause. *Obstetrics and Gynecology, 112*(1), 101–108.

Vincent, A., Barton, D. L., Mandrekar, J. N., Cha, S. S., Zais, T., Wahner-Roedler, D. L.,...Loprinzi, C.

(2007). Acupuncture for hot flashes: A randomized, sham-controlled clinical study. *Menopause, 14*(1), 45–52.

Vivekananthan, D. P., Penn, M. S., Sapp, S. K., Hsu, A., & Topol, E. J. (2003). Use of antioxidant vitamins for the prevention of cardiovascular disease: Meta-analysis of randomized trials. *Lancet, 361*(9374), 2017–2023.

Weiss, N. S., Ure, C. L., Ballard, J. H., William, A. R., & Daling, J. R. (1980). Decreased risk of fractures of the hip and lower forearm with postmenopausal use of estrogen. *New England Journal of Medicine, 303*, 1195–1198.

Willhite, L. A. (2001). Urogenital atrophy: Prevention and treatment. *Pharmacotherapy, 21*, 464–480.

Wilmoth, M. C. (1996). The middle years: Women, sexuality, and the self. *Journal of Obstetric, Gynecologic, and Neonatal Nursing, 25*(7), 615–621.

Wilson, R. (1966). *Feminine forever*. New York: Evans.

Woods, N. F., & Mitchell, E. S. (2008). Mid-life women's health. In C. I. Fogel & N. F. Woods (Eds.), *Women's health care in advanced practice nursing* (pp. 121–148). New York: Springer.

World Health Organization (WHO). (2007). *WHO FRAX Technical Report*. Retrieved from http://www.shef.ac.uk/FRAX/

Wyon, Y., Lindgren, R., Lundberg, T., & Hammar, M. (1995). Effects of acupuncture on climacteric vasomotor symptoms, quality of life, and urinary excretion of neuropeptides among postmenopausal women. *Menopause, 2*, 3–12.

Wysocki, S., Alexander, I., Schnare, S. M., Moore, A., & Freeman, S. B. (2003). Individualized care for menopausal women: Counseling women about hormone therapy. *Women's Health Care: A Practical Journal for Nurse Practitioners, 2*(12), 8–16.

14

Intimate Partner Violence

Daniel J. Sheridan
Linda A. Fernandes
Alida D. Wagner
Dawn M. Van Pelt
Jacquelyn C. Campbell

Clinicians in primary care settings can be instrumental in providing comprehensive, ongoing assessments and intervention for women experiencing intimate partner violence (IPV). Women seek primary health care for a variety of routine health issues, such as gynecologic and women's health care, contraception, and prenatal care. Primary care settings afford a unique opportunity for assessment of violence and abuse in the lives of all female patients because women are often seen in these settings for episodic health care, and they often return for periodic health maintenance and routine screening (King, 1998).

Many women who are abused say that they have had some contact with the healthcare system either for a routine examination or for treatment of one of the long-term health problems associated with IPV. This chapter identifies the most common health consequences of living in intimate partner abusive relationships and highlights the importance of IPV screening and forensic documentation. Health care of women who report experiencing IPV needs to be both thorough and objective, but does not need to be emotionally distant. Douglas and Olshaker (2001), a retired Federal Bureau of Investigation (FBI) profiler and a forensic writer, respectively, state that besides excellent medical care, caring and empathy are the two most important attributes to bring to the examination process.

Throughout this chapter, the word *patient* will be used much more frequently than the words *victim* or *survivor*. The criminal justice system primarily uses the word *victim* when describing individuals who have experienced a reported assault. Community-based women's advocacy programs often refer to women who have experienced IPV as survivors to promote their empowerment. During discussions at the International Association of Forensic Nurses (IAFN) Annual Scientific Assembly held October 2004 in Chicago, Illinois, there was consensus among most of the IAFN leaders interviewed by the primary author of this chapter that it is appropriate to use the word *patient* when discussing or documenting health care provided to individuals who report IPV.

Patients experiencing IPV have been criminally victimized and, unless murdered in the process, are survivors of the abuse. However, clinicians providing forensic-related care should keep the boundaries between the criminal justice, advocacy, and healthcare systems separate. Clinicians need to provide excellent evidence-based patient care with caring and empathy.

Definitions

IPV is an escalating pattern of abuse in which one partner in an intimate relationship controls the other through force, intimidation, or threat of violence (Saltzman, Fanslow, McMahon, & Shelley, 2002). IPV includes four categories of abuse: physical violence, sexual violence, threat of physical or sexual violence, and psychological/emotional abuse. Intimate partners may be a current or former spouse, dating partner, boyfriend, or girlfriend (Saltzman et al.). Intimate partners can be of the same or opposite sex. Physical violence includes acts such as hitting, slapping, kicking, punching, shoving, strangulation, and injuries from weapons. Sexual violence includes using physical force to make a woman engage in a sexual act against her will and abusive sexual contact. (See Chapter 15 for detailed information about sexual assault.) Some examples of emotional abuse include humiliating a woman, controlling what she can and cannot do, isolating her from friends and family, and disregarding what she wants (Saltzman et al.).

Epidemiology

In the National Violence Against Women Survey, cosponsored by the Centers for Disease Control and Prevention (CDC) and the National Institute of Justice, 25% of a nationally representative sample of 8000 U.S. women said an intimate partner had assaulted them at some time in their lives (Tjaden & Thoennes, 1998). In a more recent population-based national sample of 1800 women, 23% of women reported physical assault by an intimate partner since age 18, and 14% reported sexual assault by someone they knew (Moracco, Runyan, Bowling, & Earp, 2007). In prenatal settings, studies have identified the prevalence of abuse during pregnancy as ranging from 18.1% in a sample of adolescents and adult women (Parker, McFarlane & Soeken, 1994), to as high as 37.6% in a sample of pregnant adolescents (Curry, 1998). Empirical studies have reported that an estimated 40% to 45% of all women experiencing IPV are forced to have sex by their male partners (Campbell, 1989; Campbell & Soeken, 1999; Finkelhor & Yllo, 1997). An additional, smaller percentage of women are sexually abused by their intimate partners without any physical abuse taking place (Campbell; Campbell & Soeken).

Health Effects

Gynecologic and Chronic Health Conditions

Gynecologic problems are the most consistent, long-lasting, and widespread physical health problems experienced by women who are battered (Campbell, 2002). Increased rates of pelvic inflammatory disease (PID), heightened risks of sexually transmitted infections (STIs) including human immunodeficiency virus (HIV) and acquired immune deficiency syndrome (AIDS), unexplained vaginal bleeding, fibroids, pelvic pain, urinary tract infections, painful intercourse, decreased sexual desire, genital irritation, and other genitourinary related health problems have all been documented among women who have been battered in several population-based heathcare setting studies (Bergman & Brismar, 1991; Campbell et al., 2002; Campbell & Soeken, 1999; Chapman, 1989; Coker, Smith, Bethea, King, & McKeown, 2000; Ebby, Campbell, Sullivan, & Davidson, 1995; McCauley et al., 1995; Plichta, 1996; Plichta & Abraham, 1996). Anytime a woman presents with one or more of these gynecologic conditions, it is crucial that she be screened for IPV. Additionally, women who are abused are at a significantly higher risk for chronic health problems such as neurologic, gastrointestinal, and chronic pain symptoms (Campbell, 2002; Campbell et al., 2002; Coker et al.; McCauley et al.; Plichta; Plichta & Abraham).

A U.S. population-based study of self-reported data found the odds of having a gynecologic problem were three times higher for patients who experienced IPV (McCauley et al., 1995). Gynecologic health problems could stem from forced anal, vaginal, or other abusive sex practices, such as unsafe sex by partners outside of the relationship (Campbell et al., 2002; Ebby et al., 1995). Clinicians should explore the possibility of sexual assault or forced sexual intercourse for all women presenting with gynecologic symptoms. This is especially true for women who present with multiple or persistent gynecologic symptoms. Campbell et al. (2002) found that 30% of women who were sexually abused as adults, either with or without other forms of physical abuse, reported three or more gynecologic health problems, compared with 8% of women who experienced only physical abuse, and 6% of those who were never abused. Asking a patient about forced sex from her partner or her partner's sexual practices has to be conducted in a very professional, nonjudgmental, caring, sensitive manner, and in a private and safe environment. Women are often too embarrassed or afraid to volunteer such information, or they may not link their health problems to the abuse in their lives.

Mental Health Conditions

Post-traumatic stress disorder (PTSD) can occur when a person has experienced or witnessed a traumatic or life-threatening event. Repeated domestic assault is very traumatic and can lead to PTSD. Many patients experiencing IPV meet the four major criteria for diagnosing PTSD: (1) experiencing a traumatic event, (2) reexperiencing the traumatic event, (3) numbness and avoidance, and (4) hypervigilance (Woods & Campbell, 1993). Campbell

(2002) reports that women who have been battered experience PTSD more frequently than women who have not been in a violent relationship.

According to Campbell (2002), women who have experienced PTSD may use drugs and alcohol as coping mechanisms to deal with certain symptoms of PTSD—namely, intrusion, avoidance, and hyperarousal. Substance abuse may also begin during the abusive relationship, as the woman seeks a way to escape from the reality of her situation. Substance abuse creates additional problems for patients who are experiencing IPV because they are more likely to experience repeated patterns of partner abuse (Schornstein, 1997). In addition, it can often be difficult to find a women's shelter willing to admit a patient with a substance abuse problem, which creates difficulties when a clinician is assisting a woman to arrange a safety plan.

Women who have been battered are also prone to developing depression (Campbell, Kub, & Rose, 1996). Physical, emotional, and sexual abuse are strongly associated with depression (Hegarty, Gunn, Chondros, & Small, 2004). All women with depression should be screened for IPV; conversely, all women experiencing IPV should be evaluated for depression.

Screening

Guidelines developed by an interdisciplinary team of healthcare experts in IPV recommend that women be screened for IPV in primary care settings during their periodic examinations, especially gynecologic visits, and at all visits for a new concern (Family Violence Prevention Fund, 1999). Clinicians should routinely consider IPV as a possible diagnosis for women who present with gynecologic problems, especially multiple problems, chronic stress-related symptoms, and central nervous system (CNS) symptoms. In addition to the effects of stress and mental distress, patients experiencing IPV usually present with physical health problems as well.

Most women who have been battered do not come to healthcare facilities with obvious trauma or injuries, although women who have been battered and who present to an emergency department usually have more injuries to the head, neck, face, thorax, breasts, and abdomen than women who have not been physically abused (Campbell, 2002). When there is a question of IPV, either past or present, it is important for the clinician to obtain a focused history and to perform a systematic physical examination to assess the severity and timing of trauma, injuries, gynecologic conditions, CNS disorders, and chronic stress-related problems.

With a general understanding of the relationships and patterns associated with partner violence, the clinician can begin to understand the development of stress-related illnesses and mental disorders in women who have been battered. When a woman presents for health care, her symptoms may be very general and vague, including generalized concerns such as unexplained pain or malaise. Clinicians often have preconceived notions that these women may have some other psychological disorder, or are perhaps displaying drug-seeking behaviors. Based on the authors' extensive clinical experiences, this behavior can many times be attributed to the woman's cry for help, or as an attempt to prove to her batterer that she is afflicted with some medical disorder as a way to prevent future violence or receive sympathy. For a variety of reasons, including fear of further abuse and embarrassment, a woman who has been abused is not always forthcoming about her abuse. As a consequence, it is important for clinicians to identify signs of IPV.

Theories

Lenore Walker (1979) was the first researcher to recognize the patterns or cycles in abusive relationships. Walker developed a basic three-part cycle of violence theory to describe these patterns of violence: (1) the tension-building phase, (2) the acute-battering incident, and (3) the calm or loving phase. The tension-building phase often includes verbal put-downs by the batterer, increased arguing, and, in some cases, the woman trying to appease her batterer. The acute battering phase can include sexual assault, hitting, kicking, strangulation, and use of weapons. During the calm phase, often referred to as the *honeymoon phase*, the batterer may apologize, promise it will never happen again, or even deny the violence occurred. As time goes on, the calm phase may disappear altogether. As early as 1980, clinicians were beginning to recognize that women were often seeking treatment during the tension-building phase for stress-related symptoms or immediately after the battering phase for physical injuries (Schornstein, 1997).

While Walker's cycle of violence theory is useful in understanding some IPV situations, it is no longer viewed as the best model of IPV. Instead, to better understand the dynamics associated with the intimate partner cycle of violence, a brief discussion of Heise's (1998) framework of violence is helpful. Heise's theory is based on a social ecological framework and includes four categories to describe factors that contribute to a violent relationship: personal history, microsystem, exosystem, and macrosystem. This framework is illustrated as four concentric circles with personal history in the center and, moving outward, by the microsystem, exosystem, and macrosystems (**Figure 14-1**).

The factors influencing the personal history include witnessing marital violence as a child, being abused oneself as a child, and an absent or rejecting father. The second category, the microsystem, may consist of male dominance in the family, male control of wealth in the family, use of alcohol, and marital and verbal conflicts. The factors influencing the third category, the exosystem (i.e., formal and

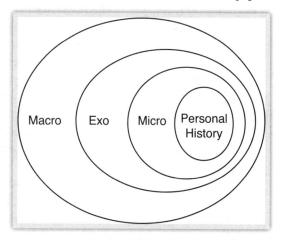

FIGURE 14-1 Heise's framework of violence.

Source: Reprinted by permission of Sage Publications, Inc., from Heise, L. L. (1998). Violence against women: An integrated, ecological framework. *Violence Against Women,* 4(3), 262–290.

informal social structures), are low socioeconomic status or unemployment, isolation of the woman and family, and delinquent peer associations. The fourth category, the macrosystem, encompasses the attitude and view of the public; it includes male entitlement or ownership of women, masculinity linked to aggression and dominance, rigid gender roles, acceptance of interpersonal violence, and acceptance of physical chastisement (Heise, 1998). These factors can be attributed to both the batterer and the victim in some circumstances.

Screening Tools

Routine screening for IPV in clinical settings is no longer an option, but rather is viewed as a standard of care, with failure to screen and document the clinician's findings being grounds for litigation (Sheridan, 2003). In 1992, the American Medical Association published guidelines that indicate physicians must be willing to routinely ask all women about IPV and screen for abuse, owing to the high prevalence of IPV (Schroeder & Weber, 1998). The Surgeon Generals of the United States, and the public health objectives for Healthy People 2000 and 2010, have identified family violence as an epidemic, and have called for an organized approach to screen, treat, and prevent further violence (Poirier, 1997).

Numerous reliable and valuable IPV screening tools are effective in a variety of clinical settings. Versions of the Abuse Assessment Screen (AAS) are the screening tools used most often in published research (Helton, 1987; McFarlane, Greenberg, Weltge, & Watson, 1995; McFarlane, Parker, Soeken, & Bullock, 1992; Parker & McFarlane, 1991; Soeken, McFarlane, Parker, & Lominack, 1998). Helton developed the original nine-question AAS (**Table 14-1**) in an effort to determine if a link existed between IPV health effects on women and fetal health.

Six-question (**Table 14-2**), then three-question (**Table 14-3**), and then two-question (**Table 14-4**) versions of the AAS have been tested and demonstrated good reliability and validity (Parker & McFarlane, 1991; McFarlane et al., 1992; McFarlane et al., 1995). Based on extensive clinical experiences, the primary author of this chapter prefers to use a six-question version of the AAS, with a preface that generalizes violence in society and notes the fact that all patients are routinely screened. With any "yes" answer on any IPV screen, the primary author recommends the interviewer respond with the following: "Thank you for sharing. Can you give me an example? When was the last time?"

The three-question AAS (McFarlane et al., 1992) is probably the most widely used IPV screen. However, it does not include questions about being afraid of one's partner, nor about being emotionally abused or controlled. It is very common to hear from women who have been battered that the pain and scars from being emotionally abused take longer to heal than the pain of physical abuse. Therefore, the clinical pressures to keep IPV screens short have to be weighed against the consequences of failure to assess the significant emotional abuse and fear of a partner that could be linked to an increased risk of intimate partner homicide.

Many clinicians are reluctant to screen for IPV because they are uncertain as to what to do with a "yes" response (Sheridan, 2003). Patients who give a positive response to being involved in ongoing IPV need to complete Campbell's Danger Assessment (DA; **Table 14-5**)

TABLE 14-1 Original Nine-Question Abuse Assessment Screening Tool

1. Do you know where you would go or who could help you if you were abused or worried about abuse?

   Yes _____   No _____

   If yes, where: _____

2. Are you in a relationship with a man who physically hurts you?

   Yes _____   No _____   Sometimes _____

3. Does he threaten you with abuse?

   Yes _____   No _____   Sometimes _____

4. Has the man you are with hit, slapped, kicked, or otherwise physically hurt you?

   Yes _____   No _____   Sometimes _____

5. If yes, has he hit you since you've been pregnant?

   Yes _____   No _____   Sometimes _____

6. If yes, did the abuse increase since you've been pregnant?

   Yes _____   No _____   Sometimes _____

7. Have you ever received medical treatment for any abuse injuries?

   Yes _____   No _____   Sometimes _____

8. If you have been abused, remembering the last time he hurt you, mark the places on the body map where he hit you (see body map in **Figure 14-2**).

9. Were you pregnant at the time?

   Yes _____   No _____   Not Applicable _____

Source: Reprinted with permission from the Nursing Research Consortium on Violence and Abuse; adapted from Helton, 1987.

and Sheridan's Harassment in Abusive Relationships: A Self-Report Scale (HARASS; **Table 14-6**). All of the items on these screening instruments have been linked to an increased risk of domestic homicide. The DA is best completed in conjunction with a calendar that serves as a prompt to remind women of abusive events around certain dates. The DA and HARASS take approximately 5 to 10 minutes each to complete; they are self-report scales that can be completed by the patient. Both instruments can be read to patients who are illiterate, have language barriers, or are unable to read secondary to the nature of their injuries.

While studies of the DA instrument have provided some preliminary data to suggest cut-off scores related to risk of homicide, the DA and HARASS instruments are best used as guides to structure safety planning. In general, the more "yes" responses on the DA tool and the more positive responses to some form of harassment, the more dangerous and potentially deadly the relationship.

MARK THE AREA OF INJURY ON THE BODY MAP. SCORE EACH INCIDENT ACCORDING TO THE FOLLOWING SCALE:

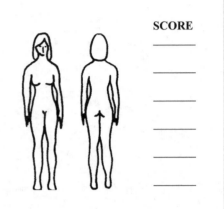

SCORE

1 = Threats of abuse including use of a weapon   _____

2 = Slapping, pushing; no injuries and/or lasting pain   _____

3 = Punching, kicking, bruises, cuts and/or continuing pain   _____

4 = Beating up, severe contusions, burns, broken bones   _____

5 = Head injury, internal injury, permanent injury   _____

6 = Use of weapon; wound from weapon   _____

If any of the descriptions for the higher number apply, use the higher number.

FIGURE 14-2 Body map.

Source: Reprinted with permission from the Nursing Research Consortium on Violence and Abuse; adapted from Parker & McFarlane, 1991.

TABLE 14-2 Six-Question Abuse Assessment Screening Tool
1. When you and your partner argue, are you ever afraid of him (her)?
2. When you and your partner verbally argue, do you think he (she) tries to emotionally hurt/abuse you?
3. Does your partner try to control you? Where you go? Who you see? How much money you can have?
4. Has your partner (or anyone) ever slapped you, pushed you, hit you, kicked you, or otherwise physically hurt you?
5. Since you have been pregnant (when you were pregnant), has your partner ever hit you, slapped you, pushed you, hit you, kicked you, or otherwise physically hurt you?
6. Has your partner ever forced you into sex when you did not want to participate?

Source: Reprinted with permission from the Nursing Research Consortium on Violence and Abuse; adapted from Parker & McFarlane, 1991.

History

Interviewing women about IPV requires that questioning be done in a sympathetic and nonjudgmental manner. Not only is this approach therapeutic, but it can also signal that someone is interested, that the woman is not alone, and that there is a safe place in which she can talk about the problem, if and when she wishes to do so. Express the belief that violence is not acceptable, no matter what she has been told by the batterer. Privacy and confiden-

TABLE 14-3 Three-Question Abuse Assessment Screening Tool

1. Within the last year have you been hit, slapped, kicked, or otherwise physically hurt by someone?
   a. Yes _____
   b. No _____
   If yes, by whom? _____
   Total number of times: _____

2. Since you have been pregnant, have you been hit, slapped, kicked, or otherwise physically hurt by someone?
   a. Yes _____
   b. No _____
   If yes, by whom? _____
   Total number of times: _____

3. Within the last year has anyone forced you to have sexual activities?
   a. Yes _____
   b. No _____
   If yes, by whom? _____
   Total number of times: _____

Source: Reprinted with permission from the Nursing Research Consortium on Violence and Abuse; adapted from McFarlane, Parker, Soeken, & Bullock, 1992.

TABLE 14-4 Two-Question Abuse Assessment Screen

1. Have you ever been hit, slapped, kicked, or otherwise physically hurt by your male partner?
2. Have you ever been forced to have sexual activities?

Source: Reprinted with permission from the Nursing Research Consortium on Violence and Abuse; adapted from McFarlane, Greenberg, Weltge, & Watson, 1995.

tiality must be guaranteed when asking questions about IPV. The most effective means of obtaining the history of abuse is to use a communication model that allows the woman to talk about the problem from her perspective, without interruption, and with enough time to relate, emphasize, and even repeat her full story (Campbell, McKenna, Torres, Sheridan, & Landenburger, 1993).

Another issue for consideration by clinicians when interviewing women about IPV is the presence of their children. IPV screening in front of children raises a variety of safety concerns. If the child talks afterward to the perpetrator about the disclosure of IPV to the clinician, it may result in retaliation for the patient, such as further abuse or prohibiting further contact with the clinician. In addition, the child may be exposed to new information or retraumatized by painful memories (Zink & Jacobson, 2003). Guidelines in the literature support the premise that screening in front of children older than three years of age should be

TABLE 14-5 Danger Assessment

DANGER ASSESSMENT

Jacquelyn C. Campbell, Ph.D., R.N.
Copyright, 2003

Several risk factors have been associated with increased risk of homicides (murders) of women and men in violent relationships. We cannot predict what will happen in your case, but we would like you to be aware of the danger of homicide in situations of abuse and for you to see how many of the risk factors apply to your situation.

Using the calendar, please mark the approximate dates during the past year when you were abused by your partner or ex partner. Write on that date how bad the incident was according to the following scale:

1. Slapping, pushing; no injuries and/or lasting pain
2. Punching, kicking; bruises, cuts, and/or continuing pain
3. "Beating up"; severe contusions, burns, broken bones
4. Threat to use weapon; head injury, internal injury, permanent injury
5. Use of weapon; wounds from weapon

(If **any** of the descriptions for the higher number apply, use the higher number.)

Mark **Yes** or **No** for each of the following. ("He" refers to your husband, partner, ex-husband, ex-partner, or whoever is currently physically hurting you.)

_____ 1. Has the physical violence increased in severity or frequency over the past year?
_____ 2. Does he own a gun?
_____ 3. Have you left him after living together during the past year?
        3a. (If have *never* lived with him, check here____)
_____ 4. Is he unemployed?
_____ 5. Has he ever used a weapon against you or threatened you with a lethal weapon?
        (If yes, was the weapon a gun?____)
_____ 6. Does he threaten to kill you?
_____ 7. Has he avoided being arrested for domestic violence?
_____ 8. Do you have a child that is not his?
_____ 9. Has he ever forced you to have sex when you did not wish to do so?
_____ 10. Does he ever try to choke you?
_____ 11. Does he use illegal drugs? By drugs, I mean "uppers" or amphetamines, speed, angel dust, cocaine, "crack", street drugs or mixtures.
_____ 12. Is he an alcoholic or problem drinker?
_____ 13. Does he control most or all of your daily activities? For instance: does he tell you who you can be friends with, when you can see your family, how much money you can use, or when you can take the car? (If he tries, but you do not let him, check here: ____)
_____ 14. Is he violently and constantly jealous of you? (For instance, does he say "If I can't have you, no one can.")
_____ 15. Have you ever been beaten by him while you were pregnant? (If you have never been pregnant by him, check here: ____)
_____ 16. Have you ever threatened or tried to commit suicide?
_____ 17. Has he ever threatened or tried to commit suicide?
_____ 18. Does he threaten to harm your children?
_____ 19. Do you believe he is capable of killing you?
_____ 20. Does he follow or spy on you, leave threatening notes or messages on answering machine, destroy your property, or call you when you don't want him to?

_____ Total "Yes" Answers

**Thank you. Please talk to your nurse, advocate or counselor about
what the Danger Assessment means in terms of your situation.**

Source: Campbell, J. C., Webster, D. W., & Glass, N. E. (2009). The Danger Assessment: Validation of a lethality risk assessment instrument for intimate partner femicide. *Journal of Interpersonal Violence, 24,* 653–674. www.dangerassessment.org

TABLE 14-6 HARASS Instrument

H arassment in

A busive

Many women are harassed in relationships with their abusive partners, especially if the women are trying to end the relationship. You may be experiencing harassment. This instrument is designed to measure harassment of women who are in abusive relationships or who are in the process of leaving abusive relationships. By completing this questionnaire, you may better understand harassment in your life. If you have any questions, please talk with the service provider who gave you this tool.

R elationships:

A

Harassment is defined as: *a persistent pattern of behavior by an intimate partner that is intended to bother, annoy, trap, emotionally wear down, threaten, frighten, terrify and/or coerce a woman with the overall intent to control her choices and behavior about leaving an abusive relationship.*

S elf-report

There are no right or wrong answers. Do not put your name on the form. The instrument takes about 10 minutes to complete.

S cale

For each item, circle the number that best describes how often the behavior occurred. Next, rate how distressing the behavior is to you. If the behavior has never occurred, circle 0 (NEVER) and go to the next question. If the question does not apply to you, circle NA (NOT APPLICABLE). If you are still in the relationship please circle below MY PARTNER. If you have left the relationship, please circle below MY FORMER PARTNER.

THE BEHAVIOR MY PARTNER MY FORMER PARTNER (circle one)	0 = Never 1 = Rarely 2 = Occasionally 3 = Frequently 4 = Very Frequently NA = Not applicable **How often does it occur?**						0 = Not at all distressing 1 = Slightly distressing 2 = Moderately distressing 3 = Very distressing 4 = Extremely distressing NA = Not applicable **How distressing is this behavior to you?**					
1. Frightens people close to me	0	1	2	3	4	NA	0	1	2	3	4	NA
2. Pretends to be someone else in order to get to me	0	1	2	3	4	NA	0	1	2	3	4	NA
3. Comes to my home when I don't want him there	0	1	2	3	4	NA	0	1	2	3	4	NA
4. Threatens to kill me if I leave or stay away from him	0	1	2	3	4	NA	0	1	2	3	4	NA
5. Threatens to harm the kids if I leave or stay away from him	0	1	2	3	4	NA	0	1	2	3	4	NA
6. Takes things that belong to me so I have to see him to get them back	0	1	2	3	4	NA	0	1	2	3	4	NA
7. Tries getting me fired from my job	0	1	2	3	4	NA	0	1	2	3	4	NA
8. Ignores court orders to stay away from me	0	1	2	3	4	NA	0	1	2	3	4	NA
9. Keeps showing up wherever I am	0	1	2	3	4	NA	0	1	2	3	4	NA
10. Bothers me at work when I don't want to talk to him	0	1	2	3	4	NA	0	1	2	3	4	NA
11. Uses the kids as pawns to get me physically close to him	0	1	2	3	4	NA	0	1	2	3	4	NA
12. Shows up without warning	0	1	2	3	4	NA	0	1	2	3	4	NA

(continues)

TABLE 14-6 HARASS Instrument *(Continued)*

THE BEHAVIOR	0 = Never 1 = Rarely 2 = Occasionally 3 = Frequently 4 = Very Frequently NA = Not applicable	0 = Not at all distressing 1 = Slightly distressing 2 = Moderately distressing 3 = Very distressing 4 = Extremely distressing NA = Not applicable
MY PARTNER MY FORMER PARTNER (circle one)	**How often does it occur?**	**How distressing is this behavior to you?**
13. Messes with my property (For example: sells my stuff, breaks my furniture, damages my car, steals my things)	0　1　2　3　4　NA	0　1　2　3　4　NA
14. Scares me with a weapon	0　1　2　3　4　NA	0　1　2　3　4　NA
15. Breaks into my home	0　1　2　3　4　NA	0　1　2　3　4　NA
16. Threatens to kill me if I leave or stay away from him	0　1　2　3　4　NA	0　1　2　3　4　NA
17. Makes me feel like he can again force me into sex	0　1　2　3　4　NA	0　1　2　3　4　NA
18. Threatens to snatch or have the kids taken away from me	0　1　2　3　4　NA	0　1　2　3　4　NA
19. Sits in his car outside my home	0　1　2　3　4　NA	0　1　2　3　4　NA
20. Leaves me threatening messages (for example: puts scary notes in the car, sends me threatening letters, sends me threats through family and friends, leaves threatening messages on the telephone answering machine)	0　1　2　3　4　NA	0　1　2　3　4　NA
21. Threatens to harm our pet	0　1　2　3　4　NA	0　1　2　3　4　NA
22. Calls me on the telephone and hangs up	0　1　2　3　4　NA	0　1　2　3　4　NA
23. Reports me to the authorities for taking drugs when I don't.	0　1　2　3　4　NA	0　1　2　3　4　NA
Additional harassing behaviors not listed above:		
24. _____	0　1　2　3　4　NA	0　1　2　3　4　NA
25. _____	0　1　2　3　4　NA	0　1　2　3　4　NA

Please answer a few additional questions:

_____ Your age in years

Check the statement that best describes you:

_ Married, living with an abusive partner

_ Single, living with an abusive partner

_ Married, living apart from an abusive partner

_ Single, living apart from an abusive partner.

Check the statement that best describes you:

_ Asian / Pacific Islander

_ Black/African American

_ Caucasian/White

_ Hispanic

_ Native American/American Indian

_ Other _____

How long were you in the above relationship? _____

Are you still in the relationship? _ Yes _ No

If you have left the relationship, how long have you been out? _____

What is your approximate annual income? _____

How many years of school have you completed? _____

*The HARASS instrument can be used without copyright permission in any clinical setting. Anyone interested in using the HARASS instrument in a research project is requested to contact the author at dsheridan@son.jhmi.edu. *Source:* Reprinted with permission of Daniel J. Sheridan, PhD, RN.

done only with prior permission from the mother, or with only general IPV screening questions and sensitivity to the mother's nonverbal behaviors and comfort (Zink & Jacobson). General questions should avoid charged words such as "hit," "hurt," "harm," and "afraid." Clinicians need to be sensitive to the unique privacy, safety, and protection issues of mothers who are survivors of IPV.

Physical Examination

The physical examination of women suspected of being abused or battered should be conducted just like any other physical assessment of an adult female. Careful attention must be directed to any signs of injury, past and present, with exact measurement taken of even the most insignificant-looking bruises (Campbell, McKenna, et al., 1993). Because most injuries are to the face, chest, breasts, and abdomen, special attention should be paid to these areas. If the woman reports sexual violence, a pelvic examination should also be included in the physical examination. If the assault was recent, assessment by a clinician skilled in forensic evidentiary examination is warranted (see Chapter 15 for additional information). The general examination of the woman should include observations about her behavior as well as her physical appearance.

Offer all patients with visible injuries photographic documentation in the medical record after obtaining consent to photograph them (Sheridan, 2003). Certain principles of forensic photography should be followed when using any photographic system. The first photograph needs to be a facial image of the patient as an identifier (Sheridan). Photographs of each injured area need to be taken in a series from farthest away (approximately 6 feet), to a middle distance (4 feet), to close up (2 feet) (Sheridan). A scale should appear in each photograph to assist in determining the relative size of the injury. If a scale used in the photograph shields any part of the body, an additional photograph is needed of the part of the body without the scale. The photograph should be labeled on the back with a white adhesive label that includes the patient's name, date of birth, hospital chart or number, date of photograph, body part location, and the photographer's name.

Using body maps and diagrams is also recommended to accurately portray the patient's physical condition (Figure 14-2). Body maps provide pictorial diagrams of all body surfaces, including separate diagrams for external genitalia, vagina, cervix, anus, and rectum. Areas of injury should be drawn on the body maps or diagrams of the corresponding location. A description of the injury should be included with each drawing.

Documentation

It is critical that the clinician accurately document all findings in the patient's record using the correct medical forensic terms. Misuse of common forensic terms in the medical record can lead to questioning of the overall accuracy and competence of the clinician should legal proceedings ensue. The terms *laceration*, *ecchymosis*, and *hematoma* are among the most commonly misused medical forensic terms (Brockmeyer & Sheridan, 1998; Campbell & Sheridan, 2004; Sheridan, 2001, 2003). A laceration is a tear in the skin or organ caused by blunt or shearing force trauma, while a cut or incision is a sharp injury caused by the cutting of skin or an organ with a sharp object such as a scalpel, razor, or knife. Ecchymoses are not bruises, but rather discolorations under the skin from a leakage or oozing of blood; they are not caused directly by blunt force trauma. A bruise or contusion is bleeding under the skin or organ caused by trauma. A hematoma is a collection of blood that can be caused by blunt force trauma or by spontaneous bleeding. Do not use hematoma as a synonym for bruise.

The following is a useful summary of the correct usage of common terms:

- Bruise can be used interchangeably with contusion.
- Laceration is related to a partial avulsion.
- Ecchymosis is related to (senile) purpura.
- Petechia is related to purpura.
- Rug burn is more accurately described as a friction abrasion.
- Incision can be used interchangeably with cut.
- Cut can be used interchangeably with sharp injury.
- Stab wounds are penetrating, deep, sharp injuries.
- A hematoma is a collection of blood that is often, but not always, caused by blunt force trauma (Campbell & Sheridan, 2004, p. 77).

Documentation in the medical record of IPV histories needs to be as thorough and objective as possible. When quoting the patient, the clinician should use such words as "states," "says," and "reports," instead of "claims" or "alleges," which can be interpreted to mean that the patient is not a credible historian (Sheridan, 2003). If a patient gives an extremely informative and powerful statement concerning the reported abuse, quote it directly in the progress note. Avoid biased documentation by avoiding words or phrases such as "refuses," "uncooperative," or "noncompliant." For example, do not chart this statement: "Patient refused to talk with the police." Instead, make this chart entry: "Patient said she did not want to talk with the police."

Management

Clinical interventions for patients experiencing IPV should be based on four important principles: empowerment, childbearing cycle-stage specificity, abuse-stage specificity, and cultural competence (Campbell & Campbell, 1996). Abusers take power and control away from their victims by isolating them from the people and information that can help them make thoughtful choices. Therefore, it is crucial that clinicians use an empowerment model of offering information, options, and support. Clinicians must not judge an abused woman's choices, nor use any kind of tactics to get her to cooperate. An empowerment model should include the information given in the following list. Use the mnemonic device of EMPOWER to help remember these items:

- Empathic listening
- Making time to properly document findings
- Providing information about domestic violence (including in later life)
- Offering options and choices
- Working with a domestic abuse specialist (including elder domestic abuse)
- Encouraging planning for safety and support
- Referring to local services (Brandl & Raymond, 1997, p. 65)

Women in ongoing abusive relationships may choose to return to the abusive home for many reasons. Prior to leaving the clinician's office, however, all patients need to know where they can find an IPV hotline and shelter information. Wallet-sized referral cards and information posters with tear-off numbers have been effective ways for women who have been abused to access helpful numbers in a manner more easily hidden from perpetrators (Sheridan & Taylor, 1993). Abused patients need to be shown the pages of telephone books that list hotline and shelter-referral numbers. The employees and volunteers who staff the IPV hotlines and women's service programs are experts at safety planning, and they should be called not only by the victims of abuse, but also by clinicians for guidance.

Minimum safety planning by a clinician should include a brief discussion about having the patient pack an emergency bag containing some money, clothing for the patient and her children, copies of bank records, immunization records, birth certificates, and protective legal orders. Patients should be encouraged to call the police before actual abuse occurs, and most definitely after any abusive act (Sheridan, 2003). Finally, every abused patient should be encouraged to use any 24-hour health setting as a safety net if she does not have access to any other safe place (Sheridan).

Special Populations

Pregnant Women

Many people think of pregnancy as a time of celebration and planning for the unborn child's future. Health professionals, however, have long recognized that pregnancy can be a time of escalating violence in an already troubled relationship (Campbell, 1989; Campbell & Alford, 1989; McFarlane et al., 1992). Bohn and Parker (1993) report that violence during pregnancy affects more women than hypertension, gestational diabetes, or almost any other serious antepartum complication. Conversely, pregnancy may provide a period of protection for some women who suffer the ill effects of IPV (Fagen, Stewart, & Hanson, 1983; Stacey & Schupe, 1983). Despite this period of protection during pregnancy, women need to be aware that the abuse may resume, and they need to understand the implications such abuse can have for both themselves and any children born into the abusive relationship (Campbell, Oliver, & Bullock, 1993). Even if the violence does not escalate, but simply continues at the rate prior to pregnancy, there are negative health effects associated with the violence for both the woman and her unborn fetus.

Complications associated with abuse during pregnancy can be the result of trauma or side effects of the psychological or controlling effects of the abuse. Mechanisms of injury are related to direct trauma to the pregnant abdomen, leading to premature labor due to rupture of membranes, placental abruption, and uterine rupture. In addition, abusive environments are associated with indirect mechanisms leading to low-birth-weight infants. Women in abusive situations are more likely than women not in abusive relationships to use alcohol, nicotine, and prescription, over-the-counter, and illicit drugs to help deal with the stress (Curry, 1998). Low birth weight may also be due to poor maternal weight gain, anemia, an unhealthy diet, STIs, and lack of social support—all potential problems stemming from the effects of stress related to an abusive relationship. As a consequence of these mechanisms, Murphy and colleagues (2001) state that abuse should be recognized as a factor contributing to low-birth-weight infants.

Adolescents

All young women should be routinely questioned about IPV during health encounters, because one out of every eight adolescents will be involved in some form of dating violence (Furniss, 1998). Dating violence results in serious and negative health outcomes, with lifelong implications for adolescent victims, including depression, unhealthy weight control behavior, sexually risky behavior, and substance abuse (Coker et al., 2000; Sells & Blum, 1996; Silverman, Raj, Mucci, & Hathaway, 2001). Plichta (1996) reported that rates of depression; eating disorders; and drug, alcohol, and tobacco use were more than twice as high in girls who reported physical or sexual dating violence as compared to girls who had not been abused.

The simple act of asking adolescents in a private and safe location about dating violence victimization and perpetration may be an important initial step toward effective intervention and prevention strategies. Questioning teenagers in a family planning clinic, emergency department, or pediatric setting about jealous or possessive partners could provide clues to the existence of dating violence. Teenagers are often uncomfortable disclosing violence to a clinician and may present with headaches, weight loss, or other somatic clues that may signal distress (Furniss, 1998). Because many adolescents accept physical and sexual aggression as normal in dating and partner relationships, clinicians can be invaluable in providing an alternative view by talking with them about types of behavior that are appropriate in an intimate relationship.

Older Women

Family violence involving the elderly has been addressed by laws in all 50 states requiring the reporting of elder or vulnerable person abuse (Fulmer & Wetle, 1986). Clinicians are mandated by law to report a case if there is reasonable cause to suspect that an elderly patient has been the victim of abuse, neglect, or mistreatment. Estimates suggest that 500,000 to 1.5 million elders are subjected to abuse and neglect each year in the United States (Brandl, 1997;

Jogerst et al., 2003). Accurate detection and assessment of elder abuse patients are critical duties of all clinicians, especially those in ambulatory care settings.

IPV affects women of all ages, but often the literature focuses on women in the child-bearing years, ignoring the unique problems of aging women who are experiencing IPV. Often elder abuse and mistreatment is viewed from an inadequate care perspective—a view that obscures important issues. Some forms of elder abuse and mistreatment derive from inadequate care and are rooted in the dynamics of caregiving. Other forms of elder abuse and mistreatment, especially physical assaults, are, in fact, domestic violence (Phillips, 2000). Also, the notion that elder abuse is equivalent to inadequate care makes unclear the gender issues and power dynamics inherent in IPV as they apply to older women. Serious physical and emotional harm, and even death, may result from wife or partner abuse at any age, but among older women, because of their physical vulnerability that increases with age, even so-called "low-severity violence" can cause serious injury or death (Phillips).

Although injury may be the reason an older woman seeks health care, it is important to remember that the physical and mental sequelae of IPV could be more subtle, including depression, sleeplessness, chronic pain, atypical chest pain, and other kinds of somatic symptoms (Phillips, 2000). Interactions with cognitively impaired or unresponsive elderly women require that the clinician assess for nonverbal cues and focus assessment on the caregiver. Characteristics of batterers that might trigger suspicion include showing possessiveness toward and jealousy of the victim, denying or minimizing the seriousness of the violence, refusing to take responsibility for the violence, and holding a rigid view of sex roles or negative attitudes toward women.

Influences of Culture

Cultural awareness is the process that allows the clinician to interact sensitively with persons from other cultures. It requires self-examination for biases and prejudices toward other cultures, and assists the clinician in avoiding cultural imposition or the tendency to impose his or her own beliefs, values, and patterns of behavior on persons from other cultures (Campbell & Campbell, 1996). Cultural skill is a process in which the clinician learns how to assess the woman's cultural values, beliefs, and practices without solely relying on written "facts" about a specific cultural group. It enables the clinician to learn systematically from the woman her perception of her situation and what she believes can be done about it (Campbell & Campbell).

The patient experiencing IPV may assume that a clinician from a majority ethnic group will perceive either her or her whole cultural group as stigmatized if the clinician learns of the family violence. Women of color who have been battered may be particularly afraid that a clinician who is a member of another ethnic group will call the police, who have historically physically assaulted men of minority ethnic groups (Campbell & Campbell, 1996). Further, women of color who have been battered may consider IPV to be a relatively unimportant issue in comparison to a serious health problem or issues of economic survival (Campbell & Campbell). Minority cultural groups often perceive IPV to be merely an outgrowth of other community problems, such as joblessness, prejudice, or substance abuse. They may consider IPV not a particularly important problem in comparison to others, or one not to be addressed in isolation (Campbell & Campbell). The patient experiencing IPV may not see the healthcare clinician as a person who understands the complexities of family violence in her cultural context and, therefore, may prefer that the clinician concentrate on other areas of care (Campbell & Campbell).

When the clinician does not speak the primary language of the patient, assessing and intervening in the area of IPV may become very difficult. To ensure that there is not a breakdown in communication, clinicians should ask the meaning of unfamiliar words. Such requests for clarification demonstrate a willingness to learn and appreciate cultural nuances rather than pretending such differences do not exist or are related to a lack of education (Campbell & Campbell, 1996). The clinician must learn to listen with a sensitive ear and must accept the challenges and rewards inherent in effective cultural communications as the patient from a different ethnic group discloses her experiences.

References

Bergman, B., & Brismar, B. (1991). A 5-year follow-up study of 117 battered women. *American Journal of Public Health, 81*, 1486–1489.

Bohn, D. K., & Parker, B. (1993). Domestic violence and pregnancy: Health effects and implications for nursing practice. In J. C. Campbell & J. Humphreys (Eds.), *Nursing care of survivors of family violence* (pp. 156–172). St. Louis, MO: Mosby.

Brandl, B. (1997). *Developing Services for Older Abused Women*. Madison, WI: Wisconsin Coalition Against Domestic Violence.

Brandl, B., & Raymond, J. (1997). Unrecognized elder abuse victims: Older abused women. *Journal of Case Management, 6*(2), 62–68.

Brockmeyer, D. M., & Sheridan, D. J. (1998). Domestic violence: A practical guide to the use of forensic evaluation in clinical examination and documentation of injuries. In J. C. Campbell (Ed.), *Empowering survivors of abuse: Health care for battered women and their children* (pp. 23–31). Thousand Oaks, CA: Sage.

Campbell, J. C. (1989). Women's response to sexual abuse in intimate relationships. *Women's Healthcare International, 38*, 335–347.

Campbell, J. C. (2002). Health consequences of intimate partner violence. *Lancet, 359*(9314), 1331–1336.

Campbell, J. C., & Alford, P. (1989). The dark consequences of marital rape. *American Journal of Nursing, 89*, 946–949.

Campbell, J. C., & Campbell, D. W. (1996). Cultural competence in the care of abused women. *Journal of Nurse-Midwifery, 41*(6), 457–462.

Campbell, J. C., Jones, A. S., Dienemann, J., Kub, J., Schollenberger, J., O'Campo, P., et al. (2002). Intimate partner violence and physical health consequences. *Archives of Internal Medicine, 162*, 1157–1163.

Campbell, J. C., Kub, J. E., & Rose, L. (1996). Depression in battered women. *Journal of the American Medical Women's Association, 51*(3), 106–110.

Campbell, J. C., McKenna, L. S., Torres, S., Sheridan, D., & Landenburger, K. (1993). Nursing care of abused women. In J. C. Campbell & J. Humphreys (Eds.), *Nursing care of survivors of family violence* (pp. 248–289). St. Louis, MO: Mosby.

Campbell, J. C., Oliver, C., & Bullock, L. (1993). Why battering during pregnancy? In J. C. Campbell & J. A. Lewis (Eds.), *Clinical issues in perinatal and women's health nursing* (pp. 343–349). Philadelphia: Lippincott.

Campbell, J. C., & Sheridan, D. J. (2004). Domestic violence assessments. In C. Jarvis (Ed.), *Physical examination and health assessment* (4th ed., pp. 73–82). St. Louis, MO: Saunders.

Campbell, J. C., & Soeken, K. (1999). Women's response to battering over time. *Journal of Interpersonal Violence, 14*, 21–40.

Chapman, J. D. (1989). A longitudinal study of sexuality and gynecologic health in abused women. *Journal of the American Osteopathic Association, 89,* 946–949.

Coker, A. L., Smith, P. H., Bethea, L., King, M. R., & McKeown, R. E. (2000). Physical health consequences of physical and psychological intimate partner violence. *Archives of Family Medicine, 9,* 451–457.

Curry, M. A. (1998). The interrelationships between abuse, substance use, and psychosocial stress during pregnancy. *Journal of Obstetric, Gynecologic, and Neonatal Nursing, 27*(6), 692–699.

Douglas, J. E., & Olshaker, M. (2001). Perpetrators. In J. S. Olshaker, M. C. Jackson, & W. S. Smock (Eds.), *Forensic emergency medicine* (pp. 1–23). Philadelphia: Lippincott Williams & Wilkins.

Ebby, K. K., Campbell, J. C., Sullivan, C. M., & Davidson, W. S. (1995). Health effects of experiences of sexual violence for women with abusive partners. *Health Care of Women International, 16,* 563–576.

Fagen, J., Stewart, D., & Hanson, K. (1983). Violent men or violent husbands? In D. Finkelhor, R. Gelles, G. Hotaling, & M. Straus (Eds.), *The dark side of families* (pp. 49–67). Beverly Hills, CA: Sage.

Family Violence Prevention Fund. (1999). *Preventing domestic violence: Clinical guidelines on routine screening.* San Francisco: Author.

Finkelhor, D., & Yllo, K. (1997). *License to rape: The sexual abuse of wives.* New York: Holt, Reinehart, & Winston.

Fulmer, T., & Wetle, T. (1986). Elder abuse screening and intervention. *Nurse Practitioner, 11*(5), 33–38.

Furniss, K. K. (1998). Screening for abuse in the clinical setting. In J. C. Campbell (Ed.), *Empowering survivors of abuse: Health care for battered women and their children* (pp. 190–194). Thousand Oaks, CA: Sage.

Hegarty, K., Gunn, J., Chondros, P., & Small, R. (2004). Association between depression and abuse by partners of women attending general practice: Descriptive, cross sectional survey. *British Medical Journal, 328,* 621–624.

Heise, L. L. (1998). Violence against women: An integrated, ecological framework. *Violence Against Women, 4*(3), 262–290.

Helton, A. (1987). *A protocol of care for battered women.* White Plains, NY: March of Dimes Birth Defects Foundation.

Jogerst, G. J., Daly, J. M., Brinig, M. F., Dawson, J. D., Schmuch, G. A., & Ingran, J. G. (2003). Domestic elder abuse and the law. *American Journal of Public Health, 93*(12), 2131–2137.

King, M. C. (1998). Changing women's lives: The primary prevention of violence against women. In J. C. Campbell (Ed.), *Empowering survivors of abuse: Health care for battered women and their children* (pp. 177–189). Thousand Oaks, CA: Sage.

McCauley, J., Kern, D. E., Kolodner, K., Dill, L., Schroeder, A. F., DeChant, H. K., et al. (1995). The "battering syndrome": Prevalence and clinical characteristics of domestic violence in primary care internal medicine practices. *Annals of Internal Medicine, 123*(10), 737–746.

McFarlane, J., Greenberg, L., Weltge, A., & Watson, M. (1995). Identification of abuse in emergency departments: Effectiveness of a two-question screening tool. *Journal of Emergency Nursing, 21*(5), 391–394.

McFarlane, J., Parker, B., Soeken, K., & Bullock, L. (1992). Assessing for abuse during pregnancy: Severity and frequency of injuries and associated entry into prenatal care. *Journal of the American Medical Association, 267*(23), 3176–3178.

Moracco, K. E., Runyan, C. W., Bowling, J. M., & Earp, J. L. (2007). Women's experience with violence: A national study. *Women's Health Issues, 17*(1), 3–12.

Murphy, C. C., Schei, B., Myhr, T. L., & Du Mont, J. (2001). Abuse: A risk factor for low birth weight? A systematic review and meta-analysis. *Canadian Medical Association Journal, 164,* 1567–1572.

Parker, B., & McFarlane, J. (1991). Identifying and helping battered pregnant women. *Maternal Child Nursing, 16*(3), 161–164.

Parker, B., McFarlane, J., & Soeken, K. (1994). Abuse during pregnancy: Effects on maternal complications and birthweight in adult and teenage women. *Obstetrics and Gynecology, 84,* 323–328.

Phillips, L. R. (2000). Domestic violence and aging women. *Geriatric Nursing, 21*(4), 188–193.

Plichta, S. B. (1996). Violence and abuse: Implications for women's health. In M. K. Falik & K. S. Collins (Eds.), *Women's health: The Commonwealth Fund Survey* (pp. 237–270). Baltimore: Johns Hopkins University Press.

Plichta, S. B., & Abraham, C. (1996). Violence and gynecologic health in women < 50 years old. *American Journal of Obstetrics and Gynecology, 174,* 903–907.

Poirier, L. (1997). The importance of screening for domestic violence in all women. *Nurse Practitioner, 22*(5), 105–122.

Saltzman, L. E., Fanslow, J. L., McMahon, P. M., & Shelley, G. A. (2002). *Intimate partner violence surveillance: Uniform definitions and recommended data elements* (2nd printing, with revisions). Atlanta, GA: Centers for Disease Control and Prevention, National Center for Injury Prevention and Control.

Schornstein, S. L. (1997). *Domestic violence and health care: What every professional needs to know*. Thousand Oaks, CA: Sage.

Schroeder, M., & Weber, J. R. (1998). Promoting domestic violence education for nurses. *Nursing Forum, 33*(4), 13–21.

Sells, C. W., & Blum, R. W. (1996). Morbidity and mortality among US adolescents: An overview of data and trends. *American Journal of Public Health, 86*(4), 513–519.

Sheridan, D. J. (2001). Treating survivors of intimate partner abuse: Forensic identification and documentation. In J. S. Olshaker, M. C. Jackson, & W. S. Smock (Eds.), *Forensic emergency medicine* (pp. 203–228). Philadelphia: Lippincott, Williams, & Wilkins.

Sheridan, D. J. (2003). Forensic identification and documentation of patients experiencing intimate partner violence. *Clinics in Family Practice, 5*(1), 113–143.

Sheridan, D. J., & Taylor, W. K. (1993). Developing hospital-based domestic violence programs, protocols, policies, and procedures. *Association of Women's Health, Obstetrics and Neonatal Nurses Clinical Issues in Perinatal and Women's Health Nursing, 4*(3), 471–482.

Silverman, J. G., Raj, A., Mucci, L. A., & Hathaway, J. E. (2001). Dating violence against adolescent girls and associated substance use, unhealthy weight control, sexual risk behavior, pregnancy, and suicidality. *Journal of the American Medical Association, 286*(5), 572–579.

Soeken, K., McFarlane, J., Parker, B., & Lominack, M. C. (1998). The Abuse Assessment Screen: A clinical instrument to measure the frequency, severity, and perpetrator of abuse against women. In J. C. Campbell (Ed.), *Empowering survivors of abuse: Health care for battered women and their children* (pp. 195–203). Thousand Oaks, CA: Sage.

Stacey, W., & Schupe, A. (1983). *The family secret: Domestic violence in America*. Boston: Beacon Press.

Tjaden, P., & Thoennes, N. (1998, November). *Prevalence, incidence, and consequences of violence against women: Findings from the National Violence Against Women Survey*. U.S. Department of Justice, National Institute of Justice, Research in Brief. Retrieved October 20, 2004, from http://www. ncjrs.org/pdf files/172837.pdf

Walker, L. E. (1979). *The battered woman*. New York: Harper & Row.

Woods, S. J., & Campbell, J. C. (1993). Posttraumatic stress in battered women: Does the diagnosis fit? *Issues in Mental Health Nursing, 14*, 173–186.

Zink, T. M., & Jacobson, J. (2003). Screening for intimate partner violence when children are present. *Journal of Interpersonal Violence, 18*(8), 872–890.

Sexual Violence

Linda E. Ledray

The focus of this chapter is on the identification of the woman who is a victim of sexual violence, her healthcare needs related to the assault, the decisions that need to be made about treatment, and community resources and referral options. The physical and psychological effects of sexual violence are presented, along with information to assist clinicians in providing treatment according to the current standard of care.

Throughout this chapter, the term *victim* is used when referring to a woman who has recently been sexually assaulted, and the term *survivor* is used when the woman has begun to heal from the traumatic event. The term *patient* is used in describing and documenting the health care provided to a woman who has been assaulted. Although it is recognized that men, women, and children can all be victims of sexual violence, this chapter focuses primarily on the care and treatment of women who have been victims of sexual violence.

Definitions

Sexual violence (also referred to as sexual assault) is a significant worldwide healthcare issue and is both a social and public health problem. Although *sexual assault* and *intimate partner violence* (IPV) are sometimes used interchangeably, these terms are actually defined differently. Intimate partner violence is perpetrated by a person well known to the victim, whereas sexual assault includes violence perpetrated by those individuals known to the victim as well as by persons either not known or not well known to the victim, such as a complete stranger or an acquaintance (Basile & Saltzman, 2002).

No clinical definition of rape or sexual assault has gained widespread acceptance as yet (Centers for Disease Control and Prevention [CDC], 2009). The lack of a consistent definition impedes the ability to accurately monitor the incidence of sexual violence and it makes measuring risk and identifying protective measures more difficult (CDC, 2009). The CDC defines sexual violence as follows:

> Any sexual act that is forced against someone's will. These acts can be physical, verbal or psychological. (CDC, 2009)

Basile and Saltzman (2002) identify four types of sexual violence (**Table 15-1**). All types include either nonconsent or the inability to give consent.

For the purposes of this chapter, the terms *rape* and *sexual assault* are used interchangeably to refer to any unwanted contact of the sexual organs (or sexual areas) of one person by another person, regardless of age, relationship, or gender. Unwanted contact includes contact that is made without permission or by force or coercion. Contact may or may not include penetration, and penetration may be by any body part or by an inanimate object.

Legal definitions vary by state, and it is important for clinicians to be familiar with their state's statutes and mandatory reporting requirements. The National Center for the Prosecution of Violence Against Women (NCPVAW) at the American Prosecutors Resource Institute (APRI) has compiled a summary of relevant state sexual assault laws (Scalzo, 2006). The summary can be found on the NCPVAW's website (identified in Appendix 15-C). Clinicians can also obtain information about state sexual assault laws from the National Association of Attorneys General, their local law enforcement agency, the prosecutor's office, or the State Attorney General's office.

Epidemiology

An estimated 89,000 forcible rapes occurred in the United States in 2008, the lowest number in the last 20 years (U.S. Department of Justice [USDOJ], 2008). These statistics do not include abusive sexual contact and noncontact sexual violence (e.g., voyeurism), nor do they

TABLE 15-1 The Four Types of Sexual Violence

1. A completed sex act—contact between the penis and the vulva or the penis and the anus involving penetration, however slight; contact between the mouth and penis, vulva, or anus; or penetration of the anal or genital opening of another person by a hand, finger, or an object.

2. An attempted (but not completed) sex act.

3. Abusive sexual contact—intentional touching, either directly or through the clothing, of the genitalia, anus, groin, breast, inner thigh, or buttocks of any person.

4. Noncontact sexual abuse—abuse that does not involve physical contact. Examples include voyeurism, intentional exposure of an individual to exhibitionism, pornography, verbal or behavioral sexual harassment, threats of sexual violence, and taking nude photographs of a sexual nature of another person.

Source: Basile & Saltzman, 2002.

take into account the probable underreporting of rape by victims (Basile & Saltzman, 2002). Tavara (2006) suggests that globally, sexual violence affects at least one-third of all women at some time during their lives.

To further understanding about violence against women the National Institute of Justice (NIJ) and the CDC jointly sponsored a national survey that was conducted from November 1995 to May 1996. The National Violence Against Women (NVAW) survey sample included both women (n = 8000) and men (n = 8005) to provide comparable data on women's and men's experiences with violent victimization (Tjaden & Thoennes, 1998). It is noteworthy that owing to the small number of Asian/Pacific Islander women identified by the survey as having been raped and the small number of men identified for several indicators (e.g., race/ethnic categories, injuries sustained during rape), the NVAW survey can provide incidence but not prevalence statistics. Some of the findings from that report (which were published in articles by Tjaden & Thoennes, 1998, 2006) are identified here:

- Approximately 17.6% of women in the United States have survived a completed or attempted rape.
- Of the female rape survivors, 21.6% were younger than age 12 when they were first raped and 32.4% were between the ages of 12 and 17.
- Women experience significantly more IPV than men: 64% of women who reported being raped, physically assaulted, or stalked since age 18 were victimized by a current or former husband, cohabitating partner, boyfriend, or date.
- The risk of violence varies among women of various minority ethnic groups. For example, American Indian/Alaskan Native women were most likely to report rape and physical assault, while Asian/Pacific Islander women were least likely to report a rape. Hispanic women were less likely than non-Hispanic women to report rape victimization. However, these statistics must be treated with caution because of small numbers.
- Violence against women is primarily male partner violence (Tjaden & Thoennes, 1998)

Health Consequences of Sexual Assault

Nongenital Physical Injury

Data from the NVAW study revealed that women are twice as likely as men to be physically injured during a rape (Tjaden & Thoennes, 2006). Most of the injuries identified in women who reported a rape and responded to the NVAW survey were relatively minor types of injuries, such as bruises and welts (Tjaden & Thoennes). Other nongenital trauma identified in the survey included lacerations, sore muscles, muscle sprain or strain, and chipped or broken teeth (Tjaden & Thoennes).

Genital Trauma

Sommers (2007) reviewed the literature to investigate the variables related to genital injury prevalence and location following sexual assault. The majority of large scale studies have identified the posterior fourchette and labia minora as the most common areas of injury in adult females who have been sexually assaulted (Sommers). Injury prevalence reported in the literature was 10% (Sommers). Although it appears that few victims sustain significant genital trauma as a result of a sexual assault, colposcopic examination is often helpful to visualize vaginal abrasions, bruises, and tears that may be too minute to easily identify with the naked eye (Carter-Snell, Olson, Jensen, Cummings, & Wiebe, 2007; Slaughter & Brown, 1992). Because the genital area is very vascular, and because injuries in this region tend to heal rapidly without scarring, most injuries are identified in examinations completed within the first 48 hours after the assault (Carter-Snell et al., 2007). Studies indicate the likelihood of genital trauma identification without the use of a colposcope to magnify the trauma is similar to that of nongenital trauma: 1% of women have severe injury, and 10% to 30% have minor injury (Geist, 1988; Tintinalli & Hoelzer, 1985). In these studies, genital injuries were always accompanied by complaints of vaginal pain, discomfort, or bleeding (Geist; Tintinalli & Hoelzer). Riggs et al. (2000) found genital trauma more often, in 52% of the cases reviewed; however, these researchers did not specifically indicate whether a colposcope was used as part of the examination.

Although both the colposcope and the anoscope have been shown to improve the identification of anal trauma, the colposcope may be less helpful than the anoscope in such evaluations. In a study of 67 male rape victims, all of whom were examined by experienced forensic examiners, 53% had genital trauma identified with the naked eye alone (Ernst et al., 2000). This number increased only slightly (8%) when the colposcope was used, but the positive findings increased by 32% (a statistically significant result) with the anoscope. The combination of naked eye, colposcope, and anoscope resulted in a total positive finding rate in 72% of the men (Ernst et al.).

Unfortunately, there is no method currently available that enables examiners to differentiate between genital trauma from sexual assault and trauma that may result from normal sexual activities or even tampon use (Keller & Nelson, 2008). Baker and Sommers (2008) examined the association between age and genital injuries in adolescent and young adult women following rape. An overall genital injury prevalence of 62.8% was identified. In this study, younger age was not significantly associated with genital injury, although it was significantly associated with an increased number of genital injuries overall and injuries to the thighs, labia minora, periurethral area, fossa navicularis, and vagina.

Being able to identify the source of the trauma can be critical in linking evidence to injuries. There is a clear need for studies that can identify a pattern of injury in consenting and non-consenting sexual contact. What is currently known is that genital trauma does not prove sexual assault, and the absence of trauma does not prove consent.

Sexually Transmitted Infections

The most frequently diagnosed sexually transmitted infections (STIs) among women who have been sexually assaulted are trichomoniasis, bacterial vaginosis, gonorrhea, and chlamydia (CDC, 2010; Workowski & Berman, 2006). However, because the incidence of these infections is also high in sexually active women, it is not feasible to determine whether the infection is a result of the assault (CDC, 2010). Chapter 21 describes preventive therapy and follow-up guidelines for STIs.

Human immunodeficiency virus (HIV) has been a concern for women who have been raped since the early 1980s. The first case in which seroconversion (the process of going from HIV-negative to HIV-positive status) was suspected as the result of a rape occurred in 1989 (Murphy, Harris, & Forester, 1989). However, data on the risks of developing viral infections from sexual assaults remain limited (Straight & Heaton, 2007). All women who have been sexually assaulted should be offered testing and medications to prevent STIs, including prophylaxis and testing for HIV. Chapter 21 provides additional information on prophylaxis, testing, and treatment of HIV.

Pregnancy

Victims of sexual assault who are of reproductive age often fear becoming pregnant as a result of the sexual assault. The incidence of an unintended pregnancy as a result of a rape is difficult to identify because not all victims report assault, and many do not report that the pregnancy resulted from the rape. Holmes, Resnick, Kilpatrick and Best (1996) surveyed 4008 women for a period of three years and found a rape-related pregnancy rate of 5%, with the adolescents in the sample having a disproportionate number of pregnancies. This rate is believed to be the lower limit of pregnancy risk (Tavara, 2006). McFarlane et al. (2005) found the pregnancy rate following rape by an intimate partner to be 26% (n = 20).

The Compassionate Assistance for Rape Emergencies (CARE) Act of 2009 and the Prevention First Act of 2009 (H.R.463/S.21) were introduced first in 2005 and again in 2009, but have yet to be passed (Smith, Brown, & Hartman, 2009). The purpose of this legislation is to direct hospitals and emergency medicine agencies that receive federal funding to inform all women who have been sexually assaulted about emergency contraception and to make such care available to them, regardless of ability to pay (Smith et al.). Some clinicians caring for women who have been victims of sexual assault do not inform their patients about the availability of emergency contraception and its ability to prevent pregnancy. Legislation ensuring that women have easy access to emergency contraception is still desperately needed (Smith et al.). See Chapter 12 for further information on emergency contraception.

Behavioral Reactions to Sexual Assault

Some studies have revealed that victims of sexual assault may later engage in risky sexual behaviors, including unprotected sexual intercourse and sex with multiple or high-risk partners (Brener, McMahon, Warren, & Douglas, 1999; Felitti, 1998; Harlow, Quina, Morokoff, Rose, & Grimly, 1993; Irwin et al., 1995; Rheingold, Acierno, & Resnick, 2004). Holmes, Resnick, and Frampton (1998), in a study of 389 adolescent and adult rape victims returning for medical follow-up care approximately 8 weeks post rape, found that 73% of those who had been sexually active since the rape had engaged in sex without consistent partner condom use.

Sexual Dysfunction

Sexual dysfunction is a common and sometimes chronic problem after a sexual assault. It may include a periodic or constant loss of sexual desire, inability to become sexually aroused, slow arousal, pelvic pain associated with sexual activity, a lack of sexual enjoyment, inability to achieve orgasm, fear of sex, avoidance of sex, intrusive thoughts of the assault during sex, vaginismus, or abstinence. Chapter 17 provides more information on female sexual dysfunction.

Substance Abuse

The use of alcohol and other drugs is widely accepted as a factor that makes women more vulnerable to a sexual assault (Kaysen, Neighbors, Martell, Fossos, & Larimer, 2006; Ledray, 1999; Messman-Moore & Long, 2002). A number of studies using self-report and medical records have found that 50% to 74% of women who were raped used alcohol or drugs immediately prior to the rape (Ledray, 2007, 2008; Logan, Cole, & Capillo, 2007).

Conversely, sexual assault can result in substance abuse, possibly as an attempt to dull the memory and avoid thinking about the assault. Numerous studies have found an increased risk of substance abuse or dependence among victims of sexual assault when they are compared to women who were not sexually assaulted (Kilpatrick, Acierno, Resnick, Saunders, & Best, 1997; Koss, 1993). In a national sample of 3006 survivors of a sex-related assault, data showed that both alcohol and drug use increased significantly after a sexual assault, even for women with no prior substance use or abuse history (Kilpatrick et al., 1997).

Mental Health Conditions After Sexual Assault

Immediately following a sexual assault, many women experience a variety of negative psychological impacts, including fear, anxiety, depression, and symptoms of post-traumatic stress disorder (Breslau, 2009; Frazier, 2000; Kilpatrick & Veronen, 1984; Ledray, 1994, 1999; Resick & Schnicke, 1990). Although many survivors of sexual assault experience a decrease in these symptoms as time goes by, others report symptoms that persist for years.

Post-traumatic stress disorder (PTSD) was first recognized and defined by the American Psychiatric Association (APA) based on diagnostic criteria in the *Diagnostic and Statistical Manual III* in 1980 (APA, 1994) and, therefore, has been considered only in studies of rape impact designed after 1980. Rape trauma syndrome (RTS), which is not a diagnosis recognized by the APA, is often described as a specific type of PTSD (Frazier, 2000) and includes a cluster of physical and psychological behaviors that are observed in survivors of sexual violence.

TABLE 15-2 The Four Basic Elements Included in a Diagnosis of PTSD*
1. Exposure to a traumatic event
2. Reexperiencing the trauma (e.g., flashbacks, intrusive memories)
3. Symptoms of avoidance and numbing (e.g., attempts to avoid thoughts or situations that remind the survivor of the traumatic event, inability to recall certain aspect of the traumatic event, feeling disconnected from others)
4. Symptoms of increased arousal (e.g., exaggerated startle response, feeling easily irritated, constant fear of danger, physiologic response when exposed to similar events)
*PTSD = post-traumatic stress disorder.

Table 15-2 summarizes the basic elements included in a diagnosis of PTSD. Symptoms must be present for at least one month and must cause clinically significant distress or impairment to be diagnosed as PTSD (APA, 1994). The rate of PTSD in survivors of sexual abuse varies from 30% to 65%, depending on the criteria used to define sexual assault (Yuan, Koss, & Stone, 2006). In an extensive review of the literature on the impact of rape, Frazier (2000) found that 75% to 94% of rape victims met the criteria for PTSD at 2 weeks after rape; 60% to 73% met the PTSD criteria at 1 to 2 months; 47% to 70% met the criteria at 3 to 6 months; and approximately 50% to 60% continued to meet the criteria at 12 months and beyond.

The rates of successful suicides following rape are typically low, but the risk is real. Kilpatrick and colleagues (1987) found that victims of rape were nine times more likely than non-victims to attempt suicide in the immediate postassault period. For this reason, it is essential that suicide risk is considered and addressed during the initial and follow-up visits.

Self-blame is a common response of victims of sexual assault (Fanflik, 2007). Janoff-Bulman (1979) thought some self-blame might actually be beneficial to sexual assault victims, as it would foster a sense of future controllability and project a sense of safety from another sexual assault. A later study challenged this finding and found no evidence to support the notion that self-blame leads to adaptive behavior (Meyer & Taylor, 1986). In fact, Meyer and Taylor (1986) found self-blame to be associated with increased levels of fear and depression. Their findings were validated in a study by Frazier (1990), who also found that all types of self-blame were associated with more depression and poor adjustment after the rape.

Assessment

A woman who has been sexually assaulted may not seek treatment immediately following the assault, but may instead wait days or even weeks before seeing a clinician. Many women who see their clinician following a rape do not disclose the sexual assault (Ledray, 1994). The patient may blame herself or feel ashamed because she feels she did something that made her more vulnerable, such as drinking alcohol or using drugs. She may fear retaliation from the assailant, or a loss of confidentiality if she reports the assault. Subsequently she may not label the forced sexual contact as an assault, especially if she was assaulted by her husband, or someone with whom she had consensual sexual contact with in the past. Some 20% of reported rapes are committed by a relative or intimate partner, and 47% by a "friend" (National Crime Victim Survey, 2004). Chapter 14 covers IPV in more detail.

A woman's initial reason for seeking an examination following an assault may be due to concerns about STIs, pregnancy, sexual dysfunction, or vaginal or abdominal discomfort. Although clinicians are mandated by law to inquire about IPV during emergency department (ED) and routine office visits, unfortunately most do not inquire about sexual assault or unwanted sexual contact. It is important to routinely screen for unwanted or forced sexual contact because sexual violence is so common among women. Two out of three victims of sexual assault will not have any overt identifiable injuries; therefore, clinicians cannot assume that the lack of identifiable trauma means the woman was not forced to have sexual contact (Ledray, 1999). Likewise, because there may be trauma, especially tears in genital tissues after consenting sexual contact, it cannot be assumed that genital trauma indicates an assault (Slaughter, Brown, Crowley, & Peck, 1997). It is important to ask women who come for health care if they have experienced any sexual violence or IPV, and the clinician must make it safe for them to disclose all occurrences of violence. Chapter 14 describes an abuse screening tool that can be used to assess for sexual assault.

Reporting Issues and Concerns

Reporting issues must be addressed first because what the clinician does is, to a great extent, determined by the woman's decision about reporting. If the woman has not decided whether to report the assault to law enforcement, it is important to ask if reporting the assault is something she wants to consider. It is also important to discuss any fears or concerns that she may have about reporting. She needs to know that any forced sexual contact is a reportable crime. Research has shown that as a group, women who report sexual assault do better psychologically than those who do not report it (Ledray, 1994). The clinician's task at the time the woman arrives for care is based on whether the woman wants to report the assault to the police (McConkey, Sole, & Holcomb, 2001). If the patient desires to report the assault, the police are notified and requested to come to the facility and take the report. A quiet and private area should be provided during the report. It is critical for the clinician to provide emotional support throughout the visit and for all procedures. If there is a local rape crisis center, its staff often are willing to accompany a woman when she reports the assault to authorities.

It is essential that clinicians are familiar with the local state-mandated reporting laws and statutory rape laws. In most states, statutory rape (sexual contact between a minor and an adult), although against the law, is not a crime clinicians are mandated to report. However, if a patient is younger than the age of 18 and the assailant was a relative, caregiver, someone in a position of authority over the patient (e.g., teacher, coach, babysitter), or someone living in the home, clinicians are mandated to report the sexual assault to law enforcement or protective services while the patient is present (McConkey et al., 2001). Clinicians are also mandated to report the sexual assault, or suspected sexual assault, of a vulnerable adult, such as an individual with a mental disability.

If a clinician is unsure about the duty to report, he or she needs to call the local adult or adolescent protective services to find out the rules for mandated reporting. If a clinician is mandated to report, it is important to let the patient know that fact and to explain the process and clinician responsibilities to her and her family. If a child is involved, the parents should be present during this discussion.

A detailed history of the assault must be obtained as well as pertinent medical history (**Table 15-3**). All communication with the patient should be supportive and nonjudgmental. Avoid using language that is derogatory or accusatory, such as "How drunk were you?" or "Why were you in that area by yourself?" It is imperative to carefully document the details provided by the patient, even those details that may seem insignificant. An important factor in prosecuting a perpetrator of sexual assault is the consistency between assessment findings and the history about the assault (LaMonica & Pagliaro, 2006).

The Evidentiary Examination

An evidentiary examination is a physical examination to collect evidence of the crime. The purpose of such an examination is to assess, document, and collect forensic evidence, in addition to providing prophylactic treatment of STIs and emergency contraception. An evidentiary examination cannot be conducted without the patient's consent.

It is important to remember that the current standard of care must be met when a patient has been sexually assaulted. Therefore, the examination involves much more than just a physical evaluation. The needs of the patient and the clinician's role depend on a number of factors (**Table 15-4**).

Whether the woman chooses to report the assault to law enforcement, or whether this is a case in which the clinician is a mandated reporter, the patient still has the right to decline a medical examination and evidence collection. Law enforcement personnel cannot order a woman to have an examination, and they cannot order a clinician to perform one. Patients who are at least 12 years of age can decide for themselves whether to consent to an examination, to receive treatment for STIs, or to use emergency contraception. Parental consent is not required unless the state in which the clinician practices has a law requiring parental or judicial consent and notification. However, it is always a good idea to suggest that an evidentiary examination be completed in case the patient wants to make a delayed report. However, if she is certain she does not want to report, or if the assault occurred outside of the local time frame for evidence collection, the clinician is not required to complete an evidentiary examination.

The time frame within which an evidentiary examination must take place to be considered valid depends on local standards. Although the National Protocol for Sexual Assault Medical Forensic Examination (USDOJ, 2004) states that forensic medical examinations can be completed as long as 72 hours after a sexual assault, a number of communities have extended the time frame allowable for an evidentiary examination to 96 to 120 hours because of advances in DNA recovery techniques.

TABLE 15-3 Information to Obtain During the Limited Pertinent Health History When Sexual Assault Is Suspected

General Medical Information

1. Chronic or acute diseases

2. Medications the patient is currently taking

3. Allergies to medications

4. Date of last normal menstrual period
    Usual duration of menses
    Length of time between menses (cycle)

5. Present contraception use

6. Whether the patient had consensual intercourse within the past 72 to 120 hours; if yes, how many hours since the last consensual intercourse

7. Use of drugs or alcohol prior to the assault; if these substances were used, the amount of substance used and whether it is a usual amount for the patient

8. General appearance and emotional status

Assault History

1. Document the date, time, and place of the assault.

2. Identify the number and race of the assailants and any information that may help to identify them.

3. Document orifices (mouth, vagina, anus, rectum, other) involved and whether penetration was successful.

4. Were objects used during the attack and if so, in which body part were they used?

5. Was a weapon used? If yes, which type?

6. Did the attacker(s) use a condom?

7. Did the assailant(s) ejaculate and if yes, where (e.g., in vagina, on clothes)?

8. Ask the patient if she was restrained during the attack and if yes, how and with what.

9. Ask if the assailant(s) threatened the patient and if yes, what was said.

10. Ask the patient if she was kissed, bitten, or licked and if so, on which locations.

11. Inquire whether the patient has bathed, showered, urinated, or defecated since the attack.

12. Has the patient changed clothes since the attack? If not, document the status (condition) of her clothes.

13. Ask the patient about her level of consciousness during the attack. If she indicates she was unconscious, ask her to explain and document the response carefully using her words.

14. Ask her if there is any other information she would like to provide at this time.

Sources: Adapted from Ledray, 1995; McConkey, Sole, & Holcomb, 2001.

TABLE 15-4 Factors to Consider When Performing an Evidentiary Examination

1. Patient's desire to report the assault to law enforcement

2. State laws concerning mandated sexual assault reporting to law enforcement, and to adult and child protective agencies

3. Time between the sexual assault and the examination

4. Injuries sustained

5. Risk of exposure to a sexually transmitted infection (STI)

6. Risk of pregnancy

7. Possibility of a drug-facilitated sexual assault (DFSA)

8. Emotional response and the availability of an advocate

9. Patient's decision and concerns about disclosing to family or friends

During the examination, it is critical to maintain the chain of custody of all evidence collected. The chain of custody is the chronological documentation that describes the seizure, custody, control, transfer, analysis, and disposition of evidence collected, regardless of whether that evidence is physical or electronic. Evidence can be used in court to convict persons of crimes, so it must be handled in a specific and careful manner to avoid later allegations of behavior that can compromise the case of the prosecution and result in acquittal of a guilty person or overturning of a guilty verdict if there is an appeal. The purpose of the chain of custody is to establish that the evidence collected is related to the crime and was not put there by someone else to make a person appear guilty.

The clinician conducts a complete examination after obtaining a signed consent to complete the medical legal examination, collect evidence, take pictures, and release the evidence to law enforcement. The evidentiary examination should be conducted following the agency protocol and the guidelines provided in the National Protocol for Sexual Assault Medical Forensic Examination (Office of Violence Against Women [OVW], 2004). Clinicians unfamiliar with the policy in their region are encouraged to check with the local sexual assault nurse examiner (SANE) program, if one is located in the community, or the local rape crisis center. A list of SANE programs can be found at www.sane-sart.com. (Appendix 15-A provides additional discussion of the steps of the evidentiary examination.)

In some localities, the clinician may also be requested to collect pulled head hairs and/or pulled pubic hairs from the victim to be used for comparison purposes if hair is found at the crime scene. Such samples are no longer collected in most jurisdictions due to the pain involved for the patient and the unlikely nature of this evidence being useful, so it is important for clinicians to know the policy and procedures required in their locale.

It is important to inform the patient that the Violence Against Women Department of Justice Reauthorization Act of 2005 (VAWA, 2006) mandates that all adolescent and adult victims of sexual assault be provided with a medical forensic examination even if the patient does not choose to report the assault to law enforcement and participate in the criminal justice process. VAWA ensures the state pays for this examination, so that the victim bears no out-of-pocket expenses. To assess a state's ongoing efforts to comply with this mandate and determine reimbursement, visit the following website: http://www.ovw.usdoj.gov/docs/admin_contact_list.pdf. The Maryland Coalition Against Sexual Assault (MCASA) was designated to provide technical assistance in the implementation of this policy. For funding or other compliance issues, MCASA can be contacted at www.mcasa.org.

To maintain the proper chain of custody, each piece of evidence collected must be properly labeled with the patient's full name, the date and time of collection, the medical examiner's full name, and the identification of the evidence. It is then sealed and either given to law enforcement or placed into a locked refrigerator or cabinet with limited access. A signature record must also be kept of everyone who has possession of the evidence from the time it is collected until it is given to law enforcement.

Management

Patient Care and Counseling

It is important to explain the extent of the trauma or lack of identification of trauma to patients when they undergo a medical examination following a sexual assault. Typically women who have been sexually assaulted are fearful about having vaginal trauma and are reassured when they receive accurate information, even if trauma is evident (Ledray, 1999). If a video colposcope is available and used during the examination, it can be helpful to turn the screen so that the patient can also view the genital area. The examiner should disclose and explain the nature of any physical trauma associated with the sexual assault. If there are no apparent injuries, the patient should be reassured about the absence of trauma. It is also important to explain that sex-related injuries usually heal rapidly, so that within days even an experienced examiner would not be able to identify that there had previously been an injury.

From a forensic and clinical perspective, treating patients prophylactically for STIs is often preferable to performing STI tests. These tests are very expensive and time-consuming for the woman who may need to return two or three times for additional testing and, unfortunately, most women who have been assaulted do not return for follow-up care (Blair & Warner, 1992). Additionally, STI testing has not proven useful in court in either adult or adolescent cases. Testing is recommended in all sexual abuse cases involving children (younger than 12 years of age) and can be useful evidence in such circumstances (Workowski & Berman, 2006). Most clinicians and forensic examiners recommend that prophylactic treatment for STIs be a component of all examinations of adolescent and adult victims of sexual assault (American College of Emergency Physicians [ACEP], 1999; CDC, 2010; Ledray, 1999; OVW, 2004). See Chapter 21 for further information about testing and treating STIs.

Based on the recommendations from survivors of sexual assault, clinicians should, in a matter-of-fact manner, provide information about the risk of HIV, testing procedures, prevention, and safe-sex options. This presentation allows the woman to make decisions based on facts, not out of fear (Ledray, 1999). Because the rates of HIV infection vary from state to state and from community to community, the actual risk of infection also varies. The decision to offer prophylactic treatment should be based on the risk due to the sexual assault combined with HIV prevalence in the specific geographic area. The risk of HIV exposure after sexual contact is, overall, reported to be less than the risk associated with other routes of exposure such as needle sharing, mother-to-infant transmission, or blood transfusions.

The CDC (2010) recommends assessing the risk of HIV infection in the assailant as well as characteristics of the assault that might increase the risk of HIV transmission. A sexual assault would be considered high risk if it involved rectal contact or vaginal contact with ejaculation, with vaginal tears or existing vaginal STIs that have caused ulcerations or open sores disrupting the integrity of the vaginal mucosa. It would also be considered high risk if the victim had some reason to know or suspect that the assailant was an intravenous drug user, HIV positive, or bisexual. It is important to inform the woman of the known toxicities of the antiretroviral drugs, and to clarify that close follow-up is recommended. Victims of assault must also be informed that there may be additional unknown benefits to treatment. This information enables the patient to make an educated decision. PEP must be initiated within 72 hours of the sexual assault to be effective (CDC).

The best approach to dealing with the issue of HIV is complicated and controversial (Blair & Warner, 1992). If the offender is HIV infected, the probability of a rape victim contracting HIV from a sexual assault will depend on the type of sexual intercourse, the presence of trauma in the involved orifice, if there was exposure to ejaculate, the viral load of the ejaculate, and the presence of other STIs (CDC, 2010; Workowski & Berman, 2006). In most instances, it is impossible to determine the HIV status of the offender in a timely fashion and, therefore, it is important for the forensic examiner to know the local infection rates.

All women who have been sexually assaulted need to be informed of the risk of conception and the availability of emergency contraception. This recommendation is supported by the American Medical Association (AMA), the American College of Obstetricians and Gynecologists, the American Public Health Association (APHA), and ACEP (Smith et al., 2009; Womack, 2008). For more information on emergency contraception, see Chapter 12.

The importance of offering complete care to sexual assault victims, including care to prevent pregnancy when requested by the victim, was affirmed by the successful lawsuit against a New York City hospital that did not ensure that a victim receive a prescription for emergency contraception to prevent pregnancy (Chivers, 2000). The National Conference of Catholic Bishops (1995) has agreed that "a female who has been raped should be able to defend herself against a potential conception from the sexual assault. If, after appropriate testing there is no evidence that conception has occurred already, she may be treated with medication that would prevent ovulation or fertilization" (p. 16).

Many states now have laws requiring all hospitals that see sexual assault victims to provide emergency contraception information or to offer emergency contraception medications. These medications include levonorgestrel emergency contraceptive pills (ECPs) (Plan

B, Plan B One-Step, Next Choice), combined ECPs (various combined oral contraceptives [COCs] can be used), and ulipristal acetate (ella). See Chapter 12 for information about these medications.

Because research clearly indicates that women can be sexually assaulted more than once, it is important to address the issue of vulnerability to prevent future abuse. Typically clinicians caring for victims of sexual assault are hesitant to discuss vulnerability because they do not want to appear to be blaming the victim for the assault. Although that may be a valid concern, all too often it results in the clinician doing nothing. Chapter 8, for example, provides alcohol misuse screening recommendations for all women.

The clinician's role encompasses addressing all aspects of the biopsychosocial needs of all patients. Clinicians must be able to provide emotional support and crisis intervention, and work as a member of the team and in concert with the assault advocate (if one is present) as well as with other professionals providing care for the woman (Ledray, Faugno, & Speck, 2001). It is the attending clinician's role to make an initial assessment of the survivor's psychological functioning sufficient to determine suicidal ideation; orientation to person, place, and time; or need for further referral for follow-up support, evaluation, or treatment.

Whenever possible, a sexual assault advocate or counselor should be available to talk with the victim when she makes the initial report and for follow-up. Because women who have been victimized by perpetrators of sexual assault are more likely than others to not take the initiative to make an initial appointment or to not show for appointments, it is important for the advocate or counselor to contact them for follow-up. Clinicians can assist the advocate by obtaining the patient's permission to give her contact information to the advocate or counselor and permission to have the advocate or counselor contact the patient.

Standard of Care

Only recently have healthcare facilities begun to recognize their responsibility to have trained staff available to provide specialized care for victims of sexual assault. Treating injuries alone is not sufficient. Since 1992, the guidelines of The Joint Commission (formerly JCAHO, the Joint Commission on Accreditation of Healthcare Organizations) have required emergency and ambulatory care facilities to have protocols on rape, sexual molestation, and IPV. In 1997, The Joint Commission began requiring healthcare facilities to develop and train their staff to use specified criteria to assist with the identification of possible victims of physical assault, rape, other sexual molestation, IPV, and abuse or neglect of older adults and children (The Joint Commission, 1997). The 2004 Joint Commission standards required not only that staff be educated in how to identify whether a woman being seen for care had been abused, but also that the medical care provided include the preservation of evidence to support future legal action (The Joint Commission, 2004).

The Sexual Assault Nurse Examiner

A sexual assault nurse examiner (SANE) is a registered nurse (RN) who has advanced education in forensic examination of sexual assault victims. SANE education includes a 40-hour didactic SANE training program with specified content, plus clinical experience (Ledray, 1999). In April 2002, the first adult and adolescent certification program was established (SANE-A), followed by introduction of the pediatric certification program in 2004 (SANE-P). The certification examination is offered through the International Association of Forensic Nurses (IAFN). The SANE performs the complete medical forensic examination, as outlined in the management section of this chapter.

While it is not necessary to be certified as a SANE to complete a sexual assault evidentiary examination, this specialized training is valuable for all medical personnel who may be completing the sexual assault examination. For more information about the education, certification, and role of the SANE, the reader is referred to the IAFN website at www.iafn.org.

When forced sexual contact is identified, further evaluation and care is necessary and includes:

- Discussion of law enforcement reporting options and mandates with the woman
- Evaluation, documentation, and treatment of injuries
- Assessment of the risk for STIs and provision of preventive care
- Pregnancy prevention and testing
- Evidence collection, maintaining the chain of custody
- Information, supportive counseling, and advocacy

Agencies should have a policy in place to ensure that a sexual assault examination is completed by a SANE or other properly trained clinician.

Special Considerations

Circumstances around sexual assault that deserve special consideration include the age of the victim (children, adolescents, elderly), disabled victims, mentally handicapped victims, and the gender and sexual orientation of the victim.

The age of the victim is important for many reasons. The very young and very elderly may both have difficulty describing the incident and relating symptoms (LaMonica & Pagliaro, 2006). Because children who are victims of sexual abuse are often subjected to the abuse over long periods of time, the collection of forensic evidence may not be possible at the time of the examination (LaMonica & Pagliaro). Elderly women may experience more injuries due to their physical fragility (LaMonica & Pagliaro). Specialized equipment may be required to examine both children and elderly victims of sexual assault. Most states have mandatory reporting laws for children and elderly victims of abuse, including sexual assault. Clinicians should ensure that they are familiar with the laws in the state in which they practice.

Although intervention and prevention of sexual violence has grown during the last few decades, the needs of lesbian, gay, bisexual, and transgender (LGBT) individuals who have been subjected to sexual assault represent a gap in the research (Gentlewarrior, 2009). Similar to other victims of sexual assault, many LGBT individuals who are sexually assaulted do not report the assault. The failure or resistance to reporting in such cases may not only reflect fear of judgment by police, but also fear of rejection by the gay community (LaMonica

& Pagliaro, 2006). Contrary to popular belief, both gays and lesbians are more frequently assaulted by heterosexual males (LaMonica & Pagliaro). Little is known about the prevalence of sexual violence in the LGBT communities; consequently, there is a dearth of information about how best to meet the needs of LGBT individuals who are survivors of sexual assault. "Bias related to homophobia, transphobia and biphobia is often directed at LGBT adults in the form of sexual violence" (Gentlewarrior, p. 5). Dunbar (2006) notes that crimes against LGBT individuals are likely to be more violent than crimes motivated by race, ethnicity, or religion. It is critically important for clinicians to develop LGBT affirmative knowledge and practice skills (Gentlewarrior). It is also critical for clinicians to appreciate the diversity of LGBT individuals so that care focuses on the needs of the person. Chapter 10 provides an in-depth discussion of health care for gender minorities.

Individuals with physical, mental, and communication disabilities must also be given special consideration because they may have limited cognition or be unable to explain exactly what happened (LaMonica & Pagliaro, 2006). It is best if the clinician is experienced in interviewing individuals with disabilities, or if the agency has support individuals with specialized interviewing skills. Reporting of sexual abuse of disabled persons is mandated in every state (LaMonica & Pagliaro).

Summary

It is recommended that clinicians have a written policy in place that is carefully followed for all cases of suspected or known sexual abuse. Collect forensic medical evidence using a sexual assault evidence collection kit if the victim presents within 72 to 120 hours after the assault (depending on local guidelines) and desires this type of evaluation. Provide crisis intervention, support, and the information the patient needs to make educated choices about her care. If possible, a sexual assault advocate or counselor should be present. Make follow-up referrals: It is important for every clinician to identify sexual assault victims they may see in their practice, even if the patient does not initially disclose the assault. Providing high-quality medical care and meeting all the health needs of sexual assault victims includes addressing the issues of physical injury, STI (including HIV) risk evaluation and prevention, pregnancy risk evaluation and prevention, and the collection and preservation of evidence, including documenting the history of the assault provided by the patient (Ledray, 1995, 2007). What the clinician does immediately can make a significant positive difference for the woman who has suffered a sexual assault. The clinician's role can be instrumental in the road to recovery and the woman's ability to survive sexual assault.

References

American College of Emergency Physicians (ACEP). (June 1999). *Evaluation and management of the sexually assaulted or sexually abused patient.* Dallas: Author.

American Psychiatric Association (APA). (1994). *Diagnostic and statistical manual of mental disorders* (4th ed.). Washington, DC: Author.

Baker, R., & Sommers, M. (2008). Relationship of genital injuries and age in adolescent and young adult rape survivors. *Journal of Obstetric, Gynecology and Neonatal Nursing, 37*, 282–289.

Basile, K. C., & Saltzman, L. E. (2002). *Sexual violence surveillance: Uniform definitions and recommended data elements.* Atlanta, GA: National Center for Injury Prevention and Control, Centers for Disease Control and Prevention. Retrieved from http://www.cdc.gov/violenceprevention/pdf/SV_Surveillance_Definitionsl-2009-a.pdf

Blair, T., & Warner, C. (1992). Sexual assault. *Topics in Emergency Medicine, 14*(4), 58–77.

Brener, N. D., McMahon, P. M., Warren, C. W., & Douglas, K. A. (1999). Forced sexual intercourse and associated health-risk behaviors among female college students in the United States. *Journal of Consulting and Clinical Psychology, 67*, 252–259.

Breslau, N. (2009). The epidemiology of trauma, PTSD, and other post trauma disorders. *Trauma, Violence & Abuse, 10*, 198–210.

Carter-Snell, C., Olson, K., Jensen, L., Cummings, G., & Wiebe, N. (2007, October). *Women's risk of injuries during sexual assault.* Paper presented at the meeting of IAFN Scientific Assembly, Salt Lake City, UT.

Centers for Disease Control and Prevention (CDC). (2010). *Sexually transmitted diseases treatment guidelines.* Retrieved from http://www.cdc.gov/std/treatment/2010/default.htm

Centers for Disease Control and Prevention (CDC). (2009). *Sexual violence prevention scientific information: Definitions.* Retrieved from http://www.cdc.gov/ncipc/dvp/SV/svp-definitions.htm

Chivers, C. J. (2000, August 6). In sex crimes, evidence depends on game of chance in hospitals. *The New York Times*, pp. 1–6.

Dunbar, E. (2006). Race, gender, and sexual orientation in hate crime victimization: Identity politics or identity risk? *Violence and Victims, 21*(3), 323–337.

Ernst, A., Green, E., Ferguson, M., et al. (2000). The utility of anoscopy and colposcopy in the evaluation of male sexual assault victims. *Annals of Emergency Medicine, 36*(5), 432–436.

Fanflik, P. (2007). *Victim responses to sexual assault: Counterintuitive or simply adaptive?* National District Attorneys Association. Retrieved from http://www.ndaa.org/pdf/pub_victim_responses_sexual_assault.pdf

Felitti, V. (1998). Long-term medical consequences of incest, rape, and molestation. *Southern Medical Journal, 84*(3), 328–331.

Frazier, P. (1990). Victim attributions and post-rape trauma. *Journal of Personality & Social Psychology, 59*(2), 298–304.

Frazier, P. (2000). The scientific status of research on rape trauma syndrome. In D. L. Faigman, D. H. Kay, M. J. Sakes, & J. Sanders (Eds.), *Modern scientific evidence: The law and science of expert testimony* (pp. 14–23). St. Paul, MN: West Group.

Geist, R. F. (1988). Sexually related trauma. *Emergency Medicine Clinics of North America, 6*(3), 439–466.

Gentlewarrior, S. (2009). *Culturally competent service provision to lesbian, gay, bisexual and transgender survivors of sexual violence* (National Online Resource Center on Violence Against Women publication No. 5U1V/CE324010-05). Washington, DC: U.S. Government Printing Office.

Harlow, L. L., Quina, K., Morokoff, P. J., Rose, J. S., & Grimly, D. M. (1993). HIV risk in women: A multifaceted model. *Journal of Applied Behavioral Research, 1*, 3–38.

Holmes, M., Resnick, H. S., & Frampton, D. (1998). Follow-up of sexual assault victims. *American Journal of Obstetrics and Gynecology, 179*, 336–342.

Holmes, M., Resnick, H., Kilpatrick, D., & Best, C. (1996). Rape related pregnancy: Estimates and descriptive characteristics from a national sample of women. *American Journal of Obstetrics & Gynecology, 175*, 320–324.

Irwin, K. L., Edlin, B. R., Wong, L., Faruque, S., McCoy, H. V., Word, C., et al (1995). Urban rape survivors: Characteristics and prevalence of human immunodeficiency virus and other sexually transmitted infections. *Obstetrics and Gynecology, 85*, 330–336.

Janoff-Bulman, R. (1979). Characterological versus behavioral self-blame: Inquiries into depression and rape. *Journal of Personality and Social Psychology, 37*, 1798–1809.

The Joint Commission. (1997). *Comprehensive accreditation manual for hospitals: The official handbook.* Oakbrook Terrace, IL: Author.

The Joint Commission. (2004). *Standard PC 3.10.10.* Oakbrook Terrace, IL: Author.

Kaysen, D., Neighbors, C., Martell, J., Fossos, N., & Larimer, M. E. (2006). Incapacitated rape and alcohol use: A prospective analysis. *Addictive Behaviors, 31*, 1820–1832.

Keller, P., & Nelson, J. (2008). Injuries to the cervix in sexual trauma. *Journal of Forensic Nursing, 4*, 130–137.

Kilpatrick, D., Acierno, R., Resnick, H., Saunders, B., & Best, C. L. (1997). A 2-year longitudinal analysis of the relationship between violent assault and substance use in women. *Journal of Consulting and Clinical Psychology, 65*(5), 834–847.

Kilpatrick, D., Saunders, B., Veronen, L., Best, C. L., & Von, J. M. (1987). Criminal victimization: Lifetime prevalence reporting to police, and psychological impact. *Crime Delinquency, 33*, 479–489.

Kilpatrick, D., & Veronen, L. (1984). *Treatment of fear and anxiety in victims of rape* (Final Report, Grant No. R01NG29602). Rockville, MD: National Institute of Mental Health.

Koss, M. (1993). Rape. Scope, impact, interventions, and public policy. *American Psychologist, 48*(10), 1062–1069.

LaMonica, P., & Pagliaro, E. (2006). Sexual assault intervention and the forensic examination. In R. Hammer, B. Moynihan, & E. Pagliaro (Eds.), *Forensic nursing* (pp. 547–578). Sudbury, MA: Jones and Bartlett.

Ledray, L. E. (1994). *Recovering from rape* (2nd ed.). New York: Henry Holt.

Ledray, L. E. (1995). Sexual assault: Clinical issues: Sexual assault evidentiary exam and treatment protocol. *Journal of Emergency Nursing, 21*, 355–359.

Ledray, L. E. (1999). Sexual assault: Clinical issues: Date rape drug alert. *Journal of Emergency Nursing, 17*(1), 1–2.

Ledray, L. E. (2007). *2 SART Model Final Report.* Washington, DC: U.S. Department of Justice, Office of Justice Programs.

Ledray, L. E. (2008). Alcohol and sexual assault: What can/should we do in the emergency department? *Journal of Forensic Nursing, 4*, 91.

Ledray, L., Faugno, D., & Speck, P. (2001). Sexual assault: Clinical issues. SANE: Advocate, forensic technician, nurse? *Journal of Emergency Nursing, 27*(1), 91–93.

Logan, T., Cole, J., & Capillo, A. (2007). Differential characteristics of intimate partner, acquaintance, and stranger rape survivors examined by a sexual assault nurse examiner (SANE). *Journal of Interpersonal Violence, 22*(8), 1066–1076.

MacFarlane, E., & Hawley, P. (1993). Sexual assault: Coping with crisis. *Canadian Nurse, 89*, 21–24.

McConkey, T., Sole, M., & Holcomb, L. (2001). Assessing the female sexual assault survivor. *Nurse Practitioner, 26*, 28–39.

McFarlane, J., Malecha, A., Watson, K., Gist, J., Battern, E., Hall, I., & Smith, S. (2005). Intimate partner sexual assault against women: Frequency, health consequences, and treatment outcomes. *Obstetrics & Gynecology, 105*, 99–108.

Messman-Moore, T., & Long, P. (2002). Alcohol and substance use disorders as predictors of child to adult sexual revictimization in a sample of community women. *Violence & Victims, 17*(3), 319–340.

Meyer, C., & Taylor, S. (1986). Adjustment to rape. *Journal of Personality and Social Psychology, 30*, 1226–1234.

Murphy, S., Harris, V., & Forester, S. (1989). Rape and subsequent seroconversion to HIV. *British Medical Journal, 299*, 718.

National Conference of Catholic Bishops. (1995). *Ethical and religious directives for Catholic health care services* [Pamphlet], pp. 14–17.

National Crime Victim Survey. (2004). Retrieved from www.stoprapevermont.org/stats/adult.html

Office of Violence Against Women (OVW). (2004). *National protocol for sexual assault medical forensic examination.* Washington, DC: U.S. Department of Justice Office on Violence Against Women.

Resick, P., & Schnicke, M. (1990). Treating symptoms in adult victims of sexual assault. *Journal of Interpersonal Violence, 5*(4), 488–506.

Rheingold, A. A., Acierno, R., & Resnick, H. S. (2004). Trauma, posttraumatic stress disorder, and health risk behaviors. In P. O. Schnurr & B. L. Green (Eds.), *Trauma and health* (pp. 217–243). Washington, DC: American Psychological Association.

Riggs, N., Houry, D., Long, G., Markovchick, V., & Feldhaus, K. (2000). Analysis of 1,076 cases of sexual assault. *Annals of Emergency Medicine, 35*(4), 358–362.

Scalzo, T. (2006). Rape and sexual assault reporting laws. *American Prosecutors Research Institute, 1*(3). Retrieved from www.ndaa.org/pdf/the_voice_vol_1_no_3_2006.pdf

Slaughter, L., & Brown, C. R. (1992). Colposcopy to establish physical findings in rape victims. *American Journal of Obstetrics & Gynecology, 176*(3), 83–86.

Slaughter, L., Brown, C. R., Crowley, S., & Peck, R. (1997). Patterns of genital injury in female sexual assault victims. *American Journal of Obstetrics & Gynecology, 176*(3), 609–616.

Smith, S., Brown, P., & Hartman, E. (2009). *Emergency contraception and sexual assault: Why compassionate care should be a standard of care.* Retrieved from http://www.center4research.org/wmnshlth/2006/ec.html

Sommers, M. (2007). Defining patterns of genital injury from sexual assault: A review. *Trauma Violence Abuse, 8,* 270. doi: 10.1177/1524838007303194. Retrieved from http://tva.sagepub.com/cgi/content/abstract/8/3/270

Straight, J., & Heaton, P. (2007). Emergency department care for victims of sexual offense. *American Journal of Health System Pharmacology, 64,* 1845–1850.

Tavara, L., (2006). Sexual violence. *Best Practice & Research Clinical Obstetrics & Gynecology, 20,* 395–408. doi: 10.1016/j.bpobgyn.2—6.01.01

Tintinalli, J., & Hoelzer, M. (1985). Clinical findings and legal resolution in sexual assault. *Annals of Emergency Medicine, 14*(5), 447–453.

Tjaden, P., & Thoennes, N. (1998). *Prevalence, incidence, and consequences of violence against women survey.* National Institute of Justice, Centers for Disease Control and Prevention Research Brief. Retrieved from http://www.ncjrs.gov/pdffiles/172837.pdf

Tjaden, P., & Thoennes, N. (2006). *Extent, nature and consequences of rape victimization: Findings from the National Violence Against Women survey.* Washington, DC: U.S. Department of Justice, Office of Justice Programs.

U.S. Department of Justice (USDOJ). (2004). *A national protocol for sexual assault medical forensic examinations: Adults/pediatrics* (DOJ Publication No. NCJ 206554). Retrieved from http://www.ncjrs.gov/pdffiles1/ovw/206554.pdf

U.S. Department of Justice (USDOJ), Federal Bureau of Investigation. (2008). *Forcible rape.* Retrieved from http://www.fbi.gov/ucr/cius2008/offenses/violent_crime/forcible_rape.html

Violence Against Women and Department of Justice Reauthorization Act of 2005, Pub. L. No. 109-162, H.R. 3402. (2006).

Womack, K. (2008). Emergency contraception to avoid unintended pregnancy following sexual assault. *Women's Health Care: A Practical Journal for Nurse Practitioners, 7,* 18–20.

Workowski, K., & Berman, S. (2006). *Sexually transmitted disease treatment guidelines, 2006* (Report 55(RR11); 1–94). Retrieved from http://www.cdc.gov/mmwr/preview/mmwrhtml/rr5511a1.htm

Yuan, N., Koss, M., & Stone, M. (2006). *The psychological consequences of sexual trauma.* Retrieved from the National Online Resource Center on Violence against Women website: http://www.vawnet.org

Steps of the Evidentiary Examination

1. *Collect clothing.* If the patient has not changed clothes, all clothing should be collected. If the patient has changed clothes, the undergarments should be collected. Each piece of clothing is placed in a separate paper bag and sealed with evidence tape.

2. *Evaluate and document injuries.* The body should be examined for any injury, however slight, that may have occurred as a result of the sexual assault. Whenever an injury is identified, it should be described in words in the examination documentation, by taking a picture with and without a measuring instrument, and by marking the location of the injury on a body drawing.

3. *Swab the involved orifices (mouth, vagina, and/or anus) and other areas.* A minimum of two swabs should always be collected from each site. Swabs from each site should be placed in separate envelopes. Whenever vaginal or anal swabs are collected, it is recommended to also collect perineal swabs. If there appears to be saliva, seminal fluid, or perspiration on the patient's body, these areas should be swabbed as well. When taking a swab from a dry area, moisten the swabs with a small amount of sterile water prior to swabbing the area. If the patient reports scratching the assailant, swab under her fingernails with a swab moistened with sterile water. When vaginal or anal contact occurred, comb the victim's pubic hair (to obtain any of the assailant's pubic hair that may have been transferred). If there is any matted pubic hair (e.g., possible seminal fluid) cut the matted hair and place it in an envelope, properly labeled as "debris from pubic area." If other debris is identified, it should be collected in a separate envelope and properly labeled.

4. *Obtain a sample of the victim's DNA.* Depending on the local protocol, this sample may consist of a buccal swab, saliva, tube of blood, or blood from a finger prick collected on special absorbent paper.

5. *Label each envelope.* Document the following items on the envelope:
   - The patient's full name
   - The likely contents (e.g., "possible saliva from area where patient reports she was bitten by assailant")
   - Where it was collected from (e.g., "left forearm")
   - Clinician's full name printed clearly and then signed
   - Date and time evidence was collected

15-B

Evidence Collection

The sexual assault evidence collection will vary depending on the local protocol and the choice of kits. It typically includes at least the following items:

1. Collection of swabs from the orifices involved in the sexual assault to look for sperm, acid phosphatase, and, most importantly, the offender's DNA.
2. Collection of swabs from the skin that may have body fluids of the assailant, including blood, saliva, or seminal fluid.
3. Buccal swabs or blood from the survivor to identify DNA. If the victim was assaulted orally, buccal swabs should not be used, as the oral cavity may be contaminated with the suspect's DNA.
4. Collection of blood or urine for possible drug screen (especially in suspected drug-facilitated sexual assault).
5. Pubic hair combing to look for the assailant's pubic hair.
6. Collection of debris from anywhere on the victim's body or clothing.

Most SANE programs no longer collect pulled head hair or pubic hair, as this is seldom useful evidence and the collection is very painful. When such samples are needed, they can be obtained in those few cases at a later time.

Website Resources

American Prosecutors' Research Institute: http://www.ndaa.org/apri

CDC Treatment Guidelines 2006: http://www.cdc.gov/std/treatment/2006/sexual-assault.htm

National District Attorneys' Association/National Center for the Prosecution of Violence Against Women: http://www.ndaa.org/ncpvaw_home.html

National Sexual Violence Resource Center: http://www.nsvrc.org

Summary of laws relevant to rape and sexual assault reporting for the victimization of competent adults: http://www.ndaa.org/pdf/rape_rept_summary.pdf

Website to identify your state's rape and domestic violence reporting requirements, and state statutes: http://www.ndaa.org/publications/apri/violence_against_women.html

The following are a selection of other websites that provide statistics related to violence against women:

Bureau of Justice, Crime and Victim Statistics: http://www.ojp.usdoj.gov/bjs/cvict.htm

Department of Justice's Office on Violence Against Women: http://www.ovw.usdoj.gov

Family Violence Prevention Fund: http://endabuse.org/content/news/detail/1092

Rape, Abuse, and Incest National Network: http://www.rainn.org/statistics

Violence Against Women: http://www.vaw.umn.edu/library/sexassault

World Health Organization, Gender-Based Violence: http://www.who.int/gender/violence/en

Other resources can be found at the following sites:

Legal issues and resources: http://www.ndaa.org/apri/programs/vawa/legal_issues_resources.html

A National Protocol for Sexual Assault Forensic Medical Examination: http://www.ncjrs.gov/pdffiles1/ovw/206554.pdf

National Association of Attorneys General: http://www.naag.org

Statistics, Government Studies plus Insightful Articles: http://www.ndaa.org/apri/programs/vawa/statistics_gov_studies.html#govsexualassault

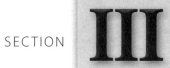

Women's Gynecologic Healthcare Management

Breast Conditions

Heather M. Aliotta
Nancy J. Schaeffer

Women rarely have neutral feelings about their breasts because, for most women, breasts are an important part of their self-image (Young, 1998). Breasts are an outward sign of being female and, depending on the culture, they may be considered taboo, worshipped, or exploited (Jones, 2004). Women may feel that they are judged and evaluated by the size and shape of their breasts because these characteristics are often associated with sexual attractiveness (Jones; Young). The importance of breast appearance is underscored by the availability of surgical procedures that offer an idealized breast size and shape. Breasts can provide both sexual pleasure and nourishment, which may engender the belief that a woman's breasts belong not only to her, but also to her sexual partner and to her baby (Jones). The meaning of her breasts to a woman will greatly influence how she reacts to having a breast condition.

The presence of symptoms in the breasts that may be associated with pathology causes understandable concern for women. A woman may have an underlying fear, which may not be articulated or even conscious, that she has breast cancer. Providing adequate emotional support when a woman presents with a breast condition is as important as ensuring accurate assessment, diagnosis, and management of the condition. The breast conditions that are the focus of this chapter are mastalgia, nipple discharge, benign breast masses, and breast cancer.

Mastalgia

Mastalgia, or breast pain, is one of the most common breast concerns for which women seek health care. Breast pain is a significant cause of anxiety, even though mastalgia is benign in 90% of cases (Meisner, Fekrazad, & Royce, 2008). Mastalgia is classified as cyclic or noncyclic, depending on whether its presence is related to the menstrual cycle. The majority of breast pain is cyclic and occurs premenstrually. As many as 70% of women experience cyclic mastalgia, and 11% to 22% of women have moderate to severe breast pain (Ader & Browne, 1997; Ader, South-Paul, Adera, & Deuster, 2001). Noncyclic mastalgia is less common, and its exact incidence is unknown.

Etiology and Pathophysiology

Mild cyclic mastalgia is considered a normal, physiologic condition caused by the hormonal changes of the menstrual cycle (Meisner et al., 2008; Olawaiye, Witham-Leitch, Danakas, & Kahn, 2005). Mastalgia can also be caused by certain medications, including combined estrogen and progestin contraceptives (i.e., pills, vaginal ring, and transdermal patch; see Chapter 12), hormone therapy (HT; see Chapter 13), antidepressants, digoxin, methyldopa, spironolactone, oxymetholone, and chlorpromazine (Meisner et al.).

Fibrocystic breast changes are common among women with mastalgia, although not all women with fibrocystic breast changes experience pain and not all women with mastalgia have fibrocystic breast changes (Olawaiye et al., 2005). Fibrocystic breast changes were originally called fibrocystic breast disease, but the associated constellation of symptoms has become increasingly recognized as common to many women; thus, these symptoms are no longer considered to constitute a disease. These changes include tender, nodular, and swollen breast tissue.

Clinical Presentation

Cyclic mastalgia typically begins in the luteal phase and subsides with menses. The pain is usually bilateral, poorly localized, and described as soreness or aching. Cyclic mastalgia most commonly occurs in women who are 30 to 50 years old (Rodden, 2009).

In contrast, noncyclic mastalgia may be constant or intermittent, and is unrelated to the menstrual cycle. Noncyclic mastalgia is more likely to cause unilateral, localized pain that is sharp or burning in nature and occurs most frequently in women aged 40 years and older (Rodden, 2009). Women with macromastia (very large breasts) may report shoulder grooving, neck pain, and back pain in addition to breast pain (Smith & Kent, 2002).

Assessment

History The clinician must determine whether the mastalgia is cyclic or noncyclic and eliminate nonbreast causes of the discomfort, such as chest wall pain. Ask the woman about the timing (especially in relation to the menstrual cycle), frequency, location, nature, severity, and mitigating factors of the pain as well as its effects on her functioning (Carmichael, Bashayan, & Nightingale, 2005). The use of an instrument to rate pain, such as a visual analog scale, may be helpful in evaluating mastalgia and monitoring the response to treatment. Prospective evaluation of pain with a daily diary has been found to be more accurate than retrospective reporting (Tavaf-Motamen, Ader, Browne, & Shriver, 1998) and can be useful in differentiating cyclic and noncyclic mastalgia. In addition, the clinician should ask the woman about other breast symptoms, such as nipple discharge or breast mass, and whether there is a previous history of any type of breast disease or surgery. Menstrual, pregnancy, lactation, and general medical histories are necessary for a comprehensive assessment. Note current medications, including exogenous hormones. Ask about the amount of caffeine and fatty food intake. Caffeine contains a chemical called *methylxanthine* that causes blood vessels to dilate, leading to distention in the breasts, sometimes resulting in mastalgia. Diets high in fat content are also thought to increase the risk for breast pain, although the reason for this relationship is unclear. Also obtain a family history, particularly regarding breast and ovarian cancer. A complete review of systems is helpful in eliminating nonbreast causes (see the discussion of differential diagnoses).

Physical Examination Perform a comprehensive breast examination, that includes inspection and palpation of the breasts with the woman in both the upright and supine positions, and evaluate the lymph nodes (see Chapter 6). Assess for skin changes, nipple discharge, and breast masses. If the pain can be reproduced with examination, note its location. The chest wall structures should also be examined for nonbreast causes of pain.

Diagnostic Testing Pregnancy testing should be performed if indicated by the woman's history because mastalgia can be a sign of pregnancy. Diagnostic imaging is frequently used in the evaluation of breast conditions, and information about these tests is provided in **Table 16-1**. A mammogram can be ordered if the woman is of appropriate age for screening with mammography; however, diagnostic imaging is helpful only to rule out the unlikely diagnosis of cancer because there are no radiologic findings associated with mastalgia (Olawaiye et al., 2005). Mammography should also be considered for women with focal breast pain

TABLE 16-1 Diagnostic Imaging Tests

Test	Source of Images	Best for Detecting	Limitations of Test
Mammogram	X-rays	Calcifications, densities, and architectural distortion	Cannot show if density is solid or cystic; has lower sensitivity in younger women
Ultrasound	Sound waves	Differentiation of solid and cystic masses	Cannot show calcifications
Magnetic resonance imaging (MRI)	Magnetic fields, may be enhanced with gadolinium contrast	Tissue with increased blood flow such as tumors	Expensive; limited to specific indications; high rate of false-positive results

who have a family history of early breast cancer or other breast cancer risk factors (Smith, Pruthi, & Fitzpatrick, 2004). If a breast mass is discovered during the evaluation of mastalgia, it needs to be evaluated appropriately, as described later in this chapter.

Differential Diagnoses

Extramammary or nonbreast causes of pain are important differential diagnoses. If the pain is reproducible with palpation of the chest wall, costochondritis or Tietze syndrome should be suspected (Smith et al., 2004). Costochondritis consists of inflammation of the costochondral or chondrosternal joints. The second through the fifth costochondral junctions are most likely to be affected. Tietze syndrome is differentiated from costochondritis by the presence of swelling with or without erythema. Nonsteroidal anti-inflammatory drugs (NSAIDs) can be helpful in relieving the symptoms of both conditions. Other potential etiologies of breast pain include pleuritis, mastitis, and shingles (Olawaiye et al., 2005).

Mastalgia is rarely the principal sign of a developing breast cancer, but the possibility of cancer increases when the mastalgia occurs postmenopause in the absence of HT or when the breast pain is accompanied by skin changes or a palpable abnormality (Smith & Souba, 1995). Mastalgia related to breast cancer usually occurs in only one area of one breast and is unrelated to a cyclic pattern (Smith et al., 2004).

Management

Once a clinician has ruled out malignancy and nonbreast causes of mastalgia, attention turns to reassuring the woman that she does not have a serious illness and relieving her symptoms. Nonpharmacologic, complementary, and alternative therapies are often successful in the treatment of mastalgia. Severe breast pain can be chronic and relapsing, and may require pharmacologic treatment.

Nonpharmacologic Therapies Reassurance is the first-line treatment for mastalgia; this practice has been found to be effective for as many as 85% of women, with more success in women with mild or moderate symptoms than those with severe mastalgia (Barros, Mottola, Ruiz, Borges, & Pinotti, 1999). Wearing a supportive bra is frequently recommended and was shown to be more effective than pharmacologic therapy in one study (Hadi, 2000). Reductions in caffeine and dietary fat have shown mixed results; however, neither of these dietary recommendations is likely to be harmful, and they may have other health benefits as well (Olawaiye et al., 2005). Supplementation with vitamins A, B, or E has not consistently demonstrated effectiveness in relieving mastalgia (Gumm, Cunnick, & Mokbel, 2004; Millet & Dirbas, 2002).

Pharmacologic Therapies Modifying the dose or route of HT may be helpful in reducing breast pain in a woman who is postmenopausal. Some women report increased mastalgia with use of hormonal contraception. Trying a different contraceptive method or delivery system, such as changing from combined oral contraceptives to a nonoral combined method (i.e., the ring or patch), may prove helpful in reducing pain. Conversely, some women report an improvement in mastalgia with use of hormonal contraception.

Danazol, tamoxifen, and bromocriptine are the primary pharmacologic therapies for mastalgia, and a meta-analysis of randomized trials found that all three of these medications offer significant relief from mastalgia (Srivastava et al., 2007). All of these medications can produce significant side effects, however, and relapses after discontinuation of therapy are common (Olawaiye et al., 2005). Danazol is the only medication approved by the U.S. Food and Drug Administration (FDA) for the treatment of mastalgia as of this writing. In a recent randomized trial that compared cabergoline with bromocriptine in 140 women with premenstrual mastalgia, researchers found that two-thirds of participants responded positively to treatment (66.6% in the bromocriptine group and 68.4% in the cabergoline group), but women in the cabergoline group had significantly less vomiting, nausea, and headache (Aydin, Atis, Kaleli, Uluga, & Goker, 2010).

Localized therapies have also been evaluated for the treatment of mastalgia. Topical use of the NSAID diclofenac diethyl ammonium gel three times daily for six months was found to be superior to a placebo for relieving the pain of both cyclical and noncyclical mastalgia in one study (Colak, Ipek, Kanik, Ogetman, & Aydin, 2003). In another study, women with noncyclical mastalgia were offered injection of 1 mL of 2% lidocaine and 40 mg of methyl prednisone at the area of maximum tenderness. Participants who were given an injection experienced greater relief of symptoms than those who were treated with either reassurance or oral or topical NSAIDs. Recurrence of symptoms occurred in 16% of the women who had an injection, and all elected to receive a second injection (Khan, Rampaul, & Blamey, 2004).

Complementary and Alternative Therapies The herbal product known as evening primrose oil (EPO) is frequently recommended for the treatment of mastalgia; however, a meta-analysis of four randomized controlled trials found EPO to be ineffective compared to placebo (Srivastava et al., 2007). The herbal treatment *Agnus castus* appears to be effective for many women with cyclic mastalgia and is well tolerated (Carmichael, 2007). Isoflavones—naturally occurring phytoestrogens—have also been proposed as a treatment for mastalgia. A small, randomized, controlled trial found that women taking isoflavones had a greater reduction in pain than women taking a placebo (Ingram, Hickling, West, Mahe, & Dunbar, 2002).

Surgical Therapies Surgery is rarely indicated in the treatment of mastalgia. Potential surgical candidates include women with macromastia whose symptoms warrant reduction mammoplasty and women with refractory mastalgia who resort to mastectomy after nonsurgical options have been unsuccessful. Mastectomy should be reserved for refractory cases and may not be curative (Davies, Cochrane, Stansfield, Sweetland, & Mansel, 1999; Salgado, Mardini, & Chen, 2005). As with any surgery, the risks and benefits of the procedure must be considered.

Special Considerations

Mastalgia is common during pregnancy and lactation. In such cases, the pain is attributed to the proliferation of breast tissue and hormonal influences on that tissue. Mastitis is the most likely diagnosis when breast pain in a lactating woman is accompanied by inflammation, chills, myalgia, and fever. Mastitis is estimated to occur in as many as 33% of breastfeeding mothers (Barbosa-Cesnik, Schwartz, & Foxman, 2003). Abscesses can also develop and should be suspected when mastitis is unresponsive to antibiotic therapy and the breast pain is worsening.

Nipple Discharge

Nipple discharge is another breast symptom that causes women to seek care, although its incidence in the general population is unknown. Concern can range from minor embarrassment to fear and anxiety about underlying pathology. Nipple discharge can be classified as normal lactation; galactorrhea unrelated to childbearing; and non-milky discharge, which is sometimes referred to as pathologic discharge (Pearlman & Griffin, 2010). Non-milky discharge that is spontaneous, unilateral, from a single duct (uniductal), and clear or bloody in color, is more likely to be associated with cancer than discharge that occurs with nipple manipulation (squeezing the nipple), is bilateral, comes from multiple ducts (multiductal), and is white, yellow, green, brown, or black in color (Rodden, 2009). (See **Color Plate 9** for an example of nipple discharge.) Nipple discharge is usually the result of a benign process, but malignancy must always be considered in the evaluation.

Etiology, Pathophysiology, and Clinical Presentation

Numerous etiologies of nipple discharge exist. Among the most common are pregnancy and lactation, galactorrhea, intraductal papilloma, mammary duct ectasia, and cancer. During pregnancy, women begin having bilateral, milky discharge that can continue as long as one year after birth or stopping breastfeeding. Clear nipple discharge during pregnancy, particularly in the third trimester, usually consists of colostrum. Bloody nipple discharge during pregnancy or lactation can occur as well, as a result of the increased vascularity of the breasts and changes in the epithelium (Sabate et al., 2007); however, evaluation is warranted if bloody discharge during pregnancy or lactation is unilateral or lasts more than 2 weeks (Pearlman & Griffin, 2010).

Galactorrhea is milky nipple discharge in a woman who has not been pregnant or lactated in the last 12 months. This type of discharge is usually bilateral and multiductal, and it may occur spontaneously or only with nipple or breast manipulation. Galactorrhea is not caused by breast pathology (Hussain, Policarpio, & Vincent, 2006; Pearlman & Griffin, 2010). Instead, it results from hyperprolactinemia, which may be caused by pituitary prolactin-secreting tumors, medications, hypothyroidism, stress, trauma, chronic renal failure, hypothalamic lesions, previous thoracotomy, and herpes zoster. In addition to galactorrhea, pituitary tumors can cause headaches and visual disturbances. Numerous medications can cause galactorrhea, including combined contraceptives containing estrogen and progestin, phenothiazines and other antipsychotics, tricyclic antidepressants, selective serotonin reuptake inhibitors, monoamine oxidase inhibitors, metoclopramide, domperidone, methadone, methyldopa, reserpine, verapamil, cimetidine, calcium-channel blockers, and amphetamines (Hussain et al.; Pearlman & Griffin; Rodden, 2009). Hyperprolactinemia can also interfere with the normal menstrual cycle, resulting in anovulation, oligomenorrhea or amenorrhea, and infertility (Fritz & Speroff, 2011).

Intraductal papilloma and mammary duct ectasia are the most common causes of nonmilky nipple discharge. Intraductal papilloma occurs most frequently in women aged 45 to 50 and results from a small, benign growth in the duct. The discharge is typically bloody, unilateral, and uniductal (Hussain et al., 2006). Mammary duct ectasia usually occurs in women older than age 50 and results from dilation of the ducts with surrounding inflammation and fibrosis. Nipple discharge with mammary duct ectasia is typically bilateral; multiductal; and green, brown, or black in color (Falkenberry, 2002; Hussain et al.). Both intraductal papilloma and mammary duct ectasia may be accompanied by a palpable mass.

While women with nipple discharge are often concerned they have cancer, such pathology is the least likely etiology, although it certainly must be considered carefully during assessment. Cancer is more likely if the nipple discharge is accompanied by a palpable mass or abnormal mammogram, and the woman is older than age 50 (Hussain et al., 2006). Approximately 10% to 15% of women with nipple discharge have breast cancer (Hussain et al.).

Assessment

History Ask the woman about the duration and color of her nipple discharge, as well as whether it occurs spontaneously or only with manipulation of the nipple or breast, whether it is unilateral or bilateral, and whether it comes from one or more ducts. Review the medications she is taking and determine whether any of these agents could be causing galactorrhea. Note other breast symptoms, such as mastalgia or breast mass, and identify any history of any type of breast disease or surgery. Ask about symptoms of hypothyroidism (e.g., fatigue, weight gain, cold intolerance), hyperthyroidism (e.g., nervousness, weight loss despite increased appetite, heat intolerance), pituitary tumor (e.g., headaches, visual problems), and hyperprolactinemia (e.g., irregular menses, infertility, decreased libido) (Hussain et al., 2006). Menstrual, pregnancy, lactation, general medical, and family histories should be obtained. Any family history of breast and ovarian cancer should be noted.

Physical Examination Perform a comprehensive breast examination that includes inspection and palpation with the woman in both the upright and supine positions, and palpation of the lymph nodes (see Chapter 6). If the nipple discharge is able to be reproduced, note the color, consistency, unilateral versus bilateral locations, and the number of ducts involved.

Assess for skin changes, breast masses, and tenderness. Additional examination may be warranted based on the patient's history, such as thyroid palpation if symptoms of a thyroid disorder are present or examination of the visual fields for women with galactorrhea who are not pregnant or breastfeeding.

Diagnostic Testing If the woman has bilateral, milky discharge, perform a pregnancy test. If this test is negative, obtain a serum prolactin level and thyroid-stimulating hormone (TSH) measurement (Pearlman & Griffin, 2010). If hyperprolactinemia is present, imaging of the sella turcica with magnetic resonance imaging (MRI) should be performed to rule out a pituitary prolactin-secreting tumor (Fritz & Speroff, 2011).

Evaluation of the woman with a non-milky discharge depends on the presence or absence of a mass and characteristics of the discharge (Pearlman & Griffin, 2010). When a palpable mass is present, it should be evaluated as described later in this chapter. If the discharge is spontaneous, unilateral, uniductal, and reproducible on examination, a mammogram and ultrasound should be performed (Pearlman & Griffin). Additional evaluation is based on imaging findings. If the discharge occurs only with manipulation, is multiductal, and is yellow, green, gray, or black in color, the woman can be observed and advised to avoid nipple stimulation, with a follow-up examination in 3 to 4 months. Women fitting this description should have mammography if they are 40 years or older and not had a mammogram in the past year (Pearlman & Griffin).

Guaiac testing and cytology are generally not recommended because they do not change the management of galactorrhea (Pearlman & Griffin, 2010). Additional diagnostic modalities that assist in ruling out malignancy include duct excision, ductoscopy, and ductography. Excision of the affected duct or ducts allows for definitive evaluation and may also be therapeutic. A fiber-optic ductoscope can be used to visualize the ducts and may prove helpful both in the diagnosis and as a guide for duct excision (Hussain et al., 2006). Ductography allows visualization of the ductal pattern through the use of dye instilled into the nipple. This test may reveal a filling defect that is due to carcinoma, papilloma, or other blockage. Although visualization of a filling defect in the duct may be helpful, the information does not significantly change the management of nipple discharge (Pearlman & Griffin). The limited availability of ductoscopy and ductography may preclude their use.

Differential Diagnoses

In addition to the conditions already described, sexual stimulation, infection or abscess, and Paget's disease (described in the section on breast cancer later in this chapter) can cause nipple discharge.

Management

Women who express colostrum during pregnancy should be reassured that the discharge is benign and advised that avoiding nipple stimulation will generally cause the discharge to resolve. The treatment of galactorrhea unrelated to pregnancy or lactation depends on the etiology. Pituitary tumors may be treated surgically, with medications, or expectantly in certain circumstances (Fritz & Speroff, 2011). Discontinuing a medication that causes galactorrhea or treating hypothyroidism if it is present may resolve the galactorrhea. Bromocriptine and cabergoline can be used to treat galactorrhea, but symptoms often recur upon discontinuation of these medications; thus long-term therapy is usually required (Fritz & Speroff). Intraductal papilloma is treated with duct excision (Pearlman & Griffin, 2010). Mammary duct ectasia can be expectantly managed or surgically treated with removal of the subareolar duct system, if symptoms are severe. If breast cancer is diagnosed, appropriate management should be initiated according to the disease stage, as is discussed in the breast cancer section later in this chapter.

Benign Breast Masses

A breast mass can be alarming for the woman as well as her clinician. Fortunately, most breast masses are benign; however, malignancy must always be considered in the evaluation of a breast mass. The likelihood of malignancy increases with age and risk factors for breast cancer, which are detailed in the breast cancer section later in this chapter.

Incidence, Etiology, and Clinical Presentation

The most common benign breast masses are fibroadenomas and cysts. Lipomas, fat necroses, phyllodes tumors, hamartomas, and galactoceles may also be encountered.

Fibroadenomas, which are composed of dense epithelial and fibroblastic tissue, are usually nontender, encapsulated, round, movable and firm. They are the most common type of breast mass in adolescents and young women. Their incidence decreases with increasing age, but they still account for 12% of masses in menopausal women (Pearlman & Griffin, 2010). Multiple fibroadenomas occur in 10% to 15% of cases (Miltenburg & Speights, 2008). A proposed etiology for formation of these masses is the effect of estrogen on susceptible tissue (Marchant, 2002).

Cysts are fluid-filled masses that are most commonly found in women 35 to 50 years of age (Berg, Sechtin, Marques, & Zhang, 2010). They are thought to result from cystic lobular involution (Marchant, 2002).

A lipoma is an area of fatty tissue that may occur in the breast or other areas of the body, including the arms, legs, and abdomen. Lipomas typically occur in the later reproductive years (Marchant, 2002). Fat necrosis is usually the result of trauma to the breast, whether as a result of external force against the tissue or subsequent to surgical manipulation of tissue (Miltenburg & Speights, 2008).

Phyllodes tumors form from periductal stromal cells of the breast and present as a firm, palpable mass. These typically large and fast-growing masses account for less than 1% of all breast neoplasms. Phyllodes tumors can range from a benign mass to a sarcoma, and they are usually seen in women aged 30 to 50 years (Pearlman & Griffin, 2010). Hamartomas are composed of glandular tissue, fat, and fibrous connective tissue, and the average age at presentation is 45 years (Lee, Sheen-Chen, Chi, Huang, & Ko, 2008).

Galactoceles are milk-filled cysts that usually occur during or after lactation. Galactoceles result from duct dilation and often have an inflammatory component (Sabate et al., 2007). See **Color Plate 10** for an example of a breast mass.

Assessment

A woman may present with a breast mass found on self-examination, or a mass may be discovered on clinical breast examination.

History If the woman found the mass, determine when she first noticed it and any changes she has noticed since that time. Ask about other breast symptoms, such as mastalgia or nipple discharge, and determine whether the woman has a history of any type of breast disease or surgery. Menstrual, pregnancy, lactation, and general medical histories should be taken. A family history of breast and ovarian cancer is particularly important.

Physical Examination Perform a comprehensive breast examination that includes inspection and palpation with the woman in both the upright and supine positions, and evaluation of the lymph nodes (see Chapter 6). If a mass is palpable, identify the size in centimeters, the shape, and the consistency or texture. Determine whether the mass is discrete (well-delineated, distinct edges) or poorly differentiated, tender to palpation, and mobile or fixed. Assess for skin changes, nipple discharge, and lymphadenopathy. When documenting the location of a mass, it may be helpful to draw a sketch of the breast with the site of the mass marked or to describe the position of the mass on the breast relative to a clock face, such as "at seven o'clock." Typical physical examination findings for benign breast masses are described in **Table 16-2**.

Diagnostic Testing If the physical examination suggests a benign mass, order an ultrasound if the patient is younger than age 30, and a mammogram with or without an ultrasound if she is 30 years or older. If the mass is suspicious on physical examination, order a mammogram and ultrasound (Pearlman & Griffin, 2010). Ultrasound helps to distinguish a cystic mass from a solid mass, but is not as accurate as tissue sampling. Mammography can be used to detect nonpalpable abnormalities if a woman is of appropriate screening age or has a solid mass. Palpable breast masses may not be visible with diagnostic imaging tests, however, so these tests cannot rule out malignancy.

Biopsy is required to definitively ascertain whether a mass is solid versus cystic, and benign versus malignant. A fine-needle aspiration (FNA) biopsy is a minimally invasive way to differentiate solid and cystic masses, and provides cytologic evaluation of a palpable mass. FNA biopsy may also be therapeutic if the mass is filled with fluid. Tissue sample findings for benign breast masses are described in Table 16-2. If cytologic evaluation does not yield definitive findings, a more invasive method of tissue sampling (**Table 16-3**) is required to

TABLE 16-2 Features of Benign Breast Masses

Type of Mass	Typical Physical Examination Findings	Tissue Sampling Findings
Fibroadenoma	Discrete, smooth, round or oval, nontender, mobile	Ductal epithelium, dense stroma, numerous elongated nuclei without fat
Cyst	Discrete, tender, mobile, size may fluctuate with the menstrual cycle	Cyst fluid and inflammation
Lipoma	Discrete, soft, nontender, may or may not be mobile	Fatty tissue
Fat necrosis	Ill defined, firm, nontender, nonmobile	Necrotic fat with inflammation
Phyllodes tumor	Discrete, firm, round, mobile, findings similar to a fibroadenoma but mass is usually larger, may observe stretching of skin due to rapid tumor growth	Stromal hypercellularity with glandular and ductal elements
Hamartoma	Discrete, nontender, nonmobile, may be nonpalpable with incidental diagnosis on imaging studies	Glandular tissue, fat, and fibrous connective tissue
Galactocele	Discrete, firm, sometimes tender	Fat globules

rule out breast cancer or to determine the type of tumor if the mass is benign (Kerlikowske, Smith-Bindman, Ljung, & Grady, 2003).

Differential Diagnoses

In addition to the types of breast masses already discussed, differential diagnoses for breast masses include fibrocystic changes, infection or abscess, and malignancy. Women with fibrocystic breast tissue may present having found what is perceived as a mass, though these changes are typically associated with nodularity or thickening rather than a discrete mass.

Management

Management of benign breast masses depends on the type of mass. A fibroadenoma that has been definitively diagnosed by cytologic analysis does not need to be removed. Instead, it can be expectantly managed and removed only if the mass becomes enlarged (Miltenburg

TABLE 16-3 Breast Tissue Sampling Procedures

Procedure	Description	Breast Target
Fine-needle aspiration biopsy	• Tissue for cytologic evaluation aspirated with a small needle • Differentiates solid and cystic masses	Palpable breast mass or thickening
Stereotactic core needle biopsy	• Large-bore needle used to obtain cores of tissue for histologic examination • Stereotactic mammography used for localization and targeting	Density or calcification seen on mammogram
Ultrasound-guided core needle biopsy	• Large-bore needle used to obtain cores of tissue for histologic examination • Ultrasound used for localization and targeting	Solid lesion seen on ultrasound
Magnetic resonance imaging (MRI)–guided needle biopsy	• MRI with intravenous contrast material used for localization and targeting	Lesions visible only with MRI
Needle-localized breast biopsy	• Use of a wire to localize an occult mammographic abnormality prior to excisional biopsy	Density or calcification seen on mammogram in a location that cannot be effectively assessed with core biopsy
Excisional breast biopsy	• Surgical procedure that requires a skin excision • Mass or mammographic abnormality is removed with a surrounding margin of normal-appearing tissue	Palpable breast mass, thickening or skin change Only used for initial diagnosis when needle biopsy is not feasible

& Speights, 2008). Fibroadenomas usually decrease in size over time, and many resolve completely (American College of Obstetricians and Gynecologists, 2006).

Asymptomatic cysts do not require intervention. Aspiration can be used to treat large or painful cysts (Berg et al., 2010).

Excision of a lipoma is not required if a breast mass is consistent with lipoma on clinical examination and tissue sampling, and if there are no suspicious findings at the site on mammography and ultrasound. If these conditions are not met, then excision should be performed (Lanng, Eriksen, & Hoffman, 2004). Fat necroses typically resolve spontaneously (Miltenburg & Speights, 2008).

Excisional biopsy is recommended for suspected phyllodes tumor, and typically a wide margin of normal surrounding tissue is also removed due to the tendency for such masses to recur (Pearlman & Griffin, 2010). Hamartomas may require excision for diagnosis, but otherwise do not have to be removed and may be expectantly managed. Aspiration of a galactocele allows for diagnosis and treatment (Sabate et al., 2007).

When benign breast masses are expectantly managed, the patient should be advised to report any new symptoms and encouraged to follow up with her clinician for examinations and diagnostic testing as recommended.

Special Considerations

Adolescents In approximately two-thirds of adolescents presenting with a breast mass, the diagnosis is a fibroadenoma. Ultrasound is the best diagnostic imaging test for this age group. Mammography is not indicated, and aspiration for diagnostic purposes should be avoided (American College of Obstetricians and Gynecologists, 2006). Breast cancer in women younger than 20 years of age is very rare (American College of Obstetricians and Gynecologists).

Pregnant and Lactating Women Evaluation of palpable findings in pregnant and lactating women is complicated by the complex breast parenchyma. Nevertheless, appropriate diagnostic imaging and breast tissue sampling should not be deferred, with the exception of mammography, which is not generally used during pregnancy because physiologic changes in the breast result in poor sensitivity for such imaging (Sabate et al., 2007). Fibroadenomas may increase in size and become symptomatic during pregnancy (Sabate et al.).

Older Women The likelihood of malignancy increases with age. Among women aged 55 years and older, 85% of breast masses are malignant. Masses in postmenopausal women are presumed malignant until proven otherwise (Osuch, 2002).

Breast Cancer

Breast cancer is one of the most feared diseases among women, even though treatment of this condition has become increasingly successful in prolonging women's lives after diagnosis. From the Halsted radical mastectomy of the 1890s to breast-sparing surgery in conjunction with other treatment modalities, the management of breast cancer has evolved dramatically over time. With increased public awareness and earlier detection, comprehensive treatment can be initiated promptly for this disease process.

Incidence

More than 230,000 new cases of invasive breast cancer and more than 55,000 new cases of in situ breast cancer are diagnosed in women in the United States each year (American Cancer

Society [ACS], 2011). A woman's lifetime risk of being diagnosed with breast cancer is 1 in 8 (Feuer et al., 1993). The risk increases gradually with age, from 1 in 233 for women ages 30 to 39 to 1 in 29 for women ages 60 to 69 (National Cancer Institute, 2010a). Breast cancer is the second leading cause, after lung cancer, of cancer deaths in women (ACS).

Etiology

Two challenging aspects of breast cancer are that many of the risk factors are nonmodifiable, and that most women with breast cancer (85%) have no identifiable risk factors other than age (Fritz & Speroff, 2011). Known risk factors for developing breast cancer are listed in **Box 16-1**.

The discovery of the *BRCA1* and *BRCA2* genetic mutations was a monumental step in the understanding of breast cancer, because mutations of these genes account for 5% to 10% of breast cancer cases (ACS, 2011). These mutations are also associated with an increased

---

BOX 16-1 *Risk Factors for Breast Cancer*

Female

Advancing age

Early menarche (before age 12 years)

Late menopause (after age 55 years)

Current combined oral contraceptive use (likely due to detection bias of regular screening)

Use of combined estrogen and progestogen hormone therapy

Nulliparity

First pregnancy after the age of 30 years

High breast tissue density

High bone mineral density

Biopsy-confirmed hyperplasia

High-dose radiation to chest, typically related to cancer treatment

Personal history of breast cancer

Family history of breast cancer

Inherited genetic mutations (less than 1% of the population)

Weight gain after age 18 years

Being overweight or obese

Physical inactivity

Consumption of one or more alcoholic beverages per day

Sources: Adapted from American Cancer Society, 2011; Fritz & Speroff, 2011.

risk of developing ovarian cancer. The risk of ovarian cancer is 39% to 46% in women with the *BRCA1* mutation and 12% to 20% in women with the *BRCA2* mutation (American College of Obstetricians and Gynecologists, 2009). Given the growing knowledge base about the genetic link to the development of breast cancer, the genetic counselor has a significant role working in collaboration with the medical team in the care of women with breast cancer.

Other potential risk factors for breast cancer include cigarette smoking and shift work, particularly at night (ACS, 2011). Studies have yielded conflicting results about other putative risk factors, and research in this area is ongoing. Although sometimes cited as a risk factor, induced abortion does not increase the risk of breast cancer (Beral et al., 2004). Breastfeeding protects a woman from developing breast cancer, and this effect increases with longer duration of lactation (Collaborative Group on Hormonal Factors in Breast Cancer, 2002). Moderate or vigorous physical activity and maintaining a normal weight are also protective against breast cancer (ACS, 2011).

Pathophysiology

Breast cancer occurs when there is erratic cell growth and proliferation in the breast tissue. Which hormones are most critical in the development of breast cancer and why a large percentage of women who develop breast cancer have no identified risk factors remain unclear (Donegan & Spratt, 2002). While the discovery of pertinent genetic factors has clarified the predisposition toward developing breast cancer in some women, there remains a significant amount of ongoing research dedicated to understanding more about the development of this disease.

Clinical Presentation and Types of Breast Cancer

Breast cancer may be detected by identification of a palpable lesion or by screening mammography. Skin changes can also be the initial manifestation of breast cancer. The types of breast cancer include carcinoma in situ, invasive breast cancer, Paget's disease, and inflammatory carcinoma. Breast cancer is further classified based on whether it originated in the ducts or lobules (see Chapter 5 for a discussion of breast anatomy and physiology).

Carcinoma in Situ Ductal carcinoma in situ (DCIS), or intraductal carcinoma, is the earliest manifestation of breast cancer and involves abnormal cells that are confined to the ducts. This condition is usually diagnosed in association with microcalcifications seen on mammography; it is rare to find a palpable mass in such cases. DCIS is sometimes referred to as a precancerous condition, although the likelihood of DCIS progressing to invasive cancer is unknown.

With lobular carcinoma in situ (LCIS), the abnormal cells are limited to the breast lobules. LCIS is a noninvasive lesion that does not always progress to invasive cancer; thus the term *lobular neoplasia* is often recommended to describe this condition. LCIS may be bilateral and is often an incidental finding noted during biopsy for another lesion (Simpson, Reis-Filho, & Lakhani, 2010).

Invasive Breast Cancer Invasive or infiltrating ductal carcinoma is the most common malignancy of the breast. Invasive ductal carcinoma usually presents as a discrete, solid mass with malignant cells escaping the confines of the ducts and infiltrating the breast parenchyma. The most common sites of metastatic spread of invasive breast cancer are the lymph nodes, bones, liver, and lungs (Meisner et al., 2008).

Invasive or infiltrating lobular carcinoma is less common and may present as a discrete mass. The mass may be characterized only by thickening or induration, with margins that are diffuse and ill defined, both on physical examination and on mammogram. Invasive lobular carcinoma is characterized by bilateral involvement more frequently than other types of breast cancer and is associated with unusual spread of metastases, including carcinomatous meningitis, intra-abdominal metastases with intestinal and ureteral obstruction, and metastases to the uterus and ovaries (Dillon, Guidi, & Schnitt, 2010).

Paget's Disease Paget's disease is a rare form of breast cancer that causes eczematous nipple changes as well as ulceration, itching, erythema, and nipple discharge. As many as half of all women with Paget's disease present with a palpable mass that is usually an underlying DCIS or invasive ductal carcinoma. Controversy exists regarding whether the nipple involvement arises from infiltration from an underlying breast tumor or is a separate process involving the nipple epidermis (Hansen, 2010).

Inflammatory Carcinoma Inflammatory breast carcinoma is a rapidly progressive type of breast cancer. This type of carcinoma causes diffuse inflammatory changes of the breast skin with erythema, edema, warmth, skin thickening, and peau d'orange (fine dimpling that makes the breast skin appear similar to the skin of an orange). There may or may not be a distinct palpable mass (Merajver, Iniesta, & Sabel, 2010).

Assessment

History The initial history for a woman with a breast mass is the same as that described in the earlier section on benign breast masses. If the cancer is already diagnosed and classified as a T3 or T4 lesion (**Table 16-4**), the woman should be asked about symptoms of metastases such as bone pain, arthralgias, cough, jaundice, abdominal pain, headaches, visual disturbances, malaise, loss of appetite, weight loss, fever, and fatigue. Clinicians should remain vigilant for symptoms of metastases in any woman with a history of breast cancer.

Physical Examination Perform a comprehensive breast examination (see Chapter 6). Note any skin changes, palpable masses, and nipple discharge. A suspicious lesion is usually hard, is painless, and has irregular borders that may be immobile and fixed to the skin or sur-

TABLE 16-4 TNM Classification of Breast Cancers

Primary Tumor (T)	
TX	Primary tumor cannot be assessed
T0	No evidence of primary tumor
Tis	Carcinoma in situ: ductal carcinoma in situ, lobular carcinoma in situ, or Paget's disease of the nipple with no associated invasive carcinoma or carcinoma in situ (Paget's disease with a tumor is classified according to tumor size)
T1	Tumor 2 cm or smaller in greatest dimension (may be subdivided into T1mi, T1a, T1b, and T1c depending on the exact size of the tumor)
T2	Tumor larger than 2 cm but not larger than 5 cm in greatest dimension
T3	Tumor larger than 5 cm in greatest dimension
T4	Tumor of any size with direct extension to the chest wall (T4a), skin (T4b), or both (T4c); inflammatory carcinoma (T4d)
Regional Lymph Nodes (N)	
NX	Regional lymph nodes cannot be assessed (e.g., previously removed)
N0	No regional lymph node metastases
N1	Metastases in movable ipsilateral axillary node(s)
N2	Metastases in ipsilateral axillary lymph nodes that are clinically fixed or matted (N2a), or in clinically detected (by imaging studies or clinical examination) ipsilateral internal mammary nodes in the absence of clinically evident axillary lymph node metastases (N2b)
N3	Metastases in ipsilateral infraclavicular lymph node(s) with or without axillary lymph node involvement (N3a), or in clinically detected (by imaging studies or clinical examination) apparent ipsilateral internal mammary lymph node(s) with clinically evident axillary lymph node metastasis (N3b), or metastases in ipsilateral supraclavicular lymph node(s) with or without axillary or internal mammary lymph node involvement (N3c)
Distant Metastases (M)	
M0	No clinical or radiographic evidence of distant metastases
M1	Distant detectable metastases

Source: Adapted from Edge et al., 2010.

rounding breast tissue. Palpate for the axillary, cervical, and supraclavicular lymph nodes. Enlargement of any of these nodes is suspicious. Examination of the lungs, abdomen, and neurologic system should also be performed to detect signs of metastases.

Diagnostic Testing Diagnostic testing for breast cancer includes imaging studies and tissue sampling. The diagnostic imaging tests most frequently used in the evaluation of breast cancer are mammography and ultrasound (Table 16-1).

Mammography can identify breast cancers that are too small to palpate on physical examination. Mammograms can also detect both benign and malignant calcifications. Benign calcifications are identified by their large, coarse, and scattered appearance. Malignant-appearing calcifications are much smaller, appearing as grains of sand. With digital mammography, a wider range of tissue contrast can be seen, subtle contrast differences can be amplified, and the images are immediately available. Mammography also identifies densities that ultrasound can further characterize as solid or fluid filled. Solid masses require further intervention, whereas simple fluid-filled cysts generally do not.

MRI is recommended for screening women at high risk for breast cancer (20% to 25% or greater lifetime risk), but evidence does not support the use of this modality for screening women at average risk (Griffin & Pearlman, 2010; Saslow et al., 2007). MRI is helpful in identifying occult breast cancer when there are axillary node metastases but no visible carcinoma on mammogram or ultrasound. This imaging technology can also assist with staging and therapy evaluation (National Comprehensive Cancer Network, 2011). MRI should be used judiciously due to its expense, high false-positive rate, and the fact that it may be unnecessary depending on findings of other imaging studies.

Breast tissue sampling procedures are described in Table 16-3.

Further Assessment When Breast Cancer Is Diagnosed Several factors guide appropriate treatment options and also serve as prognostic indicators when breast cancer is diagnosed. Malignancies are staged using the TNM system, which refers to the size of tumor, lymph node involvement, and metastatic spread (Table 16-4). Tumors can be graded and are also assessed for estrogen and progesterone receptors (ER/PR) and *HER2/neu*. The *HER2/neu* oncogene is closely related to the human epidermal growth factor. Grading the tumor indicates its differentiation, or how closely the cells resemble normal tissue. A well-differentiated tumor has a more favorable prognosis than a poorly differentiated lesion (Chang & Hilsenbeck, 2010). ER/PR-positive tumors are more likely to respond to hormonal manipulation, whereas ER/PR-negative tumors have a less favorable prognosis (Chang & Hilsenbeck). Overexpression of *HER2*, which occurs in 20% to 25% of breast cancers, is associated with more aggressive tumor cells and a poorer prognosis (Yaziji et al., 2004).

The status of the axillary lymph nodes is critical in determining treatment options for women with invasive breast cancer. For those patients with early-stage tumors less than 5 cm in size and no palpable axillary lymph nodes, the sentinel node biopsy provides necessary staging information without the associated morbidities of a full dissection, such as lymphedema, immobility of the upper extremity, and accompanying diminished quality of life. With this technique, dye is injected into the region surrounding the tumor to identify the first node draining the breast. This node, which is termed the sentinel axillary node, is then removed (Hsueh, Hansen, & Giuliano, 2000). If the sentinel node is positive, dissection of the Level I and II axillary lymph nodes is needed, although FNA or core biopsy should be considered first to confirm malignancy and the need for dissection (National Comprehensive Cancer Network, 2011).

Additional tests are performed to detect metastases. These routinely include a complete blood count, liver function tests, and a chest radiograph. Brain imaging, a bone scan, and abdominal computed tomography (CT), MRI, or ultrasound are not routine but may be warranted if metastases are suspected due to the tumor's clinical stage or signs and symptoms (National Comprehensive Cancer Network, 2011). Positron emission tomography (PET) scan may also be indicated when considering metastatic disease.

Differential Diagnoses

A palpable breast mass can be caused by any of the benign conditions discussed earlier in this chapter. The most likely differential diagnosis for invasive lobular carcinoma is fibrocystic disease. The differential diagnoses for Paget's disease include eczema, psoriasis, contact dermatitis, and, rarely, squamous cell carcinoma in situ arising in the skin (Bowen's disease). The differential diagnoses for inflammatory carcinoma include breast abscess, infection, and mastitis. The presence of any of these conditions in a woman who is not lactating is highly suspicious for malignancy.

Prevention

Two selective estrogen receptor modulators (SERMs), tamoxifen (Nolvadex) and raloxifene (Evista), as well as aromatase inhibitors, such as anastrazole (Arimidex), are used to prevent breast cancer in women who are at high risk for developing the disease; this indication is known as preventive therapy or chemoprevention (Cuzick et al., 2011; Vogel et al., 2006). All of these medications have potentially serious side effects, including thromboembolic events and endometrial cancer for SERMs and decreased bone mineral density that can increase fracture risk for aromatase inhibitors (National Cancer Institute, 2011a). Evidence supporting the use of particular agents is rapidly evolving, and the choice of agent should be made by an expert after careful consideration of patient factors and current data.

Those women who are at very high risk for breast cancer may elect to undergo prophylactic mastectomy. Salpingo-oophorectomy may also be performed in women with *BRCA1* or *BRCA2* mutations (National Comprehensive Cancer Network, 2011). The benefits of risk reduction and decreased anxiety about the possibility of developing cancer must be weighed with the risks of the surgery itself. Although it is uncommon, women must be advised that breast cancer can develop in the chest wall after prophylactic mastectomy (Dowdy, Stefanek, & Hartmann, 2004).

Management

Suspected or diagnosed breast cancer requires collaborative care with breast cancer specialists, such as a surgeon or medical oncologist. The primary treatment strategies for breast cancer include surgery, chemotherapy, radiation, hormonal therapy, and the monoclonal antibody trastuzumab (Herceptin). A combination of these modalities is often used, and the specific therapies employed must be individualized based on a variety of patient factors (e.g., cancer stage; age and menopausal status; ER, PR, and *HER2* results).

Breast-conserving surgery—that is, lumpectomy or partial mastectomy—removes the cancer but not the breast itself. In addition to removal of breast tissue alone (total or simple mastectomy), mastectomy may include removal of the breast and Level I and II lymph nodes (modified radical mastectomy). Radical mastectomy, which includes removal of the breast, pectoralis major and minor muscles, and Level I to III lymph nodes, is no longer performed, as it is associated with severe morbidities and does not offer any survival advantage over less radical surgery. Breast-conserving surgery may be performed instead of mastectomy depending on the disease stage. Studies comparing surgical treatment outcomes in women for 20 years after the procedures indicate that breast-conserving surgeries do not increase the future risk of death from recurrent disease when compared to mastectomy (Fisher et al., 2002; Veronesi et al., 2002). When mastectomy is performed, breast reconstruction is an option.

Chemotherapy may be administered after surgery (adjuvant therapy) or preoperatively (neoadjuvant therapy) to decrease the size of a large tumor prior to surgery. Radiation therapy is used regularly following breast-sparing surgery and may also be administered after mastectomy. In addition, radiation is useful for treatment of locally advanced disease of the chest wall or breast, for palliation for bone pain from bone metastases, or to strengthen a region that contains bony disease that is at risk for pathologic fracture.

The SERM tamoxifen and the aromatase inhibitors letrozole (Femara), exemestane (Aromasin), and anastrazole (Arimidex) are the hormonal therapies used in breast cancer treatment when ER/PR receptors are positive. The optimal duration of tamoxifen therapy appears to be five years, although studies regarding this aspect of care are ongoing (National Cancer Institute, 2011b).

Ductal Carcinoma in Situ Until recently, DCIS was treated with mastectomy, but this can be more radical surgery than is necessary for a carcinoma that may not progress to invasive carcinoma (Morrow & Harris, 2010). Current options for DCIS treatment include breast-conserving surgery, with or without radiation, and total mastectomy. Tamoxifen therapy after surgery may be recommended, especially for women who are ER positive. The treatment strategy depends on patient characteristics, the extent of disease, and patient preferences (Morrow & Harris; National Cancer Institute, 2011b; National Comprehensive Cancer Network, 2011).

Lobular Carcinoma in Situ Optimal management of LCIS must balance the fact that this condition is a risk factor for cancer yet is not malignant per se. Risk of cancer with LCIS is increased in both breasts (Kilbride & Newman, 2010). Treatment options include careful observation with clinical examination and mammography, preventive therapy/chemoprevention with tamoxifen, participation in breast cancer prevention trials, and bilateral prophylactic mastectomy for those patients deemed to be at high risk for breast cancer (Kilbride & Newman; National Cancer Institute, 2011b; National Comprehensive Cancer Network, 2011).

Invasive Breast Cancer Treatment of invasive carcinoma depends on multiple factors, including the size and grade of the tumor, the involvement of lymph nodes, the presence of metastases, first-time diagnosis versus recurrent disease, and the results of ER/PR and *HER2* testing. A combination of treatments including surgery, chemotherapy, radiation, hormone therapies, bisphosphonates such as zoledronic acid (Reclast, Zometa) and pamidronate (Aredia), and monoclonal antibodies (MAbs) may be used. FDA-approved MAbs for use in treatment of cancer include bevacizumab (Avastin), cetuximab (Erbitux), panitumumab (Vectibix), and trastuzumab (Herceptin). When the cancer has metastasized, the goal of treatment is control or palliative, rather than curative (National Cancer Institute, 2011b; National Comprehensive Cancer Network, 2011).

Paget's Disease Suspicion for Paget's disease should be high in any woman with nipple symptoms, as diagnosis of this disease is often delayed. Breast-conserving surgery with complete excision of the nipple and areola to clear margins, followed by radiation, is recommended if margins are negative. Mastectomy should be considered if the margins are positive or if disease is multicentric or extends beyond the central portion of the breast. Tamoxifen therapy after surgery may be recommended (Hansen, 2010; National Comprehensive Cancer Network, 2011). Use of zoledronic acid may also be useful in treatment of Paget's disease.

Inflammatory Carcinoma Women with signs and symptoms of inflammatory breast carcinoma may initially be treated with antibiotics. If a 7- to 10-day course of antibiotic coverage does not result in complete resolution of symptoms, or if the cutaneous findings are highly suspicious, immediate mammography and referral for skin biopsy are indicated. Treatment of inflammatory carcinoma involves multiple modalities including surgery, chemotherapy, radiation, hormonal therapy, aromatase inhibitors, and monoclonal antibodies (Merajver et al., 2010).

Emerging Evidence That May Change Practice

Recommendations regarding breast cancer screening, diagnostic techniques, and management are constantly evolving. A search of the National Cancer Institute's website in July 2011 identified more than 400 ongoing clinical trials related to breast cancer treatment alone. These trials will inevitably change clinical practice related to breast cancer, and clinicians must keep up-to-date with new developments. In addition, women at high risk for breast cancer, or who already have breast cancer, should be encouraged to participate in clinical trials, as these interventions are considered the best management (National Comprehensive Cancer Network, 2011).

Special Considerations

Pregnant Women The incidence of breast cancer in pregnancy is difficult to estimate. One of the largest attempts to date to study this issue involved a retrospective review that included more than 4.8 million births in California from 1991 to 1999. In this study, 1.93 per 10,000 women were diagnosed with breast cancer during pregnancy or up to 12 months postpartum (Smith, Danielsen, Allen, & Cress, 2003). The incidence of breast cancer in pregnant and postpartum women is likely to increase with the trend of delayed childbearing (National Cancer Institute, 2010a, 2010b).

Delays in diagnosis in this population are common because breast abnormalities can be difficult to detect in the presence of the normal breast changes that occur during pregnancy and lactation. Mammography, with appropriate abdominal shielding during pregnancy, and ultrasound are both appropriate technologies for evaluation of a mass or other abnormality on clinical examination (Litton & Theriault, 2010). Any palpable mass should be biopsied regardless of imaging results (Litton & Theriault; National Cancer Institute, 2010a).

Management of breast cancer during pregnancy must take into account the benefits and risks for both the mother and the fetus, and can involve making complex decisions. Surgery, either mastectomy or lumpectomy, can be performed during pregnancy. Chemotherapy can be used during the second and third trimesters but is stopped at 35 weeks or 3 weeks prior to planned birth. Radiation is contraindicated during pregnancy (Litton & Theriault, 2010; National Comprehensive Cancer Network, 2011)

References

Ader, D. N., & Browne, M. W. (1997). Prevalence and impact of cyclic mastalgia in a United States clinic-based sample. *American Journal of Obstetrics and Gynecology, 177*, 126–132.

Ader, D. N., South-Paul, J., Adera, T., & Deuster, P. A. (2001). Cyclical mastalgia: Prevalence and associated health and behavioral factors. *Journal of Psychosomatic Obstetrics and Gynecology, 22*, 71–76.

American Cancer Society (ACS). (2011). *Cancer facts and figures 2011.* Atlanta, GA: Author. Retrieved from http://www.cancer.org/Research/CancerFactsFigures/CancerFactsFigures/cancer-facts-figures-2011.

American College of Obstetricians and Gynecologists. (2006). Breast concerns in the adolescent. ACOG Committee Opinion No. 350. *Obstetrics & Gynecology, 108*, 1329–1336.

American College of Obstetricians and Gynecologists. (2009). Hereditary breast and ovarian cancer syndrome. ACOG Practice Bulletin No. 103. *Obstetrics & Gynecology, 113*, 957–966.

Aydin, Y., Atis, A., Kaleli, S., Uluga, S., & Goker, N. (2010). Cabergoline versus bromocriptine for symptomatic treatment of premenstrual mastalgia: A randomised, open-label study. *European Journal of Obstetrics & Gynecology and Reproductive Biology, 150*, 203–206.

Barbosa-Cesnik, C., Schwartz, K., & Foxman, B. (2003). Lactation mastitis. *Journal of the American Medical Association, 289*, 1609–1612.

Barros, A. C., Mottola, J., Ruiz, C. A., Borges, M. N., & Pinotti, J. A. (1999). Reassurance in the treatment of mastalgia. *Breast Journal, 5*, 162–165.

Beral, V., Bull, D., Doll, R., Peto, R., Reeves, G., & Collaborative Group on Hormonal Factors in Breast Cancer. (2004). Breast cancer and abortion: Collaborative reanalysis of data from 53 epidemiological studies, including 83,000 women with breast cancer from 16 countries. *Lancet, 363*, 1007–1016.

Berg, W. A., Sechtin, A. G., Marques, H., & Zhang, Z. (2010). Cystic breast masses and the ACRIN 6666 experience. *Radiologic Clinics of North America, 48*(5), 931–987.

Carmichael, A. R. (2007). Can Vitex *Agnus castus* be used for the treatment of mastalgia? What is the current evidence? *Evidence-Based Complementary and Alternative Medicine, 5*, 247–250.

Carmichael, A. R., Bashayan, O., & Nightingale, P. (2005). Objective analyses of mastalgia in breast clinics: Is breast pain questionnaire a useful tool in a busy breast clinic? *The Breast, 15*, 498–502.

Chang, J. C., & Hilsenbeck, S. G. (2010). Prognostic and predictive markers. In J. R. Harris, M. E. Lippman, M. Morrow, & C. K. Osborne (Eds.), *Diseases of the breast* (4th ed., pp. 443–457). Philadelphia: Lippincott Williams & Wilkins.

Colak, T., Ipek, T., Kanik, A., Ogetman, Z., & Aydin, S. (2003). Efficacy of topical nonsteroidal antiinflammatory drugs in mastalgia treatment. *Journal of the American College of Surgeons, 196*, 525–530.

Collaborative Group on Hormonal Factors in Breast Cancer. (2002). Breast cancer and breastfeeding: Collaborative reanalysis of individual data from 47 epidemiological studies in 30 countries, including 50,302 women with breast cancer and 96,973 women without the disease. *Lancet, 360*, 187–195.

Cuzick, J., DeCensi, A., Arun, B., Brown, P. H., Castiglione, M., Dunn, B., et al. (2011). Preventive therapy for breast cancer: A consensus statement. *Lancet Oncology, 12*, 496–503.

Davies, E. L., Cochrane, R. A., Stansfield, K., Sweetland, H. M., & Mansel, R. E. (1999). Is there a role for surgery in the treatment of mastalgia? *The Breast, 8*, 285–288.

Dillon, D. A., Guidi, A. J., & Schnitt, S. J. (2010). Pathology of invasive breast cancer. In J. R. Harris, M. E. Lippman, M. Morrow, & C. K. Osborne (Eds.), *Diseases of the breast* (4th ed., pp. 374–407). Philadelphia: Lippincott Williams & Wilkins.

Donegan, W., & Spratt, J. (Eds.). (2002). *Cancer of the breast* (5th ed.). St. Louis, MO: Saunders.

Dowdy, S. C., Stefanek, M., & Hartmann, L. C. (2004). Surgical risk reduction: Prophylactic salpingo-oopherectomy and prophylactic mastectomy. *American Journal of Obstetrics and Gynecology, 191*, 1113–1123.

Edge, S. B., Byrd, D. R., Compton, C. C., Fritz, A. G., Greene, F. L., & Trotti, A. (2010). *AJCC cancer staging manual* (7th ed.). New York: Springer.

Falkenberry, S. S. (2002). Nipple discharge. *Obstetrics and Gynecology Clinics of North America, 29*, 21–29.

Feuer, E. G., Wun, L. M., Boring, C. C., Flanders, W. D., Timmel, M. J., & Tong, T. (1993). The lifetime risk of developing breast cancer. *Journal of the National Cancer Institute, 85*, 892–897.

Fisher, B., Anderson, S., Bryant, J., Margolese, R. G., Deutsch, M., Fisher E. R., et al. (2002). Twenty-year follow-up of a randomized trial comparing total mastectomy, lumpectomy, and lumpectomy plus irradiation for the treatment of invasive breast cancer. *New England Journal of Medicine, 347*, 1233–1242.

Fritz, M. A., & Speroff, L. (2011). *Clinical gynecologic endocrinology and infertility* (8th ed.). Baltimore: Lippincott Williams & Wilkins.

Griffin, J. L., & Pearlman, M. D. (2010). Breast cancer screening in women at average risk and high risk. *Obstetrics & Gynecology, 116*, 1410–1421.

Gumm, R., Cunnick, G. H., & Mokbel, K. (2004). Evidence for the management of mastalgia. *Current Medical Research and Opinion, 20*, 681–684.

Hadi, M. S. (2000). Sports brassiere: Is it a solution for mastalgia? *Breast Journal, 6*, 407–409.

Hansen, N. M. (2010). Paget's disease. In J. R. Harris, M. E. Lippman, M. Morrow, & C. K. Osborne (Eds.), *Diseases of the breast* (4th ed., pp. 793–799). Philadelphia: Lippincott Williams & Wilkins.

Hsueh, E., Hansen, N., & Giuliano, A. (2000). Intraoperative lymphatic mapping and sentinel lymph node dissection in breast cancer. *CA: A Cancer Journal for Clinicians, 50*, 279–288.

Hussain, A. N., Policarpio, C., & Vincent, M. T. (2006). Evaluating nipple discharge. *Obstetrical and Gynecological Survey, 61*(4), 278–283.

Ingram, D. M., Hickling, C., West, L., Mahe, L. J., & Dunbar, P. M. (2002). A double-blind randomized controlled trial of isoflavones in the treatment of cyclical mastalgia. *Breast, 11*, 170–174.

Jones, D. P. (2004). Cultural views of the female breast. *Association of Black Nursing Faculty Journal, 15*, 15–21.

Kerlikowske, K., Smith-Bindman, R., Ljung, B., & Grady, D. (2003). Evaluation of abnormal mammography results and palpable breast abnormalities. *Annals of Internal Medicine, 139*, 274–284.

Khan, H. N., Rampaul, R., & Blamey, R. W. (2004). Local anaesthetic and steroid combined injection therapy in the management of non-cyclical mastalgia. *The Breast, 13*, 129–132.

Kilbride, K. E., & Newman, L. A. (2010). Lobular carcinoma in situ: Clinical management. In J. R. Harris, M. E. Lippman, M. Morrow, & C. K. Osborne (Eds.), *Diseases of the breast* (4th ed., pp. 341–348). Philadelphia: Lippincott Williams & Wilkins.

Lanng, C., Eriksen, B. Ø., & Hoffman, J. (2004). Lipoma of the breast: A diagnostic dilemma. *The Breast, 13,* 408–411.

Lee, W., Sheen-Chen, S., Chi, S., Huang, H., & Ko, S. (2008). Hamartoma of the breast: An underrecognized disease? *Tumori, 94,* 114–115.

Litton, J. K., & Theriault, R. L. (2010). Breast cancer during pregnancy and subsequent pregnancy in breast cancer survivors. In J. R. Harris, M. E. Lippman, M. Morrow, & C. K. Osborne (Eds.), *Diseases of the breast* (4th ed., pp. 808–816). Philadelphia: Lippincott Williams & Wilkins.

Marchant, D. J. (2002). Benign breast disease. *Obstetrics and Gynecology Clinics of North America, 29,* 1–20.

Meisner, A. L. W., Fekrazad, M. H., & Royce, M. E. (2008). Breast disease: Benign and malignant. *Medical Clinics of North America, 92,* 1115–1151.

Merajver, S. D., Iniesta, M. D., & Sabel, M. S. (2010). Inflammatory breast cancer. In J. R. Harris, M. E. Lippman, M. Morrow, & C. K. Osborne (Eds.), *Diseases of the breast* (4th ed., pp. 762–773). Philadelphia: Lippincott Williams & Wilkins.

Millet, A. V., & Dirbas, F. M. (2002). Clinical management of breast pain: A review. *Obstetrical and Gynecological Survey, 57,* 451–461.

Miltenburg, D. M., & Speights, V. O. (2008). Benign breast disease. *Obstetrics and Gynecolgic Clinics of North America, 35*(2), 258–300.

Morrow, M., & Harris, J. R. (2010). Ductal carcinoma in situ and microinvasive carcinoma. In J. R. Harris, M. E. Lippman, M. Morrow, & C. K. Osborne (Eds.), *Diseases of the breast* (4th ed., pp. 349–362). Philadelphia: Lippincott Williams & Wilkins.

National Cancer Institute. (2010a). *Breast cancer and pregnancy (PDQ®).* Retrieved from http://www.cancer.gov/cancertopics/pdq/treatment/breast-cancer-and-pregnancy/HealthProfessional

National Cancer Institute. (2010b). *Probability of breast cancer in women.* Retrieved from http://www.cancer.gov/cancertopics/factsheet/detection/probability-breast-cancer

National Cancer Institute. (2011a). *Breast cancer prevention (PDQ): Health professional version.* Retrieved from http://www.cancer.gov/cancertopics/pdq/prevention/breast/HealthProfessional

National Cancer Institute. (2011b). *Breast cancer treatment (PDQ): Health professional version.* Retrieved from http://www.cancer.gov/cancertopics/pdq/treatment/breast/HealthProfessional

National Comprehensive Cancer Network. (2011). *Breast cancer. Clinical practice guidelines in oncology—v.1.2004.* Retrieved from http://www.nccn.org/professionals/physician_gls/PDF/breast.pdf

Olawaiye, M. D., Witham-Leitch, M., Danakas, G., & Kahn, K. (2005). Mastalgia: A review of management. *Journal of Reproductive Medicine, 50,* 933–939.

Osuch, J. R. (2002). Breast health and disease over a lifetime. *Clinical Obstetrics and Gynecology, 45,* 1140–1161.

Pearlman, M. D., & Griffin, J. L. (2010). Benign breast disease. *Obstetrics & Gynecology, 116*(3), 747–758.

Rodden, A. M. (2009). Common breast concerns. *Primary Care: Clinics in Office Practice, 36*(1), 103–113.

Sabate, J. M., Clotet, M., Torrubia, S., Gomez, A., Guerrero, R., de Las Heras, P., & Lerma E. (2007). Radiologic evaluation of breast disorders related to pregnancy and lactation. *Radiographics, 27,* S101–S124.

Salgado, C. J., Mardini, S., & Chen, H. C. (2005). Mastodynia refractory to medical therapy: Is there a role for mastectomy and breast reconstruction? *Plastic & Reconstructive Surgery, 116,* 978–983.

Saslow, D., Boetes, C., Burke, W., Harms, S., Leach, M. O., Lehman, C. D., et al. (2007). American Cancer Society guidelines for breast screening with MRI as an adjunct to mammography. *CA: A Cancer Journal for Clinicians, 57,* 75–89.

Simpson, P. T., Reis-Filho, J. S., & Lakhani, S. R. (2010). Lobular carcinoma in situ: Biology and pathology. In J. R. Harris, M. E. Lippman, M. Morrow, & C. K. Osborne (Eds.), *Diseases of the breast* (4th ed., pp. 333–340). Philadelphia: Lippincott Williams & Wilkins.

Smith, B. L., & Souba, W. W. (1995). Breast disease. Algorithm and explanation: Assessment and management of breast complaints. *Scientific American Surgery, VIII,* 1–16.

Smith, L. H., Danielsen, B., Allen, M. E., & Cress, R. (2003). Cancer associated with obstetric delivery: Results of linkage with the California cancer registry.

American Journal of Obstetrics and Gynecology, 189, 1128–1135.

Smith, M., & Kent, K. (2002). Breast concerns and lifestyles of women. *Clinical Obstetrics and Gynecology, 45,* 1129–1139.

Smith, R. L., Pruthi, S., & Fitzpatrick, L. A. (2004). Evaluation and management of breast pain. *Mayo Clinic Proceedings, 79,* 353–372.

Srivastava, A., Mansel, R. E., Arvind, N., Prasad, K., Dhar, A., & Chabra, A. (2007). Evidence-based management of mastalgia: A meta-analysis of randomized trials. *The Breast, 16,* 503–512.

Tavaf-Motamen, H., Ader, D. N., Browne, M. W., & Shriver, C. D. (1998). Clinical evaluation of mastalgia. *Archives of Surgery, 133,* 211–213.

Veronesi, U., Cascinelli, N., Mariani, L., Greco, M., Saccozzi, R., Alberto, L., et al. (2002). Twenty-year follow-up of a randomized study comparing breast-conserving surgery with radical mastectomy for early breast cancer. *New England Journal of Medicine, 347,* 1227–1232.

Vogel, V. G., Costantino, J. P., Wickerham, D. L., Cronin, W. M., Cecchini, R. S., Atkins, J. N., et al. (2006). Effects of tamoxifen vs raloxifene on the risk of developing invasive breast cancer and other disease outcomes: The NSABP study of tamoxifen and raloxifene (STAR) P-2 trial. *Journal of the American Medical Association, 295,* 2727–2741.

Yaziji, H., Goldstein, L. C., Barry, T. S., Werling, R., Hwang, H., Ellis, G. K., et al. (2004). HER-2 testing in breast cancer using parallel tissue-based methods. *Journal of the American Medical Association, 291,* 1972–1977.

Young, I. (1998). Breasted experience. In R. Weitz (Ed.), *The politics of women's bodies: Sexuality, appearance, and behavior* (pp. 125–136). Oxford, UK: Oxford University Press.

16-A

Online Resources

The *CRICO/RMF Breast Care Management Algorithm: Improving Breast Patient Safety* includes risk assessment and screening recommendations; algorithms for management of screening mammogram results, nipple discharge, palpable mass, and breast pain; and discussion points for providing breast care. *http://www.rmf.harvard.edu/files/documents/cricormf_bca.pdf*

The California Department of Public Health, Cancer Detection Section, has a website that offers multiple clinician resources, including forms for recording the results of a breast-related history and physical examination as well as diagnostic algorithms for management of a palpable mass, abnormal screening mammogram results, nipple discharge, breast skin changes, breast pain, and breast biopsy results. *http://qap.sdsu.edu/resources/tools/index.html*

The National Cancer Institute's Breast Cancer page includes information about screening and testing, prevention, genetics, causes, treatment, clinical trials, cancer literature, research, and statistics. Materials for health professionals and patients are available. *http://www.cancer.gov/cancertopics/types/breast*

The National Comprehensive Cancer Network provides detailed guidelines and algorithms for breast cancer screening, diagnosis, risk reduction, and treatment. *http://www.nccn.org/professionals/physician_gls/f_guidelines.asp*

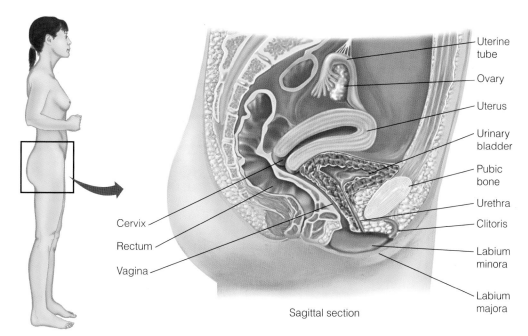

Uterine tube

Ovary

Uterus

Urinary bladder

Pubic bone

Urethra

Clitoris

Labium minora

Labium majora

Cervix

Rectum

Vagina

Sagittal section

COLOR PLATE 1 Midsagittal view of a woman's pelvic organs.

COLOR PLATE 2 The woman's external genitalia.

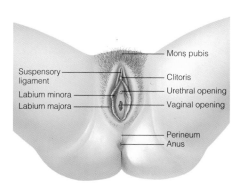

Mons pubis

Suspensory ligament

Clitoris

Urethral opening

Labium minora

Labium majora

Vaginal opening

Perineum

Anus

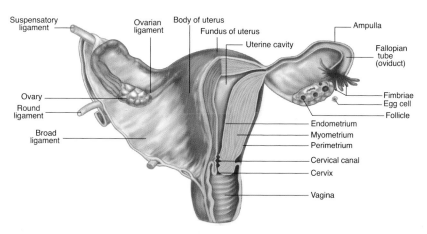

Suspensatory ligament

Ovarian ligament

Body of uterus

Fundus of uterus

Uterine cavity

Ampulla

Fallopian tube (oviduct)

Ovary

Round ligament

Broad ligament

Fimbriae

Egg cell

Follicle

Endometrium

Myometrium

Perimetrium

Cervical canal

Cervix

Vagina

COLOR PLATE 3 An anterior view of the female reproductive organs showing the relationships of the ovaries, fallopian tubes, uterus, cervix, and vagina.

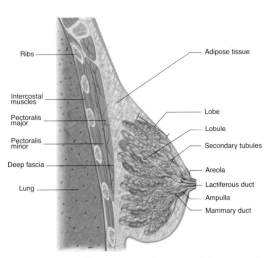

Ribs
Intercostal muscles
Pectoralis major
Pectoralis minor
Deep fascia
Lung

Adipose tissue
Lobe
Lobule
Secondary tubules
Areola
Lactiferous duct
Ampulla
Mammary duct

COLOR PLATE 4 The structure of a woman's breast and mammary glands: sagittal section.

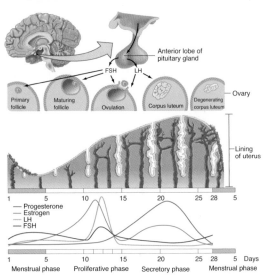

Anterior lobe of pituitary gland
FSH   LH
Primary follicle
Maturing follicle
Ovulation
Corpus luteum
Degenerating corpus luteum
Ovary

Lining of uterus

1   5   10   15   20   25 28   5
— Progesterone
— Estrogen
— LH
— FSH

1   5   10   15   20   25 28   5 Days
Menstrual phase Proliferative phase Secretory phase Menstrual phase

COLOR PLATE 5 Influence of steroid hormones on the ovaries and endometrium.

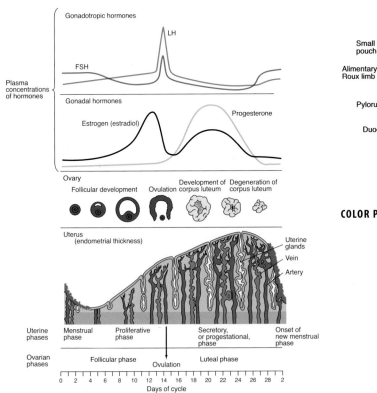

Gonadotropic hormones
LH
FSH

Plasma concentrations of hormones

Gonadal hormones
Estrogen (estradiol)
Progesterone

Ovary
Follicular development   Ovulation Development of Degeneration of
corpus luteum corpus luteum

Uterus (endometrial thickness)
Uterine glands
Vein
Artery

Uterine phases   Menstrual phase   Proliferative phase   Secretory, or progestational, phase   Onset of new menstrual phase

Ovarian phases   Follicular phase   Ovulation   Luteal phase

0 2 4 6 8 10 12 14 16 18 20 22 24 26 28 2
Days of cycle

COLOR PLATE 6 Ovarian phases and endometrial development.

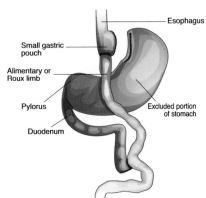

Esophagus
Small gastric pouch
Alimentary or Roux limb
Pylorus
Duodenum
Excluded portion of stomach

COLOR PLATE 7 Roux-en-Y bypass.

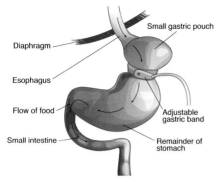

COLOR PLATE 8 Gastric banding.

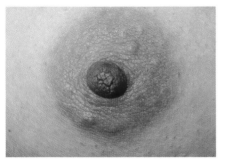

COLOR PLATE 9 An example of nipple discharge.
© Dr. H. C. Robinson/Science Photo Library

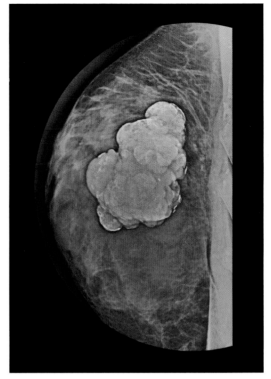

COLOR PLATE 10 An example of a breast mass.
© CNRI/Photo Researchers, Inc.

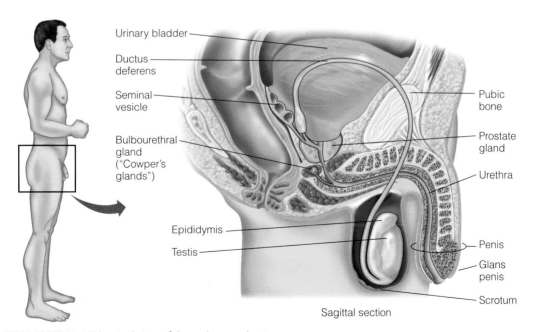

Sagittal section

COLOR PLATE 11 Midsagittal view of the male reproductive system.

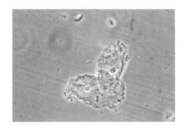

COLOR PLATE 12 A micrograph of bacterial vaginosis.
Courtesy of CDC/M. Rein

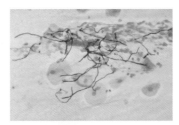

COLOR PLATE 13 A micrograph of vulvovaginal candidiasis.
Courtesy of CDC

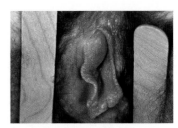

COLOR PLATE 14 Bartholin's cyst.
Courtesy of CDC/Susan Lindsley

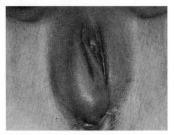

COLOR PLATE 15 Bartholin's abscess.
Reprinted from Ozdegirmenci, O., Kayikcioglu, F., & Haberal, A. (2009). Prospective randomized study of marsupialization versus silver nitrate application in the management of Bartholin gland cysts and abscesses. *Journal of Minimally Invasive Gynecology, 16*(2), 149–152.

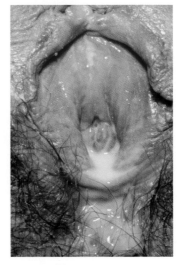

COLOR PLATE 16 An example of vaginal discharge from trichomoniasis.
© National Medical Slide Bank/Custom Medical StockPhoto

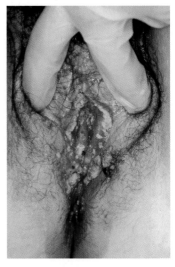

COLOR PLATE 17 Genital warts.
Courtesy of CDC/Joe Millar

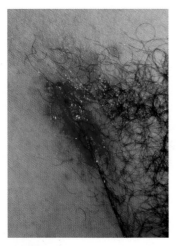

COLOR PLATE 18 Genital herpes lesions.
© Dr. P. Marazzi/Photo Researchers, Inc.

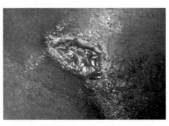

COLOR PLATE 19 Chancroid lesion.
Courtesy of CDC/J. Pledger

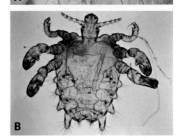

COLOR PLATE 20 Pediculosis pubis (A) is caused by *Phthirus pubis* (B).
(A) Courtesy of CDC/Joe Miller;
(B) Courtesy of CDC/W.H.O.

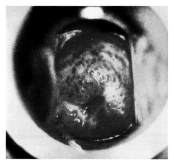

COLOR PLATE 21 Cervical petechiae with trichomoniasis (strawberry cervix).
Courtesy of CDC

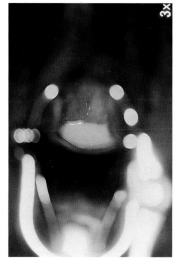

COLOR PLATE 22 Chlamydial mucopurulent cervical discharge.
Courtesy of CDC

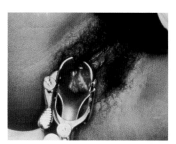

COLOR PLATE 23 Gonorrheal mucopurulent cervical discharge.
Courtesy of CDC

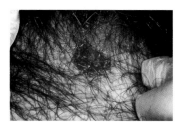

COLOR PLATE 24A Syphilitic chancre (primary syphilis).
Courtesy of CDC/Joe Miller/ Dr. N.J. Fiumara

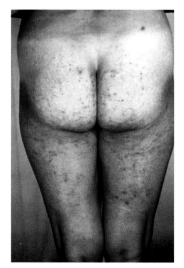

COLOR PLATE 24B Syphilitic rash (secondary syphilis)
Courtesy of CDC/J. Pledger, BSS/VD

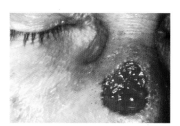

COLOR PLATE 24C A gumma is a soft, noncancerous growth resulting from the tertiary stage of syphilis.
Courtesy of J. Pledger/CDC

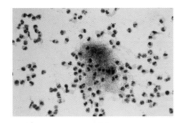

COLOR PLATE 25 Urine microscopy for a UTI.
© Dr. Frederick Skvara/Visuals Unlimited, Inc.

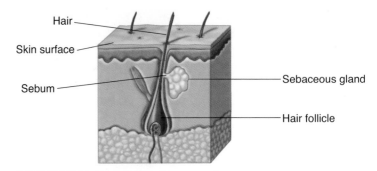

COLOR PLATE 26 Normal pilosebaceous unit.
Reprinted with permission from National Institute of Arthritis and Musculoskeletal and Skin Diseases. (2010). *Questions and answers about acne* (NIH Publication No. 06-4998). Bethesda, MD: Author.

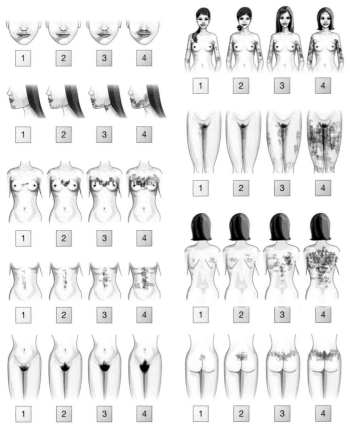

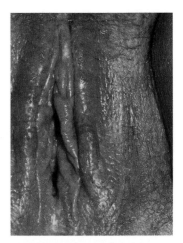

COLOR PLATE 28 Irritant contact dermatitis.
Reprinted from Stewart, K. M. (2010). Clinical care of vulvar pruritis, with emphasis on one common cause, lichen simplex chronicus. *Dermatologic Clinics, 28*(4), 669–680.

COLOR PLATE 27 Modified Ferriman–Gallwey hirsutism scale. This is a visual method of scoring hair growth in women, modified from the original scale reported by Ferriman and Gallwey in 1961. Each of the nine areas is given a score ranging from 0 (no hair) to 4 (extensive terminal hair). The scores for each of the nine areas are totaled, and a score of 8 or greater indicates hirsutism.

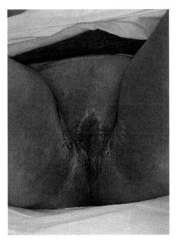

COLOR PLATE 29 Allergic contact dermatitis.
Reprinted from Schlosser, B. J. (2010). Contact dermatitis of the vulva. *Dermatologic Clinics, 28*(4), 697–706.

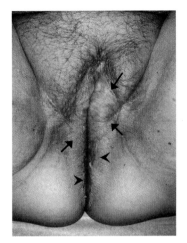

COLOR PLATE 30 Lichen sclerosus.
Reprinted from Goldstein, A. T., Thaçi, D., & Luger, T. (2009). Topical calcineurin inhibitors for the treatment of vulvar dermatoses. *European Journal of Obstetrics & Gynecology and Reproductive Biology, 146*(1), 22–29.

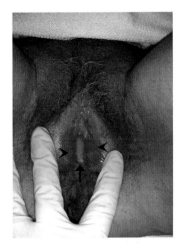

COLOR PLATE 31 Erosive lichen planus.
Reprinted from Goldstein, A. T., Thaçi, D., & Luger, T. (2009). Topical calcineurin inhibitors for the treatment of vulvar dermatoses. *European Journal of Obstetrics & Gynecology and Reproductive Biology, 146*(1), 22–29.

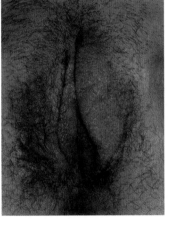

COLOR PLATE 32 Lichen simplex chronicus.
Reprinted from Stewart, K. M. (2010). Clinical care of vulvar pruritis, with emphasis on one common cause, lichen simplex chronicus. *Dermatologic Clinics, 28*(4), 669–680.

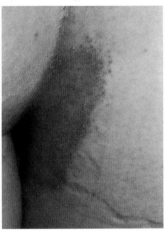

COLOR PLATE 33 Vulvar psoriasis.
Reprinted from Stewart, K. M. (2010). Clinical care of vulvar pruritis, with emphasis on one common cause, lichen simplex chronicus. *Dermatologic Clinics, 28*(4), 669–680.

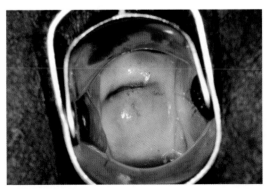

COLOR PLATE 34 Nabothian cyst.
© Dr. P. Marazzi/Photo Researchers, Inc.

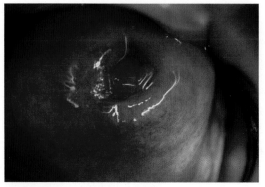

COLOR PLATE 35 Cervical polyp.
© Dr. P. Marazzi/Photo Researchers, Inc.

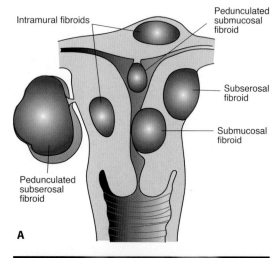

A

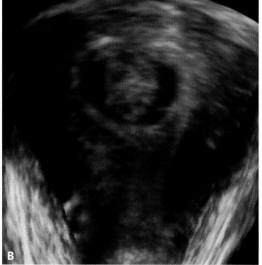

B

COLOR PLATE 36 Uterine fibroids: A. Classifications by location; B. Ultrasound image.
(B) © Dr. Najeeb Layyous/Photo Researchers, Inc.

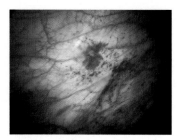

COLOR PLATE 37 Adenomyosis.
© Biophoto Associates/Photo Researchers, Inc.

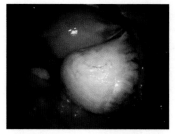

COLOR PLATE 38 Endometriosis.
© Dr. Najeeb Layyous/Photo Researchers, Inc.

COLOR PLATE 39 Ovarian cyst.
© Dr. Najeeb Layyous/Photo Researchers, Inc.

17

Female Sexual Dysfunction

Susan Chasson

We live in a society where men, women, and children are constantly bombarded with messages about the importance of sexuality. Unfortunately, these messages create a limited view of sexuality, usually emphasizing physical desirability to a partner and a person's ability to achieve orgasm. When society has a limited view of sexuality, there is the potential for using a limited approach to solve sexual problems. With the advent of sildenafil (Viagra) and other drugs for treating erectile dysfunction, many clinicians have expressed concerns that the treatment of sexual dysfunction is becoming too medicalized. The greatest concern is that researchers are spending the majority of their time looking for a magic pill that will cure female sexual dysfunction and are not looking at the complex and multiple factors that may be causes of sexual dysfunction.

When examining sexuality and sexual dysfunction, it is important to look at a broad definition of sexuality. Poorman (1988) gives us a definition of sexuality that goes beyond basic sexual function, allowing us to examine sexuality in a more holistic and comprehensive manner:

> Sexuality is interwoven with every aspect of human existence, and in its broadest sense, sexuality is defined as a desire for contact, warmth, tenderness, or love (Aletkey, 1980). Humans express and live their sexuality in their daily lives. Sexuality is not limited to an act of seduction or intercourse but encompasses every area in our lives: the way we relate to others, our friends, our family, and our work. It is evident in what we believe, how we behave, and the way we look. (p. 1)

Using a broader definition of sexuality allows the clinician to look at sexual problems in the context of both the patient as an individual and as a member of a larger society.

Evaluating and treating sexual dysfunction is a challenging area of women's health care. Composed of a complex combination of physical, psychological, and cultural components, our sexuality is shaped from conception by influences as diverse as genetics, religion, family, and the media (Morley & Kaiser, 2003). To provide care to women with sexual problems, the clinician must begin her or his practice with a correct understanding of female genital anatomy and physiology. For example, many clinicians are unaware that the clitoris is a wishbone-shaped structure measuring between 9 and 11 centimeters in length, because most medical textbooks describe the glans of the clitoris as the entire structure (Berman & Berman, 2001). The clinician must also be comfortable talking about sexual issues in a nonjudgmental fashion when dealing with the sexual problems of a patient.

Definitions of Sexual Dysfunction

Various definitions of sexual dysfunction have been proposed. This chapter follows the structure developed by an international committee sponsored by the American Urological Association Foundation. The definitions used in this chapter were presented at the Second International Consultation on Sexual Medicine (Basson et al., 2003) and remain the current recommendation for clinical settings according to international experts who reviewed them for the Third International Consultation on Sexual Medicine (Basson, Wierman, van Lankveld, & Brotto, 2010). These definitions attempt to incorporate the evolving conceptualization of women's sexual response cycle, which was not reflected in earlier diagnostic criteria that were based on outdated models of sexual response (Basson et al., 2003). While these definitions are imperfect and continue to be refined, they give clinicians a basis for diagnosis and management of sexual dysfunction. **Table 17-1** compares the categories used in this chapter with the female sexual dysfunction categories in the *Diagnostic and Statistical Manual of Mental Disorders, Fourth Edition, Text Revision* (*DSM-IV-TR*; American Psychiatric Association, 2000), which is another commonly used source of diagnostic criteria for sexual dysfunction.

The classification of sexual dysfunction used in this chapter identifies problems within the three phases of sexual response—desire, arousal, and orgasm—and also includes the sexual pain disorders dyspareunia and vaginismus. An important part of the evaluation of sexual problems is determining whether the patient perceives the sexual dysfunction as a problem (Basson, 2000). For example, a woman who is unable to achieve orgasm but is satisfied by the sexual relationship with her partner is not considered to have sexual dysfunction.

Scope of the Problem

Many women have concerns about sexual issues. In one of the first national U.S. surveys about sexual concerns, 43% of women reported sexual dysfunction. Of the 1486 women responding, 27% to 32% reported a lack of interest in sex, 22% to 28% were unable to achieve orgasm, 17% to 27% reported sex was not pleasurable, 18% to 27% described trouble lubricating, 8% to 21% experienced pain during sex, and 6% to 16% were anxious about perfor-

TABLE 17-1 Classification of Female Sexual Dysfunction

	International Definitions Committee Sponsored by the American Urological Association Foundation	Diagnostic and Statistical Manual of Mental Disorders, Fourth Edition, Text-Revised (DSM-IV-TR)
Desire	• Sexual interest/desire disorder	• Hypoactive sexual desire disorder
Arousal	• Subjective arousal disorder • Genital arousal disorder • Combined genital and subjective arousal disorder • Persistent sexual arousal disorder	• Female sexual arousal disorder
Orgasm	• Women's orgasmic disorder	• Female orgasmic disorder
Pain	• Vaginismus • Dyspareunia	• Vaginismus • Dyspareunia

Sources: Adapted from American Psychiatric Association, 2000; Basson et al., 2003; Basson et al., 2010.

mance (the ranges reflect variations among age groups) (Laumann, Paik, & Rosen, 1999). More recent national estimates are available from the Prevalence of Female Sexual Problems Associated with Distress and Determinants of Treatment Seeking (PRESIDE) study, which had 31,581 respondents. Nearly half of women (44%) reported having some type of sexual problem. Prevalence of specific problems was 39% for low desire, 26% for low arousal, and 21% for orgasm difficulties. Sexually related personal distress, measured with the Female Sexual Distress Scale, was present in 23% of respondents (Shifren, Monz, Russo, Segreti, & Johannes, 2008). These surveys indicate that sexual concerns are common.

Etiology

Developmental, health-related, partner, and relationship factors as well as sociocultural influences may all contribute to female sexual dysfunction (see Chapter 11). Physical and psychological etiologies are possible, and an individual woman may have multiple causes of sexual dysfunction. Women with sexual concerns may also be experiencing normal variations of sexuality—a possibility that must be considered in the assessment.

General Assessment for Sexual Concerns

This section describes the general assessment of any woman presenting with sexual concerns. Screening for sexual concerns is discussed in Chapter 11. Additional assessments specific to the different types of sexual dysfunction are detailed later in this chapter. The purpose of the assessment is to help identify all potential psychological or physical sources for the problem. When assessing a woman for sexual dysfunction, it is necessary to determine whether the problems are partner specific. Relationship stressors need to be evaluated to determine the source of sexual dysfunction. For example, if a woman is experiencing intimate partner violence, changing the time and location of sexual relations will probably not increase her sexual desire.

History

Assessment of the woman with sexual concerns requires a comprehensive health history that includes physical and psychosocial history questions as well as assessment of her sexual health. Investigation of physical concerns should include surgeries, chronic illnesses, medications, and allergies. Reports of surgeries that could affect vascular or neurologic function of the genital tract indicate a need for further investigation. Chronic illnesses that involve neurologic, endocrine, or vascular problems (e.g., thyroid disease, diabetes, and hypertension) are particularly of interest because of their potential impact on sexual function (Frank, Mistretta, & Will, 2008). A review of medications is important because several drugs are known to cause or exacerbate sexual problems (**Box 17-1**). Screening for latex allergies should be a standard part of any gynecologic examination, because latex products used both for contraception and during pelvic examinations may be a source of sexually related pain.

The psychosocial history should include information about the woman's partner(s) and relationship(s). Ask if she has a prior or present history of physical, emotional, or sexual abuse, or if she has ever been sexually assaulted. Assess for signs and symptoms of major depression and other mental health problems, such as post-traumatic stress disorder and obsessive–compulsive disorder, which may potentially affect sexual function. Life stressors, coping mechanisms, and body image should also be evaluated. In addition, it is important to inquire about the use of recreational drugs, alcohol, and cigarettes, because these habits may be factors in sexual dysfunction. Screen the woman for risk factors associated with sexual activity, including multiple sexual partners and use of contraception. Sexually transmitted infections can be a source of sexual pain, and use of combined estrogen and progestin contraceptives (i.e., pills, patch, and ring) may cause decreased desire in some women. The cultural and religious beliefs of the woman should be considered when evaluating and recommending treatment for sexual dysfunction as well. For example, if a woman is unable to

---

BOX 17-1 *Medications That Can Cause or Exacerbate Female Sexual Dysfunction*

Amphetamines	Combined estrogen and progestin contraceptives
Anticonvulsants	Digoxin
Antidepressants	Gonadotropin-releasing hormone (GnRH) agonists
Antihypertensives	Hormone therapy (estrogen and/or progestogen)
Antipsychotics	Lipid-lowering agents
Antiulcer drugs	Narcotics
Benzodiazepines	

Sources: Adapted from American College of Obstetricians and Gynecologists, 2011; Kingsberg & Althof, 2009.

achieve orgasm through intercourse, encouraging self-stimulation may not be an option if that practice conflicts with her religious or cultural beliefs.

Box 17-2 lists some open-ended questions that can be used to begin a discussion of a patient's sexual concerns. The Female Sexual Function Index (FSFI) can be helpful in assessment but should not replace a thorough sexual history. The FSFI assesses six domains: desire, arousal, lubrication, orgasm, satisfaction, and pain (Rosen et al., 2000). The FSFI questionnaire contains 19 items and is available online at http://www.fsfi-questionnaire.com.

When evaluating the woman with a sexual problem, reviewing normal sexual response may be all that is needed to reassure her that what she is experiencing is normal. The clinician may also need to evaluate the woman's understanding of normal sexual anatomy and function. One technique is to use a diagram to discuss genital anatomy and physiology. Women's sexual response cycle is often not well understood. For example, many people do not realize that the majority of women cannot achieve orgasm without direct or indirect stimulation of the clitoris. As a consequence, women who cannot achieve orgasm through intercourse often believe they have a problem. Discussing and describing sexual anatomy may give the woman enough information to allow her to understand and improve her sexual response.

Physical Examination

The physical examination should specifically look for potential health problems that could affect sexual function, such as undiagnosed diabetes or hypertension. Height, weight, and vital signs should be recorded. Neurologic and vascular systems should be examined. The genital examination should include inspection and palpation of both external and internal genital structures (see Chapter 6 for examination techniques).

Diagnostic Testing

Laboratory tests should be performed only when there is a clinical indication for them. The likelihood of laboratory tests identifying the etiology of a sexual dysfunction is low (Basson, 2006). Tests to consider include fasting glucose, a lipid profile, thyroid-stimulating hormone

---

BOX 17-2 *Initial Questions for Assessment of Sexual Concerns*

- Which sexual concerns, problems, or issues are you experiencing?
- How does this concern affect your sexual function, relationship(s), and life?
- What is the most distressing part of this problem?
- Which treatments have you used?
- What kind of conversations have you had with your partner(s) so far, and how have they gone?
- What do you think is the source of your sexual problem?

Sources: Association of Reproductive Health Professionals, 2010; Steege & Zolnoun, 2009; van Lankveld et al., 2010.

(TSH), prolactin, follicle-stimulating hormone (FSH), and estradiol (Brotto, Bitzer, Laan, Leiblum, & Luria, 2010; Hatzichristou et al., 2010). Measurement of androgen levels is considered controversial because assay methods vary in accuracy, precision, and reliability, and because the correlation between testosterone levels and sexual dysfunction has not been consistent in studies. Clinicians who obtain androgen levels must understand the specific assay being used and the limitations of testing (Brotto et al.; Rosner, Auchus, Azziz, Sluss, & Raff, 2007; Traish, Guay, Spark, & Testosterone Therapy in Women Study Group, 2007; Wierman et al., 2006). This issue is discussed in more detail in the section on women's sexual interest/desire disorder.

Differential Diagnoses

The clinician should begin by categorizing the type of sexual dysfunction into one or more of the classifications developed by the International Definitions Committee (see Table 17-1). Comorbidity—that is, the presence of two or more dysfunctions—is common (Basson et al., 2003). Using the information obtained in the history and physical examination, the clinician should then determine whether the source of the dysfunction is psychological, physical, or a combination of the two. The rest of this chapter presents specific assessment and management recommendations for each type of sexual dysfunction.

Further Assessment and Management of Specific Types of Sexual Dysfunction

Women's Sexual Interest/Desire Disorder

Women's sexual interest/desire disorder is "absent or diminished feelings of sexual interest or desire, absent sexual thoughts or fantasies, and a lack of responsive desire. Motivations (here defined as reasons/incentives) for attempting to have sexual arousal are scarce or absent. The lack of interest is considered to be beyond the normative lessening with life cycle and relationship duration" (Basson et al., 2003, p. 224). In 2000, Dr. Rosemary Basson proposed a new model for female sexual response based on a changed perspective of female sexual dysfunction and desire disorders. Instead of the traditional model of arousal, desire, orgasm, and resolution, Basson (2000) describes many women as moving from a state of sexual neutrality to a state where they become motivated to seek stimuli that will cause sexual arousal. Further discussion and a diagram of Basson's model can be found in Chapter 11.

Basson (2000) believes that many women are motivated to initiate sexual activity by things other than a desire for sexual gratification. These motivating factors for sexual relations may include "emotional closeness, increased commitment, bonding, and tolerance of imperfections in the relationship" (Basson, 2000, p. 53). If a woman achieves these non-sexual goals, she will view her sexual experience as positive, whether or not she personally experiences sexual gratification. Therefore, when assessing a woman for desire disorder, it is important to consider what motivates her desire for sexual relations.

Assessment of Women's Sexual Interest/Desire Disorder Assessment of sexual desire disorder should start with determining the duration of the problem. Has the woman always felt this way, or does her current state represent a change in her level of desire? It is important to look for any negative factors, either psychological or physical, that may affect desire. Are there conflicts about other issues in the woman's relationship with her partner? Is the woman experiencing pain with intercourse? Other social factors that may influence desire include financial stress, small children who continue to require care at night, or work schedules that make it difficult for couples to find the time or energy to plan for sexual intimacy.

Frequency of sexual relations is another important factor to evaluate. Many couples report a decrease in frequency of sexual intercourse with longer duration of a relationship (Avis et al., 2005). Instead of experiencing a lack of sexual desire caused by a physical or psychological source, the problem may be linked to a difference in expectations between the woman and her partner. In a recent national study, married women aged 25 to 69 years reported the following frequencies of sexual activity: not at all in the past year, 3.5% to 37.9%; a few times per year to monthly, 11.6% to 23.7%; a few times per month to weekly, 35.9% to 50.2%; two to three times per week, 6.2% to 35.2%; and four or more times per week, 0 to 5.1% (ranges reflect variations among age groups) (Herbenick et al., 2010). These statistics give the clinician a baseline for looking at decrease in desire as it relates to frequency of sexual activity.

It is also important to inquire about whether the change in desire has resulted in a change in sexual frequency. Does the woman continue to have sexual relations even when the encounters are unwanted? A woman who believes she does not have a choice about frequency of sexual relations may first need to deal with issues of power and control in the relationship before it can be determined whether her problem has a physical basis.

When using Basson's (2000) model, if a woman does not initiate sexual relations, it is necessary to find out if she is willing to participate in and able to enjoy sexual relations if sexual intercourse is initiated by her partner. This woman may simply need to be told that her pattern of response is normal for many women. Working with the woman, explore any changes that may have altered her satisfaction with her sexual relationship. Does the woman experience orgasm with sexual relations? Although many anorgasmic women report satisfying sexual relationships, over time the lack of physical pleasure may decrease motivation to engage in sexual relations.

Investigate the timing of sexual relations, and explore what occurs after intercourse. Although most men find sexual intercourse sedating, many women experience increased mental arousal after sexual relations. In this situation, a woman may be more concerned about the loss of sleep than achieving the feelings of closeness that may result from sexual relations.

Do the negatives that result from sexual relations outweigh the positive rewards? If a woman's need for intimacy is not being met during the sexual encounter, because of either lack of time or fatigue, then she may lose her motivation for future sexual encounters. Although the hormonal changes associated with menopause can affect desire, a woman's inability to achieve pregnancy—a previous motivating factor for sexual relations—may act as a factor in decreasing desire for sexual relations after menopause or sterilization.

Do associated physical symptoms indicate that a woman's lack of desire is the result of underlying illness? Fatigue may be related to thyroid dysfunction or sleep disorders. Does the woman have a chronic medical problem, such as arthritis or back pain, that makes sexual relations painful or uncomfortable? Desire disorders are also associated with thyroid disease, epilepsy, and renal disease. Screen the woman for use of medications (see Box 17-1) or a history of surgeries that could alter desire by changing hormone levels, particularly combined contraceptives, gonadotropin-releasing hormone (GnRH) agonists, antiestrogens, and hysterectomy or oophorectomy.

Menopause may be a time of decreased desire, and the reasons for this change may go beyond alterations in hormone levels. Decreased desire may be the result of insomnia, hot flashes, increased vaginal dryness, or decreased vaginal elasticity that results in pain (Weismiller, 2002). Androgen deficiency has also been targeted as a source of decreased desire in perimenopausal and menopausal women. This hormone deficiency may be associated with problems with arousal, genital sensation, libido, and orgasm as well as a decreased sense of well-being and increased fatigue (Bachmann et al., 2002). Although a consensus conference of international experts proposed a definition for female androgen insufficiency in 2002 (Bachmann et al.), the existence of this condition continues to be debated (Traish et al., 2007; Wierman et al., 2006).

Androgens are produced both by the ovaries and the adrenal glands. The ovaries produce testosterone and androstenedione, and the adrenal glands produce dehydroepiandrosterone (DHEA) and dehydroepiandrosterone-sulfate (DHEA-S). Testosterone levels decrease approximately 50% between the ages of 30 and 50 years, then decline another 15% after menopause—though the latter decrease is thought to be related to age rather than menopause (Mathur & Braunstein, 2010). Androgen levels can vary significantly from one woman to another, and the two main factors that can decrease androgen levels (other than age) are oophorectomy and oral estrogen therapy. Oophorectomy can result in a 50% loss of testosterone production, whereas oral estrogen therapy can increase sex hormone-binding globulin (SHBG), triggering a relative decrease in free testosterone levels. In addition to drug-related and ovarian-failure androgen deficiency, hypopituitarism and adrenal insufficiency can also cause abnormal levels of androgens (Bachmann et al., 2002).

Androgen insufficiency can be diagnosed by history and exclusion of other causes of symptoms. Measurement of androgen levels is not required to initiate testosterone therapy or to monitor this treatment's effectiveness (American College of Obstetricians and Gynecologists, 2011; Mathur & Braunstein, 2010). Indeed, testing for androgen levels in women is associated with several problems. Serum testosterone testing was initially designed for men, who have much higher blood levels of testosterone, so assays can be inaccurate in women. Free testosterone measured by equilibrium dialysis or the free testosterone index (calculated from measurement of total testosterone and SHBG) gives the most accurate androgen status in women (Mathur & Braunstein). The most accurate method for measuring total testosterone is mass spectroscopy after extraction and chromatography (Rosner, Auchus, Azziz, Sluss,

& Raff, 2007). It is important for the clinician to have a specific diagnosis prior to treating a woman with androgen medications (Bachmann et al., 2002).

Management of Women's Sexual Interest/Desire Disorder The appropriate treatment for hypoactive sexual desire disorder depends on the type of problem identified. Patients with undiagnosed or untreated physical or mental health problems require interventions to remedy the underlying illness. Consider changing any medications that may be affecting sexual desire (Box 17-1). If decreased desire is related to pain with intercourse, the source of the pain should be diagnosed and treated. If sexual dysfunction already exists, be aware of how medical interventions may cause the sexual problems to increase in severity. For example, decreased libido has been reported by as many as 80% to 90% of patients with depression (Clayton & Balon, 2009). At the same time, selective serotonin reuptake inhibitors (SSRIs) have a 36% to 43% rate of sexual dysfunction reported with their use (Clayton et al., 2002).

Women should be educated about normal alterations in desire that result from the aging process, longer duration of a relationship, and life changes such as those resulting from pregnancy, lactation, and menopause. Individual or couples counseling may help patients whose decreased desire is the result of life stressors or relationship problems. Some strategies for the primary care clinician include encouraging couples to communicate about their sexual needs and differences, having couples vary the time of day or location for sexual activities, and making sure couples set aside planned time for intimacy (Phillips, 2000). Cognitive behavioral therapy and sex therapy can also be beneficial for women with sexual interest/desire disorder (Basson, 2006).

Women who have sexual side effects from the SSRIs may be helped by taking bupropion SR (Wellbutrin) 150 mg twice a day (Clayton et al., 2004), sildenafil 50 mg to 100 mg before sexual activity (Nurnberg et al., 2008), or buspirone (BuSpar) 10 mg to 30 mg twice per day (Landen, Eriksson, Agren, & Fahlen, 1999). Switching the woman to an antidepressant that is associated with fewer sexual side effects, such as mirtazapine (Remeron), nefazodone (Serzone), or bupropion, is another option (Clayton & Balon, 2009).

Transdermal estrogen therapy may be beneficial for the woman experiencing decreased libido after menopause. If symptoms persist and all other causes of low libido have been excluded, testosterone therapy can be considered, although its use for this indication remains controversial (Mathur & Braunstein, 2010; Traish et al., 2007; Wierman et al., 2006). There are no androgen therapies approved by the U.S. Food and Drug Administration (FDA) for use in women; the agency has approved oral, injectable, and transdermal androgen preparations for men. Transdermal preparations are frequently used in women, but achieving proper dosing can be difficult because products are packaged in a dose appropriate for male replacement. Compounded androgen preparations are available but not recommended due to their lack of standardization. Known adverse effects from androgen supplementation include decreased levels of high-density lipoprotein (HDL; "good") cholesterol, hirsutism, acne, deepening of the voice, liver damage, hair loss, and enlargement of the clitoris. These potential risks must be discussed with the patient prior to prescribing androgen therapy. To date, little evidence has been published to support the efficacy and safety of androgen supplementation in premenopausal women and long-term (more than 6 months) androgen supplementation in menopausal women (American College of Obstetricians and Gynecologists, 2011; Mathur & Braunstein).

Sexual Arousal Disorders

Four types of sexual arousal disorders are distinguished:

- Genital sexual arousal disorder is "absent or impaired genital sexual arousal. Self-report may include minimal vulval swelling or vaginal lubrication from any type of sexual stimulation and reduced sexual sensations from caressing genitalia. Subjective sexual excitement still occurs from nongenital stimuli" (Basson et al., 2003, p. 225).
- Subjective sexual arousal disorder is "absence of or markedly diminished feelings of sexual arousal (sexual excitement and sexual pleasure) from any type of sexual stimulation. Vaginal lubrication or other signs of physical response still occur" (Basson et al., 2003, p. 225).
- Combined genital and subjective arousal disorder is "absence of or markedly diminished feelings of sexual arousal (sexual excitement and sexual pleasure) from any type of sexual stimulation as well as complaints of absent or impaired genital sexual arousal (vulval swelling, lubrication)" (Basson et al., 2003, p. 226).
- Persistent sexual arousal disorder is "spontaneous intrusive and unwanted genital arousal (e.g., tingling, throbbing, pulsating) in the absence of sexual interest and desire. Any awareness of subjective arousal is typically but not invariably unpleasant. The arousal is unrelieved by one or more orgasms and the feelings of arousal persist for hours or days" (Basson et al., 2003, p. 226). Persistent sexual arousal disorder is an uncommon condition that is outside the scope of this chapter. Women with symptoms consistent with this condition should be referred to an experienced sex therapist.

Assessment of Sexual Arousal Disorders Women should be asked whether they are experiencing vaginal lubrication or feelings of genital engorgement. It is important to determine whether the woman is having adequate stimulation to achieve arousal prior to her partner attempting intercourse. Women with difficulties in achieving arousal should be assessed for physiologic problems causing vascular or neurologic changes to the body. Diabetes, hypertension, and coronary artery disease can affect genital vasculature, for example. The woman should also be questioned about exercise or physical activities such as bicycle riding or gymnastics, which can result in nerve trauma (Brassil & Keller, 2002). Atrophic vaginitis and use of certain medications, particularly SSRIs, can also cause arousal disorders (American College of Obstetricians and Gynecologists, 2011). Other medications associated with arousal problems include anticholinergics, antihistamines, monoamine oxidase inhibitors (MAOIs), tricyclic antidepressants, and antihypertensives. Smoking and alcohol use can also affect a woman's ability to achieve sexual arousal.

Management of Sexual Arousal Disorders If arousal problems are the result of inadequate stimulation of the clitoris, instructing the woman in the use of artificial lubricants and clitoral stimulation may allow for adequate arousal to achieve orgasm. Vaginal lubricants may help increase stimulation. Treatments for medical conditions associated with arousal disorder are usually based on trying to restore blood flow to the genital tissues. A warm bath may also cause vasodilation. For perimenopausal and postmenopausal women with atrophic vaginitis, localized estrogen therapy may be beneficial. The FDA has also approved the Eros-CTD, a clitoral therapy device; it fits over the clitoris and increases blood flow to the area by creating gentle suction (Feldhaus-Dahir, 2010).

Complementary and alternative treatments for sexual arousal include yohimbine, L-arginine, and Zestra:

- Yohimbine, an extract from the bark of an African tree, is available as an over-the-counter (OTC) bark extract (yohimbe) and a prescription pure extract (yohimbine). Yohimbine is FDA approved for use in men but has been used on an off-label basis in women. It must be taken consistently for at least 14 days and can cause tachycardia and hypertension (Feldhaus-Dahir, 2010).
- L-Arginine is one of the ingredients in the nutritional supplement ArginMax, which has been shown to increase sexual desire, intercourse frequency, and sexual satisfaction (Ito, Polan, Whipple, & Trant, 2006). Topical products with L-arginine are also available on an OTC basis.
- Zestra, a topical formulation, contains a blend of botanical oils and extracts. In a randomized controlled trial, women who used Zestra had significantly greater mean improvement in the desire and arousal domains of the FSFI compared to women who used placebo. Mean improvements were also greater with Zestra than with placebo in the lubrication, pain, orgasm, and satisfaction domains of the FSFI, but these results were not statistically significant (Ferguson, Hosmane, & Heiman, 2010).

Although not approved for use in women, sildenafil has been tested in clinical trials. The outcomes of these trials have produced mixed results, but sildenafil may be beneficial for women whose arousal disorder is associated with a neurodegenerative disease (Brown, Kyle, & Ferrill, 2009). Sildenafil should not be used in women with cardiovascular disease.

Other potential therapies for arousal disorder include alprostadil and tibolone. Genital application of 400 mcg alprostadil, a prostaglandin E_1, has been demonstrated to increase genital vasocongestion, physical and emotional arousal, and sexual satisfaction (Heiman et al., 2006). Tibolone is a synthetic steroid given orally that has estrogenic, androgenic, and progestogenic properties. Tibolone has been used in Europe for many years to treat menopausal symptoms, with some evidence indicating that it improves sexual function (Modelska & Cummings, 2002). Tibolone has not been approved by the FDA for use in the United States.

Women's Orgasmic Disorder

Women's orgasmic disorder is present when "despite the self-report of high sexual arousal/excitement, there is either lack of orgasm, markedly diminished intensity of orgasmic sensations, or marked delay of orgasm from any kind of stimulation" (Basson et al., 2003, p. 226).

Assessment of Women's Orgasmic Disorder Assessment of orgasmic disorder begins with determining the duration and extent of the problem. Has the woman ever experienced an orgasm? If so, did she reach orgasm through self-stimulation or with a partner? Which sexual activities led to orgasm in the past? Inability to achieve orgasm is often related to lack of sufficient stimulation. As noted previously, many people are unaware that most women need clitoral stimulation to reach orgasm. Other causes of orgasmic disorders include trauma and abuse, particularly for women who have never had an orgasm; chronic illness, such as multiple sclerosis, chronic kidney disease, or fibromyalgia; pelvic disorders or surgery; use of medications—most notably SSRIs but also other antidepressants, antipsychotics, and mood stabilizers; alcohol and illicit drug use; relationship issues; inadequate communication between partners; and cultural, religious, or familial beliefs or inhibitions (American College of Obstetricians and Gynecologists 2011; IsHak, Bokarius, Jeffrey, Davis, & Bakhta, 2010). Inhibition of the orgasmic reflex may also occur for psychological reasons or as a response to genital pain.

Management of Women's Orgasmic Disorder As part of the management process, it is critical to address any underlying cause of the orgasmic disorder. For example, consider referring women who have been abused for counseling and switching medications for women whose orgasmic disorder seems to be drug related.

There is no specific method for a woman to achieve orgasm. For the woman who has never experienced orgasm, the clinician should begin by using a diagram to demonstrate genital anatomy to the woman. It is important to explain to the woman that, as noted earlier, most women can achieve orgasm only through direct or indirect stimulation of the clitoris. Women should be asked to try self-exploration of their genital area to determine which type of touching achieves the best response. Practicing Kegel exercises allows the woman to control her muscular tension, which may decrease inhibition of her orgasmic response. For some women, the use of a vibrator will produce the required stimulation to achieve orgasm. Women who are uncomfortable with self-stimulation may be able to instruct their partners to provide direct clitoral stimulation either manually or with a vibrator to achieve orgasm. *Becoming Orgasmic* (Heiman & Lopiccolo, 1988) is an excellent self-help guide for women who need more coaching to achieve orgasm. Cognitive-behavioral therapy or sexual therapy may be useful for women with orgasmic disorder that does not resolve with self-help measures.

Dyspareunia and Vaginismus

Dyspareunia is "persistent or recurrent pain with attempted or complete vaginal entry and/or penile vaginal intercourse" (Basson et al., 2003, p. 226). Vaginismus is "the persistent or recurrent difficulties of the woman to allow vaginal entry of a penis, a finger, and/or any object, despite the woman's expressed interest to do so. There is often (phobic) avoidance and anticipation/fear/experience of pain, along with variable involuntary pelvic muscle contraction. Structural or other physical abnormalities must be ruled out/addressed" (Basson et al., 2003, p. 226). Note that vaginal spasm has been eliminated from this definition; vaginismus as vaginal spasm has not been documented (Basson et al., 2003).

Assessment of Dyspareunia In the evaluation of sexual pain, it is important to determine the exact location of the pain. Ask about the pain onset, duration, quality, and severity as well as any factors that cause the pain to improve or worsen (van Lankveld et al., 2010). The timing of the pain in relation to the menstrual cycle should be assessed as well, especially if endometriosis is suspected (Steege & Zolnoun, 2009).

Causes of external pain may include vaginal infections, dermatologic disorders, atrophic vaginitis, allergy, and vulvar vestibulitis. Vaginal infections to consider include vulvovaginal candidiasis, trichomoniasis, bacterial vaginosis, herpes simplex virus, and human papillomavirus (van Lankveld et al., 2010). Dermatologic disorders that can cause pain with intercourse include lichen sclerosus, lichen planus, and lichen simplex chronicus (Steege & Zolnoun, 2009). A biopsy should be performed to diagnose any chronic skin conditions (see Chapter 27).

Women who are perimenopausal, postmenopausal, or lactating should be evaluated for atrophic vaginitis. Vaginal atrophy may also result from use of certain medications, including tamoxifen, danazol, medroxyprogesterone acetate, and GnRH agonists. Physical examination may demonstrate pale and dry vaginal walls with decreased rugae. In addition, vaginal pH is typically greater than 5.0 in the setting of atrophic vaginitis (Reimer & Johnson, 2011).

If the woman is using a latex barrier method for contraception, it is important to consider a latex allergy as the source of the pain. Although the condition is fairly rare, some women are sensitive to human semen. A woman with semen hypersensitivity can demonstrate localized symptoms of vaginal pain after intercourse as well as systemic symptoms of diffuse urticaria, angioedema, and malaise (Bernstein, 2011). If the clinician suspects a woman has a seminal fluid allergy, and use of latex condoms does not alleviate symptoms, the woman should be assessed for a concurrent latex allergy.

Women who report persistent pain at the vaginal introitus or inability to achieve penetration secondary to pain should be evaluated for vulvar vestibulitis (also known as localized provoked vulvodynia, vulvar vestibular syndrome, and vestibulodynia). Many of these women will describe experiencing pain while attempting to insert tampons prior to their first intercourse, but this condition can also develop in women with no previous vulvar pain. To evaluate a woman for vulvar vestibulitis, gently palpate the vestibule (see Chapter 5 for location) with a cotton swab. The woman will often describe a sharp or burning sensation when this area is touched with the swab. Pain is most often elicited at the region of six o'clock in the vulvar vestibule. Criteria for diagnosis include pain with touch or vaginal entry, localization of pain within the vestibule, and vestibular erythema (Steege & Zolnoun, 2009). The etiology of vulvar vestibulitis is unknown, though several theories have been proposed—urinary excretion of oxalates, infection, inflammation, and neuropathic changes (Haefner et al., 2005).

The woman with vaginal pain or pain after intercourse should be evaluated for chronic vaginitis, atrophic vaginitis, and allergy. Trauma related to episiotomy or obstetric lacerations may also be a source of sexual pain, with pressure during intercourse placed on the perineum or the outer third of the vagina causing pain. Signorello, Harlow, Chekos, and Repke (2001) found that 26.7% of women who had a third- or fourth-degree laceration with childbirth had pain with intercourse six months after giving birth.

Deep pelvic pain or pain with thrusting may be caused by adenomyosis, endometriosis, pelvic adhesions, or adnexal pain. Nongynecologic etiologies (e.g., Crohn's disease, irritable bowel syndrome, painful bladder syndrome, and interstitial cystitis) can also cause deep dyspareunia (Steege & Zolnoun, 2009). Trying to duplicate the pain during pelvic examination may give an indication of the source of the pain.

Management of Dyspareunia Treatment of dyspareunia will depend on the etiology of the pain. Vaginal infections should be treated with appropriate antibiotic or antifungal medication. Dermatologic disorders of the genital area are often treated with topical corticosteroids (see Chapter 27). A variety of vaginal estrogen preparations are available to treat perimenopausal and postmenopausal women with atrophic vaginitis (see Chapter 13); these products can also be used for short-term therapy in postpartum women with atrophic vaginitis. Women who dislike the discharge associated with vaginal estrogen creams often prefer to use the vaginal tablets or ring.

Women with vulvar vestibulitis are encouraged to avoid irritants to the vulvar area, wear cotton underwear, and use only water to cleanse the vulva (Haefner et al., 2005; van Lankveld et al., 2010). Nonpharmacologic treatment modalities include pelvic floor physical therapy, biofeedback, transcutaneous electrical nerve stimulation (TENS), and cognitive-behavioral therapy (Landry, Bergeron, Dupuis, & Desrochers, 2008; van Lankveld et al.). Topical 5% lidocaine ointment is effective and can be applied twice daily with a fingertip or overnight with a cotton ball (Steege & Zolnoun, 2009) as well as 30 minutes before sexual activity (Haefner et al.). Some women achieve pain relief with amitriptyline in doses as high as 150 mg per day, or gabapentin in doses as high as 3600 mg per day (Haefner et al.). For women who do not obtain relief with medical therapy, surgical removal of the vestibule can provide long-term pain relief. In a study of 126 women who underwent vestibulectomy and advancement plasty, the percentage who could have intercourse increased from 78% before surgery to 93% after surgery. Intercourse was painless after the surgery for 62% of women (Traas et al., 2006).

Treatment for pelvic pain with intercourse will depend on the source of the pain. Many women report feeling periodic sharp pain when their partner thrusts during intercourse. This pain is often the result of the penis brushing against an ovary. Teaching the woman to shift the position of her hips to change the angle of the uterus and ovaries should eliminate this type of pelvic pain. Women with pelvic infections or endometriosis should receive appropriate treatment to remedy these problems. Physical therapy that teaches the woman to relax her pelvic muscles may also be beneficial in reducing pelvic pain.

Assessment of Vaginismus Women with vaginismus are often not able to complete a pelvic examination, as involuntary contractions of the vaginal muscles can prevent insertion of a speculum or the examiner's fingers. If the woman's partner is able to insert his penis into the vagina during sexual relations, he may describe intercourse as painful because of constriction of the penis by the muscles of the vagina. Women with vaginismus may describe a history of sexual abuse or a history of pain or trauma resulting from medical procedures such as catheterization. Women with dyspareunia may also develop vaginismus in response to repeated painful stimuli.

Management of Vaginismus The treatment for vaginismus includes vaginal dilatation, progressive desensitization, and muscle relaxation (van Lankveld et al., 2010). Kegel exercises can teach a woman to control her vaginal muscles. Referral to a physical therapist can provide the woman with the opportunity to use biofeedback to learn to control the vaginal muscles. The biofeedback machines use electrodes placed externally to the vagina to measure muscle tone. The woman then learns to consciously contract and relax the vaginal muscles and receives positive reinforcement when she practices the technique correctly. Once the woman successfully controls voluntary contraction and relaxation of the muscles, a series of dilators are placed inside the vagina until the woman can accommodate an object the size of a penis. Group cognitive-behavioral therapy and individual exposure therapy may also be helpful (van Lankveld et al.).

Referral to a Therapist Specializing in Sexual Dysfunction

Clinicians who see women with sexual dysfunction should be aware of the counseling resources available in their communities. Problems that should be referred to a therapist include long-standing dysfunction, multiple dysfunctions, current or past abuse, a psychological disorder or acute psychological event, dysfunction with an unknown etiology, and dysfunction that does not respond to therapy (Phillips, 2000). The American Association of Sex Educators, Counselors, and Therapists (AASECT) is a national organization that provides certification for sex counselors and sex therapists. Sex therapists are mental health professionals with specialized training in psychotherapy for sexual problems. The AASECT website (http://www.aasect.org) can help clinicians locate a certified sex therapist in their community.

References

American College of Obstetricians and Gynecologists. (2011). Female sexual dysfunction. ACOG Practice Bulletin No. 119. *Obstetrics & Gynecology, 117*, 996–1007.

American Psychiatric Association. (2000). *Diagnostic and statistical manual of mental disorders* (4th ed., text revision). Washington, DC: Author.

Association of Reproductive Health Professionals. (2010). *Sexual health fundamentals for patient care: A report on 2010 consensus outcomes and guidance for women's health professionals.* Retrieved from http://www.arhp.org/uploadDocs/SHF_meetingreport.pdf.

Avis, N. E., Zhao, X., Johannes, C. B., Ory, M., Brockwell, S., & Greendale, G. A. (2005). Correlates of sexual function among multi-ethnic middle-aged women: Results from the Study of Women's Health Across the Nation (SWAN). *Menopause, 12*, 385–398.

Bachmann, G., Bancroft, J., Braunstein, G., Burger, H., Davis, S., Dennerstein, L., et al. (2002). Female androgen insufficiency: The Princeton consensus statement on definition, classification, and assessment. *Fertility and Sterility, 77*, 660–665.

Basson, R. (2000). The female sexual response: A different model. *Journal of Sex and Marital Therapy, 26*, 51–65.

Basson, R. (2006). Sexual desire and arousal disorders in women. *New England Journal of Medicine, 354,* 1497–1506.

Basson, R., Leiblum, S. L., Brotto, L., Derogatis, L., Fourcroy, J., Fugl-Myer, K., et al. (2003). Definitions of women's sexual dysfunctions reconsidered: Advocating expansion and revision. *Journal of Psychosomatic Obstetrics and Gynaecology, 24,* 221–229.

Basson, R., Wierman, M. E., van Lankveld, J., & Brotto, L. (2010). Summary of the recommendations on sexual dysfunctions in women. *Journal of Sexual Medicine, 7,* 314–326.

Berman, J., & Berman, L. (2001). *For women only: A revolutionary guide for overcoming sexual dysfunction and reclaiming your life.* New York: Henry Holt.

Bernstein, J. A. (2011). Human seminal plasma hypersensitivity: An under-recognized women's health issue. *Postgraduate Medicine, 123,* 120–125.

Brassil, D. F., & Keller, M. (2002). Female sexual dysfunction: Definitions, causes, and treatment. *Urologic Nursing, 22,* 237–284.

Brotto, L. A., Bitzer, J., Laan, E., Leiblum, S., & Luria, M. (2010). Women's sexual desire and arousal disorders. *Journal of Sexual Medicine, 7,* 586–614.

Brown, D. A., Kyle, J. A., & Ferrill, M. J. (2009). Assessing the clinical efficacy of sildenafil for the treatment of female sexual dysfunction. *Annals of Pharmacotherapy, 43,* 1275–1285.

Clayton, A. H., & Balon, R. (2009). The impact of mental illness and psychotropic medications on sexual functioning: The evidence and management. *Journal of Sexual Medicine, 6,* 1200–1211.

Clayton, A. H., Pradko, J. F., Croft, H. A., Montano, B., Leadbetter, R. A., Bolden-Watson, C., et al. (2002). Prevalence of sexual dysfunction among newer antidepressants. *Journal of Clinical Psychiatry, 63,* 357–366.

Clayton, A. H., Warnock, J. K., Kornstein, S. G., Pinkerton, R., Sheldon-Keller, A., & McGarvey, E. L. (2004). A placebo controlled trial of bupropion SR as an antidote for selective serotonin reuptake inhibitor-induced sexual dysfunction. *Journal of Clinical Psychiatry, 65,* 62–67.

Feldhaus-Dahir, M. (2010). Treatment options for female sexual arousal disorder: Part II. *Urologic Nursing, 30,* 247–251.

Ferguson, D. M., Hosmane, B., & Heiman, J. R. (2010). Randomized, placebo-controlled, double-blind, parallel design trial of the efficacy and safety of Zestra in women with mixed desire/interest/arousal/orgasm disorders. *Journal of Sex and Marital Therapy, 36,* 66–86.

Frank, J. E., Mistretta, P., & Will, J. (2008). Diagnosis and treatment of female sexual dysfunction. *American Family Physician, 77,* 635–642.

Haefner, H. K., Collins, M. E., Davis, G. D., Edwards, L., Foster, D. C., Hartmann, E. D., et al. (2005). The vulvodynia guideline. *Journal of Lower Genital Tract Disease, 9,* 40–51.

Hatzichristou, D., Rosen, R. C., Derogatis, L., Low, W. Y., Meuleman, E. J. H., Sadovsky, R., et al. (2010). Recommendations for the clinical evaluation of men and women with sexual dysfunction. *Journal of Sexual Medicine, 7,* 337–348.

Heiman, J. R., Gittelman, M., Costabile, R., Guay, A., Friedman, A., Heard-Davison, A., et al. (2006). Topical alprostadil (PGE_1) for the treatment of female sexual arousal disorder: In-clinic evaluation of safety and efficacy. *Journal of Psychosomatic Obstetrics and Gynaecology, 27,* 31–41.

Heiman, J. R., & Lopiccolo, J. (1988). *Becoming orgasmic.* New York: Simon & Schuster.

Herbenick, D., Reece, M., Schick, V., Sanders, S. A., Dodge, B., & Fortenberry, J. D. (2010). Sexual behaviors, relationships, and perceived health status among adult women in the United States: Results from a national probability sample. *Journal of Sexual Medicine, 7*(suppl 5), 277–290.

IsHak, W. W., Bokarius, A., Jeffrey, J. K., Davis, M. C., & Bakhta, Y. (2010). Disorders of orgasm in women: A literature review of etiology and current treatments. *Journal of Sexual Medicine, 7,* 3254–3268.

Ito, T. Y., Polan, M. L., Whipple, B., & Trant, A. S. (2006). The enhancement of female sexual function with ArginMax, a nutritional supplement, among women differing in menopausal status. *Journal of Sex and Marital Therapy, 32,* 369–378.

Kingsberg, S., & Althof, S. E. (2009). Evaluation and treatment of female sexual disorders. *International Urogynecology Journal, 20,* S33–S43.

Landen, M., Eriksson, E., Agren, H., & Fahlen, T. (1999). Effect of buspirone on sexual dysfunction in depressed patients treated with selective serotonin reuptake inhibitors. *Journal of Clinical Psychopharmacology, 19,* 268–271.

Landry, T., Bergeron, S., Dupuis, M-J., & Desrochers, G. (2008). The treatment of provoked vestibulodynia: A critical review. *Clinical Journal of Pain, 24,* 155–171.

Laumann, E. O., Paik, A., & Rosen, R. C. (1999). Sexual dysfunction in the United States: Prevalence and predictors. *Journal of the American Medical Association, 281,* 537–544.

Mathur, R., & Braunstein, G. D. (2010). Androgen deficiency and therapy in women. *Current Opinion in Endocrinology, Diabetes, & Obesity, 17,* 342–349.

Modelska, K., & Cummings, S. (2002). Tibolone for postmenopausal women: Systemic review of randomized trials. *Journal of Clinical Endocrinology and Metabolism, 87,* 16–23.

Morley, J. E., & Kaiser, F. E. (2003). Female sexuality. *Medical Clinics of North America, 87,* 1077–1090.

Nurnberg, H. G., Hensley, P. L., Heiman, J. R., Croft, H. A., Debattista, C., & Paine, S. (2008). Sildenafil treatment of women with antidepressant-associated sexual dysfunction: A randomized controlled trial. *Journal of the American Medical Association, 300,* 395–404.

Phillips, N. A. (2000). Female sexual dysfunction: Evaluation and treatment. *American Family Physician, 62,* 127–136, 141–142.

Poorman, S. G. (1988). *Human sexuality and the nursing process.* Norwalk, CT: Appleton & Lange.

Reimer, A., & Johnson, L. (2011). Atrophic vaginitis: Signs, symptoms, and better outcomes. *Nurse Practitioner, 36,* 22–28.

Rosen, R., Brown, C., Heiman, J., Leiblum, S., Meston, C., Shabsigh, R., et al. (2000). The Female Sexual Function Index (FSFI): A multidimensional self-report instrument for the assessment of sexual function. *Journal of Sex & Marital Therapy, 26,* 191–208.

Rosner, W., Auchus, R. J., Azziz, R., Sluss, P. M., & Raff, H. (2007). Utility, limitations, and pitfalls in measuring testosterone: An Endocrine Society position statement. *Journal of Clinical Endocrinology & Metabolism, 92,* 405–413.

Shifren, J. L., Monz, B. U., Russo, P. A., Segreti, A., & Johannes, C. B. (2008). Sexual problems and distress in United States women. *Obstetrics & Gynecology, 112,* 970–978.

Signorello, L. B., Harlow, B. L., Chekos, A. K., & Repke, J. T. (2001). Postpartum sexual functioning and its relationship to perineal trauma: A retrospective cohort study of primiparous women. *American Journal of Obstetrics and Gynecology, 184,* 881–890.

Steege, J. F., & Zolnoun, D. A. (2009). Evaluation and treatment of dyspareunia. *Obstetrics & Gynecology, 113,* 1124–1136.

Traas, M. A. F., Bekkers, R. L. M., Dony, J. M. J., Blom, M., van Haren, A. W. P., Hendriks, J. C. M., et al. (2006). Surgical treatment for the vulvar vestibulitis syndrome. *Obstetrics & Gynecology, 107,* 256–262.

Traish, A., Guay, A. T., Spark, R. F., & Testosterone Therapy in Women Study Group. (2007). Are the Endocrine Society's clinical practice guidelines on androgen therapy in women misguided? A commentary. *Journal of Sexual Medicine, 4,* 1223–1235.

van Lankveld, J. J. D. M., Granot, M., Weijmar Schulzt, W. C. M., Binik, Y. M., Wesselmann, U., Pukall, C. F., et al. (2010). Women's sexual pain disorders. *Journal of Sexual Medicine, 7,* 615–631.

Weismiller, D. G. (2002). The perimenopause and menopause experience: An overview. *Clinics in Family Practice, 4,* 1–12.

Wierman, M. E., Basson, R., Davis, S. R., Khosla, S., Miller, K. K., Rosner, W., et al. (2006). Androgen therapy in women: An Endocrine Society clinical practice guideline. *Journal of Clinical Endocrinology & Metabolisms, 91,* 3697–3710.

CHAPTER 18

Unintended Pregnancy

Katherine Simmonds
Frances E. Likis

Nearly half of all pregnancies in the United States are unintended. Indeed, for many women, the discovery that they are pregnant is a time of personal crisis that requires complex decision making. Clinicians who provide gynecologic health care frequently encounter these women in the clinical setting and are often responsible for providing them with diagnoses, counseling, and other needed services or referrals. These responsibilities necessitate an understanding of unintended pregnancy, the conflicts that clinicians may experience when caring for women experiencing unintended pregnancies, and the appropriate assessment and management when providing this care.

Scope of the Problem

An estimated 49% of pregnancies in the United States are unintended, and unintended pregnancies occur among women of all ages and socioeconomic groups (Finer & Henshaw, 2006). Given this rate, more than half of women in the United States will experience an unintended pregnancy by the age of 45 (Jones, Singh, Finer, & Frohwirth, 2006). Unintended pregnancy is most frequent among women who are between the ages of 18 and 24, are unmarried, are poor, are members of minority groups, or have not finished high school—all characteristics that signal significant disparities in this aspect of reproductive health (Finer & Henshaw).

Approximately 42% of unintended pregnancies end in abortion, 44% result in live births, and 14% end in miscarriage (Finer & Henshaw, 2006). An estimated 1.2 million abortions took place in the United States in 2005, continuing a general trend of decline in this rate since its peak in the early 1980s (Jones, Zolna, Henshaw, & Finer, 2008; Strauss et al., 2007). Placing the infant for adoption is an alternative to parenting for the woman who chooses to carry an unintended pregnancy to term. Comprehensive adoption statistics have not been collected in the United States for many years; thus current information about how frequently adoption is the outcome of unintended pregnancy is limited. Estimates from the 2002 National Survey of Family Growth indicate that 1% of infants born to never-married women younger than 45 years of age were relinquished for adoption between 1996 and 2002 (Jones, 2008).

Consequences of the decision to continue an unintended pregnancy and parent the child include potentially adverse effects for both women and their children. Unintended pregnancy is associated with later entry into prenatal care, a lower number of total prenatal visits, tobacco and alcohol use during pregnancy, low birth weight, infant mortality, child abuse, and insufficient resources for child development (Brown & Eisenberg, 1995). Unintended pregnancy precludes the opportunity to receive preconception care that might otherwise improve pregnancy outcomes. Women with unintended pregnancies are also at greater risk for physical abuse and depression. Couples experiencing unintended pregnancy are more likely to end their relationships, and they may forfeit their educational and professional aspirations (Brown & Eisenberg).

Historically, unintended pregnancies have been subdivided into two categories: mistimed and unwanted. Pregnancies are defined as *mistimed* if the woman wanted to have a child or another child in the future, but not at the present time. Pregnancies are considered *unwanted* if the woman never wanted to have a child or additional children. Negative effects of unintended pregnancy appear stronger among women with unwanted, rather than mistimed, pregnancies (Brown & Eisenberg, 1995).

Etiology

The most obvious reason why unintended pregnancies occur is inconsistent or incorrect use of contraceptives. Contraceptive nonuse and misuse may result from numerous causes, including lack of knowledge, barriers to access, and complex personal, interpersonal, socioeconomic, and cultural factors (Brown & Eisenberg, 1995). Inconsistent contraceptive use is another important factor that leads to unintended pregnancy: One study of more than 10,000 women who had abortions found that 54% were using a contraceptive method in the month they conceived (Jones, Darroch, & Henshaw, 2002a). Even perfect contraceptive use does not guarantee avoiding pregnancy, because inherent method failures are possible. According to the Guttmacher Institute (2000), "The typical American woman spends roughly three decades—or about 75% of her reproductive life—trying to avoid unintended pregnancy" (p. 10). Preventing pregnancy requires prolonged and concerted effort. The scale of this task, the obstacles to perfect contraceptive use, and the unavoidable failures of contraceptive methods provide insight into why unintended pregnancies are common.

Conflicts in Caring for Women with Unintended Pregnancies

Clinicians may experience complex personal responses when providing care to women with unintended pregnancies. Reactions may range from complete acceptance to deep disturbance about a woman's situation or chosen course of action, with myriad emotions between these extremes being possible. No matter what personal feelings are stirred by these clinical encounters, clinicians have professional responsibilities when providing patient care. Values clarification is a process that can help clinicians to explore the intersection of their personal beliefs and professional responsibilities, so that ultimately patients' rights are upheld (Simmonds & Likis, 2005).

Professional Responsibilities

Clinicians have professional responsibilities to uphold patient rights and autonomy, and to treat patients with respect and compassion. These responsibilities are codified by several professional organizations, including the American Academy of Physician Assistants (2008), the American College of Nurse–Midwives (1997), the American College of Obstetricians and Gynecologists (2007; reaffirmed 2011), and the National Organization of Nurse Practitioner Faculties and American Association of Colleges of Nursing (2002). These documents (**Box 18-1**) provide an ethical and legal mandate for clinicians to ensure patient access to comprehensive reproductive health services, including pregnancy options counseling. Applying these principles in the clinical setting means that women must be given the opportunity to express their concerns, desires, and need for additional information in a supportive environment. Creating such conditions can be challenging, however. Opinions about what patients "should" do may subtly or overtly influence the therapeutic relationship, particularly for clinicians who are not fully aware of the boundaries between their personal beliefs and professional responsibilities. Although a woman may make a decision that is different from what a clinician wishes or believes is best, upholding patient autonomy is paramount (Simmonds & Likis, 2005).

Values Clarification

Because unintended pregnancy and its outcomes—including such possibilities as adolescent pregnancy, single parenthood, and abortion—are socially and politically controversial, it is important for those clinicians who provide care to women of reproductive age to clarify their own values regarding these issues. Ideally, this self-assessment should take place before having a clinical encounter with a woman who is faced with an unintended pregnancy. In addition, because personal beliefs and professional work environments are dynamic, engaging in a process of ongoing values clarification benefits clinicians and the women they care for (Simmonds & Likis, 2005).

Several resources have been developed to assist clinicians to clarify their personal beliefs about pregnancy options, and to help them examine the intersection of these beliefs with their responsibilities as professionals. These materials include books, articles, and exercises that may be used either individually or in groups (**Table 18-1**). Given the heightened controversy surrounding abortion in the United States, many of these resources focus largely or exclusively on that option. Although this emphasis may be warranted, exploring beliefs about women's decisions to parent or place a child for adoption are equally impor-

BOX 18-1 *Statements of Professional Organizations*

American Academy of Physician Assistants (2008):

Reproductive Decision Making: Patients have a right to access the full range of reproductive health care services, including fertility treatments, contraception, sterilization, and abortion. Physician assistants (PAs) have an ethical obligation to provide balanced and unbiased clinical information about reproductive health care.

When the PA's personal values conflict with providing full disclosure or providing certain services such as sterilization or abortion, the PA need not become involved in that aspect of the patient's care. By referring the patient to a qualified provider who is willing to discuss and facilitate all treatment options, the PA fulfills their ethical obligation to ensure the patient's access to all legal options.

American College of Nurse–Midwives (1997):

Certified nurse–midwives (CNMs) and certified midwives (CMs) believe that every individual has the right to safe, satisfying health care with respect for human dignity and cultural variations. We support each person's right to self-determination, to complete information, and to active participation in all aspects of care. We acknowledge that the cultural, religious and ethnic diversity of CNMs and CMs and their clients allow for a variety of personal and professional choices.

Therefore, the ACNM holds the following positions:

- That every woman has the right to make reproductive choices
- That every woman has the right to access to factual, unbiased information about reproductive choices, in order to make an informed decision
- That women with limited means should have access to financial resources for their reproductive choices

American College of Obstetricians and Gynecologists (2007, reaffirmed 2011):

A pregnant woman should be fully informed in a balanced manner about all options, including raising the child herself, placing the child for adoption, and abortion. The information conveyed should be appropriate to the duration of the pregnancy. The professional should make every effort to avoid introducing personal bias.

ACOG supports access to care for all individuals, irrespective of financial status, and supports the availability of all reproductive options. ACOG opposes unnecessary regulations that limit or delay access to care.

National Organization of Nurse Practitioner Faculties and American Association of Colleges of Nursing (2002):

Upon graduation/entry into practice, women's health nurse practitioners should be able to:

- Facilitate access to reproductive health care services and provide referrals in an unbiased, timely, and sensitive manner
- Support a woman's right to make her own decisions regarding her health and reproductive choices within the context of her belief system
- Demonstrate effective communication skills in addressing sensitive topics related to sexuality, risk-taking behaviors, and abuse

TABLE 18-1 Resources for Values Clarification

Title	Type of Resource	Where to Obtain the Resource
Abortion and Options Counseling: A Comprehensive Reference	Book	The Hope Clinic for Women, Ltd. http://www.hopeclinic.com/publications .html
Caring for the Woman with an Unintended Pregnancy	CD-ROM	The Reproductive Options Education Consortium for Nursing http://www.abortionaccess.org/content /view/27/76
"Options Counseling: Techniques for Caring for Women with Unintended Pregnancies"	Article	Singer, J. (2004). Options counseling: Techniques for caring for women with unintended pregnancies. *Journal of Midwifery and Women's Health, 49*, 235–242. See Appendix A for values clarification exercises.
The Issue of Abortion in America: An Exploration of a Social Controversy	CD-ROM	Routledge http://www.routledge.com/books/The -Issue-of-Abortion-in-America-isbn 9780415184496
The Abortion Option: A Values Clarification Guide for Health Professionals	Workbook	National Abortion Federation (NAF) http://www.prochoice.org/pubs_research /publications/downloads/professional _education/abortion_option.pdf
"Induced Abortion: An Ethical Conundrum for Counselors"	Article	Millner, V. S., & Hanks, R. B. (2002). Induced abortion: An ethical conundrum for counselors. *Journal of Counseling & Development, 80*, 57–63.

tant. Unexamined personal beliefs about these options can also inadvertently affect clinical encounters. For example, a clinician may have strong personal feelings about an adolescent who reports she has decided to parent a child or about a woman who has no hesitation about placing her infant for adoption. During the values clarification process, attention to all pregnancy options is worthwhile.

The ultimate goal of values clarification is to ensure that women with unintended pregnancies receive care that is free from bias, nondirective, and without judgment. By engaging in a process of values clarification, clinicians can identify situations in which they experience conflict between their personal beliefs and professional responsibilities. Areas of perceived conflict warrant further examination.

If after an in-depth exploration of one's own beliefs the clinician determines that conflicts between her or his personal beliefs and professional responsibilities are irreconcilable, she or he must acknowledge this conflict. It is the clinician's professional obligation to make a feasible plan to ensure that women who seek care will not be denied their right to comprehensive, respectful pregnancy options counseling. Fulfilling this responsibility may require that the clinician refer patients to a colleague or to a different setting entirely. Alternative plans should not create undue hardship for women, such as necessitating long travel distances or paying out of pocket for services rendered, nor should they result in significant delays in delivery of care. Familiarity with the practices of the referral site is also essential. If women are referred to another facility for options counseling, they must be assured that the counseling offered in that site will include factual information about all of the available options and be nondirective. Clinicians who identify a high level of personal conflict in providing comprehensive pregnancy options counseling are advised not to choose to work in settings where it is a frequent job responsibility (Higginbotham, 2002).

Assessment

A pregnancy test should be performed for diagnosis or when warranted to confirm previous testing. Estimate gestational age, preferably by ascertaining the woman's last menstrual period (LMP). Bimanual examination for uterine size or ultrasound may be appropriate to determine gestational age if the LMP is unknown (see Chapter 7). Assessment of pregnancy intention is more complex and is discussed in the next section.

Management

Prevention

Ideally all pregnancies would be wanted and planned. Toward this goal, the *Healthy People 2020* objectives include increasing the percentage of pregnancies that are intended to 56% (HealthyPeople.gov, 2011). The primary way to prevent unintended pregnancy is for couples to use contraception with every act of intercourse during which they do not want to get pregnant. Improving contraception education and counseling, eliminating practice routines that impede obtaining timely services (e.g., long waits for appointments for contraceptive services, requirement for a pelvic examination prior to prescribing hormonal contraception), and removing financial barriers to contraceptive access are important strategies to reduce unintended pregnancy (Moos, 2003).

Because perfect contraceptive use is unrealistic, emergency contraception (EC) has emerged as an important method for the prevention of unintended pregnancy. EC has the potential to prevent half of the unintended pregnancies in the United States, and it is estimated to have prevented 51,000 abortions in 2000 (Finer & Henshaw, 2003; Trussell, Stewart, Guest, & Hatcher, 1992). More information about EC can be found in Chapter 12.

Pregnancy Options Counseling

Options counseling provides women faced with an unintended pregnancy with an opportunity to explore whether they will carry the pregnancy and parent the child, carry the pregnancy and place the infant for adoption, or have an abortion. Although pregnancy options counseling is sometimes referred to as abortion counseling, the two are actually quite distinct practices. Options counseling is for a woman who knows she is pregnant and needs to clarify her thoughts and feelings about her alternatives. Preabortion counseling is provided when a woman has made the decision to have an abortion but is found to have additional emotional or personal needs that warrant additional attention before or following the procedure (Baker & Beresford, 2009). Clinicians counseling women with unintended pregnancies need to understand the options available as well as the fundamental principles of pregnancy options counseling to provide adequate quality care.

It is essential for the clinician who is providing pregnancy options counseling to be nondirective in his or her approach, and to withhold personal judgment about the woman's situation and decision. Equally important is ensuring patient confidentiality. Fear that parents, a partner, or others will find out about an unintended pregnancy may prevent some women from seeking counseling.

Other essentials of providing pregnancy options counseling include establishing rapport, using neutral language, and asking open-ended questions. Options counseling is a form of crisis intervention that usually takes place during one clinician–patient interaction. As such, it is short term, addresses an immediate problem, and involves a major life crisis needing a time-limited decision (Baker, 1995).

Although every patient encounter is unique—necessitating variations in approach—the following four general steps are suggested for clinicians when providing pregnancy options counseling (Simmonds & Likis, 2005).

Explore How the Woman Feels About the Pregnancy and Her Options Asking, "How do you feel about being pregnant?" is a neutral, open-ended question that may be used to begin the counseling session, and encourages the woman to share her emotions without being directed as to what her answer should be. Avoid questions or statements that make assumptions about feelings, such as "Are you happy about the pregnancy?" or "Congratulations!" The questions "Do you know what your choices are?" and "What are your thoughts about becoming a parent? About adoption? About abortion?" help the clinician ascertain the woman's level of understanding of the available options and her feelings about each choice. Listing the risks and benefits, or pros and cons, of each option may help the woman to realistically assess her situation and make an informed decision.

Help the Woman to Identify Support Systems and Assess Risks Asking the woman whom she has told that she is pregnant, how these people have responded, and what their significance to her is allows for a greater understanding of her situation. This will help the clinician identify women who may be isolated and in need of additional support.

Assessing for risk of interpersonal violence should also be a standard component of pregnancy options counseling. Women experiencing an unintended pregnancy are at higher risk for intimate partner violence (Saltzman, Johnson, Gilbert, & Goodwin, 2003). Asking adolescents about their parents' potential reaction to the pregnancy can help identify situations where child abuse is present or possible.

Another important topic to address is the potential for coercion regarding the decision. Coercion from partners, parents, or other significant relationships may be an issue with regard to any of the options. Women may feel pressure to continue pregnancies, place children for adoption, or have abortions against their will.

Encouraging the woman to talk with those individuals whom she feels will be supportive of her decision and helping her to explore what it would be like to tell someone who may not be supportive can be valuable aspects of the counseling session, particularly in the case of adolescents. Arrange for additional follow-up for patients who report they are unable to tell anyone about the pregnancy. This step may include referral to a professional counselor.

Help the Woman to Reach a Decision or Discuss a Timetable for Decision Making Women may present for pregnancy options counseling either having just found out they are pregnant or already having been aware for some time. Some may need time to accept their situation or to discuss it with others, or both. Some may not want to discuss the matter with a clinician at all. Together with the woman, determine whether to proceed immediately with complete pregnancy options counseling, or to postpone the session until a later time. In either case, make sure that she is aware of the current estimated gestational age of the pregnancy, and that her decision is time sensitive when establishing a follow-up plan. Some women may benefit from other resources to further explore their options on their own (**Table 18-2**).

If the woman is ready to make a decision, assess whether she needs any additional information, or whether she would like to discuss any of the options further. For some women, resources that allow a better understanding or visualization of fetal development can be helpful during this stage of the decision-making process; for other women, these types of resources may not be helpful in making a decision. Accurate patient education resources on fetal development should be made available for those who express interest.

Refer or Provide the Woman with Appropriate Services Depending on what a woman chooses to do, she may be able to receive the services she needs within that setting, or she may be referred elsewhere. Knowing which resources are available for pregnant women—whether they choose to continue a pregnancy, place a child for adoption, or have an abortion—is essential. The Child Welfare Information Gateway and the National Abortion Federation (**Box 18-2**) offer information about the adoption and abortion services available in specific geographic areas. However, it is also important to consult colleagues and others in the community about the reputation and practices of any agency or clinic prior to referring patients there. Finally, when providing referrals, be sure that women understand how to access them.

Options for Women Experiencing Unintended Pregnancies

Continuing the Pregnancy

Parenting is a long-term commitment that carries immense responsibility. Optimally those who choose to parent would have the time and ability to care for a child, adequate financial resources, and support from spouses or partners, family members, and friends. Clinicians

TABLE 18-2 Patient Resources for Exploring Pregnancy Options

Title	Type	Where to Obtain the Resource	Description
http://www.pregnancyoptions.info	Website	http://www.pregnancyoptions.info	Offers online resources including exercises for the woman who is undecided about what to do about a pregnancy as well as information on all three pregnancy options.
Pregnant? Need Help? Pregnancy Options Workbook	Workbook	http://www.pregnancyoptions.info/pregnant.htm	Comprehensive workbook of information and exercises for women exploring pregnancy options. Includes all three options and addresses topics such as decision making, getting support, male partners, fetal development, and spiritual and religious concerns.
"Unsure About Your Pregnancy? A Guide To Making the Right Decision for You"	Brochure	http://prochoice.org/pubs_research/publications/downloads/are_you_pregnant/pregnancy_guide_english.pdf	Provides exercises for pregnant women who are undecided about their pregnancy. The website also provides links to information about all three options.
"Are You Pregnant and Thinking About Adoption?"	Factsheet	http://www.childwelfare.gov/pubs/f_pregna	Provides information about adoption, including community resources and considerations for fathers and relatives.

BOX 18-2 *Reproductive Options, Legislation, and Policies Resources*

Child Welfare Information Gateway
http://www.childwelfare.gov
(click on *Adoption*)

The Guttmacher Institute
http://www.guttmacher.org
Research and analysis for individual states:
http://www.guttmacher.org/statecenter

The Kaiser Family Foundation
http://www.kff.org

Specifics regarding state policies
and legislation:
http://www.statehealthfacts.kff.org
(click on *Women's Health*)

NARAL Prochoice America
http://www.naral.org

The National Abortion Federation
http://www.prochoice.org

The National Abortion Rights Action League State-by-State Guide to Legislative Bills
http://mail.naral.org/longdoc.nsf

can provide pregnant women with information about state and local programs that provide social and financial support to pregnant women and their children. Such information may prove critical in their decision-making process. Women who decide to continue a pregnancy should begin prenatal care, either in the setting where options counseling occurred, if those services are provided, or by referral to a prenatal care provider.

Adoption

Arrangements for adoption vary according to state law. Children may be placed for adoption through public or private agencies, independently using an adoption lawyer or facilitator, or directly between the birth and adoptive parents. Adoptions may be closed or open. Parents in a confidential or closed adoption do not know each other or have contact, but the adoptive parents are given relevant information about the birth parents such as medical histories. Open adoption encompasses options along a broad continuum that may range from birth parents reading about families and selecting one, to ongoing contact between the families (Smith & Brandon, 2008).

Abortion

Options for induced abortion in the United States (as of this writing) include aspiration, medication, surgical, and labor induction methods. The decision about which method is employed in an individual situation depends on several factors, including the gestational age of the pregnancy, preference of the patient, and clinician training and availability. Clinicians need to be familiar with which abortion options are available for women in their care to provide accurate counseling and referrals. In addition, nurse practitioners, nurse–midwives, and physician assistants can legally provide medical or surgical abortion in some states. The specific laws and regulations that determine whether abortion provision lies within the scope of practice of these different clinician groups vary from state to state (Taylor, Safriet, Dempsey, Kruse, & Jackson, 2009).

Aspiration Abortion   Aspiration is the most commonly used method of induced abortion in the United States, with medication abortion being the next most commonly used (Jones et al., 2008). In 2005, approximately 10% of abortions were performed by induction methods (Gamble et al., 2008). Because of their high rates of morbidity and mortality, hysterotomy and hysterectomy have fallen out of favor as techniques for abortion in this country and are rarely used (Henshaw, 2009). The most recent data on the timing of abortions indicate that 88% are performed prior to 13 weeks' gestation, and only 1.4% after 20 weeks' gestation (Gamble et al.).

Abortion may be performed as early as a pregnancy is detected, although to ensure that the pregnancy has been terminated some clinicians prefer to postpone the procedure until a gestational sac can be visualized by ultrasound or directly during postprocedure tissue examination (generally between 4 and 6 weeks' gestation). Research has demonstrated that aspiration abortion prior to 6 weeks' gestation is safe and effective, particularly if protocols that guard against missed ectopic or continuing pregnancies are followed (Edwards & Carson, 1997). Upper limits beyond which therapeutic abortion may be performed are based on legal, rather than medical restrictions, and vary from state to state. Box 18-2 describes resources that can be used to locate information on state laws.

All aspiration abortion methods involve removing the products of conception (POC) by introducing a cannula, attached to a source of suction, through the cervical os into the uterine cavity. Suction can be generated by either manual or electric pumps (MVA or EVA, respectively). MVA is generally used only for abortions earlier than 14 weeks' gestation (Meckstroth & Paul, 2009). The decision to use MVA or EVA depends on clinician preference and training as well as equipment availability.

In early abortions, evacuation of the uterus takes only a few minutes, and may be accomplished through the use of suction alone. Some clinicians choose to curette the walls of the uterus after suctioning (a process referred to as dilation and curettage [D & C]) to ensure that the procedure is complete. However, because D & C is associated with increased rates of complications and has no demonstrable benefits, the World Health Organization has recommended that this technique be replaced by suction alone for first-trimester abortions (Meckstroth & Paul, 2009).

When performing abortions after the first trimester, forceps are often used as an adjunct to suction to remove the POC. This technique is termed dilation and evacuation (D & E). Research has shown D & E to be at least as safe and less physically and emotionally stressful for patients than labor induction (Hammond & Chasen, 2009; Henshaw, 2009). In a small, randomized, controlled trial comparing D & E and labor induction, 62% of potential participants declined study enrollment primarily because of their preference for D & E (Grimes, Smith, & Witham, 2004). However, because second-trimester D & E requires more advanced training on the part of the clinician, the decision to employ labor induction instead of D & E may be based on clinician availability, rather than patient preference or medical considerations (Hammond & Chasen).

Dilation of the cervix is usually necessary to remove the POC except in very early aspiration abortions. The degree of dilation required depends on the gestational age of the pregnancy. It may be accomplished either by inserting dilating rods of increasing diameter into the cervical os immediately before inserting the cannula or by placing osmotic dilators into the cervix several hours to a day before the procedure. In general, osmotic dilators are used in later abortions, although cinician training and experience may also guide this decision. Oral or vaginal pharmacologic agents, such as misoprostol, are also used in some settings to promote cervical ripening and subsequent dilation (Meckstroth & Paul, 2009).

In the United States, women are offered various options for pain relief during and following aspiration and D & E abortions. In most settings, a paracervical block is routinely administered with a local anesthetic, such as lidocaine, prior to cervical dilation. In addition, many clinicians offer patients the options of intravenous or oral pain medications, as well as general anesthesia in some settings. Studies suggest that the use of intravenous and general anesthesia increases patient satisfaction, contributes to faster recovery and improved physiologic benefits for patients, and may positively influence operative conditions for clinicians (Nichols, Halvorson-Boyd, Goldstein, Gevirtz, & Healow, 2009). These benefits must be weighed against the inherent risks associated with the use of anesthesia. The most recent epidemiologic data available attribute 16% of all abortion-related deaths to anesthesia complications (Bartlett et al., 2004). Nonpharmacologic approaches, including positive suggestion, relaxation, and guided imagery, have also been successfully used to decrease pain, including for patients undergoing abortions (Nichols et al.).

Recovery after an abortion depends on the type of procedure done and anesthesia used, the gestational age of the pregnancy, and the existence of any complications or unusual psychosocial factors. With uncomplicated early abortions in which only local anesthesia is used, women may be able to leave as soon as 20 minutes after the procedure. Greater levels of anesthesia generally require longer periods of stabilization and monitoring. Following an abortion, women are instructed that they may resume regular activity as soon as they feel ready, although they are usually advised to not engage in sexual intercourse, rigorous exercise, or lifting of heavy objects for a few days to a week following the procedure. Evidence to support these recommendations is limited (Espey & MacIsaac, 2009).

Typically women are advised to return to the facility where the abortion was provided or to their primary care provider for a routine examination in two to three weeks to ensure a complete and uncomplicated recovery, to check their emotional well-being, and to initiate or follow up on a newly established contraceptive method. There is also little evidence to support this practice, which is costly for both women and the healthcare system. Alternative approaches for follow-up care have been suggested, including better patient education regarding self-monitoring for postabortion complications and improved delivery of contraceptive services at the time of the abortion (Grossman, Ellertson, Grimes, & Walker, 2004).

Medication Abortion Medication is a relatively new method for induced abortion in the United States, but one whose acceptance has grown steadily since the U.S. Food and Drug Administration (FDA) approved mifepristone for use in 2000. In 2005 (the most recent year for which data are available), 161,000 U.S. women obtained medication abortions, constituting 13% of all abortions; 21% of those abortions before 9 weeks' gestation (Jones et al., 2008).

Currently, the most widely used method of medication abortion in the United States is the administration of mifepristone in conjunction with misoprostol (Creinin & Danielsson, 2009). Alternative medications that can be used for effecting an early abortion include the combination of methotrexate with misoprostol, and misoprostol alone. Because of the greater frequency of mifepristone–misoprostol abortions in the United States, this method is the primary focus of this section. All methods of medication abortion are currently used only for early abortions.

Multiple studies have found mifepristone to be highly efficacious up to 63 days' gestation. Overall, success rates of 92% to 99% have been reported, with the highest rates of complete abortion occurring with vaginal or buccal (compared to oral) administration of misoprostol, and in earlier gestations (49 days or less) (Creinin & Danielsson, 2009; National Abortion Federation, 2005). Methotrexate (combined with misoprostol) abortions have been found to have similar efficacy rates with gestations of 49 days or less. Misoprostol-alone abortion has been found to be somewhat less efficacious (85% to 95%); however, studies indicate that this level of efficacy persists through the first trimester (Creinin & Danielsson).

Mifepristone works by binding to progesterone receptors more effectively than progesterone itself, thereby blocking the hormone's effects. As a result, the endometrium sloughs and the cervix softens, both of which promote expulsion of pregnancy tissue. Adding misoprostol (a prostaglandin) increases the efficacy of this regimen (Creinin & Danielsson, 2009).

Specific protocols for the use of mifepristone vary from site to site. These alternative, evidence-based options often differ from the FDA-approved protocol with regard to medication doses, their administration and timing, use of ultrasound, gestational limits, and required follow-up visits. A summary of the FDA-approved and alternative evidence-based approaches appears in **Table 18-3**.

TABLE 18-3 Comparison of Mifepristone Abortion Regimens

	FDA-Approved Regimen	**Evidence-Based Regimen***
Recommended gestational age	49 days ≤ last menstrual period	63 days ≤ last menstrual period
Mifepristone dose	600 mg orally	200 mg orally
Misoprostol dose	400 mcg orally; administered on site at the second office visit	400–800 mcg with different routes of administration (vaginal, buccal, oral); supplied at the first visit, but taken at home
Misoprostol timing	48 hours after mifepristone	15 minutes to 72 hours after mifepristone
Ultrasound use	Required	Optional
Follow-up visit	Day 14	24 hours to 2 weeks post treatment
Minimum visits	3	2

*A number of alternatives to the FDA-approved regimen for the use of mifepristone and misoprostol for medication abortion have been developed based on evidence from studies that reported fewer side effects, less expense, and/or increased patient or clinician acceptability. These evidence-based regimens vary across practice sites with regard to gestational age limits; mifepristone dose; misoprostol dose, route of administration (vaginal, buccal, or oral), patient location at administration (office vs. home), and timing of administration; use of ultrasound; and follow-up scheduling.

Source: Adapted from Creinin & Danielsson, 2009.

Currently in most settings in the United States, patients are given mifepristone (200 mg) on site following verification of gestational age via clinical examination or ultrasound. The woman is instructed to self-administer the misoprostol (400 to 800 mcg) vaginally, buccally or orally at home, which—depending on the route of administration—can be between several hours and several days later. For most women, bleeding and passage of the POC ensues within 2 to 4 hours after misoprostol administration, but can take 24 hours or longer (Creinin & Danielsson, 2009). It is common for women to continue to bleed for several weeks after the abortion; however, subsequent bleeding is usually much less than during actual pregnancy expulsion. A follow-up visit is required several days to weeks later to ensure that the pregnancy has been successfully terminated.

There are few medical contraindications to medication abortion with mifepristone–misoprostol; they include known allergies to either of the medications, chronic renal insufficiency, or long-term corticosteroid use. In addition, because of the expected bleeding, caution should be exercised in providing medication abortion (of any type) to women with severe anemia or coagulopathies, or those who use anticoagulants. Other psychosocial conditions may also render some patients inappropriate for medication abortion. Careful counseling and screening that addresses a woman's expectations of the experience, her ability to communicate with the clinician, and the need to return for follow-up are important considerations prior to providing a medication abortion. In addition, because of the potential teratogenicity of misoprostol, in the small number of cases when medication abortion fails, uterine aspiration is necessary. Therefore, all candidates must consent to this procedure before medication administration. Although research has demonstrated comparable levels of satisfaction among women following aspiration and medication abortion (Creinin & Danielsson, 2009), it is important for women to understand that medication abortion is not the optimal choice for every individual.

Medication abortion with methotrexate is similar to mifepristone with respect to the manner of service delivery, but has several distinguishing clinical features. Methotrexate is administered via intramuscular injection rather than by mouth, which may lead some women to prefer mifepristone. Perhaps the most important clinical difference lies in the timing of bleeding and expulsion of pregnancy tissue, which can take up to several weeks following medication administration. For many women, this unpredictability renders methotrexate less desirable than mifepristone. Methotrexate, however, can be used in cases when ectopic pregnancy cannot be ruled out, offers a lower-cost alternative to mifepristone, and may be available in countries where mifepristone is not available or abortion is legally restricted.

Medications can also be administered to induce an abortion after the first trimester. Current approaches generally involve administering prostaglandins, with or without the addition of mifepristone, to stimulate uterine contractions that eventually lead to expulsion of the fetus. Less commonly, oxytocin or uterine saline instillation is used for the same purpose. As previously discussed, induction methods have been found to be generally less safe and more difficult for patients than D & E and, therefore have become less commonly used in the United States. In 2005, fewer than 5% of abortions after the first trimester occurred via induction, and even after 20 weeks' gestation, only 15% were completed in this manner (Henshaw, 2009; Kapp & von Hertzen, 2009). However, because D & E requires advanced training on the part of a clinician, it may not be readily available in some settings. Because this method of abortion is less frequent and takes place in hospital settings, in-depth discussion of this technique is beyond the scope of this chapter.

Safety of Abortion Risks associated with early abortion, including death, are relatively low when procedures are carried out under modern medical conditions. Legality is an important prerequisite for such conditions to be manifest. In places where abortion is illegal or restricted, associated morbidity and mortality rates remain high. The World Health Organization (2007) estimates that 19 to 20 million unsafe abortions took place annually between 1993 and 2003, resulting in 65,000 to 70,000 deaths per year, and rendering unsafe abortion one of the leading causes of maternal mortality. In the United States, abortion mortality rates have decreased considerably since the 1970s, largely as a result of advances in technique and elimination of many legal restrictions (Shah & Ahman, 2009). The current mortality rate for legal, reported abortions in the United States is 0.7 per 100,000 (Henshaw, 2009). The risk of death increases with advancing gestational age; after 8 weeks' gestation, it increases by 38% every week (Bartlett et al., 2004). Nevertheless, given the limited number of abortions that occur after the first trimester and particularly after 20 weeks' gestation, death from abortion is relatively rare in the United States. Compared to abortion, the risk of death associated with live birth has been found to be approximately 12 times higher (Grimes, 2006).

Serious and minor complications following legal aspiration or D & E abortion are also infrequent. Possible complications (from most to least likely) include infection, missed or incomplete abortion, cervical tear, uterine perforation, hemorrhage requiring transfusion, and hematometra. Overall, minor complications are estimated to occur in fewer than 2.5% of abortions, and serious complications (i.e., those requiring hospitalization) in fewer than 0.5% (Henshaw, 2009; Tietze & Henshaw, 1996). In general, these conditions are treatable and rarely lead to long-term sequelae or death. Of particular import to many women is the fact that there is no evidence that first-trimester abortion with vacuum aspiration leads to difficulties with childbearing in the future. Secondary infertility does not increase after aspiration abortion, although unsafe abortion, as well as abortions performed with other methods (such as dilation and sharp curettage), may increase certain reproductive risks, such as midtrimester spontaneous abortions and low birth weight (Hogue, Boardman, & Stotland, 2009). To reduce potential risks, it is important for clinicians to encourage women to seek abortion services as early as possible from experienced providers.

Overall, the risk associated with medication abortion is comparable to that associated with aspiration and D & E abortions (Grimes, 2005). With medication abortion, complications attributable to instrumentation (i.e., cervical tear and uterine perforation) are avoided; however, other complications, including incomplete abortion, hemorrhage, and infection, are possible. From 2004 to 2008, six unusual, sepsis-related deaths occurred among women in the United States following the use of mifepristone–misoprostol, leading to an overall increase in the risk of death associated with this method. These infections are under investigation by the Centers for Disease Control and Prevention (CDC). At the present time, mifepristone–misoprostol abortion remains available in the United States and is generally felt to be safe for use.

Special Considerations

Adolescents

In 2001, the proportion of pregnancies that were unintended was highest among women younger than the age of 20 (Finer & Henshaw, 2006). Adolescent mothers are less likely to complete high school, are more likely to be single parents, and may have increased complications during pregnancy. Children of adolescent mothers have higher rates of low birth weight and related health problems, are more likely to be abused or neglected, and frequently have poor school performance (National Campaign to Prevent Teen and Unplanned Pregnancy, 2009).

Abortion is a more common outcome of unintended pregnancy among adolescents than among women in general. In 2002, nearly one-third (29%) of pregnancies among women younger than the age of 20 ended in abortion, compared with 21% among all women. In 34 states, minors must involve at least one of their parents or seek a judicial bypass to obtain an abortion, except in cases of medical emergency or where there is evidence of abuse or neglect (Guttmacher Institute, 2009).

In addition to abortion laws and regulations, clinicians who work with young women need to be familiar with current legislation regarding adolescent rights to confidential reproductive health services in the state where they practice. These rights are an area of great controversy in the United States, as reflected by legislative battles at both the federal and state levels. At the time of this writing, 25 states and the District of Columbia allowed minors to seek contraceptive services without the consent of a parent; the other 25 states either placed restrictions on minors (21) or had no relevant policy or case law (4) regarding this issue. Thirty-two states explicitly allow minors to consent to prenatal care without their parents' involvement, although 12 of those allow a physician to inform parents that their daughter is seeking these services if it is "in the minor's interest." Four other states allow minors to consent when they are "mature." The remaining states have no policy or case law on this subject (Guttmacher Institute, 2009). Pregnancy options counseling falls between these three aspects of reproductive health care (prenatal care and contraceptive and abortion services).

Where legislative conditions allow, reassuring adolescent patients that all counseling and follow-up related to pregnancy will be kept confidential is an important aspect of providing pregnancy options counseling to this population. Before delivering services, it is also essential to inform adolescents about clinical situations when parents or guardians may or must be informed. A full discussion of the reproductive health rights of adolescents is beyond the scope of this chapter, and readers are referred to the references cited and to the resource listing (Box 18-2) regarding laws specifically pertaining to adolescents in their practice location.

Influences of Culture

As previously discussed, notable disparities have been identified with regard to unintended pregnancy and abortion in the United States, with women between the ages of 18 and 24, unmarried, of low socioeconomic status, Latina or African American, and without a high school diploma experiencing significantly higher rates of both of these reproductive health events. In spite of this social reality, available data on unintended pregnancy and abortion reveal a complex picture. Although most women who have abortions in the United States are not married, one-fourth of married women report that their pregnancies are unintended. Among married women with unintended pregnancies, 27% have an abortion (Finer & Henshaw, 2006). The majority of women (60%) who have abortions have had one or more previous births (Jones et al., 2008). Nearly 80% of women who have an abortion report a religious affiliation. Many of these women identify themselves with religions that typically prohibit abortion: 27% are Catholic and 13% are "born-again" or evangelical (Jones, Darroch, & Henshaw, 2002b). Women who have not graduated from high school have a rate of unintended pregnancy three times higher than that of college graduates, but are far less likely to terminate their pregnancies. Nevertheless, it is important for clinicians providing pregnancy options counseling not to make assumptions about which option any individual woman will choose based on her demographic characteristics.

References

American Academy of Physician Assistants. (2008). *Guidelines for ethical conduct for the physician assistant profession.* Alexandria, VA: Author.

American College of Nurse–Midwives. (1997). *Reproductive choices* [Position statement]. Washington, DC: Author.

American College of Obstetricians and Gynecologists. (2007; reaffirmed 2011). *Abortion policy* [Policy statement]. Washington, DC: Author.

Baker, A. (1995). *Abortion and options counseling: A comprehensive reference.* Granite City, IL: Hope Clinic for Women.

Baker, A., & Beresford, T. (2009). Informed consent, patient education and counseling. In M. Paul, E. S. Lichtenberg, L. Borgatta, D. Grimes, P. Stubblefield, & M. Creinin (Eds.), *Management of unintended pregnancy and abnormal pregnancy: Comprehensive abortion care* (pp. 48–62). Chichester, UK: Wiley-Blackwell.

Bartlett, L., Berg, C., Shulman, H., Zane, S., Green, C., Whitehead, S., et al. (2004). Risk factors for legal induced abortion-related mortality in the United States. *Obstetrics and Gynecology, 103*(4), 729–737.

Brown, S. S., & Eisenberg, L. (Eds.). (1995). *The best intentions: Unintended pregnancy and the well-being of children and families.* Washington, DC: National Academy Press.

Creinin, M. D., & Danielsson, K. (2009). Medical abortion in early pregnancy. In M. Paul, E. S. Lichtenberg, L. Borgatta, D. Grimes, P. Stubblefield, & M. Creinin (Eds.), *Management of unintended pregnancy and abnormal pregnancy: Comprehensive abortion care* (pp. 208–223). Chichester, UK: Wiley-Blackwell.

Edwards, J., & Carson, S. A. (1997). New technologies permit safe abortion at less than six weeks' gestation and provide timely detection of ectopic gestation. *American Journal of Obstetrics and Gynecology, 176,* 1101–1106.

Espey, E., & MacIsaac, L. (2009). Contraception and surgical abortion aftercare. In M. Paul, E. S. Lichtenberg, L. Borgatta, D. Grimes, P. Stubblefield, & M. Creinin (Eds.), *Management of unintended pregnancy and abnormal pregnancy: Comprehensive abortion care* (pp. 157–177). Chichester, UK: Wiley-Blackwell.

Finer, L. B., & Henshaw, S. K. (2003). Abortion incidence and services in the United States in 2000. *Perspectives on Sexual and Reproductive Health, 35,* 6–15.

Finer, L. B., & Henshaw, S. K. (2006). Disparities in rates of unintended pregnancy in the United States, 1994 and 2001. *Perspectives on Sexual and Reproductive Health, 38*, 90–96.

Gamble, S. B., Strauss, L.T., Parker, W. Y., Cook, D. A., Zane, S. B., & Hamdan, S. (2008). Abortion surveillance—United States, 2005. *MMWR Surveillance Summary 2008, 57*, 1–32.

Grimes, D. A. (2005). Risk of mifepristone abortion in context. *Contraception, 71*, 161.

Grimes, D. A. (2006). Estimation of pregnancy-related mortality risk by pregnancy outcome, United States, 1991 to 1999. *American Journal of Obstetrics and Gynecology, 194*, 92–94.

Grimes, D. A., Smith, M. S., & Witham, A. D. (2004). Mifepristone and misoprostol versus dilation and evacuation for midtrimester abortion: A pilot randomised, controlled trial. *British Journal of Obstetrics and Gynaecology, 111*, 148–153.

Grossman, D., Ellertson, C., Grimes, D. A., & Walker, D. (2004). Routine follow-up visits after first trimester induced abortion. *Obstetrics and Gynecology, 103*, 738–745.

Guttmacher Institute. (2000). *Fulfilling the promise: Public policy and U.S. family planning clinics.* New York: Author.

Guttmacher Institute. (2009, July). Parental involvement in minors' abortions. *State Policies in Brief.* Retrieved from http://www.guttmacher.org/statecenter/spibs/spib_PIMA.pdf

Hammond, C., & Chasen, S. (2009). Dilation and evacuation. In M. Paul, E. S. Lichtenberg, L. Borgatta, D. Grimes, P. Stubblefield, & M. Creinin (Eds.), *Management of unintended pregnancy and abnormal pregnancy: Comprehensive abortion care* (pp. 157–177). Chichester, UK: Wiley-Blackwell.

HealthyPeople.gov (2011). *2020 topics and objectives.* Retrieved from http://www.healthypeople.gov/2020/topicsobjectives2020/default.aspx

Henshaw, S. K. (2009). Unintended pregnancy and abortion in the USA: Epidemiology and public health impact. In M. Paul, E. S. Lichtenberg, L. Borgatta, D. Grimes, P. Stubblefield, & M. Creinin (Eds.), *Management of unintended pregnancy and abnormal pregnancy: Comprehensive abortion care* (pp. 24–35). Chichester, UK: Wiley-Blackwell.

Higginbotham, E. (2002). When your beliefs run counter to care. *RN, 65*(11), 69–72.

Hogue, C. J., Boardman, L. A., & Stotland, N. (2009). Answering questions about long-term outcomes. In M. Paul, E. S. Lichtenberg, L. Borgatta, D. Grimes, P. Stubblefield, & M. Creinin (Eds.), *Management of unintended pregnancy and abnormal pregnancy: Comprehensive abortion care* (pp. 252–263). Chichester, UK: Wiley-Blackwell.

Jones, J. (2008). Adoption experiences of women and men and demand for children to adopt by women 18–44 years of age in the United States, 2002. *Vital and Health Statistics, 23*(7), 1–36.

Jones, R. K., Darroch, J. E., & Henshaw, S. K. (2002a). Contraceptive use among US women having abortions in 2000–2001. *Perspectives on Sexual and Reproductive Health, 34*, 294–303.

Jones, R. K., Darroch, J. E., & Henshaw, S. K. (2002b). Patterns in the socioeconomic characteristics of women obtaining abortions in 2000–2001. *Perspectives on Sexual and Reproductive Health, 34*, 226–235.

Jones, R. K., Singh, S., Finer, L. B., & Frohwirth, L. F. (2006). *Repeat abortion in the United States* (Occasional Report No. 29). New York: Guttmacher Institute.

Jones, R. K., Zolna, M. R., Henshaw, S. K., & Finer, L. B. (2008). Abortion in the United States: Incidence and access to services, 2005. *Perspectives on Sexual and Reproductive Health, 40*(1), 6–16.

Kapp, N., & von Hertzen, H. (2009). Medical methods to induce abortion in the second trimester. In M. Paul, E. S. Lichtenberg, L. Borgatta, D. Grimes, P. Stubblefield, & M. Creinin (Eds.), *Management of unintended pregnancy and abnormal pregnancy: Comprehensive abortion care* (pp. 178–192). Chichester, UK: Wiley-Blackwell.

Meckstroth, K., & Paul, M. (2009). First-trimester aspiration abortion. In M. Paul, E. S. Lichtenberg, L. Borgatta, D. Grimes, P. Stubblefield, & M. Creinin (Eds.), *Management of unintended pregnancy and abnormal pregnancy: Comprehensive abortion care* (pp. 135–156). Chichester, UK: Wiley-Blackwell.

Moos, M-K. (2003). Unintended pregnancies: A call for nursing action. *MCN: The American Journal of Maternal/Child Nursing, 28*, 24–30.

National Abortion Federation. (2005). *Early options: A provider's guide to medical abortion.* Washington, DC: Author.

National Campaign to Prevent Teen and Unplanned Pregnancy. (2009). *Why it matters: Teen pregnancy.* Retrieved from http://www.thenationalcampaign.org/why-it-matters/wim_teens.aspx

National Organization of Nurse Practitioner Faculties and American Association of Colleges of Nursing.

(2002). *Nurse practitioner primary care competencies in specialty areas: Adult, family, gerontological, pediatric, and women's health*. Rockville, MD: Department of Health and Human Services.

Nichols, M., Halvorson-Boyd, G., Goldstein, R., Gevirtz, C., & Healow, D. (2009). Pain management. In M. Paul, E. S. Lichtenberg, L. Borgatta, D. Grimes, P. Stubblefield, & M. Creinin (Eds.), *Management of unintended pregnancy and abnormal pregnancy: Comprehensive abortion care* (pp. 90–110). Chichester, UK: Wiley-Blackwell.

Saltzman, L. E., Johnson, C. H., Gilbert, B. C., & Goodwin, M. M. (2003). Physical abuse around the time of pregnancy: An examination of prevalence and risk factors in 16 states. *Maternal and Child Health Journal, 7,* 31–43.

Shah, I., & Ahman, E. (2009). Unsafe abortion: The global public health challenge. In M. Paul, E. S. Lichtenberg, L. Borgatta, D. Grimes, P. Stubblefield, & M. Creinin (Eds.), *Management of unintended pregnancy and abnormal pregnancy: Comprehensive abortion care* (pp. 10–23). Chichester, UK: Wiley-Blackwell.

Simmonds, K., & Likis, F. (2005). Providing options counseling for women with unintended pregnancies. *Journal of Obstetric, Gynecologic, and Neonatal Nursing, 34*(3), 373–379.

Smith, K. J., & Brandon, D. (2008). The hospital-based adoption process: A primer for perinatal nurses. *MCN, 33,* 382–388.

Strauss, L.T., Gamble, S. B., Parker, W. Y., Cook, D. A., Zane, S. B., & Hamdan, S. (2007). Abortion surveillance—United States, 2004. *Morbidity and Mortality Weekly Report: Surveillance Summaries, 56*(9), 1–33.

Taylor, D., Safriet, B., Dempsey, G., Kruse, B., & Jackson, C. (2009). *Providing abortion care: A professional toolkit for nurse–midwives, nurse practitioners, and physician assistants*. Retrieved December 19, 2009, from http://www.apctoolkit.org

Tietze, C., & Henshaw, S. K. (1996). *Induced abortion: A worldwide review* (3rd ed.). New York: Guttmacher Institute.

Trussell, J., Stewart, F., Guest, F., & Hatcher, R. A. (1992). Emergency contraceptive pills: A simple proposal to reduce unintended pregnancies. *Family Planning Perspectives, 24,* 269–273.

World Health Organization. (2007). *Unsafe abortion: Global and regional estimates of incidence of unsafe abortion and associated mortality in 2000* (5th ed.). Geneva, Switzerland: Author.

Infertility

Ellen Olshansky

Infertility is a condition that generates a variety of meanings among those experiencing it, including those who care for people with infertility, family members and friends of people with infertility, and the society in which infertility occurs. Some individuals choose infertility and specifically seek it out through surgical means, such as tubal ligation or vasectomy, whereas for many others it is an unwanted condition. Thus there is both unwanted infertility and wanted infertility.

The inability to become a mother or a father due to unwanted infertility is a profound and extremely difficult challenge for a significant portion of the population. People who desire to conceive and bear a child but are unable to do so often suffer immensely. Unwanted infertility occurs in approximately 15% of couples in the United States (Practice Committee of the American Society for Reproductive Medicine [ASRM], 2006b). It often goes unrecognized as a serious problem, however, because it is not a life-threatening illness. For those experiencing it, infertility often has a significant impact and is viewed as a major life crisis (Olshansky, 1996a).

We live in a pronatalist society, which adds to the emotionally charged nature of infertility. Definitions of femininity are socially constructed and interlaced with the ability to give birth. Many women internalize these societal expectations, seeing themselves as failures if they are unable to conceive (Olshansky, 1992).

Historically, infertility has been viewed as a woman's problem. This view is changing because of enhanced abilities to diagnose infertility, which have led to the recognition that both male and female factors cause infertility. Nevertheless, matters of reproduction, childbearing, and childrearing continue to be viewed primarily as women's issues. Many women have grown up rehearsing to be mothers, believing that their femininity and identity are interrelated with childbearing. Finding that they are unable to conceive can be both shocking and devastating to these individuals. Some women may be able to deconstruct such ideas through involvement in organizations and groups that support greater choices of lifestyles for women. Yet even women who may not feel that it is their duty to bear children may continue to desire children.

Infertility has also raised some issues and opportunities that were generally ignored before the advent of technological approaches to treat this condition. For example, treatments for cancer, such as chemotherapy and radiation, may cause a person to become infertile. Today, these individuals may preserve their fertility through the freezing of sperm or eggs. Some technological advances, however, have led to ethical dilemmas, including issues of who has the right to a frozen embryo, who is the real parent, and who is considered eligible for certain treatments.

This chapter provides an overview of the pathophysiology of infertility, including the various causes of infertility, the diagnostic procedures related to infertility, and the treatments for infertility. It also highlights the various options available beyond trying to conceive, including adoption and child-free living. Ethical issues are discussed, and the sociocultural and psychological issues related to infertility are addressed. Finally, suggestions are made for ways that clinicians can assist those experiencing infertility to have a better quality of life during and after the infertility experience.

Defining Infertility

The medical definition of infertility is "failure to achieve a successful pregnancy after 12 months or more of regular unprotected intercourse" (Practice Committee of the ASRM, 2008b, p. S60). Infertility is classified as primary or secondary according to the pregnancy history. A couple who has never been pregnant has primary infertility. Secondary infertility is "the inability to become pregnant, or to carry a pregnancy to term, following the birth of one or more biological children" (Resolve, 2008). The prevalence rate of secondary infertility is higher than that of primary infertility (Resolve).

For women older than age 35, evaluation and treatment of infertility are considered after six months of attempting pregnancy, instead of one year, for the following reasons: The remaining time for a successful pregnancy is limited, fecundity declines gradually beginning at age 32 and more rapidly after 37, the incidence of conditions that impair fertility (e.g., fibroids and endometriosis) increases, and there is a higher risk of pregnancy loss (Practice Committee of the ASRM, 2006a, 2008a, 2008b). However, maternal age cannot be considered separately from the context of the relationship between the woman and her partner, normal declining sexual activity with age, social conditions, and physical problems in the male (Hanson, 2003; Practice Committee of the ASRM, 2008a). The average maternal age is increasing because of social trends in which women have been pursuing higher education and careers and postponing marriage and childbearing (Practice Committee of the ASRM, 2006a).

Male fertility takes a much different trajectory than female fertility. The sperm count of men usually does not decrease significantly until they reach approximately age 55. Even with that decrease, men are usually able to father children throughout their lives.

From a personal perspective. however, an individual often constructs his or her own definition of infertility, which is influenced by the social context in which that person lives. For example, a couple who has been trying to conceive for three months and has many friends who have recently become pregnant with no apparent difficulty may begin to see themselves as infertile even though they are not considered infertile according to the medical definition. The couple may become very anxious and seek health care, but are turned away because they do not fit the medical definition of infertility. Meanwhile, their anxiety may increase, which could have a detrimental effect on their ability to conceive (Domar, 2002).

Conversely, a 40-year-old nulligravida may go for a routine gynecologic examination and her clinician may warn her that she should consider conceiving very soon because her childbearing years are almost over. There may be an assumption that this woman—and all women, for that matter—choose to be mothers. For this particular woman, her life goals may not include parenting. Although it was correct to provide her with information about childbearing, it would have been more appropriate to ask her, in a nonjudgmental manner, about her goals related to childbearing with the recognition that not all women choose to become mothers.

Overview of Anatomy and Physiology Related to Infertility

An understanding of the anatomy and physiology of the female and male reproductive systems as well as the processes of fertilization and implantation is crucial to understanding the etiology of infertility. Women's reproductive anatomy and physiology were discussed in Chapter 5; therefore, the discussion in this chapter is limited to an overview of men's reproductive anatomy and physiology, fertilization, and implantation.

Anatomy and Physiology of the Male Reproductive System

The anatomic components of the male reproductive system include the penis, urethra, seminal vesicles, prostate gland, vas deferens, epididymis, and testes (testicles); see **Figure 19-1**, **Color Plate 11**, and **Table 19-1**. Sperm production relies on a functioning hypothalamic–pituitary–testicular axis that has many similarities to the hypothalamic–pituitary–ovarian axis in women. The pituitary produces follicle-stimulating hormone (FSH) and luteinizing hormone (LH) in response to secretion of gonadotropin-releasing hormone (GnRH) by the hypothalamus. FSH and LH initiate testicular production of sperm and testosterone, which are also necessary for spermatogenesis. Approximately 72 days are required for spermatogenesis, after which sperm mature in the epididymis and then travel out of the vas deferens during ejaculation (Fritz & Speroff, 2011).

Fertilization and Implantation

The processes of fertilization (also known as conception) and implantation involve several steps. Sperm must be produced and deposited in the vagina, and then transported through

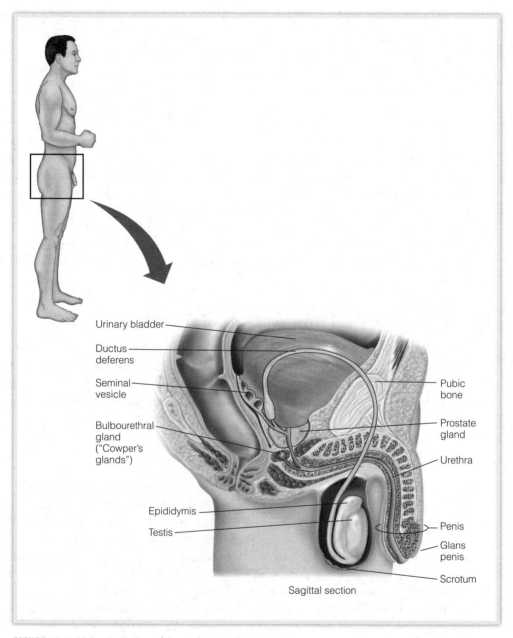

Urinary bladder

Ductus deferens

Seminal vesicle

Bulbourethral gland ("Cowper's glands")

Epididymis

Testis

Pubic bone

Prostate gland

Urethra

Penis

Glans penis

Scrotum

Sagittal section

FIGURE 19-1 Midsagittal view of the male reproductive system.

TABLE 19-1 Functions of the Male Reproductive Anatomy

Organs	Functions
Penis	External organ through which semen and urine are expelled
Urethra	Tube that carries semen and urine through the penis; its external opening is at the tip of the penis
Seminal vesicles	Two internal saclike structures that secrete fructose and other substances into the seminal fluid to promote viability of the semen
Prostate gland	Internal gland that secretes substances into the seminal fluid to nourish and increase the motility of the sperm
Vas deferens	Bilateral tubes through which sperm are propelled from each epididymis to the urethra for ejaculation
Epididymis	Stores sperm while they mature and connects the testicles to the vas deferens; each testicle has an adjacent epididymis
Testes	Produce testosterone and immature sperm; suspended externally in the scrotum
Bulbourethral gland	Two internal glands that produce an alkaline mucoid secretion that coats and lubricates the urethra

the vagina, cervix, and fallopian tubes. In the fallopian tubes, the sperm are transformed by a process called capacitation, which changes the surface characteristics of sperm. Capacitation is essential to the sperm's ability to fertilize an egg and enables the sperm to undergo acrosome reaction, to bind to the zona pellucida, and to acquire hypermotility—all of which help to increase the sperm's ability to penetrate the ovum. The ovaries must produce a mature ovum (oocyte), which requires integrated functioning along the hypothalamic–pituitary–ovarian axis. The ovum is transported from the ovary into the fallopian tube where it is fertilized by the sperm. The fertilized ovum then travels down the fallopian tube into the uterus.

Implantation is the process by which the fertilized ovum attaches to the uterine wall and penetrates the uterine epithelium and the maternal circulatory system. Implantation can occur only if there is destruction of the zona pellucida, which is the surface of the fertilized ovum.

Pathophysiology and Etiologies of Infertility

Approximately 55% of infertility cases are due to female factors, and 35% of cases are due to male factors. In 10% of all infertility cases no cause can be found (unexplained infertility) (Fritz & Speroff, 2011).

When presenting or discussing the pathophysiology of infertility, attention should be given to avoiding the use of terms that reflect negatively upon women. For example, cervical mucus that is not receptive to sperm is commonly referred to as "hostile cervical mucus," and a cervix that prematurely dilates is commonly called an "incompetent cervix." Although some may view such adjectives as innocuous, this terminology actually reflects negatively upon women, connoting blame on the woman's part for the infertility.

Female Etiologies

The majority of female infertility is due to ovulatory dysfunction and tubal and pelvic problems. Unexplained infertility, and combined or interactional infertility, which are discussed separately in this chapter, account for most other cases of infertility among women.

Ovulatory dysfunction may involve either a total lack of ovulation or the occurrence of irregular ovulation. Anovulation is usually, but not always, evidenced by irregular menstrual bleeding patterns or amenorrhea. Numerous causes of ovulatory dysfunction are possible, which can result from any interruption of the hypothalamic–pituitary–ovarian axis. Etiologies of ovarian dysfunction include hyperandrogenic disorders, physiologic anovulation at either end of the reproductive spectrum, hyperprolactinemia, pituitary tumors, thyroid disorders, eating disorders, low or high body mass index (BMI), medications, and possibly stress. Further information about etiologies of anovulation can be found in Chapters 25 and 26.

A short duration of the luteal phase can also cause female infertility and is considered a subtle form of ovulatory dysfunction. A short luteal phase is commonly referred to as luteal-phase deficiency or inadequate luteal phase, because it is associated with abnormally low levels of progesterone production by the corpus luteum. The term *luteal phase defect* is no longer used because it may reflect negatively upon women, as previously explained. The luteal phase is considered short when less than 13 days elapse between the midcycle LH surge and the onset of menses (Fritz & Speroff, 2011). This shortened duration can lead not only to infertility, but also to recurrent miscarriage.

Tubal problems are usually related to blockages within the tubes, which make it difficult or impossible for the sperm and the ovum to meet. These blockages may be anatomic, but more frequently occur as a result of sexually transmitted infections (STIs) that have progressed to pelvic inflammatory disease (PID; see Chapter 21). The STI may have been asymptomatic and, therefore, gone unrecognized and untreated, resulting in tubal scarring; however, tubal scarring may result even when STIs are treated. Tubal problems can also result from previous ectopic pregnancy or tubal surgery.

Other pelvic problems to consider when assessing women for causes of infertility include endometriosis, Asherman syndrome, and other uterine factors. Endometriosis is a condition in which menstrual tissue grows in areas outside of the uterus rather than being sloughed off with each menstrual period. Endometriosis may or may not cause pain; paradoxically, pain may not correlate with the extent of the disease process. For example, slight pain may correlate with severe endometriosis. This disease process can be elusive to diagnose and treat (see Chapter 27 for further information about endometriosis).

Asherman syndrome "results from intrauterine adhesions that obstruct or obliterate the uterine cavity" (Fritz & Speroff, 2011, p. 459). Asherman syndrome is usually caused by overzealous postpartum curettage, but can also occur after cesarean birth, myomectomy, or other uterine surgery. Hypomenorrhea, amenorrhea, or dysmenorrhea may be present in conjunction with this condition (Fritz & Speroff).

Other potential uterine causes of infertility include fibroids, endometrial polyps, and chronic endometritis. The exact effects of these factors on fertility are not known, and they are not considered a common cause of infertility. Congenital anomalies of the uterus, such as a bicornuate uterus or septate uterus, are typically associated with pregnancy loss and complications but not infertility (Fritz & Speroff, 2011).

Male Etiologies

Male factor infertility may be caused by anatomic or structural problems, abnormalities in sperm production or function, and sexual, hormonal, and genetic conditions. A structural cause of male infertility is undescended testes (cryptorchidism). The testes are normally descended by the age of two and are, therefore, external to the body; if undescended, however, they are exposed to higher temperatures that cause damage to the sperm.

Hypospadias is a congenital anomaly that results in the urethral outlet being located on the shaft of the penis rather than at the end. This type of structural problem may make it difficult to deposit semen in the woman's vagina.

Untreated or recurrent STIs in the male may result in scarring and blockage of the reproductive tract. Finally, a varicocele or varicose vein in the scrotum may affect male fertility. It is theorized that the presence of these abnormalities causes an elevation in scrotal temperature, thereby hampering spermatogenesis.

Men who contract mumps later in life, particularly after adolescence, may become infertile, because the illness can result in a condition known as orchitis or testicular inflammation. However, because the condition is usually unilateral, sterility rarely results.

Infection, particularly in the prostate gland, can cause a decreased sperm count. Decreased blood flow to the testes, which can occur from testicular torsion, can also lead to a decreased sperm count. Environmental factors may negatively affect sperm production in some men, although more research is needed in this area. Certain temporary causes of sperm abnormalities have been identified as well, such as being exposed to high temperatures due to illness accompanied by a high fever, or the use of hot tubs or saunas. In these instances, the decreased sperm count or motility will likely be improved after a three-month period of avoiding this exposure.

Other causes of male infertility are attributed to sexual difficulties—in particular, to erectile dysfunction. Hormonal problems, such as decreased testosterone production, can interfere with spermatogenesis. Genetic problems, such as Klinefelter's syndrome, can cause azoospermia. Despite the many known etiologies, male factor infertility is often idiopathic.

Combined Causes

Combined or interactional causes of infertility include the inability of sperm to survive in the woman's cervical mucus because of the presence of antisperm antibodies. These antibodies can be present in either the male or the female, and their presence causes the sperm to agglutinate or clump, which decreases their motility. Testing for antisperm antibodies is no longer performed routinely because of advances in infertility treatments; therefore, this condition may go undetected. Other interactional causes of infertility include simultaneous female and male causes of infertility that together increase the risk for infertility and sexual difficulties. Emotional problems in one or both partners may or may not contribute to infertility, and these may also occur as a result of infertility.

Unexplained Infertility

Unexplained infertility refers to situations in which no specific cause for the infertility can be found. Unexplained infertility is a diagnosis of exclusion, meaning that all other possible causes for the infertility have been ruled out. Interestingly, before the increased use of various technological means to diagnosis infertility problems, the rate of unexplained infertility was much higher. As scientific advances have enhanced clinicians' ability to diagnose an increasing number of causes of infertility, fewer people are being diagnosed with unexplained infertility.

Assessment of Infertility

A diagnosis of infertility is not made until a couple has attempted pregnancy for at least 12 months; thus evaluation is not initiated until this amount of time has elapsed. Earlier assessment is warranted for "women with 1) age over 35, 2) history of oligo/amenorrhea, 3) known or suspected uterine/tubal disease or endometriosis, or 4) a partner known to be subfertile" (Practice Committee of the ASRM, 2006b, p. S264).

Evaluation of infertility begins with a thorough history and physical examination. Clinicians who provide gynecologic care often perform limited assessment of male partners (for example, obtaining relevant history and ordering semen analysis) and then refer men to another clinician if additional evaluation is needed. Diagnostic tests for infertility are most useful and cost-effective if they proceed sequentially in a logical order.

History

Initially, it is essential that the clinician obtain an accurate and detailed history from the woman and her partner. This information includes general medical, family, social, emotional, occupational, recreational, and lifestyle histories. The clinician should identify the duration of infertility and any previous evaluation or treatment. A detailed gynecologic history, with particular attention to the menstrual and pregnancy histories as well as any previous surgeries or procedures (see Chapter 6), is crucial to the infertility evaluation. The frequency of coitus, any sexual difficulties, and history of STIs in either partner are also important pieces of information to collect. When asking about previous pregnancies, clarify whether the woman and her partner have ever become pregnant together or with other partners. If so, obtain a pregnancy history, including whether the woman had a vaginal or cesarean birth. During the review of systems, ask the woman specifically about nipple discharge, hirsutism, pelvic pain, dyspareunia, and symptoms of thyroid disorders (Practice Committee of the ASRM, 2006b).

Ideally, the woman and her partner would each be interviewed separately and then together to encourage the most complete evaluation. This may be a stressful time for the individuals or couple because an initial infertility assessment also acknowledges the problem of infertility (Devine, 2003).

Physical Examination

A complete physical examination of the woman, including a pelvic examination, should be performed (Practice Committee of the ASRM, 2006b). During the general examination, it is particularly important to note weight and BMI; the presence of acne, hirsutism, or alopecia that could indicate a hyperandrogenic disorder (see Chpater 26); thyroid abnormalities, such as enlargement, nodule, or tenderness; and nipple discharge or visual changes that could indicate a pituitary mass. The pelvic examination should focus on identifying any abnormalities of the internal genitalia, such as enlargement, tenderness, and masses, as well as evidence of gynecologic infections or STIs. If infection is suspected, microscopic examination of vaginal secretions and chlamydia and gonorrhea testing should be performed (see Chapter 6).

The male should also have a complete physical examination, with attention to the reproductive organs to rule out structural problems.

Diagnostic Testing and Procedures

The basic and simple diagnostic procedures that should be done with an initial evaluation include ovulation detection and semen analysis. More specific tests that may be warranted include laboratory testing, hysterosalpingogram, transvaginal ultrasound, hysteroscopy, laparoscopy, postcoital testing, endometrial biopsy, and sperm penetration assay. The couple's history should guide the clinician's decisions as to which testing is needed. Evaluation generally proceeds from less to more invasive tests. If a woman is ovulatory, it is preferable to organize the infertility evaluation according to the menstrual cycle. This way, many of the tests can be performed within the same month.

Ovulation Detection Women can detect ovulation by monitoring and recording their basal body temperature (BBT) each day upon awakening. A BBT thermometer is different from a fever thermometer, in that the BBT thermometer is calibrated in tenths of degrees, allowing for the detection of smaller changes in temperature. The woman should measure her temperature before eating or drinking; the measurement is most accurate if taken before rising from bed. If a woman ovulates, the biphasic cycle is indicated by temperature recordings consistently lower than 98°F during the follicular phase and consistently higher than 98°F during the luteal phase. Although fluctuations inevitably occur within each of the phases, plotting the temperatures on a graph makes a biphasic pattern evident. Usually there is a slight drop in temperature just prior to ovulation, and a surge in temperature with ovulation (**Figure 19-2**).

Recording the BBT is helpful because it provides useful data for assessment. This temperature should be recorded for at least three months because one menstrual cycle does not provide enough information; rather, it is best to have a record of at least three menstrual cycles to assess whether there is a pattern in the cycles. BBT charting is a noninvasive test that is controlled by the woman. The temperature can be oral, axillary, or rectal but should be taken the same way each time.

Although keeping a record of one's BBT provides useful information, an alternative and more accurate method of ovulation detection is available in the form of over-the-counter urine tests for LH. Women can perform these tests in their home. The presence of a surge in LH (which is noted as a color change on the test strip) in the first morning urine indicates ovulation is likely occurring. Urine LH testing may become cost-prohibitive if used for an extended period, however.

Semen Analysis Most male factor infertility is detected with semen analysis. It is important that semen analysis be performed early in the infertility evaluation so that male factor infertility can be diagnosed before the woman undergoes extensive, invasive diagnostic procedures. Semen can be collected by masturbation with ejaculation into a sterile container or by intercourse with ejaculation into a special collection condom if a man is uncomfortable with masturbation. Instructions include a defined period of abstinence of two to three

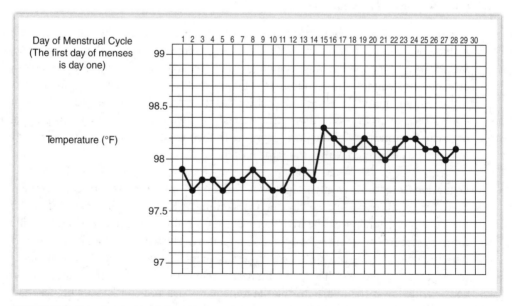

FIGURE 19-2 Sample basal body temperature chart.

days prior to sample collection. No more than one hour should elapse between collection and microscopic examination of the semen sample. The sample should be kept at room or body temperature during transport (Male Infertility Best Practice Policy Committee of the American Urological Association [AUA] & Practice Committee of the ASRM, 2006).

The World Health Organization (WHO) criteria are widely used to determine if a semen sample falls within normal ranges. These criteria were recently updated following a large study that included semen samples from more than 4500 men in 14 countries on 4 continents (Cooper et al., 2010). The reference values established prior to the current (2010) values were believed to have significant limitations because data were derived from reference populations that were not clearly defined and obtained from laboratories that had unknown comparability related to analytic methodologies (Cooper et al.). The reference limits (see **Table 19-2**) currently accepted are lower than those previously provided as the normal or accepted reference values except for the number of total sperm per ejaculate. Therefore, if the clinician is reviewing an infertility case and the semen analysis was done prior to 2010 it should be repeated and compared with the 2010 WHO reference values. The WHO semen analysis reference values are available at http://www.who.int/reproductivehealth/publications /infertility/9789241547789/en/index.html.

It is important to appreciate that these values are reference ranges—not the minimum values needed for fertilization. Thus a man whose semen falls outside the ranges can be fertile, and a man whose semen is within the ranges can be infertile. A complete male evaluation usually includes at least two semen analyses (Male Infertility Best Practice Policy Committee of the AUA & Practice Committee of the ASRM, 2006).

TABLE 19-2 World Health Organization Lower Reference Limits for Semen Characteristics

Characteristic	Lower Reference Limit	
	5th Centile	**95% CI**
Semen volume per mL	1.5	1.4–1.7
Total sperm number (10^6 per ejaculate)	39	33–46
Sperm concentration (10^6 per mL)	15	12–16
Total motility (PR + NP, %)	40	38–42
Progressive motility (PR, %)	32	31–34
Vitality (live spermatozoa, %)	58	55–63
Sperm morphology (normal forms, %)	4	3.0–4.0
pH	≥ 7.2	Not applicable

Note: CI = confidence interval; mL = milliliter; NP = nonprogressive motility; PR = progressive motility.
Sources: Data from Cooper et al., 2010; WHO, 2010.

Laboratory Testing Various infertility tests are performed on blood samples. Initial evaluation usually includes measurement of thyroid-stimulating hormone (TSH) and prolactin levels, as women can have asymptomatic thyroid disease or hyperprolactinemia. An elevated prolactin level in the absence of lactation requires imaging of the sella turcica to rule out a pituitary mass. If BBT charting or LH urine testing does not demonstrate a biphasic curve, measuring serum progesterone levels midway through the luteal phase can be helpful in detecting whether a woman is ovulating. Serial progesterone tests to detect short luteal phase are not recommended (Fritz & Speroff, 2011). Additional laboratory tests, such as FSH, LH, and testosterone measurements, may be indicated if the woman is amenorrheic or has signs and symptoms of a hyperandrogenic disorder (see Chapters 25 and 26).

Some clinicians perform assessments of "ovarian reserve" to guide infertility treatment options and predict the likelihood of success, particularly among women who are 35 years or older, have only one ovary or have had ovarian surgery, or have not responded to exogenous gonadotropin stimulation (Practice Committee of the ASRM, 2006b). One method is to obtain a serum FSH level on cycle day 3. Another protocol is the clomiphene citrate challenge, which consists of measurement of serum FSH and estradiol levels on cycle day 3, administration of clomiphene citrate (100 mg/day) from cycle days 5 to 9, and another serum FSH level on cycle day 10 (Fritz & Speroff, 2011).

Hysterosalpingogram A hysterosalpingogram (HSG) is a procedure in which a water-soluble or oil-soluble contrast is injected through the woman's cervix into her uterus. During the HSG, the transport of the contrast is observed by radiologic imaging. This procedure is ideally performed two to five days after menstruation ends to avoid interference from menstrual tissue and disruption of potential fertilization and implantation. In a normal HSG, the contrast travels unobstructed through the uterus and into the fallopian tubes. Thus this test indicates whether the fallopian tubes are patent or whether a structural abnormality is present in the uterus or tubes (Fritz & Speroff, 2011).

Transvaginal Ultrasound and Hysteroscopy Transvaginal ultrasound can help identify uterine factors associated with infertility, such as fibroids and endometrial polyps. Ultrasound evaluation of the endometrium has not proved valuable in infertility evaluation (Fritz & Speroff, 2011). Hysteroscopy can be used for definitive diagnosis and treatment of intrauterine conditions causing infertility (Fritz & Speroff).

Laparoscopy The outside surfaces of the uterus, tubes, and ovaries can be observed via a laparoscope, which is inserted into the abdomen through the umbilicus. In this procedure, the pelvic organs are examined for any abnormalities, including structural alterations, endometriosis, or pelvic adhesions. Laparoscopy can be used not only for diagnosis of endometriosis and pelvic adhesions, but also for treatment. In addition, hysteroscopy may be performed simultaneously to evaluate the uterine cavity.

Diagnostic Testing and Procedures That Are No Longer Performed Regularly Three diagnostic tests and procedures previously used in infertility assessment are now infrequently performed in clinical practice: the postcoital test, endometrial biopsy, and the sperm penetration assay.

A postcoital test (PCT) is done to evaluate the interaction of the sperm and cervical mucus around the time of ovulation. After the couple has sexual intercourse, a sample of the woman's cervical mucus is obtained by the clinician for microscopic examination. Normally, live, motile sperm will be seen. If there are fertility-related problems, such as the cervical mucus being too acidic or the man having an abnormally low sperm count, the clinician might see predominantly immotile sperm or no sperm at all in the sample. Owing to the subjectivity of PCT results and the availability of treatments that avoid cervical factors (e.g., intrauterine insemination and in vitro fertilization), routine use of the PCT is now unnecessary, and this test should be performed only when it will influence the treatment strategy (Male Infertility Best Practice Policy Committee of the AUA & Practice Committee of the ASRM, 2006; Practice Committee of the ASRM, 2006b).

Endometrial biopsy (EMB) of the uterine lining has been used in infertility assessment to evaluate endometrial development. Endometrial cells from the biopsy are microscopically examined to assess the phase of the menstrual cycle. The day of the woman's menstrual cycle is compared with the phase of the endometrial tissue to determine if the two are consistent. EMB was considered the gold standard for the diagnosis of short luteal phase for many years, but research has shown that it is not a valid diagnostic tool for this condition. Fritz and Speroff (2011) recommend calculation of the length of the luteal phase, using BBT charting or urine LH testing, as the best method for diagnosis of short luteal phase. The use of EMB in infertility assessment is now relatively rare in clinical practice.

Sometimes the cause of infertility is the inability of the sperm to penetrate the ovum. In the sperm penetration assay, sperm are exposed to hamster eggs to determine their ability to penetrate, because there is a correlation between the ability of sperm to penetrate human eggs and hamster eggs. This test is mentioned because it highlights the fact that sperm problems are sometimes better understood in interaction with the ova. This test, however, has been done less frequently as more sophisticated tests have emerged.

Differential Diagnosis

The differential diagnosis of infertility includes the etiologies detailed previously. It is important to recognize that several causes may exist simultaneously.

Prevention of Infertility

The focus in infertility has traditionally been diagnosis and treatment, but there has recently been attention to prevention. Young women can be taught to prevent STIs, or if they have symptoms or suspect they may have been exposed to infection, to seek care early to prevent PID and subsequent infertility. Paradoxically, certain contraceptive methods may protect future fertility by decreasing the risk of PID, ectopic pregnancies, and endometriosis (see Chapter 12). In addition, avoiding some environmental factors may prevent infertility, although more definitive studies are needed to clarify these risk factors.

Management of Infertility

Treatments for infertility are usually specific to the cause. Sometimes treatments are general because a specific cause of infertility cannot be determined (unexplained infertility). Approaches to treatment in these instances raise complex issues about risks and benefits.

Patient Education

Education about when a woman is fertile during the menstrual cycle and coital timing can be extremely beneficial for some patients. The infertility evaluation is also an opportune time to suggest health promotion behaviors. Behaviors that may specifically improve fertility include achieving a BMI in the range of 20 to 25 if the woman is underweight or overweight, stopping smoking, and reducing alcohol ($\leq$ 4 drinks per week) and caffeine (< 250 mg per day) consumption (Fritz & Speroff, 2011).

Ovulation Induction

If there is evidence of anovulation or infrequent ovulation, medication to induce ovulation may be prescribed. Because ovulation induction medications are so widely used and are frequently called "fertility drugs," there is a misconception by the public that these medications improve general fertility. In reality, these medications specifically help with ovulation and are usually not warranted in women who ovulate but want to improve their fertility. However, empiric treatment with clomiphene citrate is sometimes used for women with unexplained infertility, particularly those who will not or cannot seek more aggressive treatment (Practice Committee of the ASRM, 2006c).

The first choice of medication for ovulation induction is usually clomiphene citrate (Clomid, Serophene), which works by binding estrogen receptors in the pituitary gland, thereby blocking those receptors from detecting circulating estrogen. As a result, the hypothalamus increases its secretion of GnRH, which stimulates the pituitary to secrete FSH and LH. These hormones, in turn, stimulate and initiate an ovulatory menstrual cycle.

Clomiphene citrate is taken orally once a day for five consecutive days. The initial dose is usually 50 mg. The medication is typically started on the third to fifth day after menses begins spontaneously or is induced with progestin. Ovulation usually occurs 14 days after the first dose. The dose can be increased in increments of 50 mg if ovulation does not occur at the lower dose; however, most pregnancies occur at dosages of 50 to 100 mg (Practice Committee of the ASRM, 2006c). Clomiphene citrate can be administered in doses as high as 250 mg, but other approaches should be considered if continued increases in the dose prove unsuccessful. If ovulation does occur at a specific dose, the woman should remain on that dose each month, because an increased dose provides no advantage. The combination of insulin-sensitizing agents, such as metformin, with clomiphene citrate may be beneficial in women with polycystic ovary syndrome (see Chapter 26) who have not responded to either medication by itself. In addition, clomiphene citrate is sometimes combined with glucocorticoids or gonadotropins when ovulation does not occur with clomiphene citrate alone (Practice Committee of the ASRM, 2006c).

Side effects of clomiphene citrate include hot flashes, headaches, ovarian enlargement, multiple gestation, and, less frequently, nausea and visual disturbances. Multiple gestations are a frequent concern among women taking ovulation induction medications. In pregnancies that occur among women taking clomiphene citrate, 8% are multiple gestations and the vast majority of these pregnancies involve twins. Appropriate monitoring of women using clomiphene citrate includes ovulation detection with BBT charting, urine LH testing, or serum progesterone levels to determine effectiveness of the treatment. Close follow-up for ovarian enlargement is also warranted, although monthly pelvic or ultrasound examinations are no longer routinely required. Treatment is limited to six ovulatory cycles (Practice Committee of the ASRM, 2006c).

More potent ovulation induction with injectable exogenous gonadotropins can be tried for women who do not respond to clomiphene citrate. Recombinant or purified FSH (Follistim, Gonal-F) or human menopausal gonadotropins containing FSH and LH (Pergonal, Repronex) are most commonly used for this purpose. These medications work by directly stimulating development of the ovarian follicles and are used in conjunction with human chorionic gonadotropin (hCG), recombinant LH, or a GnRH agonist, which is administered in the final stages of follicle maturation to induce oocyte release. Administration of exogenous gonadotropins increases the risk of ovarian hyperstimulation and tends to result in multiple gestations—even more so than with clomiphene citrate. Careful timing of the medication used to induce oocyte release is necessary to limit this risk (Practice Committee of the ASRM, 2008d). The complex protocols and potential serious side effects of exogenous gonadotropins require careful treatment and extensive monitoring that is best performed by clinicians who are experienced in their use.

Women undergoing ovulation induction therapy must be informed about the medication, including its mechanism of action and potential side effects and risks. Exogenous gonadotropins can be very expensive, which is a consideration for many people. Some research suggests there may be a link between a woman's use of ovulation-inducing medication and later development of ovarian cancer. Although a meta-analysis found no increase in ovarian cancer among women with infertility who were treated when compared to those who were not (Kashyap, Moher, Fung, & Rosenwaks, 2004), judicious use of ovulation induction medications remains prudent.

Treatment of Short Luteal Phase

There is an association between hyperprolactinemia and short luteal phase. Treatment to normalize the prolactin level, therefore, may lengthen the luteal phase. In the absence of this identifiable cause, treatment of short luteal phase can be ambiguous.

One theory of treatment is that the follicular phase of the menstrual cycle should be enhanced with ovulation induction methods because short luteal phase is a form of ovulatory dysfunction. This concept suggests that clomiphene citrate or other ovulation induction medications might be used to remedy this problem (Fritz & Speroff, 2011). Another theory is that the luteal phase of the menstrual cycle should be enhanced by administering progesterone, thereby increasing the secretory endometrium. Progesterone is administered vaginally (200 to 600 mg/day) or by intramuscular injection (50 mg/day). If the woman conceives, she usually continues progesterone therapy throughout the first trimester, although treatment beyond 9 weeks' gestation is very likely unnecessary. The optimal route, dose, and duration of progesterone therapy are uncertain. There is no evidence to support one strategy as being more beneficial than the other (i.e., progesterone administration versus ovulation induction medications) (Practice Committee of the ASRM, 2008c).

Treatment for Male Factor Infertility

Treatment for male factor infertility depends on the specific problem. For example, certain hormonal problems respond to medical therapy, and surgical repair of a varicocele can be beneficial. Unfortunately, many causes of male factor infertility are not amenable to treatment. In such cases, pregnancy may still be achieved with artificial insemination, intrauterine insemination (IUI), or intracytoplasmic sperm injection (the last technique is discussed in the later section on assisted reproductive technologies).

Insemination procedures begin with the man masturbating to collect the semen, which is then processed in a laboratory to remove the seminal plasma, creating a more highly concentrated specimen of motile sperm. For artificial insemination, the clinician then places the semen into the woman's cervix. With IUI, the semen is placed directly into her uterus, bypassing the cervix. This approach is particularly warranted when a problem with the cervical mucus is the cause of the infertility.

Artificial and intrauterine insemination must be performed in a precisely timed manner based on the woman's menstrual cycle. These procedures can lead to increased stress for the couple, however. The man may feel greater pressure to perform by producing the semen, and the woman may feel more anxious about having intercourse at "appropriate" times and abstaining at "inappropriate" times. Intrauterine insemination is often used in conjunction with ovulation induction even if no male factors are identified. This combination of approaches is used to increase the success of the ovulation induction by enhancing the precision and accuracy of timing.

Options for Women and Men with Infertility

Technological advances have led to an increasing array of procedures for becoming pregnant, including the possibility of collaborative reproduction. Women and men may also choose adoption or child-free living. These options are presented in this section, and their psychological and ethical considerations are the focus of the next section.

Assisted Reproductive Technologies

In vitro fertilization (IVF) is the most widely used assisted reproductive technology (ART) procedure. In this technique, the ovaries are hyperstimulated with medication and then several mature ova are surgically retrieved, placed in a laboratory dish, and then mixed with sperm. Fertilization takes place in vitro and, after fertilization, one or more embryos are transferred directly into the woman's uterus for implantation. Because IVF bypasses the fallopian tubes, it is commonly attempted in women who have tubal blockage from structural problems or secondary to pelvic infection or scar tissue. It is also used when the etiology of infertility remains unknown.

Gamete intrafallopian transfer (GIFT) is another form of ART. In this case, however, fertilization occurs in vivo rather than in vitro. The egg and sperm are both placed directly into the fallopian tube via laparoscopy so that fertilization can occur. The woman must have at least one patent fallopian tube for GIFT to be successful. Women and men who are Catholic may choose this method over IVF because the Catholic Church condones GIFT, but not IVF.

Zygote intrafallopian transfer (ZIFT) is a process in which the ovaries are hyperstimulated and the ova are surgically retrieved. They are then fertilized in vitro, as with IVF. The zygotes are placed in the fallopian tube laparoscopically the day after fertilization.

Intracytoplasmic sperm injection (ICSI) is a newer technique in which the egg is directly injected with one sperm. This procedure is used when the man has a low sperm count or in other situations involving male factor infertility. Intracytoplasmic sperm injection is used in conjunction with IVF or ZIFT.

Collaborative Reproduction

Collaborative, or third-party, reproduction refers to the involvement of a person who will not be raising the child, such as a sperm or egg donor or surrogate mother. One person may donate sperm or eggs (genetic parent) and/or carry the pregnancy (gestational mother) for another person or couple who will raise the child (rearing parents). Collaborative reproduction may involve artificial or intrauterine insemination, or ART. Collaborative reproduction may be chosen when infertility treatment or ART has proved unsuccessful or is not possible because of individual factors. Women who are situationally infertile, or those who are unable to conceive by virtue of not having a male partner, may also seek donor insemination. These women may be single or may be lesbians. Insemination is a very viable option for them.

Use of donor sperm is the most common type of collaborative reproduction, but women may also become pregnant with donor eggs. For example, a known or anonymous woman may donate her eggs to an individual or couple. The eggs are fertilized in vitro with sperm, most likely from the male partner of the couple with infertility (rearing father), and then transferred to the female partner with infertility for gestation. In this instance, the egg donor is the genetic mother and the woman who becomes pregnant is the gestational and rearing mother. Surrogate mothers can be genetic and gestational mothers if they carry a fetus who is conceived from their own egg, or solely gestational mothers if they carry a fetus conceived from another couple's egg and sperm, such as from a woman who can conceive but not carry a pregnancy.

Adoption

For those couples who are able to separate pregnancy from parenting, adoption is often an ideal option. Couples who choose to adopt usually go through a home study by an adoption agency prior to being approved for adoption. Other couples work with private attorneys to find a woman who is willing to give her child up for adoption. International adoption has become increasingly popular as more people have begun to go outside of the United States to adopt children.

Although adoption is often an excellent option for individuals or couples seeking parenthood, not all cultures embrace this practice. In India, infertility is referred to as "adoption gone awry," and people seek solutions in secret, thus making adoption an unacceptable option because it is difficult to keep that secret (Bharadwaj, 2003).

Child-Free Living

Some individuals or couples eventually come to a decision to live their lives without children. The term *child-free* connotes that this state has now become a choice rather than something occurring against their will. People without children may be referred to as *childless*, but this term indicates a loss or absence. Granted, this situation was initially childlessness for those who hoped to conceive, but through the process of reconciling their loss, some people are able to come to a conclusion of their own volition to remain child-free.

Evidence for Best Practices Related to Infertility Care

Practices that offer ART are urged to follow the guidelines developed by the Practice Committee of the Society for Assisted Reproductive Technology (SART) and the Practice Committee of the ASRM (2008). These guidelines address minimum requirements for all personnel, the specialized training and experience required for personnel, minimum standards to follow for each technological procedure, ethical and experimental procedures, recordkeeping, and informed consent. The guidelines are updated periodically and are considered the standard for the delivery of ART. The ASRM regularly publishes bulletins and reports, in the journal *Fertility and Sterility*, that are helpful in clarifying other clinical aspects of infertility care.

Special Considerations

This section presents some of the controversial issues related to infertility and its treatment. Infertility can have psychosocial effects on the individuals and couples involved as well as on their larger families. The new technologies that are now used to both diagnose and treat infertility have created many ethical issues. The psychosocial and ethical issues are the focus of this section.

Psychological, Family, Relationship, and Social Issues

Extensive research suggests that many psychological issues are related to infertility, whether the psychological problems are causes or consequences of infertility. Historically, women were viewed as psychogenically infertile—a very negative term implying that women who were unable to conceive were psychologically unstable, had unresolved relationship issues with their mothers, or were hysterical or neurotic. Psychoanalytic theory in the 1950s and 1960s explained infertility as solely a woman's problem, to the exclusion of any involvement by men. A few decades later, the scientific literature developed an increasing focus on psychological problems in both women and men that occurred as a consequence of infertility rather than as a cause, mitigating the negative labels on women. A better understanding was developed about the difficulties and stresses that both women and men experienced as a result of their inability to conceive or bear a child. Recently, scientific literature has taken a more complex view, indicating that infertility has both psychological causes and consequences for women and men.

In general, infertility is profoundly distressing for those experiencing it, whether this is a cause or a consequence. Olshansky (1996a) generated a theory of identity as infertile to reflect the experience of infertility becoming so central to one's definition of self that a person begins to take on an identity as an infertile person. Other identities are pushed to the periphery as the identity as infertile becomes central.

Recent research suggests that psychological problems, such as depression and anxiety, may contribute to the development of infertility, although further study on this theory is needed. Domar (2002) found that using a mind–body approach to elicit a relaxation response helps some women conceive.

Complicated psychological issues often come to the fore surrounding a decision or inability to make a decision to stop infertility treatment. This is particularly likely with the ongoing advances in reproductive technology that are making new options continually available. The introduction of new treatments may raise hopes and make it difficult to stop treatment for fear that there will be a feeling of not having done everything possible to conceive, which could then make it difficult to resolve infertility later.

Infertility is directly intertwined with family issues because it represents the inability to expand a family. Some people even view it as an inability to have a family, implying that two people in a couple are not a family by virtue of not having children and further emphasizing a societal bent toward pronatalism. Family gatherings can be extremely difficult for persons dealing with infertility because they may be directly confronted with their inability to conceive, especially if young children are present. Family issues may extend to others, such as the parents of people with infertility who are experiencing the loss related to not being grandparents. Family members may pressure couples with infertility with comments such as "Why are they taking so long to have a baby?"

As stated earlier, women and men experience infertility within a socially pronatalist context. As a result, they are often viewed as abnormal or as not fulfilling their responsibilities to continue the human race. Women, by virtue of the general social approach to and view of women's roles, may experience feeling even more "aberrant" than do men.

Social issues may vary in different societies and in different socioeconomic groups. For example, a study in South Africa found that although infertility is a large problem, the resources for treatment are limited (Stewart-Smythe & van Iddekinge, 2003). Tubal problems are the most frequently diagnosed cause of infertility in South Africa, and the best treatment is IVF. This is an expensive technique, however, and as such is less available and accessible in the public sector of South Africa. Inhorn (2003) corroborated this problem in her case study of infertility in Egypt, where she found that even though reproductive technologies are available, many structural and cultural constraints prevent access to such technologies. She further states that more attention should be paid to preventable infertility problems, specifically infections that lead to PID.

Ethical Issues

Many of the ethical issues related to infertility occur as a result of the increasing use of technology; however, it is important to note that ethical issues existed prior to and may be independent of advances in infertility treatment. Access to infertility treatment has always been an issue, but it has been particularly compounded by the never-ending stream of technology that has been introduced into the healthcare realm. The expense of infertility treatment raises the question of whether these therapies will be limited to those with the financial means to afford them, as the costs for such treatment are frequently not covered by insurance. The ability to conceive with technology but without a partner also leads to questions regarding whether single women, single men, or lesbian or gay couples will be treated.

Other ethical issues concern who the parents are in situations where extra embryos have been frozen and the couple subsequently divorces, or when a surrogate mother decides she no longer wants to relinquish the infant. In fact, the larger issue is how the "real parent" is defined. Parties involved in various situations may include the genetic mother, the surrogate mother, the gestational mother, the adoptive or rearing mother, and the birth mother. Egg donation is one example of a treatment that raises many ethical as well as legal issues (Robertson, 1995).

Another ethical dilemma can occur when several embryos are transferred into the woman's uterus and multiple embryos survive. The presence of multiple embryos may create a high risk for all of them, and the woman may choose to selectively abort one or more to reduce this risk. This situation creates complex ethical as well as emotional issues. Limiting the number of embryos transferred is advisable (Practice Committee of the ASRM & Practice Committee of the SART, 2009).

Ethical concerns have also arisen about the ability to perform pre-implantation testing with ART. After in vitro fertilization, a cell is removed from the embryo for genetic testing. This evaluation allows couples with known inherited disorders to select nonaffected embryos for transfer, but leads to questions about genetic engineering. The sex of the embryo can also be determined, which is useful for sex-linked disorders, but is controversial when sex selection is purely for parental preference.

These are just a few of the many ethical issues that arise in relation to infertility care and treatment. There are no simple answers to these conflicts, but they warrant consideration both from a societal perspective and on the level of caring for individual patients. The ASRM regularly publishes reports, in the journal *Fertility and Sterility*, that address ethical issues in infertility.

Infertility and Cancer

Progress in medicine has provided much better prognoses for many people with a diagnosis of cancer. As a result, people who survive cancer may want to conceive. Counseling about fertility preservation options and future reproduction prior to cancer treatment is recommended (Ethics Committee of the ASRM, 2005). Conversely, some concern is raised about the possibility that infertility and its treatment may increase the risk for or development of cancer, although research has not confirmed this fear (Venn, Healy, & McLachlan, 2003).

Infertility and Women in the Later Years of Childbearing

With the increased use of technology to treat infertility, more options have been developed for women at the end of their childbearing years. Thus women in their mid-40s to even early 50s may conceive and carry a pregnancy to term. Although this flexibility provides more opportunities for women, it also creates more complex decisions for women and their families. Certain genetic risks to the fetus, such as Down syndrome, are known to be higher when women become pregnant at later ages. At the same time, there may be advantages to women and their children in parenting at older ages. More research is needed in this area.

Patient Counseling

It is crucial for clinicians to recognize that treatment for infertility involves more than physical treatment. Olshansky (1996b) noted four important aspects of care that should be included in a counseling approach to persons with infertility. Clinicians should assist patients in:

1. Confronting and analyzing the choices available to them by providing complete and accurate information while empowering them to make decisions that only they can make.
2. Focusing on and reclaiming the successful parts of their lives by helping them to see positive aspects of themselves rather than defining themselves based on their infertility.
3. Moving on with their lives by helping them to stop treatment when appropriate and seek other options.

4. Developing and maintaining healthy interpersonal relationships by emphasizing the importance of relationships to good mental health.

Incorporating these aspects into clinical care can improve patients' quality of life both during and after infertility treatment.

References

Bharadwaj, A. (2003). Why adoption is not an option in India: The visibility of infertility, the secrecy of donor insemination, and other cultural complexities. *Social Science and Medicine, 56*(9), 1867–1880.

Cooper, T. G., Noonan, E., von Eckardstein, S., Auger, J., Baker, H. W. G., Behre, H., … Vogelson, K. (2010). World Health Organization reference values for human semen characteristics. *Human Reproduction Update, 16*(3), 231–245. doi: 10.1093/humupd/dmp048

Devine, K. (2003). Caring for the infertile woman. *MCN: The American Journal of Maternal–Child Nursing, 28*(2), 100–105.

Domar, A. D. (2002). *Conquering infertility*. New York: Viking Press.

Ethics Committee of the American Society for Reproductive Medicine. (2005). Fertility preservation and reproduction in cancer patients. *Fertility and Sterility, 83*, 1622–1628.

Fritz, M., & Speroff, L. (2011). *Clinical gynecologic endocrinology and infertility* (8th ed.). Baltimore: Lippincott Williams & Wilkins.

Hanson, B. (2003). Questioning the construction of maternal age as a fertility problem. *Health Care for Women International, 24*(3), 166–176.

Inhorn, M. C. (2003). Global infertility and the globalization of new reproductive technologies: Illustrations from Egypt. *Social Science and Medicine, 56*(9), 1837–1851.

Kashyap, S., Moher, D., Fung, M. F., & Rosenwaks, Z. (2004). Assisted reproductive technology and the incidence of ovarian cancer: A meta-analysis. *Obstetrics & Gynecology, 103*, 785–794.

Male Infertility Best Practice Policy Committee of the American Urological Association (AUA) & Practice Committee of the American Society for Reproductive Medicine (ASRM). (2006). Report on optimal evaluation of the infertile male. *Fertility and Sterility, 86*(suppl 4), S202–S209.

Olshansky, E. F. (1992). Redefining the concepts of success and failure in infertility treatment. *NAACOG's Clinical Issues in Women's Health and Perinatal Nursing, 3*(2), 343–347.

Olshansky, E. (1996a). Theoretical issues in building a grounded theory: Application of a program of research on infertility. *Qualitative Health Research, 6*(3), 394–405.

Olshansky, E. (1996b). A counseling approach with persons experiencing infertility: Implications for advanced practice nursing. *Advanced Practice Nursing Quarterly, 2*(3), 42–47.

Practice Committee of the American Society for Reproductive Medicine (ASRM). (2006a). Aging and infertility in women. *Fertility and Sterility, 86*(suppl 4), S248–S252.

Practice Committee of the American Society for Reproductive Medicine (ASRM). (2006b). Optimal evaluation of the infertile female. *Fertility and Sterility, 86*(suppl 1), S264–S267.

Practice Committee of the American Society for Reproductive Medicine (ASRM). (2006c). Use of clomiphene citrate in women. *Fertility and Sterility, 86*(suppl 1), S187–S193.

Practice Committee of the American Society for Reproductive Medicine (ASRM). (2008a). Age-related fertility decline: A committee opinion. *Fertility and Sterility, 90*(suppl 1), S154–S155.

Practice Committee of the American Society for Reproductive Medicine (ASRM). (2008b). Definitions of infertility and recurrent pregnancy loss. *Fertility and Sterility, 90*(suppl 1), S60.

Practice Committee of the American Society for Reproductive Medicine (ASRM). (2008c). Progesterone supplementation during the luteal phase and in early pregnancy in the treatment of infertility: An educational bulletin. *Fertility and Sterility, 90*(suppl 1), S150–153.

Practice Committee of the American Society for Reproductive Medicine (ASRM). (2008d). Use of exogenous gonadotropins in anovulatory women: A technical bulletin. *Fertility and Sterility, 90*(suppl 1), S7–12.

Practice Committee of the American Society for Reproductive Medicine (ASRM) & Practice Committee of the Society for Assisted Reproductive Technology (SART). (2009). Guidelines on number of embryos transferred. *Fertility and Sterility, 92*, 1518–1519.

Practice Committee of the Society for Assisted Reproductive Technology (SART) & Practice Committee of the American Society for Reproductive Medicine (ASRM). (2008). Revised minimum standards for practices offering assisted reproductive technologies. *Fertility and Sterility, 90*(suppl 1), S165–168.

Resolve. (2008). *Secondary infertility*. Retrieved July 25, 2009, from http://www.resolve.org/site/Page Server?pagename=lrn_wii_si

Robertson, J. A. (1995). Legal issues in human egg donation and gestational surrogacy. *Seminars in Reproductive Endocrinology, 13*(3), 210–218.

Stewart-Smythe, G. W., & van Iddekinge, B. (2003). Lessons learned from infertility investigations in the public sector. *South African Medical Journal, 93*(2), 141–143.

Venn, A., Healy, D., & McLachlan, R. (2003). Cancer risks associated with the diagnosis of infertility. *Best Practice and Research in Clinical Obstetrics and Gynecology, 17*(2), 343–367.

World Health Organization (WHO). (2010). *WHO laboratory manual for the examination and processing of human semen* (5th ed.). Retrieved from http://www .who.int/reproductivehealth/publications/infertility/ 9789241547789/en/index.html

20

Gynecologic Infections

Catherine Ingram Fogel

G ynecologic infections, often associated with vaginal discharge, itching of the vulva and vagina, and vaginal or vulvar pain, are among the most frequent reasons a woman seeks help from a clinician. Different women perceive discharge and itching in unique ways. One woman may be extremely uncomfortable, another may feel only minor distress, a third may be very anxious, and a fourth may be mildly concerned. Women's reactions depend on many factors, including their previous experiences or knowledge; societal, religious, and cultural beliefs; and the number and severity of symptoms.

Vaginal Secretions

Normal Characteristics

Vaginal secretions are a normal, regularly occurring experience for women during their reproductive years. The numerous variations in the amount and characteristics of vaginal secretions are determined by physiology, emotions, and pathology. Women who have adequate endogenous or exogenous estrogen will have vaginal secretions. The major source of these secretions is the cervical mucosa, although small amounts are also secreted by the Bartholin's, sebaceous, sweat, and apocrine glands of the vulva. Vaginal lubrication, which is pushed through the semipermanent vaginal membrane as a result of increased vasocongestion in the spongelike tissues surrounding the vagina, occurs during sexual excitement (Ayres, 2004).

Normal vaginal secretions are clear to cloudy in appearance and may turn yellow after drying. The discharge is slightly slimy, is non-irritating, and has a mild inoffensive odor. The alkaline, shiny mucoid substance secreted by the cervix, by comparison, is more abundant than vaginal secretions and is less viscous at ovulation. Normal vaginal secretions are acidic, with a pH range of 3.8 to 4.2. Döderlein's bacilli are customarily seen in the vaginal secretions of women during their reproductive years. The amount of vaginal discharge a woman experiences is not, in itself, an indication of infection.

Life-Cycle Changes

The female newborn may have a mucous discharge for 1 to 10 days following birth as a result of in utero stimulation of the uterus and vagina by maternal estrogen. A similar mucoid discharge may be seen a few years before and after menarche as a result of increased estrogen production by the maturing ovaries. Pregnancy often substantially increases mucus production, with a resulting profuse discharge, particularly during the last few weeks before childbirth. A similar discharge may occur in a woman taking combined oral contraceptives (Hatcher et al., 2007).

Before menarche and following menopause, when estrogen levels are low, vaginal secretions are minimal. The vaginal epithelium is inactive and thin, the cells contain very little glycogen, Döderlein's bacilli are absent, and the vaginal pH is between 6 and 7. Such inactive mucosa is particularly susceptible to infection, whereas the estrogen-stimulated vaginal mucosa during the reproductive years is less vulnerable.

Vaginal secretions normally vary throughout the menstrual cycle. During the immediate postmenstrual phase, when the estrogen level is low, the mucosa is thin and relatively inactive with little cervical cell secretion present. Vaginal cells proliferate and exfoliate rapidly as estrogen production increases. At the same time, the cervical cells secrete increasing amounts of mucus. Maximal estrogen production occurs at ovulation and causes a profuse watery discharge, primarily from the cervix. Secretions then decrease until just prior to menstruation.

Vaginitis and Vaginosis

Vaginitis is an inflammation of the vagina characterized by an increased vaginal discharge containing numerous white blood cells. In contrast, vaginosis is not associated with white blood cells. Vaginitis occurs when the vaginal environment is altered, either by a microorganism (**Table 20-1**) or by a disturbance that allows the pathogens found normally in the vagina to proliferate. Factors that can disturb the vaginal environment include douches, vaginal medications, antibiotics, hormones, contraceptives, stress, sexual intercourse, and changes in sexual partners (Schaffer, 2003).

Vulvovaginitis—that is, inflammation of the vulva and vagina—may be caused by vaginal infection or copious amounts of leukorrhea, an increased amount of vaginal and cervical discharge consisting of epithelial cells and cervical mucus that can cause maceration of tissues. In addition, chemical irritants, allergens, and foreign bodies may produce inflammatory reactions. Bacterial vaginosis (BV), vulvovaginal candidiasis (VVC), and trichomoniasis are the most common causes of abnormal vaginal discharge (see Chapter 21 for a discussion of trichomoniasis). See **Color Plate 16** for an example of vaginal discharge.

TABLE 20-1 Vaginal Discharge

	Normal Discharge	Bacterial Vaginosis	Vulvovaginal Candidiasis
Vaginal pH	3.8–4.5	> 4.5	< 4.5 (usually)
Wet prep	Normal flora	With saline solution: positive for clue cells, decreased lactobacilli	With potassium hydroxide (KOH): pseudohyphae with yeast buds
Discharge	White/clear Thin/mucoid	Thin, homogenous, grayish-white, adherent	Thick or thin, white, curd-like ("cottage cheese"), adherent
Amine odor (KOH "whiff" test)	Absent	Present (fishy)	Absent
Vulvar pruritis	No	Mild if present at all	Yes, swelling, excoriation, redness
Genital ulceration	No	No	Skin may crack with severe cases
Pelvic pain	No	No	No
Dysuria	No	Occasionally	Severe cases
Dyspareunia	No	Occasionally	Occasionally
Main patient concern	None or variable	May be asymptomatic, vaginal discharge, vaginal odor that is often worse after intercourse	Vaginal itching, burning, and/or discharge
Risk of PID	No	Yes	No

Sources: Data from CDC, 2010; Eckert, 2006.

Prevention Measures

Clinicians can do much to alleviate the discomfort associated with abnormal vaginal discharge by teaching preventive measures, providing information to assist in recognizing symptoms, and suggesting self-care activities to prevent and treat vaginitis. Preventive measures are important for all types of vaginal infections, but particularly for women with recurrent episodes of vaginitis. General health promotion, including adequate rest, reduction of life stressors, and a healthy diet low in refined sugars, may help to decrease the likelihood of infection. Good personal hygiene is essential for preventing vaginal infections. The perineal area needs to be washed often to remove perspiration and smegma accumulations, and then patted dry rather than rubbed. Towels, washcloths, sponges, douching equipment, vaginal diaphragms, cervical caps, and underwear should be clean and never shared. Bathtubs should be washed after each use.

Critical to prevention efforts is teaching women the proper way to wipe after voiding and defecation. One should always wipe from front to back (never the reverse) to avoid introducing bacteria into the vagina or urethra. Sprays, powders, soaps, and deodorants that are perfumed or irritating in any way should not be used. Any chemicals that irritate the skin or vaginal mucosa, or that alter the vaginal environment, should be avoided. Clothing that is too tight, does not allow free air flow to the perineum, or traps moisture should be avoided. Underwear and pantyhose should always have a cotton crotch. Women should not douche, because douching can strip the vagina of its normal flora, introduce bacteria, and aggravate inflammation. The only exception to this rule is when medication is needed.

Women should be encouraged to change tampons, sanitary pads, and panty liners frequently. They should be counseled not to wear tampons to bed and not to use them when flow is scanty, as the tampon may adhere to the vaginal wall or cervix and cause trauma when removed. In addition, women should avoid perfumed sanitary products because they can be an allergen or chemical irritant.

Bacterial Vaginosis

Bacterial vaginosis, formerly called nonspecific vaginitis, *Haemophilus* vaginitis, or *Gardnerella*, is the most prevalent vaginal infection in women of reproductive age (Marrazzo et al., 2010). Black and Mexican American women have a greater risk of developing BV than do white women (Allsworth & Peipert, 2007).

Bacterial vaginosis (see **Color Plate 12**) is a clinical syndrome in which normal hydrogen peroxide–producing *Lactobacillus* sp. are replaced with high concentrations of anaerobic (e.g., *Prevotella*, *Peptostreptococcus*, *Eubacterium*, and *Mobiluncus* sp.) and facultative anaerobic (i.e., *Gardnerella vaginalis* and *Mycoplasma hominis*) bacteria. With the proliferation of anaerobes, the level of vaginal amines increases and the normal acidic pH of the vagina is altered. As epithelial cells slough, numerous bacteria attach to their surfaces forming clue cells. When the amines are volatilized, the characteristic fishy odor associated with BV occurs. The cause of the microbial alteration is not completely understood, but BV is not considered to be a sexually transmitted infection (STI). What is known is that BV is associated with new or multiple sex partners (male or female), douching, and a lack of vaginal lactobacilli (Centers for Disease Control and Prevention [CDC], 2010). Women who have never been sexually active are rarely affected.

Bacterial vaginosis may cause serious infections in some women, including pelvic inflammatory disease (PID) and postoperative infections, such as posthysterectomy vaginal cuff infection, postabortion endometritis, and postcesarean wound infection (Marrazzo et al., 2010). Studies suggest that BV also increases a woman's risk of acquiring STIs, including human immunodeficiency virus (HIV), and of transmitting HIV infection (Koumans, Markowitz, & Hogan, 2002; Taha, Hoover, & Dallabetta, 1998).

As many as 50% of women with BV are asymptomatic. The most common symptom is a malodorous discharge. A fishy odor may be noticed by the woman or her partner after heterosexual intercourse because semen releases the vaginal amines. When it is present, the BV discharge is usually increased, thin, white or gray, and milky in appearance. Some women also may experience mild irritation, vulvar pruritus, postcoital spotting, irregular bleeding episodes, vaginal burning after intercourse, and urinary discomfort.

Assessment

A careful history may help distinguish BV from other vaginal infections if the woman is symptomatic. Reports of fishy odor and increased thin vaginal discharge are considered the most significant findings. Reports of increased odor after intercourse are also suggestive of BV. Previous occurrences of similar symptoms, diagnoses, and treatments should be investigated, because women may experience repeat episodes associated with antibiotic use, douching, or life stresses.

A speculum examination is performed to inspect the vaginal walls and cervix. A microscopic examination of vaginal secretions is always performed with both normal saline and 10% potassium hydroxide (KOH). The presence of clue cells (vaginal epithelial cells coated with bacteria that obscure cell borders) in the saline smear is highly diagnostic because this phenomenon is specific to BV (**Figures 20-1A and 20-1B**). KOH is used to test for amine

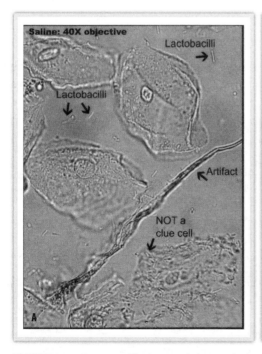 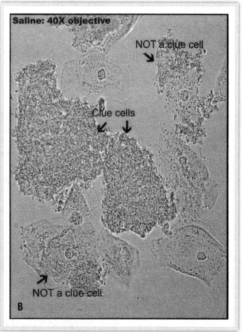

FIGURE 20-1 Wet mount findings with bacterial vaginosis. No bacterial vaginosis (a)—presence of normal epithelial cells and *Lactobacilli*. Bacterial vaginosis (b)—clue cells and absence of *Lactobacilli*.

Source: Used with permission from Washington State Department of Health STD/TB Program, Seattle STD/HIV Prevention Training Center, and Cindy Fennell, MS, MT, ASCP.

odor. A fishy odor will be released when KOH is added to vaginal secretions on a slide or on the lip of the withdrawn speculum (whiff test).

Vaginal secretions should also be tested for pH. Nitrazine paper is sensitive enough to detect a pH of 4.5 or greater. The smear should be taken from the lateral walls of the vagina, not the cervix, to ensure an accurate pH assessment. In asymptomatic women, BV can be reliably diagnosed by Gram stain as well.

Diagnosis is based on the presence of three out of four of the following Amsel criteria:

- White, thin adherent discharge
- pH > 4.5
- Positive whiff test
- Clue cells on wet mount (more than 20% of epithelial cells are clue cells)

Differential Diagnosis

The differential diagnoses for BV include trichomoniasis, vulvovaginal candidiasis, presence of a foreign body, chemical vaginitis, contact vaginitis, chlamydia, gonorrhea, genital herpes, and normal physiologic discharge (Hawkins, Roberto-Nichols, & Stanley-Haney, 2008).

Management

Table 20-2 outlines treatment guidelines for BV. Vaginal metronidazole should not be given to women with a known allergy to oral metronidazole (CDC, 2010). Clindamycin cream is

TABLE 20-2 Bacterial Vaginosis and Vulvovaginal Candidiasis Treatment

Vaginal Infection	Recommended Regimens	Alternative Regimens
Bacterial vaginosis	Metronidazole 500 mg orally twice a day for 7 days OR	Tinidazole 2 g orally once daily for 3 days OR
	Metronidazole gel 0.75%, one full applicator (5 gm) intravaginally, daily for 5 days OR	Tinidazole 1 g orally once daily for 5 days OR
	Clindamycin cream 2%, one full applicator (5 gm) intravaginally, at bedtime for 7 days	Clindamycin 300 mg orally twice a day for 7 days OR
		Clindamycin ovules 100 g intravaginally once at bedtime for 3 days
	Pregnant Women	**Pregnant Women**
	Metronidazole 500 mg orally twice a day for 7 days OR	None
	Metronidazole 250 mg orally three times a day for 7 days OR	
	Clindamycin 300 mg orally twice a day for 7 days	

TABLE 20-2 Bacterial Vaginosis and Vulvovaginal Candidiasis Treatment *(Continued)*

Vaginal Infection	Recommended Regimens	Alternative Regimens
Uncomplicated vulvovaginal candidiasis	**Over-the-Counter Intravaginal Agents** Butoconazole 2% cream 5 gm intravaginally for 3 days OR Clotrimazole 1% cream 5 gm intravaginally for 7–14 days OR Clotrimazole 2% cream 5 gm intravaginally for 3 days OR Miconazole 2% cream 5 gm intravaginally for 7 days OR Miconazole 4% cream 5 gm intravaginally for 3 days OR Miconazole 100 mg vaginal suppository, one suppository for 7 days OR Miconazole 200 mg vaginal suppository, one suppository for 3 days OR Miconazole 1,200 mg vaginal suppository, one suppository for 1 day OR Tioconazole 6.5% ointment 5 gm intravaginally in a single application **Prescription Intravaginal Agents** Butoconazole 2% cream (single dose bioadhesive product), 5 gm intravaginally for 1 day OR Nystatin 100,000-unit vaginal tablet, one tablet for 14 days OR Terconazole 0.4% cream 5 gm intravaginally for 7 days OR Terconazole 0.8% cream 5 gm intravaginally for 3 days OR Terconazole 80 mg vaginal suppository, one suppository for 3 days **Oral Agent** Fluconazole 150 mg oral tablet, one tablet in single dose	

(continues)

TABLE 20-2 Bacterial Vaginosis and Vulvovaginal Candidiasis Treatment

Vaginal Infection	Recommended Regimens	Alternative Regimens
Complicated vulvovaginal candidiasis (VVC)	**Recurrent VVC Initial Therapy** Longer duration of initial therapy, 7–14 days of topical therapy, or a 100-mg, 150-mg, or 200-mg oral dose of fluconazole every third day for a total of 3 doses (day 1, 4, and 7) **Recurrent VVC Maintenance Therapy** 100-mg, 150-mg, or 200-mg dose of oral fluconazole weekly for 6 months If oral regimen is not feasible, consider intermittent use of topical treatments **Severe VVC** 7–14 days of topical azole OR Fluconazole 150 mg in 2 sequential doses, 2nd dose 72 hours after initial dose **Non-albicans VVC** Nonfluconazole azole drug (oral or topical) for 7–14 days **Recurrent non-albicans VVC** 600 mg boric acid in gelatin capsule vaginally each day for 14 days **Pregnancy** Topical azole therapy, applied for 7 days **HIV Infection** Should not differ from that of seronegative women	

Source: Data from CDC, 2010.

preferred in case of allergy or intolerance to metronidazole or tinidazole. Treatment of sexual partners is not recommended because it does not affect a woman's response to treatment or her likelihood of relapse or recurrence (CDC). **Table 20-3** lists alternative therapies for BV.

Special Considerations

Pregnant Women Bacterial vaginosis is associated with chorioamnionitis, premature rupture of fetal membranes, preterm labor and birth, and postpartum endometritis (CDC,

TABLE 20-3 Alternative Therapies for Vaginitis

Intervention	Dosage	Administration	Use
Gentian violet	Few drops in water, 0.25% to 2%	Douche or local application	Vulvovaginal candidiasis
Vinegar (white)	1 tablespoon per pint of water	Douche every 5–7 days or twice a day for 2 days	Vulvovaginal candidiasis or trichomoniasis
	1–2 tablespoons per quart of water	Douche 1–2 times/ week	Bacterial vaginosis
Acidophilus culture	2 tablespoons per pint of water	Douche twice a day	Vulvovaginal candidiasis
Vitamin C	500 mg two to four times daily	Orally	Vulvovaginal candidiasis
Acidophilus tablet	40 million–1 billion units (1 tab) daily	Orally	Vulvovaginal candidiasis
Yogurt	1 application to labia or in vagina	Hourly as needed	Vulvovaginal candidiasis
Goldenseal	1 teaspoon in 3 cups warm water, strain and cool	Douche	Bacterial vaginosis
Garlic clove	1 peeled clove wrapped in cloth dipped in olive oil	Overnight in vagina, change daily	Bacterial vaginosis
Boric acid powder	600 mg in gelatin capsule	Every day in vagina x 14 days	Bacterial vaginosis
Sassafras bark	Steep in warm water Compress	Wash affected area	Vulvovaginal candidiasis
Cold milk, cottage cheese, yogurt	Compress or insert in vagina	Apply to affected area	Pruritis

Sources: Data from Balch & Balch, 1997; Hudson, 1999; Low Dog, 2004; Shaley, Battino, Weiner, Colodner, & Keness, 1996.

2010). However, conflicting evidence has been gathered on the question of whether treatment of asymptomatic pregnant women reduces adverse outcomes of pregnancy. Treatment is recommended for pregnant women with BV who have symptoms, and guidelines for such treatment can be found in Table 20-2. Clindamycin vaginal cream is not recommended in pregnancy because it is associated with low birth weight and neonatal infections in newborns whose mothers were treated with this medication (CDC, 2010).

Talking with the Patient The importance of completing the course of medication and of not consuming alcohol while taking metronidazole (and for 48 hours after completing the treatment) must be emphasized. Women should be informed that metronidazole can cause nausea, vomiting, and cramps even if alcohol is not consumed. In addition, women should be counseled to avoid intercourse until their symptoms cease, and to then use condoms until they complete their treatment. Women should be instructed to refrain from douching, both in general and during treatment.

Vulvovaginal Candidiasis

Vulvovaginal candidiasis (see **Color Plate 13**) or yeast infection accounts for 20% to 25% of all vaginal infections and is the second most common type of vaginal infection in the United States. Three-fourths of all women are expected to have at least one episode of VVC in their lifetimes, and 40% to 45% will have two or more episodes (CDC, 2010). It is difficult to determine the actual incidence of VVC, however, as it is not a reportable condition and the availability of over-the-counter (OTC) treatments prevents many cases from being seen by clinicians (Scharbo-DeHaan & Anderson, 2003). Most (80% to 90%) women who have VVC will have uncomplicated disease (**Table 20-4**).

The most common cause of VVC is *Candida albicans*. Indeed, 90% or more of VVC episodes in women are believed to be caused by this organism. However, VVC can also be caused by non-*albicans* species such as *Candida glabrata*, *Candida tropicalis*, *Candida parapsilosis*, and *Candida krusei* (Hawkins et al., 2008).

Numerous factors have been identified as predisposing a woman to development of VVC, including the following:

TABLE 20-4 Classification of Vulvovaginal Candidiasis (VVC)		
Uncomplicated VVC	**Complicated VVC**	**Recurrent VVC**
Sporadic or infrequent VVC	Recurrent VVC	4 or more episodes in symptomatic VVC in 1 year
OR	OR	
Mild to moderate VVC	Severe VVC	Pathogenesis of RVVC is poorly understood, and most women with RVVC have no apparent predisposing or underlying conditions
OR	OR	
Likely to be *C. albicans*	Non-albicans candidiasis	
OR	OR	
Nonimmunocompromised women	Women with uncontrolled diabetes, debilitation, and immunosuppression	Obtain vaginal cultures to confirm the clinical diagnosis and identify unusual species

Sources: Data from CDC, 2010; Scharbo-DeHaan & Anderson, 2003; Sinclair, 2004.

- Repeated courses of systemic or topical antibiotic therapy, particularly broad-spectrum antibiotics
- Diabetes, especially when uncontrolled
- Pregnancy
- Obesity
- Consumption of a diet high in refined sugars or artificial sweeteners
- Use of corticosteroids and exogenous hormones
- Immunosuppressed states, including HIV seropositivity
- Local allergic or hypersensitivity reactions

Clinical observations and research have also suggested that tight-fitting clothing and underwear or pantyhose made of nonabsorbent materials create an environment in which *Candida* can grow.

The most common symptom of VVC is vulvar and possibly vaginal pruritus (Table 20-1). The itching may be mild or intense, interfere with rest and activities, and occur during or after intercourse. Some women report a feeling of dryness. Others may experience painful urination as the urine flows over the vulva; this symptom usually occurs in women who have excoriation resulting from scratching. Most often the discharge is thick, white, and lumpy with the consistency of cottage cheese. Often the discharge is found in patches on the vaginal walls, cervix, and labia. The vulva is commonly red and swollen, as are the labial folds, vagina, and cervix. Although no characteristic odor is associated with VVC, sometimes a yeasty or musty smell occurs.

Assessment

In addition to obtaining a careful record of the woman's symptoms (their onset and course), the patient history is a valuable screening tool for identifying predisposing risk factors. The physical examination should include a thorough inspection of the vulva and vagina. A speculum examination, saline and KOH wet smears, and vaginal pH are performed. Vaginal pH is normal with VVC. If the pH is greater than 4.5, however, the clinician should suspect trichomoniasis or BV. The characteristic pseudohyphae may be seen on a wet smear done with normal saline, although they may sometimes be confused with other cells and artifacts. Pseudohyphae are best seen on the KOH wet smear (**Figures 20-2A, 20-2B, and 20-2C**). Diabetes screening should be considered for women with recurrent infections. Testing for chlamydia, gonorrhea, and HIV should be done if the patient history indicates the presence of risk factors for STIs (see Chapter 21). Vaginal cultures should be obtained in recurrent or resistant cases to confirm the diagnosis and identify unusual species, and with suspected candidiasis when the KOH prep is negative (CDC, 2010).

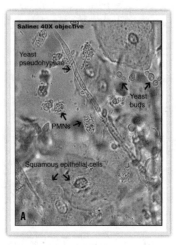 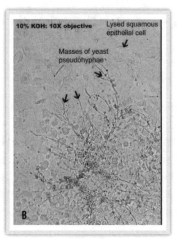 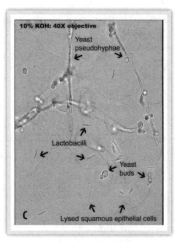

FIGURE 20-2 Wet mount findings with vulvovaginal candidiasis. PMNs = polymorphonuclear leukocytes/white blood cells.

Source: Used with permission from Washington State Department of Health STD/TB Program, Seattle STD/HIV Prevention Training Center, and Cindy Fennell, MS, MT, ASCP.

Differential Diagnosis

The differential diagnoses for VVC include BV, trichomoniasis, chemical vaginitis, contact vaginitis, chlamydia, gonorrhea, genital herpes, and normal physiologic discharge. Clinicians should also consider candidiasis secondary to diabetes, pregnancy, HIV seropositivity, and infection with non-*albicans* species such as *Candida glabrata* or *Candida tropicalis* (Hawkins et al., 2008).

Management

A number of antifungal preparations are available for the treatment of VVC (Table 20-2), and no single brand is significantly more effective than another. Women must be counseled that the creams and suppositories recommended for treatment of this condition are oil based; thus they may weaken latex condoms and diaphragms. Many of the effective topical azole drugs are available on an OTC basis. Self-treatment with OTC medications should be attempted only by women who have been previously diagnosed with VVC and who are experiencing the same symptoms. Any woman whose symptoms persist or who has a recurrence of symptoms within 2 months of treatment should be evaluated by a clinician (CDC, 2010). Unnecessary or inappropriate use of OTC preparations is common, and can lead to delays in treating other causes of vulvovaginitis.

If vaginal discharge is extremely thick and copious, vaginal debridement with a cotton swab followed by application of vaginal medication may be useful. Alternative therapies for VVC can be found in Table 20-3. Women who have extensive irritation, swelling, and discomfort of the labia and vulva may find sitz baths helpful in decreasing inflammation and increasing comfort. Adding colloidal oatmeal to the bath may also increase the woman's comfort.

Special Considerations

Pregnant Women Pregnant women who suspect they have candidiasis should be counseled not to self-treat their infection and to contact their clinician. Oral medication for VVC is not recommended in pregnancy. Only topical azole therapies, applied for 7 days, are recommended for use by pregnant women (CDC, 2010).

Talking with the Patient Bathing daily with lots of water and minimal soap may help prevent recurrent infections. Additional measures to minimize the moist environment of the vagina, which can help prevent recurrences, include not wearing underwear to bed, wearing loose-fitting slacks and jeans, wearing cotton-crotched underwear or pantyhose, and not sitting in wet bathing suits or clothing for long periods. Completing the full course of treatment prescribed is essential to removing the pathogen, and women should be instructed to continue applying the medication even during menstruation. Women should be counseled not to use tampons, as they will absorb the medication. If possible, intercourse should be avoided during treatment; if this is not feasible, the woman's partner should use a condom to prevent the introduction of more organisms. Women should be counseled to avoid feminine hygiene sprays, deodorants, scented tampons or pads, perfumed or colored toilet paper, and fabric softeners—all of which may cause irritation and allergies. Ingesting vitamin C (500 mg two to four times per day), oral acidophilous (40 million to 1 billion units daily), or live culture yogurt several times a week may also be helpful in preventing recurrences (Hawkins et al., 2008).

Toxic Shock Syndrome

Toxic shock syndrome (TSS) is "an acute, febrile illness produced by a bacterial exotoxin, with a fulminating downhill course involving dysfunction of multiple organ systems" (Eckert & Lentz, 2007, p. 596). This exotoxin is produced by certain strains of *Staphylococcus aureus*. Approximately half of TSS cases are related to menses, and TSS is more likely with use of higher-absorbency tampons, multiple days of tampon use, and leaving individual tampons in place for long periods (Eckert & Lentz). Symptoms, as shown in **Table 20-5**, include fever, rash, hypotension, myalgia, and vomiting (CDC, 2011).

Assessment

In addition to a careful history of the woman's symptoms, their onset, and the course of the infection, the history is a valuable screening tool for identifying predisposing risk factors such as menses with tampon use (usually within 5 days of onset of symptoms), history of

TABLE 20-5 CDC Case Definition for Toxic Shock Syndrome

Clinical Case Definition

An illness with the following clinical manifestations:
- Fever: temperature ≥ 102.0°F (38.9°C)
- Rash: diffuse macular erythroderma
- Desquamation: 1–2 weeks after onset of rash
- Hypotension: systolic blood pressure ≤ 90 mm Hg for adults or less than fifth percentile by age for children aged less than 16 years
- Multisystem involvement (three or more of the following organ systems):
  - Gastrointestinal: vomiting or diarrhea at onset of illness
  - Muscular: severe myalgia or creatine phosphokinase level at least twice the upper limit of normal
  - Mucous membrane: vaginal, oropharyngeal, or conjunctival hyperemia
  - Renal: blood urea nitrogen or creatinine at least twice the upper limit of normal for laboratory or urinary sediment with pyuria (≥ 5 leukocytes per high-power field) in the absence of urinary tract infection
  - Hepatic: total bilirubin, alanine aminotransferase enzyme, or asparate aminotransferase enzyme levels at least twice the upper limit of normal for laboratory
  - Hematologic: platelets < 100,000/mm^3
  - Central nervous system: disorientation or alterations in consciousness without focal neurologic signs when fever and hypotension are absent

Laboratory Criteria for Diagnosis

Negative results on the following tests, if obtained:
- Blood or cerebrospinal fluid cultures (blood culture may be positive for *Staphylococcus aureus*)
- Negative serologies for Rocky Mountain spotted fever, leptospirosis, or measles

Case Classification

Probable: A case that meets the laboratory criteria and in which four of the five clinical findings described above are present

Confirmed: A case that meets the laboratory criteria and in which all five of the clinical findings described above are present, including desquamation, unless the patient dies before desquamation occurs

Source: CDC, 2011.

TSS, and history of recent surgery, wound, or nasal packing (Shannon, 2004). Upon physical examination, dermatologic findings may differ depending on the stage of the illness. Early signs may include generalized erythematous and macular rash; generalized, nonpitting edema; and erythema of palms and soles. After the acute phase, findings may include generalized maculopapular rash and desquamation of fingers, palms, toes, and soles. Pelvic examination may reveal hyperemic vaginal mucosa and vulvar and vaginal tenderness (Eckert & Lentz, 2007). The diagnosis of TSS is made on the basis of clinical manifestations meeting the 2011 CDC case definition (Table 20-5).

Differential Diagnosis

Numerous conditions can cause fever and/or rash. Clinicians should consider TSS in any woman with unexplained fever and a rash during or immediately following menses (Eckert & Lentz, 2007).

Management

All women with a suspected case of TSS should be immediately referred to a physician. All menstruating women and others at risk for TSS should be educated about the signs and symptoms of TSS and ways to prevent its occurrence, such as using low-absorbency tampons, changing tampons frequently, alternating pad and tampon use, and removing barrier contraception within 24 hours. Women who have had TSS should be instructed not to use barrier contraceptive methods or tampons.

Bartholin's Cyst and Bartholin's Abscess

The Bartholin's glands are two mucous-secreting, nonpalpable glandular structures with duct openings within the posterolateral vulvar vestibule that provide minimal lubrication. Obstruction of a duct results in a nontender mass approximately 1 to 8 cm in size. Obstruction occurs from nonspecific inflammation or trauma. Continued fluid secretion after obstruction results in cyst formation (Eckert & Lentz, 2007). Abscess formation occurs when the cystic fluid becomes infected. Originally, it was thought that gonorrhea was the primary cause of Bartholin's abscess; however, it is now clear that most cases are not caused by STIs. Positive cultures for Bartholin's gland abscesses typically contain multiple bacteria, many of which are normal vaginal flora (Eckert & Lentz).

Most women with a Bartholin's cyst are asymptomatic. An abscess usually develops rapidly over 2 to 4 days, and most will spontaneously rupture within 3 to 4 days (Eckert & Lentz, 2007). Symptoms include varying amounts of pain or tenderness, difficulty sitting or walking, and dyspareunia. Extensive inflammation may cause systemic symptoms.

Assessment

A Bartholin's cyst (see **Color Plate 14**) may be an incidental finding during a routine pelvic examination. The cyst appears as a visible round or oval mass causing a crescent-shaped vestibular entrance. It is nontender but tense, and palpable swelling—usually unilateral and without erythema or inflammation—is apparent. A Bartholin's abscess (see **Color Plate 15**) is a very tender, edematous fluctuant mass with erythema of the overlying skin. Labial edema and distortion are observed on the affected area. The affected area is rarely larger than 5 cm in size. An area of softening or pointing suggests an impending rupture. Cultures of purulent abscess fluid and of the cervix for *N. gonorrhoeae* and *C. trachomatis* should be obtained to rule out a STI.

Differential Diagnosis

Differential diagnoses include cyst versus abscess, neoplasm, STI, mesonephric cyst of the vagina, and epithelial inclusion cyst (Eckert & Lentz, 2007).

Management

Small asymptomatic cysts do not require treatment. In contrast, treatment is indicated for a symptomatic cyst or abscess. The aim of treatment for a cyst or abscess is to create a fistulous tract from the dilated duct to the vestibule. Options include placement of a Word catheter, marsupialization, and incision and drainage (I&D). A Word catheter is a short catheter with a Foley balloon that is inflated after the catheter is inserted through an incision in the abscess. Marsupialization is a surgical procedure during which a pouch is formed for the gland to drain. Placement of a Word catheter for 4 to 6 weeks or marsupialization is preferable to incision and drainage (I&D), as recurrence can occur after I&D (Eckert & Lentz, 2007). Referral is indicated for marsupialization, recurrent cyst or abscess formation, and women older than 40 years of age to rule out neoplasm.

References

Allsworth, J. E., & Peipert, J. F. (2007). Prevalence of bacterial vaginosis: 2001–2004 National Health and Nutrition Examination Survey Data. *Obstetrics & Gynecology, 109*(1), 114–120.

Ayres, T. (2004). Sexual dysfunction. In W. Star, L. Lommel, & M. Shannon (Eds.), *Women's primary health care* (2nd ed., pp. 12-132–12-134). San Francisco: UCSF Nursing Press.

Balch, J. F., & Balch, P. A. (1997). *Prescription for prevention* (2nd ed.). Garden City Park, NY: Avery.

Centers for Disease Control and Prevention (CDC). (2010). Sexually transmitted diseases treatment guidelines 2010. *Morbidity and Mortality Weekly Report, 59*(RR-12), 1–110.

Centers for Disease Control and Prevention (CDC). (2011). *Toxic-shock syndrome (TSS): 1997 case definition.* Retrieved January 24, 2011, from http://www.cdc.gov/ncphi/disss/nndss/casedef/toxicsscurrent.htm

Eckert, L. O. (2006). Acute vulvovaginitis. *New England Journal of Medicine, 355*(12), 1244–1252.

Eckert, L. O., & Lentz, G. M. (2007). Infections of the lower genital tract: Vulva, vagina, cervix, toxic shock syndrome, HIV infections. In V. L. Katz, G. M. Lentz, R. A. Lobo, & D. M. Gershenson (Eds.), *Comprehensive gynecology* (5th ed., 569–606). St. Louis, MO: Mosby.

Hatcher, R. A., Trussell, J., Nelson, A. L., Cates, W., Stewart, F., & Kowal, D. (2007). *Contraceptive technology* (19th ed.). New York: Ardent Media.

Hawkins, J. W., Roberto-Nichols, D. M., & Stanley-Haney, J. L. (2008). *Guidelines for nurse practitioners in gynecologic settings* (9th ed.). New York: Springer.

Hudson, T. (1999). *Women's encyclopedia of natural medicine.* Los Angeles: Keats.

Koumans, E. H., Markowitz, L. E., & Hogan, V. (2002). Indications for therapy and treatment recommendations for bacterial vaginosis in nonpregnant and pregnant women: A synthesis of data. *Clinical Infectious Diseases, 35*, S152–S172.

Low Dog, T. (2004). *Women's health in complementary and alternative medicine.* St. Louis, MO: Elsevier.

Marrazzo, J. M., Martin, D. H., Watts, D. H., Schulte, J., Sobel, J. D., Hillier, S. L., et al. (2010). Bacterial vaginosis: Identifying research gaps, proceedings of a workshop sponsored by DHHS/NIH/NIAD. *Sexually Transmitted Diseases, 37*(12), 732–744.

Schaffer, S. D. (2003). Vaginitis and sexually transmitted diseases. In E. Q. Youngkin & M. S. Davis (Eds.), *Women's health: A primary care clinical guide* (3rd ed., pp. 261–290). Upper Saddle River, NJ: Pearson Prentice Hall.

Scharbo-DeHaan, M., & Anderson, D. G. (2003). The CDC 2002 guidelines for the treatment of sexually transmitted diseases: Implications for women's health care. *Journal of Midwifery & Women's Health, 48*, 96–104.

Shaley, E., Battino, S., Weiner, E., Colodner, R., & Keness, Y. (1996). Ingestion of yogurt containing *Lactobacillus* acidosis compared with pasteurized yogurt as prophylaxis for recurrent candidal vaginitis and bacterial vaginosis. *Archives of Family Medicine, 5*, 593–596.

Shannon, M. (2004). Toxic shock syndrome. In W. Star, L. Lommel, & M. Shannon (Eds.), *Women's primary health care* (2nd ed., pp. 12-147–12-150). San Francisco: UCSF Nursing Press.

Sinclair, C. (2004). *A midwife's handbook.* St. Louis, MO: Saunders.

Taha, T. E., Hoover, D. R., & Dallabetta, G. A. (1998). Bacterial vaginosis and disturbances of vaginal flora: Association with increased acquisition of HIV. *AIDS, 12*, 1699–1706.

CHAPTER

21

Sexually Transmitted Infections

Catherine Ingram Fogel

Despite more than 30 years of the U.S. Surgeon General targeting sexually transmitted infections (STIs) as a priority for prevention and control efforts (Public Health Service, 1979), these infections continue to be among the most common health problems in the United States today. Approximately 19 million new STIs occur in the United States every year (Centers for Disease Control and Prevention [CDC], 2010d). At least 50% of Americans will contract one or more STIs during their lifetime (CDC, 2010a). STIs are a direct cause of tremendous human suffering, place heavy demands on healthcare services, and cost the U.S. healthcare system as much as $16.4 billion each year (CDC, 2010d; Institute of Medicine, 1997).

An STI is not any one specific disease; rather, this term refers to "a variety of clinical syndromes caused by pathogens that can be acquired and transmitted through sexual activity" (CDC, 2010e). Common STIs are listed in **Table 21-1**. These terms have replaced the older designation of venereal disease, which primarily described gonorrhea and syphilis. STIs may be caused by a wide spectrum of bacteria, viruses, protozoa, and ectoparasites (organisms that live on the outside of the body, such as a louse). Historically, many STIs were considered to be symptomatic illnesses usually afflicting men; however, women and children can have more severe symptoms and sequelae from these infections than men.

Preventing, identifying, and managing STIs are essential components of women's health care. Clinicians can assume an essential role in promoting women's reproductive and sexual health by counseling women about the risks of STIs, including human immunodeficiency virus (HIV); encouraging sexual and other risk-reduction measures; and being familiar with assessment and management strategies related to STIs. In doing so, clinicians can assist women in avoiding STIs and in living better with the sequelae and chronic infections of STIs.

TABLE 21-1 Common Sexually Transmitted Infections

Infection	Causative Organism
Chancroid	*Haemophilus ducreyi*
Chlamydia	*Chlamydia trachomatis*
Genital herpes	Herpes simplex virus
Genital warts	Human papillomavirus (HPV)
Gonorrhea	*Neisseria gonorrhoeae*
Hepatitis	Hepatitis B virus (HBV), hepatitis C virus (HCV)
HIV infection and acquired immunodeficiency syndrome (AIDS)	Human immunodeficiency virus (HIV)
Molluscum contagiosum	Molluscum contagiosum virus
Pubic lice	*Phthirus pubis*
Syphilis	*Treponema pallidum*
Trichomoniasis	*Trichomonas vaginalis*

This chapter begins with an overview of STI transmission, screening, and detection. Topics that need to be addressed when talking with a woman who has been diagnosed with an STI are presented as well. The remaining sections address specific STIs, including human papillomavirus, genital herpes, chancroid, pediculosis pubis, trichomoniasis, chlamydia, gonorrhea, pelvic inflammatory disease (PID), syphilis, hepatitis B virus (HBV), and HIV infection.

Transmission of Sexually Transmitted Infections

The chance of contracting, transmitting, or suffering complications from STIs depends on multiple biologic, behavioral, social, and relationship risk factors (**Table 21-2**). That is, microbiologic, hormonal, and immunologic factors influence individual susceptibility and transmission potential for STIs. These factors are partially influenced by a woman's sexual practices, substance use, and other health behaviors. Health behaviors, in turn, are influenced by socioeconomic factors and other social influences.

Biologic Factors

Women are biologically more likely to become infected with STIs than men. For example, the risk of a woman contracting gonorrhea from a single act of intercourse is 60% to 90%, whereas the corresponding risk for a man is 20% to 30%. Men are two to three times more likely to transmit HIV to women than the reverse. This difference arises because the vagina

TABLE 21-2 Risk Factors for STIs and HIV

Previous or current STI
Sex with multiple or new partners
Initiating sex at a young age
Unprotected sex
Sex with high-risk partners
Sex with an HIV-infected partner
Sex in exchange for money or drugs
Sex while intoxicated
Illicit drug use
Injection drug use
Mental illness
Age younger than 25 years
Living in an area with high STI/HIV prevalence
Residing in a detention or correctional facility

Source: CDC, 2010e.

has a larger amount of genital mucous membranes exposed and is an environment more conducive for infections than the penis (Cates, Alexander, & Cates, 1998). Further, risk for trauma is greater during vaginal intercourse for women than for men (Kurth, 1998).

STIs are frequently asymptomatic in women and, therefore, are more likely to go undetected than the same diseases in men. Additionally, when or if symptoms develop, they are often confused with those of other diseases not transmitted sexually. This relative frequency of asymptomatic and unrecognized infections in women results in delayed diagnosis and treatment, chronic untreated infections, and complications. Further, it can be more difficult to diagnose STIs in a woman because the anatomy of her genital tract makes clinical examination more difficult. Lesions that occur inside the vagina and on the cervix are not readily visible, and the normal vaginal environment (a warm, moist, enriched medium) is ideal for nurturing an infection.

The prevalence rates of many STIs are highest among adolescents, whose lack of immunity and biologic susceptibility are contributing factors to their vulnerability to such infections. Seventy percent of all adolescent girls have had vaginal sex by the age of 19 years, with the end result being many young women at risk for STIs (Alan Guttmacher Institute, 2011). The earlier a woman begins to have sexual intercourse, the longer her period of sexual activity is, the greater her number of partners, and the less apt she is to use barrier contraception (Schmid, 2001). Compared to older women prior to menopause, female adolescents and young women are more susceptible to cervical infections, such as chlamydial infections, gonorrhea, and HIV, because of the ectropion of the immature cervix and resulting larger exposed surface area of cells unprotected by cervical mucus. These cells eventually recede into the inner cervix as women age. Women who are postmenopausal also are at increased risk because of the thin vaginal and cervical mucosa that occurs as estrogen levels decline. Further, women who are pregnant have higher rates of cervical ectropion (Cunningham et al., 2010).

Other biologic factors that may increase a woman's risk of acquiring, transmitting, or developing complications of certain STIs include vaginal douching, risky sexual practices, use of hormonal contraceptives, and bacterial vaginosis. Risk for contracting the infections that can lead to PID may be increased with vaginal douching, and risk for PID may also increase with greater frequency of douching (CDC, 2010e). Certain sexual practices—for example, anal intercourse, sex during menses, and vaginal intercourse without sufficient lubrication (dry sex)—may also predispose a woman to acquiring an STI; the bleeding and tissue trauma that can result from these practices facilitates invasion by pathogens. The role of oral contraceptives in the acquisition and transmission of STIs is not fully understood, however. Studies have found combined oral contraceptives to be associated with a decreased risk of developing PID but an increased risk of chlamydial infection (Morrison, Turner, & Jones, 2009; Nelson, 2007). Combined oral contraceptives do not increase the risk of HIV infection (Morrison et al.). Bacterial vaginosis is associated with multiple STIs and increases the risk for HIV and genital herpes acquisition (Atashili, Poole, Ndumbe, Adimora, & Smith, 2008; Cherpes, Meyn, Krohn, Lurie, & Hillier, 2003).

Social Factors

Preventing the spread of STIs, including HIV, is difficult without addressing community and individual issues that have a tremendous influence on prevention, transmission, and treatment of these infections. Societal factors such as poverty, lack of education, social inequity, and inadequate access to health care indirectly increase the prevalence of STIs in at-risk populations. Persons with the highest rates of many STIs are often those with the least access to health care, and health insurance coverage influences whether and where a woman obtains STI care services and preventive services. Further, even if a woman of lower socioeconomic status perceives herself to be at risk for an STI, she may not practice protective behaviors if survival is an overarching concern or if other risks appear to be more threatening or imminent (Mays & Cochran, 1988). The need to secure shelter, food, clothing, money, and safety for herself and her children may override any concerns about preventive health measures and, therefore, discourage her from changing risky behaviors (Nyamanthi & Lewis, 1991).

Social Interactions and Relationships

STIs are the only illnesses whose spread is directly caused by the human urge to share sexual intimacy and reproduce. Sexual behavior within the context of relationships is a critical risk factor for preventing and acquiring STIs, because intimate human contact is the common vehicle of transmission. Notably, the gender-power imbalance and cultural proscriptions often associated with sexual relationships can make it difficult for women to protect themselves from infection (Miller, Exner, Williams, & Ehrhardt, 2000; Mize, Robinson, Bockting, & Scheltma, 2002). Women may perceive that they have less say than men over when and under which circumstances intercourse occurs. Young women are particularly at risk in this context, as they may lack the negotiating skills, self-efficacy, and self-confidence needed to successfully negotiate for safer sex practices. Premarital and extramarital sexual activity are common practices among many women, yet because of the secrecy and cultural proscriptions surrounding such activities, women may engage in them without preparation, leading to risk for themselves and their partners.

Some women may be dependent upon an abusive male partner or a partner who places a woman at risk through his own risky behaviors (Kurth, 1998). The risk of acquiring STIs is high among women who are physically and sexually abused. Past and current experiences with violence, particularly sexual abuse, erode women's sense of self-efficacy to exercise control over sexual behaviors, engender feelings of anxiety and depression, and increase the likelihood of risky sexual behaviors (Maman, 2000). Additionally, fear of physical harm and loss of economic support may hamper women's efforts to enact protective practices. Further, past and current abuse is strongly associated with substance abuse, which also increases the risk of contracting an STI.

Risk of acquiring an STI is determined not only by the woman's actions but also by her partner's behaviors. Although prevention counseling customarily includes recommending that women identify any partner who is at high risk and the nature of their sexual practices, this advice may be unrealistic or culturally inappropriate in many relationships because of use of drugs and the presence of other medical factors. Women who engage in sexual activities only with other women may also be at risk for infection. Many women who identify themselves as lesbians have had intercourse with a man by choice, by force, or by necessity. Their female partners may also have other STI risk factors, such as injection-drug use.

Societal Norms

Relationships and sexual behavior are regulated by cultural norms that influence sexual expression in interpersonal relationships. Women are often socialized to please their partners and to place men's needs and desires first; as a consequence, they may find it difficult to insist on safer sex behaviors. Traditional cultural values associated with passivity and subordination may diminish the ability of many women to adequately protect themselves.

Power imbalances in relationships are the product of, and contribute to, the maintenance of traditional gender roles that identify men as the initiators and decision makers of sexual activities and women as passive gatekeepers (Miller et al., 2000). As long as traditional gender norms define the roles in sexual relationships as men having the dominant role in sexual decision making, women will find it difficult to negotiate with their partners about condom use. Additionally, cultural norms define talking about condoms as implying a lack of trust that runs counter to the traditional gender norm expectations for women (Maman, 2000). Women often do not request condom use because of a need to establish and maintain intimacy with partners. Urging women to insist on condom use may be unrealistic if their cultural norm includes traditional gender roles that do not encourage women to talk about sex, initiate sexual practices, or control intimate encounters.

Substance Use

The use of alcohol and drugs is associated with increased risk of HIV and STIs. For example, in many areas trends in crack use have paralleled trends in syphilis, gonorrhea, chancroid, and HIV infection incidence. This association may arise for several reasons, including social factors such as poverty and lack of educational or economic opportunities, and individual factors such as high risk-taking propensity and low self-esteem. In addition to the risk from needle sharing, use of drugs and alcohol may contribute to risk of HIV infection by undermining cognitive and social skills, thus making it more difficult for users to engage in HIV-protective actions (Harris & Kavanagh, 1995). Further, depression and other psychological problems as well as history of sexual abuse are associated with substance abuse and, therefore, contribute to risky behaviors. Being high and unable to clean drug paraphernalia can be a pervasive barrier to protective practice. Further, drug use may take place in settings where persons participate in sexual activities while using drugs. Finally, women who use drugs may be at higher risk if they exchange sex for drugs or money, and if they have higher numbers of sexual partners and encounters (Dolcini, Coates, Catania, Kegeles, & Hauck, 1995).

Past and current physical, emotional, and sexual abuse characterize the lives of many, if not most, women using drugs (Kearney, 2001; McFarlane, Parker, & Cross, 2001). For women who have experienced violence, use of alcohol and drugs can evolve into a coping mechanism by which they self-medicate to relieve feelings of anxiety, guilt, fear, and anger stemming from the violence (Grella, Anglin, & Annon, 1996). Women's drug use is strongly linked to relationship inequities and the ability of some men to mandate women's sexual behavior.

STI Screening and Detection

Prompt diagnosis and treatment are predicated on the assumption that any person who believes he or she may have contracted an STI, has symptoms of an STI, has had sexual relations with someone who has symptoms of an STI, or has a partner who has been diagnosed with an STI will seek care. To obtain prompt diagnosis and treatment, patients must know how to recognize the major signs and symptoms of all STIs and must be willing and able to obtain health care if they experience symptoms or have sexual contact with someone who has an STI. Clinicians have the responsibility of educating their patients regarding the signs and symptoms of STIs. This may be done when a woman comes in for her annual health examination, seeks contraception, or obtains preconception or prenatal care. Clinicians also must ensure that patients know where and how to obtain care if they suspect they might have contracted an STI. Many local health departments have clinics specifically designed to treat STIs, with services often available for free or at a reduced cost.

Screening

All women who are sexually active should be screened regularly through history, physical examination, and laboratory studies. To identify those at risk, specific questions should be asked during the collection of a health history (**Table 21-3** and **Table 21-4**). Risk assessment depends on a woman's willingness to self-identify risk factors that may be seen as socially unacceptable or stigmatizing. Some women may not reveal such risk factors directly to clinicians, but are willing to do so if asked to fill out a questionnaire using questions similar to those given in the Sexual Risk History (Table 21-3). Screening for specific infections is discussed in the sections later in this chapter that address individual infections. Any woman who has been diagnosed with an STI should be screened for other STIs, because comorbidity of such infections is high and many STIs can be asymptomatic.

TABLE 21-3 Sexual Risk History

Are you sexually active? Have you had sex/intercourse with anyone in the past 6 months/year?
- If no, have you had intercourse in the past?
- If yes, have your partners been men, women, or both?
  - How many people have you had sex with in the past 6 months/year?
  - How many different people are you having sex with right now?
  - Does your partner have any other partners that you know of?

Have you ever had sex with someone who had been in jail?

Have you ever had sex with someone who has had a blood transfusion or hemophilia?

Have you ever had sex with someone whom you were afraid put you at risk for HIV/STI?
- Someone who had a positive HIV test?
- Someone you think might have HIV/AIDS?
- Someone who uses drugs? IV drugs? Cocaine?
- Someone who might have had sex with a prostitute or with both men and women?

Have you ever been told that you had an STI?
- Never
- Chlamydia
- Gonorrhea
- Trichomoniasis
- Syphilis
- Other (list)

Have you ever been told that you had a pelvic infection or PID?

Many women have sex when they have drunk too much alcohol or have been using drugs. Has this happened to you?

What kinds of drugs do you use?
- Opioids: Types, route of administration, and frequency?
- Stimulants: Types, route of administration, and frequency?
- Crack cocaine: Frequency? Have you had sex in a crack house?
- Alcohol: Types and frequency?

Have you ever blacked out from alcohol or drugs, especially during sex?

Have you ever traded sex for drugs, money, food, housing, or anything else?

Do you ever have sex when you are high?

Can you tell me the kinds of sex that you have? This will help determine what your risks are.
- Mouth on penis or vulva: Protected, unprotected, or none?
- Penis in vagina: Protected, unprotected, or none?
- Penis in the rectum: Protected, unprotected, or none?
- Mouth on anus: Protected, unprotected, or none?

(continues)

TABLE 21-3 Sexual Risk History *(Continued)*

For every sexually active woman, ask:

- Are you worried about catching a sexually transmitted infection or HIV (the AIDS virus)?
- Do you do anything to prevent catching an infection?
- Have you had sex without a condom?
- When did you start using condoms?
- Have you performed oral sex on a man or woman without a barrier (dental dam, plastic wrap, condom)?

Sources: Adapted from Brown, 2004; Carcio, 1999; Fogel, 1995; Fogel & Lauver, 1990; Kurth, 1998; MacLauren, 1995; Starr, Lommel, & Shannon, 2004.

TABLE 21-4 Menstrual/Gynecologic History Questions to Assess Risk of STIs

Do you experience now or have you ever experienced:

Frequent vaginal infections

Unusual vaginal discharge/odor

Vaginal itching/burning/sores/warts

Sexually transmitted infections (ask about individual infections)

Abdominal pain

Pelvic inflammatory disease/infection of the uterus, tubes, ovaries

Rape

Physical, emotional, sexual abuse

Abnormal Pap test

Pain/bleeding with intercourse

Severe menstrual cramps occurring at end of period

Ectopic pregnancy

Assessment

The diagnosis of an STI is based on the integration of relevant history, physical, and laboratory data.

A history that is accurate, comprehensive, and specific is essential for accurate diagnosis. Generally the history should be taken first, with the woman dressed. Information should be collected in a nonjudgmental manner, avoiding assumptions of sexual preference. All partners should be referred to as "partners," rather than by gender. It is helpful to begin with open-ended questions because they often elicit information that might otherwise be missed. These queries can be followed with symptom-specific questions and relevant history. Specific areas to address include the reason why the woman has sought care and any symptoms she has noticed; a sexual history, including a description of the date and type of sexual activity; number of partners; whether she has had contact with someone who recently had an STI; and potential sites of infection (e.g., mouth, cervix, urethra, and rectum). Pertinent medical history includes anything that will influence the management plan, such as history of drug allergies, previously diagnosed chronic illnesses, and general health status. A menstrual history, including the date of the woman's last menstrual period, must always be obtained so that pregnancy may be ruled out—certain medications used to treat STIs are contraindicated in pregnancy. When indicated, an HIV-oriented systems review should be conducted. Any positive answers regarding symptoms should be followed up to elicit information about onset, duration, and specific characteristics, such as color, amount, and consistency of discharge.

Before the actual physical examination is performed, the clinician should discuss the procedure to be followed with the woman so that she is prepared. The physical examination begins with careful visualization of the external genitalia, including the perineum. Erythema, edema, distortions, lesions, trauma, and any other abnormalities are noted. Palpation can locate areas of tenderness. During the speculum examination, the vagina and cervix are inspected for edema, thinning, lesions, abnormal coloration, trauma, discharge, and bleeding. Thorough palpation of inguinal area and pelvic organs, milking of the urethra for discharge, and assessment of vaginal secretion odors are essential.

Appropriate laboratory studies will be suggested, in part, by the history and physical examination results. Additional laboratory studies may be performed in female patients because women are often infected with more than one STI simultaneously and because many are asymptomatic. These tests include microscopic examination of vaginal secretions (wet mount), chlamydia and gonorrhea testing, Venereal Disease Research Laboratory (VDRL) or rapid plasma reagin (RPR) testing for syphilis, and a hepatitis B panel. When an STI is diagnosed, testing for other STIs is essential. The woman should be notified that HIV testing will be performed unless she specifically declines such testing (see the section on HIV testing later in this chapter). Other laboratory tests, such as a complete blood count, urinalysis, or urine culture and sensitivity, should be obtained if indicated. Further, if the history or physical examination indicates pregnancy is possible, a urine human chorionic gonadotropin (hCG) test should be performed.

Reporting

Accurate identification and timely reporting of STIs are integral components of successful infection control efforts. Clinicians are required to report certain STIs to the state public health officials, who in turn report these infection rates to the CDC. Nationally notifiable

STIs include chancroid, chlamydia, gonorrhea, hepatitis, HIV, and syphilis (CDC, 2011f). The requirements for reporting other STIs differ from state to state. Additionally, individuals with STIs should be asked to identify and notify all partners who might have been exposed to the infection. Clinicians are legally responsible for reporting all cases of those infections identified as reportable and should know the requirements of the state in which they practice. The patient must be informed when a case will be reported and told why. Failure to inform the patient that the case will be reported is considered a serious breach of professional ethics.

Confidentiality is a crucial issue for many patients. When an STI is reportable, women need to be told they may be contacted by a health department representative. They should be assured that the information reported to and collected by health authorities is maintained in strictest confidence. Reports are protected by statute from subpoena in most jurisdictions. Every effort, within the limits of one's public health responsibilities, should be made to reassure patients.

Talking with the Patient

Patient counseling is an essential part of caring for a patient with an STI (**Table 21-5** and **Table 21-6**). The woman with an STI will need support in seeking care at the earliest possible stage of symptoms. Counseling women about STIs is essential for the following reasons:

- Preventing new infections or reinfection
- Increasing compliance with treatment and follow-up
- Providing support during treatment
- Assisting patients in discussions with their partners

Women must be made aware of the serious potential consequences of STIs and the behaviors that increase their likelihood of infection.

The clinician must make sure that the woman understands which infection she has, how it is transmitted, and why it must be treated. Women should be given a brief description of the infection in language they can understand. This description should include modes of transmission, incubation period, symptoms, infectious period, and potential complications.

Effective treatment of STIs necessitates a careful, thorough explanation of the treatment regimen and follow-up procedures. Comprehensive and precise instructions about medications must be provided, both verbally and in writing. Side effects, benefits, and risks of medications should be discussed. Unpleasant side effects or early relief of symptoms may sometimes discourage women from completing their medication course. All patients should be strongly urged to continue taking their medication until the full regimen is finished, regardless of whether their symptoms diminish or disappear in a few days. Comfort measures that decrease symptoms such as pain, itching, or nausea should be suggested. Providing written information is a useful strategy because this is a time of high anxiety for many women, and they may not be able to hear or remember what they were told. A number of booklets

---

TABLE 21-5 Patient Information

The only certain way to prevent STIs is to avoid sexual contact with others. If you choose to be sexually active, there are things you can do to decrease your risk of developing an STI:

- Have sex with only one person who doesn't have sex with anyone else and who has no infections.
- Always use a condom and use it correctly.
- Use clean needles if you inject any drugs.
- Prevent and control other STIs to decease your susceptibility to HIV infection and to reduce your infectiousness if you are HIV positive.
- Wait to have sex for as long as possible. The younger you are when you have sex for the first time, the more likely you are to catch an STI. The risk of acquiring an STI also increases with the number of partners you have over a lifetime.

Anyone who is sexually active should do the following:

- Always use protection unless you are having sex with only one person who doesn't have sex with anyone else and who has no infections.
- Have regular checkups for STIs even if you have no symptoms and especially when having sex with a new partner.
- Learn the common symptoms of STIs. Seek health care immediately if any suspicious symptoms develop, even if they are mild.
- Avoid having sex during menstruation. Women with HIV are probably more infectious, and women without HIV are probably more susceptible to becoming infected during that time.
- Avoid anal intercourse, but if practiced, use a condom.
- Avoid douching. It removes some of the normal protective bacteria in the vagina and increases the risk of getting some STIs.

Anyone diagnosed as having an STI should do the following:

- Be treated to reduce the risk of transmitting an STI to another person.
- Notify all recent sex partners and urge them to get a checkup as soon as possible to decrease the risk of catching the infection again from them.
- Follow the clinician's recommendations and complete the full course of medication prescribed. Have a follow-up test if necessary.
- Avoid all sexual activity while being treated.

---

on STIs are available, or the clinician may wish to develop literature specific to the practice setting and patient population.

In general, women will be advised to refrain from intercourse until all treatment is finished. After treatment, women should be urged to continue using condoms to prevent recurring infections, especially if they have had PID or continue to have intercourse with new partners. Women may wish to avoid having sex with partners who have many other sexual partners. All women who have contracted an STI should be taught safer sex practices, if this education has not been provided already. Follow-up appointments should be made as needed.

TABLE 21-6 Sexual Risk Practices

Safest	Low Risk	Possibly Risky (Possible Exposure)	High Risk (Unsafe)
Behavior	*Behavior*	*Behavior*	*Behavior*
Abstinence	Wet kissing	Cunnilingus	Unprotected anal intercourse
Self-masturbation	Vaginal intercourse with condom	Fellatio	Unprotected vaginal intercourse
Monogamous (both partners and no high risk activities)	Anal intercourse with condom	Mutual masturbation with skin breaks	Oral–anal contact
Hugging*, massage*, touching*	Fellatio interruptus	Vaginal intercourse after anal contact without new condom	Fisting
Dry kissing	Urine contact with intact skin		Multiple sexual partners
Mutual masturbation		*Prevention*	Sharing sex toys, douche equipment
Drug abstinence	*Prevention*	Dental dam or female condom with cunnilingus	Sharing needles
	Avoid exposure to potentially infected body fluids	Use condom with fellatio	
Prevention			*Prevention*
Avoid high risk behaviors	Consistently use condom & spermicide	Use latex gloves	Avoid exposure to potentially infected body fluids
	Avoid anal intercourse		Consistently use condom & spermicide
			Avoid anal penetration
			If having anal penetration, use condom with intercourse, latex glove with hand penetration
			Avoid oral–anal contact
			Do not share sex toys, needles, douching equipment
			If sharing needles, clean with bleach before and after use

*Assumes no breaks in skin.
Sources: Adapted from Fogel, 1995; Star, 2004.

Addressing the psychosocial component of STIs is essential. Be aware that a woman may be afraid or embarrassed to tell her partner and ask him or her to seek treatment, or she may be concerned about confidentiality. The effect of a diagnosis of an STI on a committed relationship for the woman, who is now faced with the necessity of dealing with uncertain monogamy, can be significant. In other instances, the woman may be afraid that telling her partner about the STI may place her in danger of escalating abuse. The potential consequences of talking with her partner must be discussed with each patient.

In most situations involving STIs, sexual partners should be examined; thus the woman is asked to identify and notify all partners who might have been exposed (partner notification). Often, she will find this step difficult to do. Empathizing with the woman's feelings and suggesting specific ways of talking with partners will help decrease her anxiety and assist in efforts to control infection. For example, the clinician might suggest that the woman say, "I care about you and I'm concerned about you. That's why I'm calling to tell you that I have a sexually transmitted infection. My clinician is _____ and she will be happy to talk with you if you would like." Offering literature and role-playing situations with the woman may also be of assistance. It is often helpful to remind the woman that, although this may be a potentially embarrassing situation, most persons would rather know than not know they have been exposed to an STI. Clinicians who take the time to counsel their patients on how to talk with their partners can improve compliance and case finding.

In situations when patient referral may not be effective or possible, health departments should be prepared to assist the woman—through either contact referral or clinician referral. Contact referral is the process by which a woman agrees to notify her partners by a certain time. If her partners do not obtain medical evaluation and treatment within the given time period, then clinician referral is implemented. Clinician referral is the process by which partners named by identified patients are notified and counseled by health department clinicians (CDC, 2010e).

Human Papillomavirus and Genital Warts

Human papillomavirus (HPV) infection is now the most common STI in the United States (CDC, 2010a). Its exact incidence is not known, because clinicians are not required to report these cases. However, it is estimated that as many as 6 million people become newly infected with HPV each year, and at least 50% of sexually active men and women will have HPV at some point in their lives (CDC).

HPVs are a group of double-stranded DNA viruses with more than 100 known serotypes, of which more than 40 can infect the genital tract, including the external genitalia, vagina, urethra, and anus (American College of Obstetricians and Gynecologists, 2005, reaffirmed 2009). Most HPV infections are asymptomatic, subclinical, or unrecognized, and many HPV infections clear spontaneously. More seriously, HPV can cause genital warts and cervical cancer. Most (90%) genital warts are caused by HPV types 6 and 11, which carry a low risk for triggering invasive cancer. Some other types (i.e., 16, 18, 31, 33, and 35) that are occasionally found in genital warts are associated with cervical intraepithelial neoplasia (CDC, 2010e). Two high-risk HPV types, 16 and 18, cause 70% of cervical cancers (Munoz et al., 2003).

Although the period of communicability is unknown, as many as 75% of all persons exposed to genital warts, also known as condylomata acuminata or condyloma, will subsequently develop them (American College of Obstetricians and Gynecologists, 2005, reaffirmed 2009). Genital warts in women are most frequently seen in the posterior part of the introitus; however, lesions can also be found on the buttocks, vulva, vagina, anus, and cervix. Typically the lesions present as small (2 to 3 mm in length, 10 to 15 mm in height), soft, papillary swellings occurring singularly or in clusters on the genital and anal–rectal region (**Color Plate 17**). Warts are usually flesh colored or slightly darker on Caucasian women, black on African American women, and brownish on Asian women. Infections of long duration may appear as a cauliflower-like mass. In moist areas such as the vaginal introitus, the lesions may appear to have multiple, fine, fingerlike projections. Vaginal lesions often appear as multiple warts. Flat-topped papules, 1 to 4 mm in diameter, are sometimes seen on the cervix; often these lesions are visualized only under magnification. Although they are usually painless, the lesions may sometimes be uncomfortable, particularly when very large, inflamed, or ulcerated. Chronic vaginal discharge, pruritus, or dyspareunia can occur as well.

Assessment

A woman with HPV lesions may have symptoms such as a profuse, irritating vaginal discharge, itching, dyspareunia, or postcoital bleeding. She may also report "bumps" on her vulva or labia. History of known exposure is important because of the potentially long latency period for HPV infection and the possibility of subclinical infections in men. Nevertheless, the lack of a history of known exposure cannot be used to exclude a diagnosis of HPV infection.

Physical inspection of the vulva, perineum, anus, vagina, and cervix is essential whenever HPV lesions are suspected or seen. Speculum examination of the vagina may block some lesions; thus it is important to rotate the speculum blades until all areas are visualized. When lesions are visible, the characteristic appearance previously described is considered diagnostic. In many instances, however, cervical lesions are not visible; moreover, some vaginal or vulvar lesions may be unobservable to the naked eye. Gloves should be changed between vaginal and rectal examinations to prevent the potential spread of vulvar or vaginal lesions to the anus. Diagnosis is made by careful, thorough clinical examination of visible genital warts or by biopsy of cervical lesions and (rarely) of lesions at other sites if the diagnosis is not clear. Perform testing for other STIs when genital warts are present.

Women with genital warts should have cervical cancer screening according to the standard recommendations (see Chapter 8); more frequent screening is not recommended (CDC, 2010e). HPV DNA testing should be performed only for women aged 21 years and older with a Pap test result of atypical squamous cells of undetermined significance (ASC-US) or for women aged 30 years and older in conjunction with Pap testing for cervical cancer screening. HPV DNA testing is inappropriate for STI screening, adolescents (women 20 years and younger), abnormal Pap results other than ASC-US (e.g., atypical squamous cells cannot rule out a high-grade lesion [ASC-H], low-grade squamous intraepithelial lesion [LSIL], and high-grade squamous intraepithelial lesion [HSIL]), routine screening in women younger than age 30, and women considering vaccination against HPV (American Society for Colposcopy and Cervical Pathology, 2009).

Differential Diagnoses

HPV lesions must be differentiated from molluscum contagiosum, condylomata lata, and carcinoma. Molluscum contagiosum lesions are half-domed, smooth, and flesh-colored to pearly white papules with depressed centers. Condylomata lata are a form of secondary syphilis and generally are flatter and wider than genital warts. Cancers to be ruled out include squamous cell carcinoma, carcinoma in situ, and malignant melanoma. An extensive list of other differential diagnoses for vulvar lesions can be found in Chapter 27.

Prevention

The most clinically significant HPV types can now be prevented with vaccination. Both the bivalent vaccine (HPV2, Cervarix) and the quadrivalent vaccine (HPV4, Gardasil) protect against HPV types 16 and 18, which cause the majority of cervical cancers. In addition, the quadrivalent vaccine prevents HPV types 6 and 11, which cause the majority of genital warts, and it provides some protection against vulvar and vaginal cancers and precancers (CDC, 2010b, 2010e).

Routine HPV vaccination is recommended for girls aged 11 to 12 years. HPV vaccines can be given to girls as young as age 9 and are also recommended for adolescents and women aged 13 to 26 years who were not vaccinated or did not complete the series earlier. Ideally, vaccination should occur before the adolescent or woman becomes sexually active and, therefore, has the potential for HPV exposure. Vaccination is recommended for women who have evidence of existing HPV infection, such as Pap test abnormalities or genital warts, to provide protection against HPV types that have not yet been acquired. Vaccination will not treat existing HPV infection, cervical cytologic abnormalities, or genital warts (American College of Obstetricians and Gynecologists, 2010b; CDC, 2010b).

Both vaccines are given in a series of three intramuscular injections. The second dose is given 1 to 2 months (and at least 4 weeks) after the first dose. The third dose is given 6 months (and at least 12 weeks) after the second dose. The series does not need to be restarted if the second and third doses are delayed. When possible, the same vaccine (bivalent or quadrivalent) should be given for all three doses. HPV testing prior to vaccination is not recommended (CDC, 2010b).

The HPV vaccines are not recommended during pregnancy but can be given during lactation. Routine pregnancy testing prior to vaccination is not recommended. If a woman is found to be pregnant after the vaccine is given, the remaining vaccines in the series should be delayed until after she gives birth, and the clinician should report the exposure to the vaccine manufacturer (Merck at 800-986-8999 for the quadrivalent vaccine and GlaxoSmithKline at 888-452-9622 for the bivalent vaccine). No intervention is needed. Both vaccines are contraindicated for women with hypersensitivity to any vaccine component. The quadrivalent vaccine is also contraindicated for women with yeast hypersensitivity. Women with anaphylactic latex allergy who are receiving the bivalent vaccine should be given the vaccine from a single-dose vial rather than using a prefilled syringe, as the latter contains latex (CDC, 2010b).

Management

The primary goals of treatment of visible genital warts are removal or reduction of warts and relief of signs and symptoms—not the eradication of HPV. If left untreated, genital warts may resolve, remain unchanged, or increase in size and number (CDC, 2010e). Treatment of genital warts can be difficult. The patient often must make multiple office visits if clinician-administered regimens are used, and recurrence is common.

Treatment of genital warts should be guided by preference of the woman, available resources, and experience of the clinician. None of the treatments is superior to any of the others, and no one treatment is ideal for all women or all warts (CDC, 2010e). Available treatments are outlined in **Table 21-7**. Any concurrent vaginal infections or STIs should also be treated.

Women who are experiencing discomfort associated with genital warts may find that bathing with an oatmeal solution and drying the area with a hair dryer on a lower setting will provide some relief. Keeping the area clean and dry will also decrease the growth of warts. Cotton underwear and loose-fitting clothes that decrease friction and irritation also

TABLE 21-7 Treatment of External Genital Warts

Patient-Applied Regimens	Clinician-Administered Regimens	Alternative Regimens
Podofilox 0.5% solution or gel **or** Imiquimod 5% cream **or** Sinecatechins 15% ointment	Cryotherapy with liquid nitrogen or cryoprobe, repeat applications every 1–2 weeks **or** Podophyllin resin 10%–25% in a compound tincture of benzoin **or** Trichloroacetic acid (TCA) or bichloracetic acid (BCA) 80%–90% **or** Surgical removal by tangential scissor excision, tangential shave excision, curettage, or electrosurgery	Intralesional interferon **or** Photodynamic therapy **or** Topical cidofovir

Source: CDC, 2010e.

may decrease discomfort. Women should be advised to maintain a healthy lifestyle to aid the immune system. Women can also be counseled regarding diet, rest, stress reduction, and exercise. All women who smoke should be counseled in smoking-cessation techniques.

Talking with the Patient

Counseling messages for women with HPV infection and genital warts are outlined in **Table 21-8**. The partners of women with genital warts should be evaluated and treated if lesions are present. Condoms should be used until both partners are lesion free and for as long as

---

TABLE 21-8 Counseling Messages for Women with Human Papillomavirus and Genital Warts

The CDC recommends that the following key counseling points be conveyed to all persons with HPV:

- Genital HPV infection is very common and can be passed through vaginal, anal, or oral sexual contact.
- Most sexually active adults will get HPV at some point in their lives, although most will never know it because HPV infection usually has no signs or symptoms.
- HPV infection usually clears spontaneously without causing health problems, but some infections progress to genital warts, precancerous conditions, and cancers. The types of HPV that cause genital warts are not the same as the types that can cause cancer.
- A diagnosis of HPV in one sex partner is not indicative of sexual infidelity in the other partner.
- Treatments are available for genital warts but not for eradicating the actual virus.
- HPV does not affect female fertility or the ability to carry a pregnancy to term.
- Correct and consistent condom use might lower the chances of giving or getting genital HPV, but condom use is not fully protective because HPV can infect areas that are not covered by a condom. The only way to definitively avoid giving and getting HPV is to abstain from sexual activity.
- Tests for HPV are available to screen for cervical cancer in certain women.
- Two HPV vaccines are available, both of which protect against the HPV types that cause 70% of cancers. One of the vaccines also provides protection against the HPV types that cause 90% of genital warts. Both vaccines are most effective when all doses are administered before sexual contact.

The following key counseling points are for persons diagnosed with genital warts and their partners:

- Genital warts are not life threatening. If they are not treated, genital warts might go away, stay the same, or increase in size or number. It is very unusual for genital warts to turn into cancer.
- It is difficult to determine how or when a person became infected with HPV. Genital warts can be transmitted even when no visible signs of warts are present, even after warts are treated.
- It is not known how long a person remains contagious after warts are treated or whether informing subsequent sexual partners about a history of genital warts is beneficial to their health.
- Genital warts commonly recur after treatment, especially in the first three months.
- Women with HPV do not need more frequent Pap tests.
- HPV testing is unnecessary in sexual partners of persons with genital warts. However, STI screening for both sex partners is beneficial if one partner has genital warts.
- Persons with genital warts should inform their current sex partner(s) because warts can be transmitted to other partners. They should refrain from sexual activity until the warts are gone or removed.

Source: CDC, 2010e.

nine months after the appearance of lesions, as subclinical HPV may remain infectious. All sexually active women with multiple partners or a history of HPV should be encouraged to use latex condoms during intercourse to decrease HPV acquisition or transmission. Women with HPV infection may radically alter their sexual practices both out of fear of transmission of the virus to or from a partner, and owing to genital discomfort associated with treatment, which may have a negative effect on their sexual relationships. Unless the partner accepts and understands the necessary precautions, it may be difficult for the woman to follow the treatment regimen. The clinician can offer to discuss feelings that the woman may have and, when indicated, joint counseling can be suggested.

Genital Herpes

Genital herpes is a recurrent, incurable viral infection characterized by painful vesicular eruption of the skin and mucosa of the genitals. Two types of herpes simplex virus (HSV) have been identified as causing genital herpes: HSV-1 and HSV-2. HSV-2 is usually transmitted sexually, whereas HSV-1 is transmitted nonsexually. Although HSV-1 is more commonly associated with gingivostomatitis and oral ulcers (fever blisters), and HSV-2 with genital lesions, both types are not exclusively associated with those sites. HSV-2 infection increases the risk of women acquiring HIV by at least threefold (Freeman et al., 2006).

Genital herpes is one of the most common STIs in the United States, but its exact prevalence is unknown because HSV is not a reportable infection. In the National Health and Nutrition Examination Survey (NHANES) 2005–2008, among those 7,293 participants aged 14 to 49 years who had HSV-2 testing, seroprevalence was 20.9% in women and 11.5% in men. HSV-2 seroprevalence was three times higher in black women than in white women (48.0% versus 15.9%, respectively). Prevalence also increased with a higher number of lifetime sex partners: Seroprevalence was 5.4% in women with one lifetime sex partner, 18.8% in women with two to four lifetime partners, 21.8% in women with five to nine lifetime partners, and 37.1% in women with 10 or more lifetime partners. Among all study participants who were positive for HSV-2, 81.1% reported they had never had a clinician tell them they had genital herpes (CDC, 2010c).

In fact, most people who have HSV-2 have never been diagnosed with genital herpes. Despite their mild or unrecognized infections, they intermittently shed the HSV-2 virus in the genital tract. As a result, most genital herpes infections are transmitted by individuals who do not know they have HSV-2 or who do not have symptoms at the time of transmission (CDC, 2010e).

An initial or primary genital herpes infection characteristically has both systemic and local symptoms and lasts approximately three weeks. Women generally have a more severe clinical course than do men. Flu-like symptoms with fever, malaise, and myalgia first appear about a week after exposure, peak within four days, and subside over the next week. Multiple genital lesions develop at the site of infection, usually the vulva. Other commonly affected sites are the perianal area, vagina, and cervix. The lesions begin as small painful blisters or vesicles that become "unroofed," leaving ulcerated lesions (**Color Plate 18**). Individuals with primary herpes often develop bilateral, tender, inguinal lymphadenopathy; vulvar edema; vaginal discharge; and severe dysuria.

Ulcerative lesions last 4 to 15 days before crusting over. New lesions may develop over a period of 10 days during the course of the infection. Cervicitis is also common with initial HSV-2 infections. The cervix may appear normal, or it may be friable, reddened, ulcerated, or necrotic. A heavy, watery to purulent vaginal discharge is common. Extragenital lesions may be present because of autoinoculation. Urinary retention and dysuria may occur secondary to autonomic involvement of the sacral nerve root.

Women experiencing recurrent episodes of genital herpes typically develop only local symptoms that are usually less severe than those associated with the initial infection. Systemic symptoms are usually absent, although the characteristic prodromal genital tingling is common. Recurrent lesions are unilateral, are less severe than the original lesions, and usually last 7 to 10 days without prolonged viral shedding. Lesions begin as vesicles and progress rapidly to ulcers. Very few women with recurrent disease have cervicitis.

Assessment

In making the diagnosis of genital herpes, a history of exposure to a person with HSV infection is important, although infection from an asymptomatic individual is common. A history of viral symptoms, such as malaise, headache, fever, or myalgia, is suggestive of HSV infection. Local symptoms such as vulvar pain, dysuria, itching, or burning at the site of infection, and painful genital lesions that heal spontaneously also are very suggestive of HSV infection. The clinician should also ask about prior history of a primary infection, prodromal symptoms, vaginal discharge, dysuria, and dyspareunia.

During the physical examination, assess for inguinal and generalized lymphadenopathy and elevated temperature. Carefully inspect the entire vulvar, perineal, vaginal, and cervical areas for vesicles or ulcerated or crusted areas. A speculum examination may be very difficult for the patient because of the extreme tenderness often associated with genital herpes. Any genital lesion that is extremely tender should be tested for HSV even if the appearance is not consistent with the classic herpes lesions.

Although a diagnosis of HSV infection may be suspected from the history and physical examination, it can be confirmed only by laboratory studies. Isolation of HSV in cell culture or by polymerase chain reaction (PCR) is the preferred test in women who have genital ulcers or other mucocutaneous lesions. Viral culture is less sensitive than PCR. The culture yield is best during a primary infection or if the specimen is taken during the vesicular stage of the disease because the sensitivity of a culture declines rapidly as lesions begin to heal. Culture and PCR can be negative in a person with HSV infection because the virus is shed intermittently (CDC, 2010e).

Type-specific serologic tests are useful in confirming a clinical diagnosis because false-negative HSV cultures are common, especially with healing lesions or recurrent infection. Antibodies are present within the first several weeks after infection and persist indefinitely. Clinicians should be certain to specifically request serologic type-specific glycoprotein G (gG)–based assays. Serologic test options include laboratory-based assays and point-of-care tests using capillary blood or serum during a clinic visit. The sensitivity of these tests varies from 80% to 98%, and false-negative results can occur, especially in early stages of infection. The specificity of these assays is 96% or greater, and false-positive results can occur in patients with a low likelihood of HSV infection. Serologic screening for HSV is not recommended for the general population but should be considered in women who experience recurrent or atypical genital symptoms with negative HSV cultures, have a clinical diagnosis of genital herpes without laboratory confirmation, present for STI evaluation (especially if they have multiple sexual partners), or have HIV. Testing should also be considered for asymptomatic partners of patients with HSV infection (CDC, 2010e). All patients with genital herpes should be tested for other STIs, including chlamydia, gonorrhea, syphilis, and HIV.

Differential Diagnoses

Differential diagnoses include syphilis, chancroid, lymphogranuloma venereum, granuloma inguinale, as well as non-STI vulvar lesions (see Chapter 27).

Management

Genital herpes is a chronic and recurring disease for which there is no known cure. Systemic antiviral drugs partially control the symptoms and signs of HSV infections when used for the primary or recurrent episodes, or when used as daily suppressive therapy. These drugs do not cure the infection, however, nor do they alter subsequent risk, frequency, or rate of recurrences after discontinuation. Three antiviral medications provide clinical benefits for genital herpes: acyclovir, valacyclovir, and famciclovir. Treatment recommendations are given in **Table 21-9**. Topical antiviral therapy is not recommended due to its minimal benefits (CDC, 2010e).

Systemic antiviral therapy should be given to all patients experiencing their first genital herpes episode. Most people with a symptomatic first episode of genital HSV-2 infection will experience recurrent episodes of genital lesions; by comparison, recurrence is less common with genital HSV-1 infection. Lifelong, intermittent, asymptomatic, genital shedding occurs in those persons infected with HSV-2. Recurrent genital herpes can be treated with daily suppressive therapy, which decreases the frequency of recurrences and the risk of transmitting HSV, or episodic therapy may be implemented when lesions occur to help them heal more quickly. Episodic therapy should be started within one day of when the lesion begins or during the prodromal symptoms if present. Patients using episodic therapy should be provided with a prescription or medication in advance to facilitate immediate treatment of outbreaks (CDC, 2010e).

Cleaning lesions twice a day with a saline solution will help prevent secondary infection. Coexisting bacterial infections must be treated with appropriate antibiotics. Oral analgesics, such as aspirin or ibuprofen, may be used to relieve pain and systemic symptoms associated

TABLE 21-9 Treatment of Genital Herpes

*Primary Infection**

Acyclovir 400 mg orally three times a day for 7–10 days

or

Acyclovir 200 mg orally five times a day for 7–10 days

or

Famciclovir 250 mg orally three times a day for 7–10 days

or

Valacyclovir 1 gm orally twice a day for 7–10 days

*Treatment can be extended if healing is incomplete after 10 days of therapy

Recurrent Infection

Acyclovir 400 mg orally three times a day for 5 days

or

Acyclovir 800 mg orally twice a day for 5 days

or

Acyclovir 800 mg orally three times a day for 2 days

or

Famciclovir 125 mg orally twice a day for 5 days

or

Famciclovir 1000 mg orally twice a day for 1 day

or

Famciclovir 500 mg orally once, followed by 250 mg twice a day for 2 days

or

Valacyclovir 500 mg orally twice a day for 3 days

or

Valacyclovir 1 gm orally once a day for 5 days

Suppressive Therapy

Acyclovir 400 mg orally twice a day

or

Famciclovir 250 mg orally twice a day

or

Valacyclovir 500 mg orally once a day (may be less effective than other valacyclovir or acyclovir dosing regiments in patients who have 10 or more episodes per year)

or

Valacyclovir 1 gm orally once a day

Source: CDC, 2010e.

with initial infections. Any topical agents should be used with caution, because the mucous membranes affected by herpes are very sensitive. Ointments containing cortisone should be avoided. Women should be informed that occlusive ointments may prolong the course of infections.

Complementary measures that may increase comfort for women when lesions are active include warm sitz baths with baking soda; keeping lesions warm and dry by using a hair dryer set on cool or patting dry the area with a soft towel; wearing cotton underwear and loose clothing; applying cold milk or witch hazel compresses followed by aloe vera gel or Burrow's solution (Domeboro) to lesions four times a day for 30 minutes; oatmeal baths; applying cool, wet, black tea bags to lesions; and applying compresses with an infusion of cloves or peppermint oil and clove oil to lesions (Collins-Bride & Murphy, 2004; Sinclair, 2004).

Many complementary and alternative products are used for genital herpes, though the evidence supporting the effectiveness of most of these products is absent or limited (Perfect, Bourne, Ebel, & Rosenthal, 2005). The amino acid L-lysine has been used for active lesions and suppression. It is thought that L-lysine has an inhibitory effect on the amino acid arginine, which supports HSV infection. Minimizing consumption of the following foods, which contain arginine, may help as well: coffee, grains, chicken, chocolate, corn, dairy products, meat, peanut butter, nuts, and seeds. Avoiding citrus foods may also be helpful (Balch & Balch, 1997; Page, 2000; Sinclair, 2004).

A number of herbal remedies may also help with the discomforts of herpes infections and possibly expedite healing of lesions. Zinc may be taken orally or applied via a topical solution or intravaginal sponges. Honey, propolis, and aloe vera are applied as creams or ointments (Perfect et al., 2005). Liquid Burdock can be applied as a compress or taken orally (Griffith, 2000; Nissim, 1996; Page, 2000; Stapleton & Tiran, 2000). Calendula comes in an ointment or infused oil that can be applied locally, as a tea that can be used to make a sitz bath, and as a tincture that is diluted with water and applied to lesions with a cotton swab (Cummings & Ullman, 1997; Griffith; Nissim; Page; Sinclair, 2004; Singingtree, 1993; Stapleton & Tiran). Echinacea extract has antiviral properties, stimulates the body's immune system, and may be taken orally or applied locally to reduce inflammation and pain; it should be used at the first indication of a herpes outbreak (Balch & Balch, 1997; Griffith; Page). Goldenseal may be taken by capsule, tea, or extract, or applied locally to decrease inflammation and pain (Balch & Balch; Griffith; Page). Myrrh can be applied locally as a diluted tincture or as a compress to decrease pain and inflammation. When applied to the lesions, diluted tincture of myrrh has a drying effect, although it stings (Balch & Balch; Page; Stapleton & Tiran). Tea tree oil stimulates the immune system and can be applied locally or added to bath water (Page; Sinclair; Stapleton & Tiran).

Talking with the Patient

Women should be advised that viral shedding—and, therefore, transmission of HSV to a partner—is most likely with active lesions, but can occur even when they are asymptomatic. Therefore, all current and future sex partners should be informed that the woman has genital HSV infection. Women whose partners do not have HSV infection should refrain from sexual contact from the onset of the prodrome until the complete healing of lesions. During asymptomatic periods, condoms and suppressive therapy can be used to reduce the risk of transmission to partners who do not have HSV infection. Women should be taught how to examine themselves for herpetic lesions using a mirror and good light source to look, and a wet cloth or finger covered with a finger cot to rub lightly over the labia. The clinician should ensure that patients understand that when lesions are active, sharing intimate articles (e.g., washcloths, wet towels) that come into contact with the lesions should be avoided. Women should be educated about the risk of neonatal HSV infection and advised that if they become pregnant, they need to be certain to disclose their history of genital herpes to the clinicians providing their prenatal care and care for their newborn (CDC, 2010e).

Chancroid

Chancroid is a bacterial infection of the genitourinary tract caused by the gram-negative bacteria known as *Haemophilus ducreyi*. Chancroid is uncommon in the United States, with only 28 cases being reported in the country in 2009. This number may be an underestimate, however, reflecting the fact that the causative organism of chancroid is difficult to culture (CDC, 2010d). Chancroid is a genital ulcer; thus it is a risk factor for HIV transmission. The major way chancroid is acquired is through sexual contact and trauma. Infection through autoinoculation of fingers or other sites occasionally occurs. The incubation period, though not well established, usually ranges from four to seven days but may be as long as three weeks.

Typically the woman presents with a history of a painful macule on the external genitalia that rapidly changes to a pustule and then to an ulcerated lesion (**Color Plate 19**). The patient may develop enlarged unilateral or bilateral inguinal nodes known as buboes. After one to two weeks, the skin overlying the lymph node becomes erythematous, the center necroses, and the node becomes ulcerated.

Assessment

A probable diagnosis of chancroid can be made when one or more painful genital ulcers are present; there is no evidence of syphilis (per dark-field examination of ulcer exudate or serologic testing at least seven days after ulcer onset); the clinical presentation, ulcer appearance, and regional lymphadenopathy (if present) are typical for chancroid; and HSV testing of the exudate is negative. Definitive diagnosis of chancroid is difficult because the organism can be identified only by culture on a special medium that is not used routinely; even when this technique is used, the test's sensitivity is less than 80% (CDC, 2010e). Testing for HIV and syphilis should be performed at the time of diagnosis and repeated in three months.

Differential Diagnoses

Differential diagnoses include syphilis, HSV, lymphogranuloma venereum, folliculitis, metastatic genital cancer (cervical, vagina, vulvar), and other vulvar lesions (see Chapter 27).

Management

The recommended treatments for chancroid are azithromycin, 1 gm orally in a single dose; ceftriaxone, 250 mg IM in a single dose; ciprofloxacin, 500 mg orally twice a day for three days; or erythromycin base, 500 mg orally four times a day for seven days (CDC, 2010e). Women with comorbid HIV infection may require repeated or longer therapy.

Patients should be reexamined three to seven days after beginning therapy. If treatment is successful, symptomatic improvement should be apparent within three days of starting therapy, although it may take more than two weeks for complete healing of large ulcers. All sexual partners who have had sexual contact within 10 days preceding the onset of symptoms with a person diagnosed with chancroid should be evaluated regardless of whether symptoms are present.

Pediculosis Pubis

Pediculosis is a parasitic infection caused by the following three species of lice:

- *Pediculosis humanus capitis* (head louse infecting the scalp)
- *Pediculosis humanus corporus* (body or clothing louse infecting the trunk)
- *Phthirus pubis* (pubic lice or "crabs")

P. pubis inhabit the genital area but may also be found in other hair-bearing areas of the body, including the axillae, chest, thighs, eyelashes, and head. A woman may be infected through contact with infected clothing or bedding, and by sexual transmission.

Assessment

A patient usually presents with pruritus, caused by the lice ingesting saliva, and then depositing digestive juices and feces into the skin. Women may report seeing the lice or known exposure to a household member or sexual partner with head, body, or pubic lice. A history of shared clothing, bathing equipment, or bedding may also be given. Diagnosis is made by direct examination of the egg cases (nits) in the involved area (**Color Plate 20**). Although the nits are usually visible to the naked eye, a hand lens and light can be helpful in identifying them. Black dots (excreta) may be visible on the surrounding skin and underclothing, and crusts or scabs may be seen in the pubic area. Women with pediculosis pubis should be tested for other STIs.

Differential Diagnoses

Differential diagnosis includes anogenital eczema and pruritus, seborrheic dermatitis, pruritus vulvae, folliculitis, tinea cruris, and scabies. Other concomitant STIs should be ruled out.

Management

Recommended treatments for pediculosis pubis are permethrin 1% cream rinse or pyrethrins with piperonyl butoxide. These medications are applied to the affected areas and washed off after 10 minutes. If symptoms do not resolve within one week and treatment failure is thought to be due to drug resistance, an alternative regimen consists of Malathion 0.5% lotion applied for 8 to 12 hours and washed off. Oral ivermectin (250 mcg/kg) repeated in 2 weeks is another alternative regimen, although research supporting the efficacy of this therapy is limited (CDC, 2010e). Advise patients to wash all clothing, bed linens, and towels in hot water and to dry these items thoroughly on the hot cycle to destroy lice and nits.

Trichomoniasis

Trichomoniasis is caused by *Trichomonas vaginalis*, an anaerobic one-celled protozoan with characteristic flagellae. The organism most commonly lives in the vagina in women, and in the urethra in men. Among women presenting with vaginitis symptoms, 4% to 35% will have trichomoniasis. In the NHANES 2001 to 2004 data, the prevalence of *T. vaginalis* infection was found to be 3.1% among 3754 women aged 14 to 49 years who provided self-collected vaginal swab specimens. The prevalence of *T. vaginalis* was 10 times higher in black women than in white women (13.3% versus 1.3%, respectively), and 85% of the women with infection were asymptomatic (Sutton et al., 2007). Trichomoniasis is sexually transmitted during vaginal–penile intercourse or vulva-to-vulva contact. Nonsexual transmission is possible but rare. Trichomoniasis is believed to facilitate HIV transmission (Sutton et al.).

Although trichomoniasis may be asymptomatic, women commonly experience a characteristically yellow to greenish, frothy, mucopurulent, copious, malodorous discharge. Inflammation of the vulva, vagina, or both may be present, and the woman may have irritation, pruritus, dysuria, or dyspareunia. Typically, the discharge worsens during and after menstruation.

Assessment

In addition to the history of current symptoms, a careful sexual history, including information on the last intercourse and last sexual contact, should be obtained. Any history of similar symptoms in the past and treatment used should be noted. The clinician should determine whether the woman's partners were treated and whether she has engaged in subsequent relations with new partners. Additional important information includes the last menstrual period, method of contraception, and other medications.

Inspect the external genitalia for excoriation, erythema, edema, ulceration, and lesions. On speculum examination, note the quantity, color, consistency, and any odor of the vaginal discharge. Often the cervix and vaginal walls will demonstrate characteristic "strawberry spots," or tiny petechiae (**Color Plate 21**), and the cervix may bleed on contact. In severe infections, the vaginal walls, the cervix, and occasionally the vulva may be acutely inflamed. The pH of vaginal discharge is elevated.

Diagnosis is usually made by wet prep visualization of the typical one-celled flagellate trichomonads (**Figure 21-1**). This method has a sensitivity of only approximately 60% to 70%, however, and the slide must be viewed immediately to ensure optimal results. Microscopic examination of the wet mount may also reveal increased numbers of white blood cells. Point-of-care tests are also available with higher sensitivity (more than 83%) and specificity (more than 97%).

Culture is a sensitive and highly specific method of diagnosis, but is not routinely performed. Culture should be performed when trichomoniasis is suspected but cannot be con-

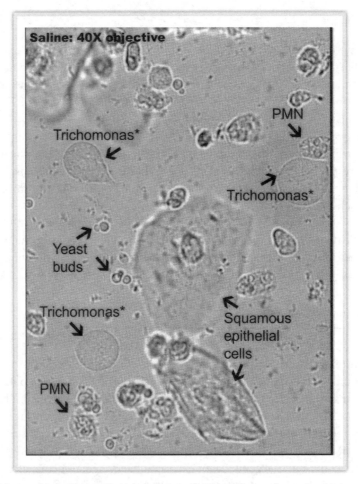

FIGURE 21-1 Wet mount findings with trichomoniasis. PMNs = polymorphonuclear leukocytes/white blood cells. Trichomonads must be motile for conclusive diagnosis.

Source: Used with permission from Washington State Department of Health STD/TB Program, Seattle STD/HIV Prevention Training Center, and Cindy Fennell, MS, MT, ASCP.

firmed with microscopy. Pap test sensitivity for *T. vaginalis* is better with liquid-based testing than the traditional Papanicolaou smear, but confirmatory testing may still be needed (CDC, 2010e). All patients with trichomoniasis should be tested for other STIs, including chlamydia, gonorrhea, syphilis, and HIV.

Differential Diagnoses

Differential diagnoses for trichomoniasis include other conditions that cause vaginal discharge (see Chapter 20), such as vulvovaginal candidiasis, bacterial vaginosis, chlamydia, and gonorrhea.

Management

The recommended treatment for trichomoniasis is metronidazole 2 gm orally in a single dose or tinidazole 2 gm orally in a single dose. Topical metronidazole is not recommended. If single-dose metronidazole treatment fails and reinfection is excluded, metronidazole 500 mg orally twice a day for 7 days should be prescribed. If infection persists, consider metronidazole or tinidazole 2 gm orally for 5 days. If infection persists, consultation with a specialist is warranted (CDC, 2010e).

When taking metronidazole or tinidazole, the patient is advised not to drink alcoholic beverages, or she will experience severe abdominal distress, nausea, vomiting, and headache. Abstinence from alcohol should continue 24 hours after completing metronidazole treatment and 72 hours after completing tinidazole treatment. Sex partners of patients with trichomoniasis should be treated as well, and patients should abstain from sex until both partners have been treated and are asymptomatic (CDC, 2010e).

Chlamydia

Chlamydia, which is caused by the bacterium *Chlamydia trachomatis*, is the most commonly reported nationally notifiable disease in the United States. Nearly 1.25 million cases were reported to the CDC in 2009, with at least that many more estimated to have gone undetected (CDC, 2010d). Sexually active adolescents and women aged 14 to 24 years of age have nearly three times the prevalence of chlamydia as women aged 25 and 39 years. The prevalence of chlamydia is five times higher in black women than in white women (CDC, 2011a). Risk factors for this infection include multiple sexual partners and failure to use barrier methods of contraception. The most serious complication of chlamydial infections for women is PID (see the section on PID later in this chapter).

Assessment

When assessing patients for chlamydia, in addition to obtaining information about any risk factors, inquire about the presence of any symptoms—while recognizing that chlamydia is usually asymptomatic. Women experiencing symptoms may report spotting or postcoital bleeding, mucoid or purulent cervical discharge, urinary frequency, dysuria, lower abdominal pain, or dyspareunia. Bleeding results from inflammation and erosion of the cervical columnar epithelium.

Physical examination findings of guarding, referred pain, or rebound upon abdominal examination should raise suspicion for PID. Cervical friability may be detected with the speculum examination. Discharge, if present, is characteristically mucopurulent (**Color Plate 22**). During the bimanual examination, a woman may report pain with cervical movement, and the examiner may detect adnexal fullness and uterine tenderness. These findings are also suggestive of PID.

The CDC has expanded recommendations for chlamydia screening among asymptomatic women. All sexually active women aged 25 years and younger should be screened for chlamydia annually (CDC, 2010e). Women older than age 25 years with risk factors (e.g., new or multiple partners) should also be screened. Chlamydia testing can be performed using urine or swab specimens from the endocervix or vagina. Screening procedures for chlamydial infection include nucleic acid amplification tests (NAATs), cell culture, direct immunofluorescence, enzyme immunoassay (EIA), and nucleic acid hybridization tests. NAATs are the preferred technique because they provide the highest sensitivity (see Chapter 6). Women with a positive urine test should have a pelvic examination to identify complications, such as PID. All patients with chlamydia should be tested for other STIs, including gonorrhea, syphilis, and HIV.

Differential Diagnoses

Differential diagnoses include gonorrhea, trichomoniasis, PID, appendicitis, and cystitis.

TABLE 21-10 Treatment of Chlamydial Infections

Recommended Regimens
Azithromycin 1 gm orally in a single dose
or
Doxycycline 100 mg orally twice a day for 7 days
Alternative Regimens
Erythromycin base 500 mg orally four times a day for 7 days
or
Erythromycin ethylsuccinate 800 mg orally four times a day for 7 days
or
Levofloxacin 500 mg orally once daily for 7 days
or
Ofloxacin 300 mg orally twice a day for 7 days
Source: CDC, 2010e.

Management

Recommendations for treatment of chlamydial infections are found in **Table 21-10**. Treatment of current and recent sexual partners is imperative. A test of cure (3 to 4 weeks after treatment) is not necessary unless a woman is pregnant, has persistent symptoms, or may have reinfection. A high prevalence of reinfection is observed in women who have had chlamydial infections in the preceding several months, usually from reinfection by an untreated partner. Patients should be advised to abstain from sex until their sexual partners are treated and to wait 7 days after single-dose treatment or until completion of a 7-day regimen before resuming sexual activity. Clinicians should advise all patients with chlamydia to be rescreened 3 months after treatment (CDC, 2010e).

Gonorrhea

Gonorrhea, which is caused by the aerobic, gram-negative diplococcus *Neisseria gonorrhoeae*, is the second most commonly reported bacterial STI after chlamydia. In 2009, 301,174 cases of gonorrhea were reported in the United States. The rate of infection was slightly higher in women than in men (105.5/100,000 versus 90.8/100,000, respectively). Gonorrhea rates are highest among adolescents and young adults aged 15 to 24 years, and 71% of the women who had gonorrhea in 2009 were members of this age group. The rate of gonorrhea in black women is more than 15 times the rate in white women (CDC, 2010d).

Gonorrhea is almost exclusively transmitted by sexual activity, primarily through genital-to-genital contact; however, it is also spread by oral-to-genital and anal-to-genital contact. Sites of infection in females include the cervix, urethra, oropharynx, Skene's glands, and Bartholin's glands. In addition to age, other risk factors for this infection include early onset of sexual activity and multiple sexual partners.

The main complication of gonorrheal infections is PID. Women may also develop a pelvic abscess or Bartholin's abscess. Disseminated gonococcal infections (DGI) are a rare (0.5% to 3%) complication of untreated gonorrhea. DGI occurs in two stages: The first stage is characterized by bacteremia with chills, fever, and skin lesions; it is followed by the second stage during which the patient experiences acute septic arthritis with characteristic effusions, most commonly of the wrists, knees, and ankles (Star & Deal, 2004a).

Assessment

Women with gonorrhea often remain asymptomatic. When symptoms are present, they are often less specific than the symptoms in men. Women may report dyspareunia, a change in vaginal discharge, unilateral labial pain and swelling, or lower abdominal discomfort. Later in the infection's course, women may describe a history of purulent, irritating vaginal discharge, or rectal pain and discharge. Menstrual irregularities may be the presenting symptom, with longer, more painful menses being noted. Women may also report chronic or acute lower abdominal pain. Unilateral labial pain and swelling may indicate Bartholin's gland infection (see Chapter 20), and periurethral pain and swelling may indicate inflamed Skene's glands. Infrequently, dysuria, vague abdominal pain, or low backache prompts women to seek care. Later symptoms may include fever (possibly high), nausea, vomiting, joint pain and swelling, or upper abdominal pain (liver involvement).

Women may develop a gonococcal rectal infection following anal intercourse and report symptoms of profuse purulent anal discharge, rectal pain, and blood in the stool. Rectal itching, fullness, pressure, and pain are also common symptoms. Women with gonococcal pharyngitis may appear to have viral pharyngitis, as some individuals will have a red, swollen uvula and pustule vesicles on the soft palate and tonsils similar to streptococcal infections.

Physical examination is individualized based on the woman's presenting symptoms. Obtain vital signs and perform a general skin inspection for signs of classic DGI lesions, which are painful necrotic pustules on an erythematous base, approximately 1 mm to 2 cm in diameter. Inspect the pharynx and oral cavity for erythema, edema, and lesions. Assess for cervical lymphadenopathy. Palpate the abdomen for masses, tenderness, and rebound tenderness. During the speculum examination, inspect the vaginal walls for discharge and redness, and examine the cervix for mucopurulent discharge, ectopy, and friability (**Color Plate 23**). During the bimanual examination, observe for cervical motion tenderness, uterine tenderness, adnexal tenderness, and adnexal masses—which are all findings associated with PID.

Gonorrhea testing can be performed by culture, nucleic acid hybridization tests, and NAATs. Endocervical swabs are required for culture and nucleic acid hybridization tests. NAATs can be performed using urine or swab specimens from the endocervix or vagina. Although the FDA has not formally approved NAATs for use in the rectum or pharynx, some laboratories have established performance specifications for using NAATs with specimens from these sites. NAAT products vary, however, and clinicians must be certain that the test they are using is appropriate for the specimen type (CDC, 2010e). All patients with gonorrhea should be tested for other STIs, including chlamydia, syphilis, and HIV.

Differential Diagnoses

Differential diagnoses for gonorrhea include chlamydia, trichomoniasis, PID, appendicitis, and cystitis.

Management

Recommended therapies for gonorrhea are listed in **Table 21-11**. Treatment of current and recent sexual partners is imperative. Patients who are treated for gonorrhea should be concomitantly treated for chlamydia because coinfection rates are high, and dual therapy may help hinder the development of antimicrobial-resistant *N. gonorrhoeae*. Quinolones are no longer used to treat gonorrhea because of the high rate of quinolone-resistant strains of the organism (CDC, 2010e).

TABLE 21-11 Treatment of Uncomplicated Gonococcal Infections of the Cervix, Urethra, and Rectum

Ceftriaxone 250 mg IM in a single dose

If ceftriaxone is not an option:

Cefixime 400 mg orally in a single dose

or

Other single-dose injectable cephalosporin regimens (ceftizoxime 500 mg IM, cefoxitin 2g IM with probenecid 1 gm orally, or cefotaxime 500 mg IM)

plus

Azithromycin 1 gm orally in a single dose (preferred)

or

Doxycycline 100 mg orally twice a day for 7 days

Sources: CDC, 2010e, 2011b.

A test of cure (3 to 4 weeks after treatment) is not necessary (CDC, 2010e). Decreased susceptibility of the infectious organism to cefixime has been reported, which has raised concerns about the potential for development of cephalosporin-resistant strains.

Clinicians must be vigilant for treatment failures (CDC, 2011b). Patients whose symptoms do not resolve after treatment should have a culture, with any gonococci that are isolated being tested for antimicrobial susceptibility. All patients with gonorrhea should be retested three months after treatment due to the high rate of reinfection (CDC, 2010e).

Pelvic Inflammatory Disease

Pelvic inflammatory disease occurs in the upper female genital tract and includes any combination of endometritis, salpingitis, tubo-ovarian abscess, and pelvic peritonitis (CDC, 2010e). Each year more than 750,000 women in the United States will have an episode of acute PID (Sutton, Sternberg, Zaidi, St. Louis, & Markowitz, 2005). These estimates do not include women who have PID that is undiagnosed because it is asymptomatic or presents atypically (Soper, 2010). Adolescents have the highest risk of developing PID because of their decreased immunity to infectious organisms and increased risk of gonorrhea and chlamydia (Star & Deal, 2004a).

Multiple organisms have been found to cause PID, and most cases are associated with infection by more than one organism. Common causative agents are *N. gonorrhoeae* and *C. trachomatis*. In addition to the pathogens that cause gonorrhea and chlamydia, a wide variety of anaerobic and aerobic microorganisms, including some found in the vaginal flora, are associated with PID (CDC, 2010e). Bacterial vaginosis is common in women with PID and may facilitate the ascent of microorganisms into the upper genital tract (Soper, 2010).

Major medical complications are associated with PID. Short-term consequences include tubo-ovarian abscess and Fitz-Hugh-Curtis syndrome (perihepatitis). Long-term sequelae from PID may include chronic pelvic and abdominal pain, increased risk of ectopic pregnancy, infertility, and recurring PID (Soper, 2010).

As noted earlier, PID may be caused by a wide variety of infectious agents, and it encompasses a wide variety of pathologic processes; therefore, the infection can be acute, subacute, or chronic, and may be associated with a wide range of symptoms. Diagnosis of PID is difficult because almost all of the most common signs and symptoms could accompany other urinary, gastrointestinal, or gynocologic tract problems. Accurate and prompt diagnosis is crucial to minimize long-term sequelae; thus clinicians should maintain a high suspicion for PID and a low threshold for its diagnosis.

Assessment

When PID is suspected, the history taking must be comprehensive. Relevant history includes recent pelvic surgery, abortion, childbirth, dilatation of the cervix, or IUD insertion (within the last month). A thorough sexual risk history should be obtained, including current or most recent sexual activity, number of partners, and method of contraception; this information will assist the clinician in identifying possible increased risk for STI exposure. The severity and extent of symptoms that women with PID experience vary widely. Commonly reported symptoms include abdominal, pelvic, and low back pain; abnormal vaginal discharge; intermenstrual or postcoital bleeding; fever; nausea and vomiting; and urinary frequency (Soper, 2010). Women may report levels of pain ranging from minimal discomfort to dull, cramping, and intermittent pain to severe, persistent, and incapacitating pain. Pelvic pain is usually exacerbated by the Valsalva maneuver, intercourse, or movement. Symptoms of STIs in a woman's partners also should be noted.

As part of the assessment for PID, obtain vital signs and perform a complete physical examination. While fever may be present, the majority of women with PID have a normal temperature at evaluation (Soper, 2010). Physical examination may reveal adnexal tenderness, abdominal tenderness, uterine tenderness, and tenderness with cervical movement. Pelvic tenderness is usually bilateral. There may or may not be a palpable adnexal swelling or thickening. A pelvic mass suggests tubo-ovarian abscess.

There is no single laboratory test that can be used to detect upper genital tract infections. A pH test and wet mount of the vaginal secretions should be performed, along with tests for chlamydia and gonorrhea, although negative results do not rule out these infections' presence in the upper genital tract. Other laboratory tests that are not needed for diagnosis but are recommended for women with clinically severe PID are a complete blood count (CBC) and erythrocyte sedimentation rate (ESR) (Soper, 2010). All patients with PID should be tested for syphilis and HIV as well. Laboratory data are useful only when considered in conjunction with the history and physical examination findings. Pelvic ultrasound should be performed in patients requiring hospitalization and those with a pelvic mass found on examination (Soper, 2010).

Clinical diagnosis of PID is imprecise; nevertheless, most diagnoses of PID are made clinically because laparoscopy and biopsy are too expensive and invasive to be practical screening tools. In 2002, the CDC established new minimum criteria for beginning treatment of PID (**Table 21-12**), in recognition of the fact that delay in diagnosis and treatment of PID is associated with severe sequelae. In addition, a diagnosis of PID should be considered in a woman with any of the common symptoms of PID.

Differential Diagnoses

Symptoms of PID may mimic those associated with other disease processes such as ectopic pregnancy, endometriosis, ovarian cyst with torsion, pelvic adhesions, inflammatory bowel disease, and acute appendicitis.

Management

Perhaps the most important action a clinician can take is prevention counseling. Primary prevention is education about avoiding STIs, whereas secondary prevention involves prompt treatment of lower genital tract infections to prevent ascension of the disease to the upper

TABLE 21-12 Diagnosing PID

Empiric treatment of PID should be initiated in sexually active young women and other women at risk for STIs if they are experiencing pelvic or lower abdominal pain, if no cause for the illness other than PID can be found, and if one or more of the following minimum criteria are present on pelvic examination:

- Cervical motion tenderness
- Uterine tenderness
- Adnexal tenderness

One or more of the following additional criteria can be used to enhance the specificity of the minimum criteria and support a diagnosis of PID:

- Oral temperature > 101°F (> 38.3°C)
- Abnormal cervical or vaginal mucopurulent discharge
- Presence of abundant numbers of white blood cells on saline microscopy of vaginal fluid
- Elevated erythrocyte sedimentation rate
- Elevated C-reactive protein level
- Laboratory documentation of cervical infection with *N. gonorrhoeae* or *C. trachomatis*

The most specific criteria for diagnosing PID include the following conditions:

- Endometrial biopsy with histopathologic evidence of endometritis
- Transvaginal sonography or magnetic resonance imaging techniques showing thickened, fluid-filled tubes with or without free pelvic fluid or tubo-ovarian complex, or Doppler studies suggesting pelvic infection (e.g., tubal hyperemia)
- Laparoscopic abnormalities consistent with PID

Source: CDC, 2010e.

genital tract. Instructing women in self-protective behaviors such as practicing safer sex and using barrier contraceptive methods is critical. Also important is the detection of asymptomatic gonorrheal and chlamydial infections through routine screening of women with risk factors. Partner notification when an STI is diagnosed is essential to prevent reinfection.

In the past, the majority of women with PID were hospitalized so that bed rest and parenteral therapy could be started. Today, most women with PID are not hospitalized. A randomized controlled trial of 831 women with mild to moderate PID found no difference in short-term improvement and long-term reproductive outcomes (e.g., pregnancy rates, PID recurrence, chronic pelvic pain, and ectopic pregnancy) between those treated in inpatient and outpatient settings (Ness et al., 2002). The decision of whether to hospitalize a patient should be based on each woman's individual circumstances. To guide clinicians' decisions regarding hospitalization, the CDC (2010e) has developed specific criteria for hospitalization, including the need to rule out surgical emergencies (e.g., appendicitis); pregnancy; no clinical response to oral antimicrobial therapy; inability to follow or tolerate an outpatient oral regimen; severe illness, nausea and vomiting, or high fever; and tubo-ovarian abscess. At present, no data exist to suggest that adolescents would benefit from hospitalization for treatment.

Although treatment regimens vary with the infecting organism, a broad-spectrum antibiotic is generally administered. Several antimicrobial regimens have proved to be effective, and no single therapeutic regimen appears to be superior to the others **(Table 21-13)**. Substantial clinical improvement should occur within 72 hours of beginning treatment. Women who have not responded in this time frame should be reevaluated to confirm the diagnosis of PID; they may also need hospitalization (if the woman is being treated on an outpatient basis), additional testing, and surgical intervention. Women who do not respond to oral therapy and have a confirmed diagnosis of PID should be treated with an inpatient or outpatient parenteral regimen. Women on parenteral regimens can usually be transitioned

TABLE 21-13 Treatment of Pelvic Inflammatory Disease

Parenteral Regimens	Oral Regimens
Parenteral Regimen A	*Oral Regimen A*
Cefotetan 2 gm IV every 12 hours	Ceftriaxone 250 mg IM in a single dose
or	**plus**
Cefoxitin 2 gm IV every 6 hours	Doxycycline 100 mg orally twice a day for 14 days
plus	**with or without**
Doxycycline 100 mg orally or IV every 12 hours	Metronidazole 500 mg orally twice a day for 14 days
Parenteral Regimen B	*Oral Regimen B*
Clindamycin 900 mg IV every 8 hours	Cefoxitin 2 gm IM in a single dose and probenecid 1 gm orally administered concurrently in a single dose
plus	
Gentamicin loading dose IV or IM (2 mg/kg of body weight), followed by a maintenance dose (1.5 mg/kg) every 8 hours. Single-day dosing (3–5 mg/kg) may be substituted.	**plus**
	Doxycycline 100 mg orally twice a day for 14 days
	with or without
	Metronidazole 500 mg orally twice a day for 14 days
Alternative Parenteral Regimen	*Oral Regimen C*
Ampicillin/sulbactam 3 gm IV every 6 hours	Other parenteral third-generation cephalosporin (e.g., ceftizoxime or cefotaxime)
plus	
Doxycycline 100 mg orally or IV every 12 hours	**plus**
	Doxycycline 100 mg orally twice a day for 14 days
	with or without
	Metronidazole 500 mg orally twice a day for 14 days

Source: CDC, 2010e.

to oral therapy 24 hours after they begin to show clinical improvement. If a woman with an IUD develops PID, there is insufficient evidence to recommend that the IUD be removed. Close clinical follow-up is required if the IUD is left in place (CDC, 2010e).

Minimal pelvic examinations should be done during the acute phase of the disease, and analgesics can be given for pain. During the recovery phase, the woman should restrict her activity and make every effort to obtain adequate rest and consume a nutritionally sound diet. Women with PID who have gonorrhea or chlamydia should have repeat testing for these pathogens 3 to 6 months after treatment (CDC, 2010e).

Health education is central to effective management of PID. Clinicians should explain to women the nature of their infection and should encourage them to comply with all therapy and prevention recommendations, emphasizing the necessity of taking all medication, even if symptoms resolve. Any potential problems that would prevent a woman from completing a course of treatment, such as lack of money for prescriptions or lack of transportation to return to a clinic for follow-up appointments, should be identified and the importance of follow-up visits emphasized. The woman's sex partners should be evaluated and treated as well. The woman diagnosed with PID will need supportive care, because PID is so closely tied to sexuality, body image, and self-concept. Her feelings need to be discussed, and her partners included in the counseling when appropriate.

Syphilis

Syphilis is a systemic disease caused by *Treponema pallidum*, a motile spirochete. There are an estimated 45,000 cases of syphilis, including 14,000 cases of primary and secondary syphilis, in the United States each year. Syphilis rates are higher for black and Hispanic women than they are for white women. In 2009, the male-to-female ratio for primary and secondary syphilis was 5.6, a difference that is primarily due to the number of men who have sex with men who have syphilis. In contrast to other bacterial STIs that affect mostly adolescents and adults younger than age 25 years, syphilis persists into the 30s and 40s in both men and women (CDC, 2010d).

Syphilis is characterized by periods of active symptoms and periods of asymptomatic latency. The disease can affect any tissue or organ in the body. Transmission is thought to be by entry into the subcutaneous tissue through microscopic abrasions that can occur during sexual intercourse. The infection can also be transmitted through kissing, biting, or oral–genital sex.

Syphilis is a complex infection that can lead to serious systemic disease and even death when untreated. Infection manifests itself in distinct stages with different symptoms and clinical manifestations (**Table 21-14**).

Primary syphilis is characterized by a primary lesion, or a chancre, which often begins as a painless papule at the site of inoculation and then erodes to form a nontender, shallow, indurated, clean ulcer that is several millimeters to a few centimeters in size (**Color Plate 24A**). The chancre is loaded with spirochetes and is most commonly found on the genitalia, although it may also occur on the cervix, perianal area, or mouth.

TABLE 21-14 Stages of Syphilis

	Primary	**Secondary**	**Early Latent**	**Late Latent**	**Tertiary**
Time After Exposure	3–90 days (average 21)	4–10 weeks	≤ 1 year	> 1 year	Years (usually 15 to 30)
Infectious Routes	Sexual Vertical Chancre	Sexual Vertical	Sexual Vertical	Vertical	None
Clinical Symptoms In addition, neurosyphilis (central nervous system infection) can occur at any stage	Chancre Regional lymphadenopathy	Chancre may still be present Skin lesions (papular rash of soles and palms, patchy alopecia, condylomata lata) Symptoms of systemic illness (fever, malaise, anorexia, weight loss, headache, myalgias) Lymphadenopathy	None	None	Cardiovascular syphilis (aortitis) Skin lesions (gumma)

Sources: CDC, 2010e, 2011g; Kent & Romanelli, 2008.

Secondary syphilis is characterized by a widespread, symmetrical maculopapular rash on the palms and soles (**Color Plate 24B**) and generalized lymphadenopathy. The woman may also experience fever, headache, and malaise. Condylomata lata (wartlike lesions) may develop on the vulva, perineum, or anus.

If the patient is untreated, she enters a latent phase that is asymptomatic for the majority of individuals. At this point, if the disease is still not treated, approximately one-third of patients will develop tertiary syphilis. Cardiovascular (chest pain, cough), dermatologic (multiple nodules or ulcers; **Color Plate 24C**), skeletal (arthritis, myalgia, myositis), and neurologic (headache, irritability, impaired balance, memory loss, tremor) symptoms can develop in this stage. Neurologic complications are not limited to tertiary syphilis; rather, a variety of syndromes (e.g., meningitis, meningovascular syphilis, general paresis, and tabes dorsalis) may span all stages of the disease. In recent years, evidence indicates that the disease is shifting from the more traditional symptomatic forms of neurosyphilis to asymptomatic central nervous system involvement with subtler, less well-defined syndromes (Star & Deal, 2004b).

Assessment

Women with primary syphilis may be asymptomatic, or they may report an anogenital lesion that is typically raised, painless, and indurated. Seventy percent of women with secondary syphilis will give a history of flu-like symptoms, including sore throat, malaise, headache, fever, myalgias, arthralgias, hoarseness, and anorexia. These women may also report skin rashes on the trunk, extremities, palms, and soles that may be pruritic (Star & Deal, 2004b). Approximately 25% of patients will report a persistent primary chancre. Some women will experience alopecia and have a "moth-eaten" look or lose the lateral one-third of an eyebrow. Occasionally women will have a history of low-grade fever. When syphilis is suspected, a comprehensive sexual risk history should be obtained.

The physical examination includes a general examination of the skin for alopecia, rash on the feet and palms, and condylomata lata. Additionally, the clinician should conduct a pharyngeal examination and inspect for enlarged inguinal nodes. Inspect the external genitalia for vulvar lesions and chancre at the point of inoculation. A speculum examination is performed to inspect for lesions on the vaginal walls and cervix and for vaginal and cervical discharge. A bimanual examination is conducted to assess uterine size, shape, consistency, mobility, and tenderness, and to palpate for adnexal masses and tenderness. When history and clinical findings suggest the need, a neurologic examination may be performed as well.

Dark-field examination and direct fluorescent antibody for *T. pallidum* (DFA-TP) of lesion exudates or tissue will provide a definitive diagnosis of early syphilis. The availability of these tests is limited, however, and their sensitivity is low. Thus they are rarely used (Kent & Romanelli, 2008).

The ability to confirm the diagnosis of syphilis depends on serology results obtained during the disease's latency and late infection phases. Any test for antibodies may not be reactive in the presence of active infection, as it takes time for the body's immune system to develop antibodies to any antigens. A presumptive diagnosis is possible with the use of two serologic tests: nontreponemal and treponemal.

Nontreponemal antibody tests such as the VDRL and RPR are used as screening tests, and are relatively inexpensive, sensitive, moderately nonspecific, and fast. False-positive results are not unusual with these tests, and can occur in the setting of increased age, autoimmune disorders, malignancy, pregnancy, injection-drug use, and recent vaccination (Kent & Romanelli, 2008). Sequential serologic tests should be obtained by using the same method (VDRL or RPR), preferably by the same laboratory (CDC, 2010e). A high titer (more than 1:16) usually indicates active disease. A fourfold change in the titer (e.g., from 1:16 to 1:4 or from 1:8 to 1:32) is considered clinically significant. Treatment of syphilis usually causes a progressive decline in the pathogen's presence that may result in a negative VDRL or RPR, but low titers may persist. Rising titer (fourfold) or failure of titer to decrease fourfold within 6 to 12 months suggests reinfection or treatment failure (Kent & Romanelli).

The treponemal tests—that is, the fluorescent treponemal antibody absorbed (FTA-ABS) test and the *T. pallidum* passive particle agglutination (TP-PA) assay—are used to confirm positive nontreponemal test results. Patients with early primary or incubating syphilis may have negative test results. Seroconversion usually takes place 6 to 8 weeks after exposure, so testing should be repeated in 1 to 2 months when a suspicious genital lesion exists. Treponemal antibody tests frequently stay positive for the remainder of the patient's life regardless of treatment or disease activity; therefore, treatment is monitored by VDRL or RPR titers of the VDRL or RPR. Tests for concomitant STIs, including HIV, should be performed as well.

Cerebrospinal fluid (CSF) testing may assist in confirming the diagnosis of neurosyphilis. Both a CSF-VDRL and CSF FTA-ABS can be performed, although routine CSF analysis in patients with primary or secondary syphilis is not recommended. Instead, testing of the CSF should be performed in specific situations—for example, in patients with symptoms or signs of neurologic or ophthalmic disease, in patients with persistent or recurring signs or symptoms, when titers increase fourfold, with high initial titers (1:32 or greater) that fail to decrease fourfold, in patients with symptomatic late syphilis, and when evidence of active tertiary syphilis is found (CDC, 2010e).

Management

Parenteral penicillin G is the preferred drug for treating patients with all stages of syphilis (**Table 21-15**). It is the only proven therapy that has been widely used for patients with neurosyphilis, congenital syphilis, and syphilis during pregnancy. Single-dose therapy is used to treat primary, secondary, and early latent syphilis. Women who have late latent, tertiary, or unknown-duration syphilis require weekly treatment for 3 weeks. Women with primary or secondary syphilis should have repeat clinical evaluation and serologic testing at 6 and 12 months after treatment. Women with latent or unknown-duration syphilis should have repeat clinical evaluation and serologic testing at 6, 12, and 24 months after treatment. Information on follow-up of patients with tertiary syphilis is limited. Partner treatment is imperative, and management depends on the stage of the patient's infection and the timing of partner's exposure. Detailed recommendations can be found in the CDC treatment guidelines (CDC, 2010e).

Hepatitis B

Hepatitis B virus (HBV) is a bloodborne pathogen transmitted by percutaneous or mucosal exposure to infectious blood or body fluids (e.g., semen, saliva). In 2007, 4519 cases of acute, symptomatic hepatitis B were reported in the United States. After accounting for asymptomatic infections and underreporting, the CDC estimated that there were 38,000 new infections in this country in 2007. The overall incidence (1.5/100,000) currently reported is the lowest ever recorded and has declined 82% from the rate found in 1990 (8.5/100,000) (CDC, 2009). The widespread use of HBV vaccination has contributed to this decline.

Hepatitis B infection is caused by a large DNA virus and is associated with three antigens and their antibodies. Thus screening for active or chronic disease or disease immunity is based on testing for these antigens and their antibodies (**Table 21-16**). HBV is more

TABLE 21-15 Treatment of Syphilis for Women Who Are HIV-Negative and Not Pregnant	
Recommended	*Primary, secondary, and early latent syphilis:*
	Benzathine penicillin G 2.4 million units IM in a single dose
	Late latent syphilis, latent syphilis of unknown duration, and tertiary syphilis:
	Benzathine penicillin G 7.2 million units total, administered as three doses of 2.4 million units IM each at 1-week intervals
Alternatives if penicillin allergic*	*Primary, secondary, and early latent syphilis:*
	Doxycycline 100 mg orally twice a day for 14 days
	or
	Tetracycline 500 mg orally four times daily for 14 days
	Late latent syphilis or latent syphilis of unknown duration:
	Doxycycline 100 mg orally twice a day for 28 days
	or
	Tetracycline 500 mg orally four times daily for 28 days
	Tertiary syphilis:
	Consult an infectious diseases specialist

*There are limited data to support these regimens, so close follow-up is essential. Penicillin desensitization and treatment should be considered for persons with a penicillin allergy whose compliance with therapy or follow-up cannot be ensured.

Source: CDC, 2010e.

TABLE 21-16 Parameters of Hepatitis B Testing	
HBsAg	Hepatitis B surface antigen
	Indicates the patient has acute or chronic HBV infection and can transmit it to others
Anti-HBs	Hepatitis B surface antibody
	Indicates the patient has immunity resulting from vaccination or previous infection
Anti-HBc	Total hepatitis B core antibody
	Indicates the patient has previous or ongoing infection
IgM anti-HBc	IgM antibody to hepatitis B core antigen
	Indicates the patient has had an acute infection within the past six months

infectious than HIV and hepatitis C virus (HCV), with HBV being able to survive outside the body for at least seven days (CDC, 2010e, 2011c). HBV infection may be transmitted both parenterally and through intimate contact. In particular, hepatitis B surface antigen (HBsAg) has been found in blood, saliva, sweat, tears, vaginal secretions, and semen. Perinatal transmission does occur, but the fetus is not at risk of contracting the infection until the child makes contact with contaminated blood at birth. HBV has also been transmitted by artificial insemination.

Factors considered to place a woman at increased risk for HBV are those associated with STI risk in general (e.g., history of multiple sexual partners, multiple STIs), injection-drug use, history of hemodialysis or blood transfusions, occupational exposure to blood and body fluids (e.g., public safety workers exposed to blood in the workplace, healthcare workers), individuals who live in households with persons who have chronic HBV infection, and persons born in or traveling to a country with a high incidence of HBV infection (CDC, 2011c). Although HBV can be transmitted via blood transfusion, the incidence of such infections has decreased significantly since testing of blood for the presence of HBsAg became possible.

HBV infection is a disease that affects primarily the liver. It remains asymptomatic in as many as half of the persons with the infection. When symptoms occur, they begin an average of 90 days after HBV exposure and usually last for several weeks. Symptoms of HBV infection include arthralgias, fatigue, anorexia, nausea, vomiting, fever, abdominal pain, clay-colored stools, dark urine, and jaundice. Approximately 5% of adults with HBV infection become chronically infected, and 15% to 25% of individuals with chronic HBV infection will die prematurely from liver cancer or cirrhosis (CDC, 2010e, 2011c).

Assessment

Components of the history to be obtained when hepatitis B is suspected include symptoms of the disease and risk factors. Physical examination includes inspection of the skin for rashes, inspection of the skin and conjunctiva for jaundice, and palpation of the liver for enlargement and tenderness. Weight loss, fever, and general debilitation should be noted.

Interpretation of test results for hepatitis B is complex (Table 21-16). Women who have negative HBsAg, anti-HBc, and anti-HBs tests are susceptible to infection, and vaccination should be considered (see the next section on management). A woman with a positive anti-HBs test with negative HBsAg and anti-HBc tests has immunity from vaccination. A woman with a negative HBsAg test and positive anti-HBc and anti-HBs tests has immunity from previous infection that is now resolved. A woman with acute hepatitis B infection will have positive HBsAg, anti-HBc, and IgM anti-HBc tests and a negative anti-HBs test. A woman with chronic hepatitis B infection will have positive HBsAg and anti-HBc tests and negative IgM anti-HBc and anti-HBs tests. A woman with a positive anti-HBc test and negative HBsAg and anti-HBs tests should be referred for further evaluation, as this result has multiple interpretations, including resolved infection, false-positive anti-HBc, low-level chronic infection, and resolving acute infection (CDC, 2011c).

Women who have hepatitis B should be prepared to undergo repeat testing, as HBV serologic markers may also be used to monitor the progression of the disease. Testing for other STIs, including HIV, should be performed.

Management

All nonimmune women at risk of hepatitis B should be informed of the existence of a hepatitis B vaccine. Vaccination is recommended for all individuals who have had more than one sex partner within the past 6 months as well as for anyone being evaluated or treated for an STI. In addition, all children younger than 19 years of age; injection-drug users; residents and staff of facilities for developmentally disabled persons; individuals who have a sexual partner or household contact who is HBsAg positive; individuals with end-stage renal disease, chronic liver disease, or HIV; persons whose occupation exposes them to blood or body fluids; travelers to areas with high rates of HBV infection; and anyone who wants protection from HBV infection should be vaccinated (CDC, 2010e). Multiple vaccinations are available, including one that protects against both the hepatitis B and hepatitis A viruses. Clinicians should consult current immunization schedules (http://www.cdc.gov/vaccines /recs/schedules/default.htm) and product information to determine the appropriate vaccine, dose, and frequency based on the patient's age; individual factors, such as immunocompromised status; and need to complete the vaccine series. The vaccine should be given in the deltoid muscle.

Women with a definite exposure to hepatitis B should be given hepatitis B immunoglobulin intramuscularly in a single dose as soon as possible, and preferably within 24 hours after exposure. There is no specific treatment for acute hepatitis B; recovery is usually spontaneous. Education about preventing transmission of HBV to others is paramount. Women with chronic HBV should be referred to a specialist.

Human Immunodeficiency Virus

In the early summer of 1981, the occurrence of several rare illnesses such as *Pneumocystis carinii* pneumonia, *Mycobacterium* and *M. intracellulare* infections, cryptosporidiosis, Kaposi's sarcoma, and non-Hodgkin's lymphoma in a cluster of gay and bisexual men represented a medical mystery that was solved by the identification of a single infectious agent that was destroying the immune system of infected persons—the human immunodeficiency virus (CDC, 1981). Although the earliest identified victims of the HIV/AIDS epidemic were typically homosexual men, symptoms of the syndrome were identified in a woman within two months of the earliest reports of the disease in men. Within the first year of the epidemic, female partners of hemophiliacs infected with HIV, women using injection drugs, and female partners in heterosexual relationships in poor countries, notably Haiti, were diagnosed with HIV/AIDS.

Deeply ingrained social and cultural forces that tend to devalue women, and particularly poor women of color, perpetuated the tendency for HIV and AIDS to be considered a "men's disease," and more specifically, a disease of homosexual men; as a consequence, this disease has typically been underdiagnosed in women. However, the rapid spread of HIV among women is indisputable, with the percentage of AIDS cases among U.S. women and female adolescents (age 13 and older) increasing from 7% in 1985 to 27% in 2007 (CDC, 2011e). One-fourth of the estimated 56,300 new cases of HIV in the United States in 2006 occurred in women (Hall et al., 2008). Black women are disproportionately affected by this disease, having an HIV incidence rate that is nearly 15 times as high as the rate in white women and nearly four times the rate in Hispanic/Latino women (CDC, 2008).

As of 2006, there were more than 275,000 women living with HIV in the United States. Most (72.4%) of these women acquired HIV through heterosexual contact. The remaining infections were attributed to injection-drug use (26.3%) or other factors, such as hemophilia, blood transfusion, or unreported or unknown transmission (CDC, 2008).

The Effect of HIV on the Immune System

The human immune system functions to protect the body from invasion by a variety of microbes and tumor cells. The immune system is composed of two arms: humoral immunity, involved with antibody production, and cellular immunity, effected largely through T-helper lymphocytes (also known as CD4 cells). Central components of the cellular arm of the immune system are macrophages and CD4 cells. HIV specifically targets CD4 cells, binding to the cell surface protein known as the CD4 receptor. The virus affects the cells in two ways: (1) the absolute numbers of these cells are depleted and (2) the function of the remaining cells is impaired, resulting in a gradual loss of immune function. Progressive depletion of CD4 cells in peripheral blood occurs with advancing HIV disease, and CD4 cell counts are used to estimate the cumulative immunologic damage caused by HIV (Anderson, 2005). If its course is unimpeded, HIV can destroy as many as 1 billion CD4 cells per day. In addition to its aggressive destruction, HIV is genetically highly variable, mutating with apparent ease.

HIV Transmission Issues Specific to Women

As noted earlier in this chapter, several factors increase women's risk for acquiring HIV. In addition to the anatomically driven susceptibility of the female genitalia, the integrity of the tissues of the lower genital tract influence HIV transmission risk. Trauma during intercourse, STI-related inflammation or cervicitis, and an STI lesion (e.g., HSV ulcer or syphilis chancre) increase susceptibility to HIV infection, as does any activity or condition that disrupts the tissues of the vagina.

HIV can also be transmitted through receptive oral sex with ejaculation. Any condition that interrupts the integrity of oral tissues, including periodontal disease, increases the risk of HIV transmission in this manner.

Women who have sex with women have a small risk of transmission, especially in sexual activities that may result in some level of vaginal trauma. However, clinicians must be careful not to assume that a woman is at very low risk for HIV because she has an expressed sexual preference for women. Lesbians may have a history of sexual intercourse with men or other risk factors for HIV infection.

Assessment

HIV Screening and Reporting The CDC now recommends HIV screening be a routine part of clinical care for patients aged 13 to 64 years in all healthcare settings (Branson et al., 2006). Patients presenting for STI treatment should be screened for HIV at each visit where they have new symptoms. Individuals at high risk for HIV should be tested for the presence of the virus at least once a year. Patients must be informed orally or in writing that HIV testing will be performed unless they decline (opt-out screening). Consent for HIV testing should be incorporated into the general consent for care. A separate consent form specific for HIV screening is not required or recommended (Branson et al.).

All 50 states collect HIV surveillance data using confidential name-based reporting standards. Some states offer only confidential testing, whereas others also offer anonymous testing (CDC, 2011d). State laws regarding HIV testing vary, and clinicians must be fully informed of regulations where they practice. The National HIV/AIDS Clinicians' Consultation Center maintains a compendium of state HIV testing laws that is a helpful reference for clinicians (http://www.nccc.ucsf.edu/consultation_library/state_hiv_testing_laws).

Diagnostic Tests HIV infection is diagnosed by testing for HIV antibodies in a person's blood or oral fluid. HIV screening is conducted with standard enzyme-linked immunosorbent assay (ELISA) or enzyme immunoassay (EIA) tests that are sent to a laboratory or with newer rapid HIV tests that can be performed at the point of care and yield results within minutes (Greenwald, Burstein, Pincus, & Branson, 2006). If the screening test is reactive, then a more specific confirmatory test such as the Western blot (WB) or an immunofluorescence assay (IFA) is conducted. Although a negative antibody test usually indicates that a person is not infected, these tests cannot detect a recent infection. A patient with a negative test who has known or suspected exposure to HIV should be retested at three months after the exposure.

Post-test Counseling The CDC recommendations no longer require prevention counseling as part of a screening program (Branson et al., 2006). Nevertheless, prevention counseling is strongly encouraged for patients who are seronegative for HIV but at risk for infection. Patients who are at high risk for HIV or who have known or suspected exposure to the virus should also be counseled about the need for repeat testing.

If a screening test is positive for HIV, the clinician must explain the need for confirmatory testing. If confirmatory testing is positive for HIV, the woman must be given time to react emotionally. She must assimilate a lot of information at the time of this visit. Allowing her to express her feelings prior to discussing issues related to partner notification, treatments, and other issues may allow her to take in some of the important information that must be conveyed at this time. Women with HIV must understand that although they may exhibit no signs or symptoms of HIV disease, they are still infectious, and will remain so for life. Basic information regarding minimizing transmission risk must be relayed to the patient at the time of diagnosis.

A plan for treatment must be established, which includes prompt referral to a clinician with HIV expertise. Unless the patient is clearly immunocompromised and in need of immediate treatment for opportunistic infection, there is likely to be an interval between diagnosis and treatment decisions. This time can be used by the woman to begin to adapt emotionally and psychologically to her diagnosis. She can make decisions about who must be told about her infection, and institute behaviors that are required of her to minimize the risk of transmitting the virus to others. Sensitive and nonjudgmental care at this time can assist the woman to make healthy accommodations in the face of her HIV diagnosis.

Management

Effective management and treatment of the patient with HIV involves the use of antiretroviral therapy (ART) to "reduce HIV-associated morbidity and prolong the duration and quality of survival, restore and preserve immunologic function, maximally and durably suppress plasma HIV viral load, and prevent HIV transmission" (Panel on Antiretroviral Guidelines for Adults and Adolescents, 2011, p. 24). Six classes of HIV ARTs exist:

- Nucleoside reverse transcriptase inhibitors (NRTIs)
- Nonnucleoside reverse transcriptase inhibitors (NNRTIs)
- Protease inhibitors (PIs)
- Fusion inhibitors (FIs)
- CCR5 antagonists
- Integrase strand transfer inhibitors (INSTIs)

Combination therapy with multiple ARTs is recommended (Panel on Antiretroviral Guidelines for Adults and Adolescents, 2011). Detailed treatment of HIV is beyond the scope of this chapter and is best provided by clinicians experienced in HIV management. Research and development activities directed toward new therapies and the testing of different combinations of therapies can quickly change the state of the science. The AIDSinfo website (www.aidsinfo.nih.gov) contains the most current recommendations for HIV/AIDS management. Clinicians with questions about HIV/AIDS management can contact the National HIV Telephone Consultation Service (Warmline) at 800-933-3413. This service is free of charge and available Monday through Friday from 8 a.m. to 8 p.m. Eastern time.

Clinicians providing gynecologic care to women with HIV must be aware of the fact that the infection may necessitate adjustments to the usual standards of care (American College of Obstetricians and Gynecologists, 2010a). For instance, HIV infection affects the recommendations for cervical cancer screening and management of abnormal Pap test results (American College of Obstetricians and Gynecologists; Wright et al., 2007). HIV infection and treatment must be also considered when a woman is choosing a contraceptive method (CDC, 2010f).

Women with HIV who develop vaginal infections and STIs may require different treatment regimens and follow-up (CDC, 2010e).

Very few diseases in history have been associated with the high levels of stigmatization that may accompany an HIV diagnosis. Many persons with HIV choose to keep their diagnosis a secret from family, friends, and coworkers. Although this decision means they must hide clinic visits, medications, and HIV-related illnesses, they may feel this course of action is preferable to experiencing the stigma that accompanies this diagnosis. Persons with HIV may face the dissolution of important relationships when and if the diagnosis becomes known. Clinicians can assist patients in identifying supportive persons who can be helpful as the patient adapts to the diagnosis and treatment.

Clinicians can help patients reframe their understanding of HIV, particularly in terms of understanding it as a chronic disease that can be managed, rather than as a terminal illness. Viewing HIV as a manageable illness, taking care of her physical and emotional health, staying connected with others in supportive relationships, and nurturing her spiritual well-being can assist the woman with HIV to regain a sense of control and hope (Barroso, 1999). Clinicians are in a unique position to understand the multiplicity of factors and issues that confront persons with HIV. Awareness of these factors can enhance health care by improving both the physical and mental health of patients, as well as the long-term health outcomes for women with HIV.

Sexually Transmitted Infections During Pregnancy

Perinatal outcomes can be affected by various STIs because pregnant women may transmit the infection to their fetus, newborn, or infant through vertical transmission (via the placenta, during vaginal birth, or after birth through breastfeeding) or horizontal transmission (close physical or household contact). Some STIs (e.g., syphilis) cross the placenta and infect the fetus in utero. Other STIs (e.g., gonorrhea, chlamydia, hepatitis B, and genital herpes) can be transmitted as the baby passes through the birth canal. HIV can cross the placenta during pregnancy, be transmitted during the birth process and, unlike most other STIs, can infect the infant during breastfeeding. The harmful effects of STIs may potentially include stillbirth, low birth weight, conjunctivitis, pneumonia, neonatal sepsis, neurologic damage, blindness, deafness, acute hepatitis, meningitis, chronic liver disease, and cirrhosis. Many of these problems can be prevented if the woman is screened and treated for STIs during pregnancy.

All pregnant women should be screened for HIV, syphilis, hepatitis B surface antigen, and *C. trachomatis* at the first prenatal visit. Women at risk for gonorrhea or hepatitis C should also be screened for these infections. Repeat testing for STIs later in pregnancy is warranted for some women. Clinicians should refer to the CDC treatment guidelines (2010e) and state laws for guidance. The treatment recommendations presented in this chapter are for women who are not pregnant. Because many STI treatment regimens differ during pregnancy, clinicians should consult the most current CDC treatment guidelines when caring for pregnant women.

Conclusion

STIs are among the most common health problems of women in the United States and around the world. Women experience a disproportionate amount of the burden associated with these illnesses, including complications of infertility, perinatal infections, poor pregnancy outcomes, chronic pelvic pain, genital tract neoplasms, and potentially death. Additionally, these infections interfere with a woman's lifestyle and cause considerable distress, both emotional and physical. Clinicians can help to ameliorate the misery, morbidity, and mortality associated with STIs and other common infections by providing accurate, safe, sensitive, and supportive care.

Knowledge of STIs is constantly increasing and changing, with new and improved prevention, diagnostic, and treatment modalities being developed and reported on an ongoing basis. All clinicians have a responsibility to stay up-to-date on these developments by reviewing journals, attending conferences, and being knowledgeable about recommendations and bulletins from the CDC. Furthermore, it is important that clinicians be aware of policies, recommendations, and guidelines of the state in which they practice, which also may change frequently.

References

Alan Guttmacher Institute. (2011). *Facts on American teens' sexual and reproductive health*. Retrieved from http://www.guttmacher.org/pubs/FB-ATSRH.html

American College of Obstetricians and Gynecologists. (2005, reaffirmed 2009). Human papillomavirus. ACOG Practice Bulletin No. 61. *Obstetrics & Gynecology, 105*, 905–918.

American College of Obstetricians and Gynecologists. (2010a). Gynecologic care for women with human immunodeficiency virus. ACOG Practice Bulletin No. 117. *Obstetrics & Gynecology, 116*, 1492–1509.

American College of Obstetricians and Gynecologists. (2010b). Human papillomavirus vaccination. Committee Opinion No. 467. *Obstetrics & Gynecology, 116*, 800–803.

American Society for Colposcopy and Cervical Pathology. (2009). *HPV genotyping clinical update*. Retrieved from http://www.asccp.org/Portals/9 /docs/pdfs/Consensus%20Guidelines/clinical _update_20090408.pdf

Anderson, J. R. (Ed.). (2005). *A guide to the clinical care of women with HIV*. Rockville, MD: U.S. Department of Health and Human Services, Health Resources and Service Administration, HIV/AIDS Bureau.

Atashili, J., Poole, C., Ndumbe, P. M., Adimora, A. A., & Smith, J. S. (2008). Bacterial vaginosis and HIV acquisition: A meta-analysis of published studies. *AIDS, 22*, 1493–1501.

Balch, J. F., & Balch, P. A. (1997). *Prescription for prevention* (2nd ed.). Garden City Park, NY: Avery.

Barroso, J. (1999). Long-term nonprogressors with HIV disease. *Nursing Research, 48*(5), 242–249.

Branson, B. M., Handsfield, H. H., Lampe, M. A., Janssen, R. S., Taylor, A. W., Lyss, S. B., et al. (2006). Revised recommendations for HIV testing of adults, adolescents, and pregnant women in health-care settings. *Morbidity and Mortality Weekly Report, 55*, 1–17.

Cates, J., Alexander, L., & Cates, W. J. (1998). Prevention of sexually transmitted diseases in an era of managed care: The relevance for women. *Women's Health Issues, 8*(3), 169–186.

Centers for Disease Control and Prevention (CDC). (1981). *Pneumocystis* pneumonia—Los Angeles. *Mortality and Morbidity Weekly Review, 30*, 250–252.

Centers for Disease Control and Prevention (CDC). (2008). Subpopulation estimates from the HIV incidence surveillance system—United States, 2006. *Morbidity and Mortality Weekly Report, 57*, 985–989.

Centers for Disease Control and Prevention (CDC). (2009). Surveillance for acute viral hepatitis—United States, 2007. *Morbidity and Mortality Weekly Report, 58*(SS-3), 1–27.

Centers for Disease Control and Prevention (CDC). (2010a). *Fact sheet: Genital HPV.* Retrieved from http://www.cdc.gov/std/hpv/hpv-fact-sheet.pdf

Centers for Disease Control and Prevention (CDC). (2010b). FDA licensure of bivalent human papillomavirus vaccine (HPV2, Cervarix) for use in females and updated HPV vaccination recommendations for the Advisory Committee on Immunization Practices (ACIP). *Morbidity and Mortality Weekly Report, 59,* 456–459.

Centers for Disease Control and Prevention (CDC). (2010c). Seroprevalence of herpes simplex virus type 2 among persons aged 14–49 years in the United States, 2005–2008. *Morbidity and Mortality Weekly Report, 59,* 626–629.

Centers for Disease Control and Prevention (CDC). (2010d). *Sexually transmitted disease surveillance 2009.* Atlanta, GA: U.S. Department of Health and Human Services. Retrieved from http://www.cdc.gov/std/stats09/default.htm

Centers for Disease Control and Prevention (CDC). (2010e). Sexually transmitted diseases treatment guidelines, 2010. *Mortality and Morbidity Weekly Report, 59*(RR-12), 1–110. Retrieved from http://www.cdc.gov/STD/treatment/2010/default.htm

Centers for Disease Control and Prevention (CDC). (2010f). U.S. medical eligibility criteria for contraceptive use, 2010: Adapted from the World Health Organization medical eligibility criteria for contraceptive use, 4th edition. *Morbidity and Mortality Weekly Report, 59,* 1–86.

Centers for Disease Control and Prevention (CDC). (2011a). CDC grand rounds: Chlamydia prevention: Challenges and strategies for reducing disease burden and sequelae. *Morbidity and Mortality Weekly Report, 60,* 370–373.

Centers for Disease Control and Prevention (CDC). (2011b). Cephalosporin susceptibility among *Neisseria gonorrhoeae* isolates—United States, 2000–2010. *Morbidity and Mortality Weekly Report, 60,* 873–877.

Centers for Disease Control and Prevention (CDC). (2011c). *Hepatitis B FAQs for health professionals.* Retrieved from http://www.cdc.gov/hepatitis/HBV/HBVfaq.htm

Centers for Disease Control and Prevention (CDC). (2011d). *HIV infection reporting.* Retrieved from http://www.cdc.gov/hiv/topics/surveillance/reporting.htm

Centers for Disease Control and Prevention (CDC). (2011e). *HIV surveillance in women.* Retrieved from http://www.cdc.gov/hiv/topics/surveillance/resources/slides/women/index.htm

Centers for Disease Control and Prevention (CDC). (2011f). *Nationally notifiable conditions.* Retrieved from http://www.cdc.gov/osels/ph_surveillance/nndss/phs/infdis.htm

Centers for Disease Control and Prevention (CDC). (2011g). *Syphilis (Treponema pallidum): 1996 case definition.* Retrieved from http://www.cdc.gov/osels/ph_surveillance/nndss/casedef/syphiliscurrent.htm

Cherpes, T. L., Meyn, L. A., Krohn, M. A., Lurie, J. G., & Hillier, S. L. (2003). Association between acquisition of herpes simplex virus type 2 in women and bacterial vaginosis. *Clinical Infectious Diseases, 37,* 319–325.

Collins-Bride, G. M., & Murphy, J. R. (2004). Genital herpes simplex virus. In W. L. Star, L. L. Lommel, & M. T. Shannon (Eds.), *Women's primary health care* (2nd ed.). San Francisco: UCSF Nursing Press.

Cummings, S., & Ullman, D. (1997). *Everybody's guide to homeopathic medicines.* New York: Putman.

Cunningham, F. G., Leveno, K. J., Bloom, S. L., Hauth, J. C., Rouse, D. J., & Spong, C. Y. (2010). *Williams obstetrics* (23rd ed.). New York: McGraw-Hill.

Dolcini, M., Coates, T. J., Catania, J. A., Kegeles, S. M., & Hauck, W. W. (1995). Multiple sexual partners and their psychosocial correlates: The population-based AIDS in multiethnic neighborhoods (AMEN) study. *Health Psychologist, 14*(2), 22–31.

Fogel, C. I. (1995). Sexually transmitted diseases. In C. I. Fogel & N. F. Woods (Eds.), *Women's health care.* Thousand Oaks, CA: Sage.

Freeman, E. E., Weiss, H. A., Glynn, J. R., Cross, P. L., Whitworth, J. A., & Hayes, R. J. (2006). Herpes simplex virus 2 infection increases HIV acquisition in men and women: Systematic review and meta-analysis of longitudinal studies. *AIDS, 20,* 73–83.

Greenwald, J. L., Burstein, G. R., Pincus, J., & Branson, B. (2006). A rapid review of rapid HIV antibody tests. *Current Infectious Disease Reports, 8,* 125–131.

Grella, C. E., Anglin, M. D., & Annon, J. J. (1996). HIV risk behaviors among women in methadone maintenance treatment. *Substance Abuse & Misuse, 31*(3), 277–301.

Griffith, H. W. (2000). *Healing herbs: The essential guide.* Tucson, AZ: Fisher Books.

Hall, H. I., Song, R., Rhodes, P., Prejean, J., An, Q., Lee, L. M., et al. (2008). Estimation of HIV incidence in the United States. *Journal of the American Medical Association, 300,* 520–529.

Harris, R. M., & Kavanagh, K. H. (1995). Perception of AIDS risk and high-risk behaviors among women in methadone maintenance treatment. *AIDS Education and Prevention, 7*(5), 415–428.

Institute of Medicine. (1997). *The hidden epidemic: Confronting sexually transmitted diseases.* Washington, DC: National Academy Press.

Kearney, M. H. (2001). *Perinatal impact of alcohol, tobacco and other drugs* (2nd ed.). White Plains, NY: Educational Services, March of Dimes.

Kent, M. E., & Romanelli, F. (2008). Reexamining syphilis: An update on epidemiology, clinical manifestations, and management. *Annals of Pharmacotherapy, 42,* 226–236.

Kurth, A. (1998). Promoting sexual health in the age of HIV/AIDS. *Journal of Nurse-Midwifery, 43*(3), 162–181.

Maman, S. C. (2000). The intersections of HIV and violence: Directions for future research and interventions. *Social Science & Medicine, 50,* 459–478.

Mays, V. M., & Cochran, S. D. (1988). Issues in the perception of AIDS risk and risk reduction activities by black and Hispanic/Latina women. *American Psychology, 43,* 949–957.

McFarlane, J., Parker, B., & Cross, B. (2001). *Abuse during pregnancy: A protocol for prevention and intervention* (2nd ed.). White Plains, NY: Educational Services, March of Dimes.

Miller, S., Exner, T. M., Williams, S. P., & Ehrhardt, A. A. (2000). A gender-specific intervention for at-risk women in the USA. *AIDS Care, 13*(3), 603–612.

Mize, S. J. S., Robinson, B. E., Bockting, W. O., & Scheltma, K. E. (2002). Meta-analysis of the effectiveness of HIV prevention interventions for women. *AIDS Care, 14*(2), 163–180.

Morrison, C. S., Turner, A. N., & Jones, L. B. (2009). Highly effective contraception and acquisition of HIV and other sexually transmitted infections. *Best Practice & Research: Clinical Obstetrics & Gynaecology, 23,* 263–284.

Munoz, N., Boxch, F. X., de Sanjose, S., Herrero, R., Castellsaque, X., Shah, K. V., et al. (2003). Epidemiologic classification of human papillomavirus types associated with cervical cancer. *New England Journal of Medicine, 348,* 518–527.

Nelson, A. L. (2007). Combined oral contraceptives. In R. A. Hatcher, J. Trussell, A. L. Nelson, W. Cates, F. Stewart, & D. Kowal (Eds.), *Contraceptive technology* (19th ed., pp. 193–270). New York: Ardent Media.

Ness, R. B., Soper, D. E., Holley, R. L., Peipert, J., Randall, H., Sweet, R. L., et al. (2002). Effectiveness of inpatient and outpatient treatment strategies for women with pelvic inflammatory disease: Results from the Pelvic Inflammatory Disease Evaluation and Clinical Health (PEACH) randomized trial. *American Journal of Obstetrics and Gynecology, 186,* 929–937.

Nissim, R. (1996). *Natural healing in gynecology: A manual for women.* San Francisco: HarperCollins.

Nyamanthi, A. M., & Lewis, C. E. (1991). Coping of African American women at risk for AIDS. *Women's Health Issues, 1*(2), 53–62.

Page, L. (2000). *Healthy healing* (11th ed.). Carmel Valley, CA: Healthy Healing.

Panel on Antiretroviral Guidelines for Adults and Adolescents. (2011). *Guidelines for the use of antiretroviral agents in HIV-1–infected adults and adolescents.* Retrieved from http://www.aidsinfo.nih.gov /ContentFiles/AdultandAdolescentGL.pdf

Perfect, M. M., Bourne, N., Ebel, C., & Rosenthal, S. L. (2005). Use of complementary and alternative medicine for treatment of genital herpes. *Herpes, 12,* 38–41.

Public Health Service. (1979). *Healthy people: The Surgeon General's report on health promotion and disease prevention.* Washington, DC: U.S. Government Printing Office.

Schmid, G. P. (2001). Epidemiology of sexually transmitted infections. In S. Faro & D. E. Soper (Eds.), *Infectious diseases in women.* Philadelphia: Saunders.

Sinclair, C. (2004). *A midwife's handbook.* St. Louis, MO: Saunders.

Singingtree, D. (1993). Herbal helps. *Midwifery Today, 26,* 16.

Soper, D. E. (2010). Pelvic inflammatory disease. *Obstetrics & Gynecology, 116,* 419–428.

Stapleton, H., & Tiran, D. (2000). Herbal medicine. In D. Tiran & S. Mack (Eds.), *Complementary therapies for pregnancy and childbirth* (2nd ed., pp. 105–128). Edinburgh, UK: Bailliere Tindall.

Star, W. (2004). Sexually transmitted diseases. In W. L. Star, L. L. Lommel, & M. T. Shannon (Eds.), *Women's primary health care* (2nd ed.). San Francisco: UCSF Nursing Press.

Star, W., & Deal, M. (2004a). Gonorrhea. In W. L. Star, L. L. Lommel, & M. T. Shannon (Eds.), *Women's primary health care* (2nd ed.). San Francisco: UCSF Nursing Press.

Star, W., & Deal, M. (2004b). Syphilis. In W. L. Star, L. L. Lommel, & M. T. Shannon (Eds.), *Women's primary health care* (2nd ed.). San Francisco: UCSF Nursing Press.

Sutton, M., Sternberg, M., Koumans, E. H., McQuillan, G., Berman, S., & Markowitz, L. (2007). The prevalence of *Trichomonas vaginalis* infection among reproductive-age women in the United States, 2001–2004. *Clinical Infectious Diseases, 45,* 1319–1326.

Sutton, M. Y., Sternberg, M., Zaidi, A., St. Louis, M. E., & Markowitz, L. E. (2005). Trends in pelvic inflammatory disease hospital discharges and ambulatory visits, United States, 1985–2001. *Sexually Transmitted Diseases, 32,* 778–784.

Wright, T. C., Massad, L. S., Dunton, C. J., Spitzer, M., Wilkinson, E. J., & Solomon, D., for the 2006 ASCCP-Sponsored Consensus Conference. (2007). 2006 consensus guidelines for the management of women with abnormal cervical screening tests. *Journal of Lower Genital Tract Disease, 11*(4), 201–222.

22

Urinary Tract Infection in Women

Mickey Gillmor-Kahn

U rinary tract infection (UTI) continues to be a major health problem for women world-wide. Bacteria ascend from the colonized urethra into the bladder and can continue to ascend into the kidneys. If left untreated, UTIs can cause lasting damage to the kidneys, severe morbidity, and even mortality. Few UTIs arrive through the bloodstream. Women are afflicted with UTIs much more often than men, owing to women's pelvic anatomy and shorter urethras.

Scope of the Problem

Clinicians who provide women's gynecologic health care will frequently diagnose and treat UTIs regardless of the type of healthcare setting. Half of all women have experienced a UTI by age 32 (Foxman & Brown, 2003). The burden of disease on women and on society is great. The Urologic Diseases in America Project (Litwin et al., 2005) found 6.8 million office or hospital outpatient clinic visits with a primary diagnosis of UTI in the United States in 2000. In addition, the researchers identified 1.3 million hospital emergency department visits and more than 245,000 hospital stays for UTI. Litwin et al. estimate a total expenditure of $2.5 billion related to UTI in 2000 alone. Whatever clinicians can do to treat UTI rapidly and inexpensively will reduce these burdens. Of course, prevention would be even better, but unfortunately knowledge of effective strategies for prevention remains in its infancy.

Etiology

Urinary tract infection requires a susceptible host and an active pathogen. At least 50% of UTIs in nonhospitalized women can be ascribed to *Escherichia coli* (Foxman & Brown, 2003).

In fact, some strains of *E. coli* are specifically adapted to growth in the bladder and, therefore, are designated as uropathogenic *E. coli*. In addition to *E. coli*, many other pathogens grow well in the bladder and can cause a symptomatic infection. These organisms include *Staphylococcus saprophyticus*, which may account for as many as 15% of UTIs (Foster, 2008); *Enterobacter* species; *Pseudomonas* species; and *Proteus mirabilis*. In addition to the presence of a uropathogen, the bladder epithelium must provide a hospitable environment for growth of the pathogen. There is reason to believe that part of that hospitable environment includes a genetic predisposition toward developing UTI.

Women's increased susceptibility to UTI derives from their anatomy. The female urethra is short; there is a short distance between the urethra and the anus; and the perineal environment is moist, encouraging migration of bacteria from the rectum to the urethra (Foxman & Brown, 2003). Women whose mothers have had frequent UTIs also seem to be more susceptible to these infections. **Box 22-1** lists risk factors for UTI.

Types of Urinary Tract Infections

Urinary tract infections can be divided into two general classifications: cystitis, a relatively simple infection involving only the urinary bladder, and upper tract infection or pyelonephritis, an infection involving one or both kidneys (see **Box 22-2**). Many women also experience transient asymptomatic bacteriuria that either may eventually lead to infection or may resolve on its own. Even symptomatic UTIs may spontaneously resolve without treatment, although several studies have found that outcome to be unlikely (Falagas, Kotsantis, Vouloumanou, & Rafailidis, 2009).

Cystitis

Acute bacterial cystitis is the most common type of UTI affecting women. Symptoms typically include dysuria with urinary frequency and urgency. Usually there is no fever, no costovertebral angle tenderness, and no flank pain. Uncomplicated cystitis occurs in a woman who is not pregnant, has not had any recent treatment with antibiotics, has not had another UTI in the last 6 months (or two UTIs in the last 12 months), has no decreased immunity due to other conditions, and has no signs of upper tract infection. Uncomplicated acute bacterial cystitis can be treated without a culture; in fact, it can be treated without a urinalysis in women who have had UTIs frequently in the past and have classic symptoms (American College of Obstetricians and Gynecologists, 2008, reaffirmed 2010).

Complicated bacterial cystitis occurs in women who are pregnant, have had recent antibiotics, have had another UTI within the last 6 months (or two other UTIs in the past 12 months), or have decreased immunity from another condition. These women require culture and sensitivity tests for diagnosis and to determine the appropriate treatment.

Asymptomatic bacteriuria, by definition, does not cause the patient to experience any symptoms, but a coincidental urinalysis shows bacteria in the urine. Treatment is not needed

---

BOX 22-1 *Possible Risk Factors for Urinary Tract Infection in Premenopausal and Postmenopausal Women*

Premenopausal Women
- Previous UTI
- Frequent, vigorous, or recent sexual activity
- Diaphragm contraceptive use
- Use of vaginal spermicidal agents
- Maternal history of UTI
- UTI as a child
- Diabetes mellitus
- Obesity
- Sickle cell trait
- Anatomic congenital abnormalities
- Urinary tract calculi
- Neurologic disorders or medical conditions requiring indwelling or repetitive bladder catheterization

Postmenopausal Women
- History of any previous UTI
- Diabetes
- Sexual activity
- Vaginal atrophy
- Incomplete bladder emptying
- Urinary incontinence
- Rectocele, cystocele, urethrocele, or uterovaginal prolapse
- ABO blood group non-secretor status

Sources: Adapted from American College of Obstetricians and Gynecologists, 2008, reaffirmed 2010; Wagenlehner, Weidner, & Naber, 2009.

BOX 22-2 *Types of Urinary Tract Infections*

Asymptomatic bacteruria: Bacteria present in the urine with no symptoms

Bacterial cystitis: Involves only the urinary bladder

- Uncomplicated
- Complicated

Pyelonephritis: Involves one or both kidneys

- Uncomplicated
- Complicated

---

unless the woman is pregnant. By the same token, screening of asymptomatic women who are not pregnant should be avoided (Gross & Patel, 2007; Nicolle, 2006).

Pyelonephritis

When infection in the bladder ascends to the kidneys, the patient has pyelonephritis. Some authors distinguish between pyelitis (an infection in the renal pelvis that does not extend into the parenchyma) and pyelonephritis (an infection extending into the renal parenchyma). This discussion here uses the term *pyelonephritis* for both conditions because they are impossible to differentiate clinically. Rarely, upper tract infection will arrive by descending through the bloodstream rather than ascending from the bladder. As in lower tract infection, upper UTI is most commonly the result of colonization with *E. coli*, although other organisms can also be involved (Ramakrishnan & Scheid, 2005).

Pyelonephritis is similarly divided into uncomplicated and complicated infections. Uncomplicated pyelonephritis occurs in a woman who has symptoms of upper tract infection, but is not pregnant and is not nauseated or vomiting. Most of these infections can be treated on an outpatient basis. Patients who are pregnant, vomiting, hypotensive, or immunodeficient should usually be hospitalized for treatment.

Good studies of the incidence of pyelonephritis, the organisms responsible for this type of UTI, the relative efficacy of inpatient and outpatient treatment, and epidemiology are all lacking (Foxman, Ki, & Brown, 2007). One epidemiologic study suggests that many cases of pyelonephritis are actually treated without culture, but this practice is not recommended (Czaja, Scholes, Hooton, & Stamm, 2007).

Symptoms of pyelonephritis typically include fever, chills, back pain, costovertebral angle tenderness, and flank pain. Some women will have dysuria, urinary frequency, and urgency as well. Occasionally, pyelonephritis will be silent until the patient presents with hypotension and even septic shock. Some patients experience nausea, vomiting, and/or diarrhea. Silent pyelonephritis should be considered in any woman who presents with illness and has a history of repeated UTI, especially if the UTI ascended to the kidneys. Untreated pyelonephritis may lead to kidney damage, including secondary hypertension and renal failure (Piccoli et al., 2008).

Assessment

History

Uncomplicated, nonrecurrent bacterial cystitis can be treated based on the patient's history alone; no laboratory testing is required. The clinician can diagnose by history alone in a reliable patient, as the differential diagnosis of uncomplicated UTI is brief. A report of nonrecurrent dysuria, frequency, and urgency is adequate to diagnose lower UTI. To rule out upper tract infection or a complicated UTI, other history must be elicited, however (see **Box 22-3**).

Physical Examination

Physical examination of the woman with urinary symptoms is useful primarily to rule out more complicated disease. Some women with simple UTI have suprapubic tenderness. Flank pain may be present, but usually is not with simple UTI. Its presence would raise the index of suspicion for pyelonephritis. Typically, the woman with pyelonephritis feels acutely ill. She may have fever, chills, nausea, vomiting, and costovertebral angle tenderness, as well

BOX 22-3 *Questions to Ask to Rule Out Complicated Cystitis and Upper Urinary Tract Infection*

1. Are you or could you be pregnant?
2. Have you had any fever or chills?
3. Do you have any flank pain or back pain?
4. Are you nauseated or have you vomited?
5. Have you ever had a bladder infection before? If so, when? How was it treated?
6. Have you taken any medicines recently? Antibiotics? Pain relievers? Over-the-counter products?
7. Do you have any other medical problems?
8. Do you take any medications on a regular basis?
9. Are you having any vaginal discharge or other vaginal problems?

as the symptoms of cystitis—namely, dysuria, frequency, urgency, and suprapubic pain (Ramakrishnan & Scheid, 2005).

Laboratory Testing

In the event that the clinician cannot rule out a complicated UTI or an upper tract infection by history alone, laboratory testing is necessary. Tools available include the urine dipstick, microscopic urinalysis, and urine culture with sensitivities. Each has its place in the diagnostic process.

The urine dipstick is an inexpensive screening tool that may be used to confirm the UTI diagnosis if the history is ambiguous. A concentrated first voided specimen is most reliable, but not always available. A dipstick that is positive for leukocyte esterase or nitrite is 75% sensitive and 82% specific for UTI (American College of Obstetricians and Gynecologists, 2008, reaffirmed 2010). Symptomatic women with a negative dipstick should have a microscopic urinalysis and/or a urine culture and sensitivity test because the dipstick may be falsely negative for a number of reasons—usually because the sample is too dilute.

Leukocyte esterase on dipstick indicates that leukocytes are present in the urine, but cannot determine whether the leukocytes came from the bladder or from the vagina. While clinicians have long requested a clean midstream voided sample, studies have found little difference in contamination from vaginal and perineal secretions between women who washed prior to voiding and those who did not (Blake & Doherty, 2006). Extensive teaching about perineal cleansing prior to collecting a midstream sample is not necessary. With this change in practice, it is possible to collect the first part of the urine stream to use in nucleic acid amplification testing (NAAT) or polymerase chain reaction (PCR) testing for gonorrhea and chlamydia, and the second midstream part for urine culture.

Nitrites are produced in the urine when bacteria present in the urine convert the normally present nitrates to nitrites. Although *E. coli*, the most common uropathogen, does

BOX 22-4 *Indications for a Urine Culture in a Woman with Urinary Tract Infection Symptoms*

- Pregnancy
- Signs of upper tract infection
- Recent urinary tract infection
- Recent antibiotic treatment
- Chronic disease affecting the immune system

convert nitrates to nitrites, not all uropathogens do so. Therefore, failure to identify nitrites on dipstick or urinalysis does not rule out a UTI.

Urine microscopy for the woman with pyelonephritis will usually reveal red blood cells, white blood cells, and white blood cell casts (**Color Plate 25**). Samples from patients with cystitis alone usually do not show casts.

Urine culture is the reference standard for diagnosis of a UTI. Sensitivities to antibiotics ascertained at the time of the culture will guide appropriate treatment. Culture and sensitivity tests are expensive and time-consuming, however, and empiric treatment should not be delayed to wait for these results. Urine culture is not needed for symptomatic women who meet the criteria for uncomplicated bacterial cystitis (American College of Obstetricians and Gynecologists, 2008, reaffirmed 2010); these patients can be treated based on history alone. **Box 22-4** lists indications for urine culture. Increasing concern about empiric treatment with antibiotics and the development of resistant uropathogens may mean that in the future urine culture or at least dipstick diagnosis will again be recommended prior to treatment (Wagenlehner, Weidner, & Naber, 2009).

A urine culture and sensitivity test is indicated in any woman with a complicated cystitis or symptoms of upper tract disease. Empiric treatment must be initiated prior to obtaining the culture and sensitivity results and then modified if the results indicate resistance or the patient is not improving. Blood cultures have not been shown to be useful unless the diagnosis is uncertain, the patient is immunocompromised, or there is evidence of descending infection from the blood to the kidney (American College of Obstetricians and Gynecologists, 2008, reaffirmed 2010).

Differential Diagnoses

The differential diagnosis of dysuria/urgency/frequency in women includes bacterial cystitis, pyelonephritis, interstitial cystitis/painful bladder syndrome, and urethritis related to a sexually transmitted infection—usually gonorrhea or chlamydia. The differential diagnosis for a woman with pyelonephritis symptoms should also include nephrolithiais. Usually fever associated with pyelonephritis will resolve within 72 hours of treatment with appropriate antibiotics. Failure to resolve may indicate abscess, obstruction, or a resistant organism.

Management

Cystitis

Antibiotic Treatment Treatment of an uncomplicated lower UTI will depend largely on resistance patterns in the community, if known, and on patient history and allergies. **Table 22-1** shows the treatment regimens recommended by the American College of Obstetricians and Gynecologists for an uncomplicated acute bacterial cystitis.

TABLE 22-1 Treatment Regimens for Uncomplicated Acute Bacterial Cystitis

Antimicrobial Agent	Dose	Adverse Events
Trimethoprim–sulfamethoxazole	One tablet (160 mg trimethoprim + 800 mg sulfamethoxazole), twice daily for 3 days	Fever, rash, photosensitivity, neutropenia, thrombocytopenia, anorexia, nausea and vomiting, pruritus, headache, urticaria, Stevens-Johnson syndrome, and toxic epidermal necrosis
Trimethoprim	100 mg, twice daily for 3 days	Rash, pruritus, photosensitivity, exfoliative dermatitis, Stevens-Johnson syndrome, toxic epidermal necrosis, and aseptic meningitis
Ciprofloxacin	250 mg, twice daily for 3 days	Rash, confusion, seizures, restlessness, headache, severe hypersensitivity, hypoglycemia, hyperglycemia, and Achilles tendon rupture (in patients older than 60 years)
Levofloxacin	250 mg, once daily for 3 days	Same as for ciprofloxacin
Norfloxacin	400 mg, twice daily for 3 days	Same as for ciprofloxacin
Gatifloxacin	200 mg, once daily for 3 days	Same as for ciprofloxacin
Nitrofurantoin macrocrystals	50–100 mg, four times daily for 7 days	Anorexia, nausea, vomiting, hypersensitivity, peripheral neuropathy, hepatitis, hemolytic anemia, and pulmonary reactions
Nitrofurantoin monohydrate macrocrystals	100 mg, twice daily for 7 days	Same as for nitrofurantoin macrocrystals
Fosfomycin tromethamine	3 g dose (powder) single dose	Diarrhea, nausea, vomiting, rash, and hypersensitivity

Source: Reprinted with permission from the American College of Obstetricians and Gynecologists, 2008, reaffirmed 2010.

Indiscriminate prescribing of antibiotics has led to resistance patterns in many communities. Given this fact, clinicians should consult infectious disease experts in their communities, if available, to become aware of the prevalence of resistance and alter prescribing as needed. Frequent review of these patterns is appropriate, because resistance changes over time. Whenever possible, however, clinicians should prescribe the least expensive and narrowest-spectrum drug to avoid increasing the problem of microbial resistance and to decrease costs for both patients and the health system (American College of Obstetricians and Gynecologists, 2008, reaffirmed 2010; Fihn, 2003; Gross & Patel, 2007).

Although 7-day treatment has been the norm in the past, research has shown equal effectiveness with 3-day regimens of many of these drugs; thus the latter regimens are now recommended (see Table 22-1). Over-prescribing leads to unnecessary costs to both the patient and the health system (American College of Obstetricians and Gynecologists, 2008, reaffirmed 2010; Kahan, Chinitz, & Kahan, 2004).

Treatment of Pain An acute UTI can be extremely painful and cause significant disruption in a woman's life. Symptoms should resolve within 72 hours of the initiation of antibiotic treatment. If they do not, the clinician must consider a change in therapy or another diagnosis. Some women will desire treatment of the dysuria for one or two days with phenazopyridine, which is now available in the United States on an over-the-counter basis. This drug will color the urine orange and is associated with numerous adverse effects, including gastrointestinal upset, headaches, rash, hemolysis in those with glucose-6-dehydrogenase deficiency, and nephrotoxicity (Fihn, 2003; Scheurer, 2006). Patients should be cautioned against chronic use of phenazopyridine. Those choosing to use this agent should also be made aware of the danger associated with its accidental ingestion by children (Gold & Bithoney, 2003).

Pyelonephritis

Uncomplicated pyelonephritis occurs in the woman who has clinical evidence of upper tract disease, but is not pregnant, is able to tolerate oral treatment, and has no concurrent conditions leading to immunocompromise. Most authorities agree that uncomplicated pyelonephritis may be treated on an outpatient basis if the woman is likely to be able to complete outpatient treatment and is able to return for follow-up. Treatment for 10 to 14 days is recommended, usually with a fluoroquinolone if resistance to this antibiotic does not exceed 10% in the community (American College of Obstetricians and Gynecologists, 2008, reaffirmed 2010; Ramakrishnan & Scheid, 2005; Wagenlehner et al., 2009). Knowledge of local patterns of resistance should guide initial treatment, followed by evaluation of treatment results and the culture and sensitivity test. Severely ill women with pyelonephritis may need hospitalization to receive parenteral antibiotics. Piccoli et al. (2006), in an extensive review of randomized controlled trials of pyelonephritis treatment, found little solid evidence for determining what the ideal length of treatment is, which drugs are better, or even whether renal scarring post pyelonephritis results in negative long-term effects.

Hospitalization is appropriate when parenteral treatment is needed, other conditions warrant increased surveillance, or the woman is unable to manage an outpatient regimen (Wagenlehner et al., 2009); **Box 22-5** summarizes these criteria. Decisions about hospitalization for pregnant women will depend on the woman's social support, age, and degree of illness. Most clinicians prefer at least a brief period of hospitalized observation while initial doses or parenteral antibiotics are given to the pregnant woman, along with monitoring for preterm contractions and respiratory sufficiency. Daily prophylaxis with nitrofurantoin throughout the remainder of the pregnancy may be appropriate (Hill, Sheffield, McIntire, & Wendel, 2005).

Patient Education

Clinicians treating women with UTIs can share with them what is known and unknown about prevention of UTIs. While forcing fluids is not recommended, drinking to alleviate thirst can be helpful as well as not delaying voiding. The importance of completing the treatment regimen even if symptoms resolve before all medications are taken should be emphasized to avoid the development of resistant organisms. Most importantly, a woman who has been diagnosed with a UTI should be advised to contact the clinician if her symptoms persist after 48 hours of antibiotic treatment.

Prevention

Many women suffer frequent UTIs. In fact, as many as 20% to 30% of women with a UTI will have at least one additional infection within 12 months (Albert et al., 2004). Risk factors for UTI should be investigated and altered where that is possible. Recurrent UTI is defined as three or more UTIs in a 12-month period (Albert et al.).

Clinicians and the lay public have promoted many recommendations regarding how to avoid a UTI, but there is little evidence that most of them are effective. Increasing fluids, wiping front to back, and avoidance of delayed urination have not been adequately studied. These simple measures will, no doubt, still be recommended by many clinicians, because they make empiric sense and are inexpensive. Aggressive hydration could, however, be harmful if

---

BOX 22-5 *Indications for Hospitalizing a Woman with Pyelonephritis*

- Severe illness
- Pregnancy—at least for observation, to rule out preterm labor
- Immunocompromise
- Inability to tolerate oral treatment due to vomiting
- Inability to comply with oral treatment or return for follow-up due to age, living situation, or lack of social support

large volumes of urine encourage retrograde flow into the ureters. Similarly, no studies have demonstrated the efficacy of postcoital voiding in women whose UTIs appear to be associated with sexual activity (Fihn, 2003).

Most UTIs derive from intestinal and/or vaginal bacteria. On the theory that ingestion of lactobacilli could potentially change the flora of the intestine or the vagina, various forms of lactobacilli have been suggested as a preventive measure. The use of lactobacilli vaginal suppositories has been studied in several small randomized, controlled trials. In one study, no preventive effect was demonstrated (Barrons & Tassone, 2008). In another study, ingestion of a probiotic beverage (a cultured milk product) was compared to cranberry/lingonberry juice and to placebo; no UTI preventive effect was found with the probiotic beverage (Kontiokari et al., 2001).

The use of cranberry products, by comparison, has some solid research behind it. The previously mentioned study by Kontiokari et al. (2001) found a relationship between ingestion of cranberry/lingonberry juice and a reduction in recurrent UTIs compared to controls and compared to those subjects drinking the probiotic beverage. Other studies have confirmed the association between ingestion of cranberry products and decreased rates of UTIs (Dugoua, Seely, Perri, Mills, & Koren, 2008; Jepson & Craig, 2008). Cranberry products contain several substances that may help to prevent UTIs. Early theories focused on the conversion of quinic acid in the cranberries to hippuric acid, which would then inhibit growth of bacteria. Measurement of the levels of hippuric acid in the bladder after ingestion of cranberry does not bear out this theory, however. Current theories suggest that the fructose in cranberries keeps *E. coli* from adhering to the bladder cell walls or that substances called proanthrocyanidins do the same by a different process. In vitro studies have demonstrated inhibition of *E. coli* attachment for both fructose and proanthrocyanidins (Jepson & Craig).

Antibiotic prophylaxis has been studied in the form of a number of different regimens. Single-dose postcoital antibiotics may be helpful for women who find an association between sexual activity and UTIs. Trimethoprim–sulfamethoxazole (TMP/SMX), trimethoprim alone, nitrofurantoin, and a fluoroquinolone have all been shown to be effective for this purpose. Alternatively, continuous prophylaxis with nitrofurantoin, TMP/SMX, or a fluoroquinolone decreases recurrence rates. Some women will prefer to self-initiate a 3-day course of treatment only if symptoms develop. Concerns regarding resistance patterns and the promotion of increased resistance as previously described for acute treatment apply equally to prophylactic uses of these drugs. Additionally, concerns have been raised about the use of sulfonamides in early pregnancy.

Special Considerations

Adolescents

Because of the association between sexual activity and UTI, a UTI in a teenager may indicate the initiation of sexual activity. A discussion of pregnancy risk and sexually transmitted infection prevention is appropriate. Whether an adolescent with pyelonephritis needs to be hospitalized will depend on the clinician's judgment of whether she will be able to comply with outpatient treatment.

Postmenopausal Women

The strongest predictor of UTI in a study of postmenopausal women was premenopausal lifetime history of more than six UTIs (Jackson et al., 2004). Although one early study (Raz & Stamm, 1993) showed a decreased incidence with intravaginal estrogen treatments, this finding has not been verified in subsequent studies (Jackson et al., 2004)

Pregnant Women

Anatomic and physiologic changes related to pregnancy place the pregnant woman at increased risk of UTI, including pyelonephritis. In addition, UTI increases the risk of pre-term labor (Nicolle, 2006). For this reason, a urine culture is recommended for all women at the first prenatal visit, regardless of symptoms, and bacteriuria should be treated whether symptomatic or not (Hill et al., 2005). Many clinicians will choose to hospitalize the pregnant woman with pyelonephritis to monitor for preterm labor and assure adequate treatment.

Influences of Culture

Women in professions where frequent urination is impeded have higher rates of UTIs. Nurses, teachers, and factory workers where voiding on demand is restricted or difficult are all susceptible to such infections, for example. Education about the need for voiding when the urge is present can decrease the incidence of UTIs in these women. They should also be cautioned against limiting fluids to decrease the need to urinate. Some who have worked under these conditions for a long time will no longer feel a need to urinate until the bladder is already overdistended. For them, timed voiding may be helpful in reestablishing normal bladder responsivity (Su, Wang, Lu, & Guo, 2006).

References

Albert, X., Huertas, I., Pereiró, I. I., Sanfélix, J., Gosalbes, V., & Perrota, C. (2004). Antibiotics for preventing recurrent urinary tract infection in non-pregnant women. *Database of Systematic Reviews, 3*, CD001209. doi: 10.1002/14651858.CD001209.pub2

American College of Obstetricians and Gynecologists. (2008, reaffirmed 2010). ACOG Practice Bulletin No. 91: Treatment of urinary tract infections in nonpregnant women. *Obstetrics & Gynecology, 111*, 785–794.

Barrons, R., & Tassone, D. (2008). Use of *Lactobacillus* probiotics for bacterial genitourinary infections in women: A review. *Clinical Therapeutics, 30*(3), 453–468. doi: 10.1016/j.clinthera.2008.03.013

Blake, D. R., & Doherty, L. F. (2006). Effect of perineal cleansing on contamination rate of mid-stream urine culture. *Journal of Pediatric & Adolescent Gynecology, 19*(1), 31–34. doi: 10.1016/j.jpag.2005.11.003

Czaja, C. A., Scholes, D., Hooton, T. M., & Stamm, W. E. (2007). Population-based epidemiologic analysis of acute pyelonephritis. *Clinical Infectious Diseases, 45*(3), 273–280. doi: 10.1086/519268

Dugoua, J., Seely, D., Perri, D., Mills, E., & Koren, G. (2008). Safety and efficacy of cranberry (*Vaccinium macrocarpon*) during pregnancy and lactation. *Canadian Journal of Clinical Pharmacology, 15*(1), e80–e86.

Falagas, M. E., Kotsantis, I. K., Vouloumanou, E. K., & Rafailidis, P. I. (2009). Antibiotics versus placebo in the treatment of women with uncomplicated cystitis: A meta-analysis of randomized controlled trials. *Journal of Infection, 58*, 91–102. doi: 10.1016/j.jinf.2008.12.009

Fihn, S. D. (2003). Clinical practice: Acute uncomplicated urinary tract infection in women. *New England Journal of Medicine, 349*, 259–266. doi: 10.1056/NEJMcp030027

Foster, R. T. (2008). Uncomplicated urinary tract infections in women. *Obstetrics and Gynecology Clinics of North America, 38*, 235–248. doi: 10.1016/j.ogc.2008.03.003

Foxman, B., & Brown, P. (2003). Epidemiology of urinary tract infections: Transmission and risk factors, incidence, and costs. *Infectious Disease Clinics of North America, 17*(2), 227–241. doi: 10.1016/S0891-5520(03)00005-9

Foxman, B., Ki, M., & Brown, P. (2007). Antibiotic resistance and pyelonephritis. *Clinical Infectious Diseases, 45*(3), 281–283. doi: 10.1086/519267

Gold, N. A., & Bithoney, W. G. (2003). Methemoglobinemia due to ingestion of at most three pills of pyridium in a 2-year-old: Case report and review. *Journal of Emergency Medicine, 25*(2), 143–148. doi: 10.1016/S0736-4679(03)00162-8

Gross, P. A., & Patel, B. (2007). Reducing antibiotic overuse: A call for a national performance measure for not treating asymptomatic bacteriuria. *Clinical Infectious Diseases, 45*(10), 1335–1337. doi: 10.1086/522183; PMid:17968830

Hill, J. B., Sheffield, J. S., McIntire, D. D., & Wendel, G. D. (2005). Acute pyelonephritis in pregnancy. *Obstetrics & Gynecology, 105*(1), 18–23.

Jackson, S. L., Boyko, E. J., Scholes, D., Abraham, L., Gupta, K., & Fihn, S. D. (2004). Predictors of urinary tract infection after menopause: A prospective study. *American Journal of Medicine, 117*, 903–911.

Jepson, R. G., & Craig, J. C. (2008). Cranberries for preventing urinary tract infections. *Cochrane Database of Systematic Reviews, 1*, CD001321. doi: 10.1002/14651858.CD001321.pub4

Kahan, N. R., Chinitz, D. P., & Kahan, E. (2004). Longer than recommended empiric antibiotic treatment of urinary tract infection in women: An avoidable

waste of money. *Journal of Clinical Pharmacology & Therapeutics, 29*(1), 59–63. doi: 10.1111/j.1365-2710.2003.00537.x

Kontiokari, T., Sundqvist, K., Nuutinen, M., Pokka, T., Koskela, M., & Uhari, M. (2001). Randomised trial of cranberry–lingonberry juice and *Lactobacillus* GG drink for the prevention of urinary tract infections in women. *British Medical Journal, 322*(7302), 1571. doi: 10.1136/bmj.322.7302.1571

Litwin, M. S., Saigal, C. S., Yano, E. M., Avila, C., Geschwind, S. A., Hanley, J. M., … Wang, M. (2005). Urologic Diseases in America Project: Analytical methods and principal findings. *Journal of Urology, 173*, 933–937. doi: 10.1097/01.ju.0000152365.43125.3b

Nicolle, L. E. (2006). Asymptomatic bacteriuria: Review and discussion of the IDSA guidelines. *International Journal of Antimicrobial Agents, 28S*, S42–S48. doi: 10.1016/j.ijantimicag.2006.05.010

Piccoli, B. G., Cresto, E., Ragni, F., Veglio, V., Scarpa, R. M., & Frascisco, M. (2008). The clinical spectrum of acute "uncomplicated" pyelonephritis from an emergency medicine perspective. *International Journal of Antimicrobial Agents, 31*(suppl 1), S46–S53. doi: 10.1016/j.ijantimicag.2007.09.017

Piccoli, G. B., Consiglio, V., Colla, L., Mesiano, P., Magnano, A., Burdese, M., … Piccoli, G. (2006). Antibiotic treatment for acute "uncomplicated" or "primary" pyelonephritis: A systematic, "semantic revision." *International Journal of Antimicrobial Agents, 28S*, S49–S63. doi: 10.1016/j.ijantimicag.2006.05.017

Ramakrishnan, K., & Scheid, D. C. (2005). Diagnosis and management of acute pyelonephritis in adults. *American Family Physician, 71*, 933–942.

Raz, R., & Stamm, W. E. (1993). A controlled trial of intravaginal estriol in postmenopausal women with recurrent urinary tract infections. *New England Journal of Medicine*, 753–756. doi: 10.1056/NEJM199309093291102

Scheurer, D. B. (2006). An over-the-counter omission. *Southern Medical Journal, 99*, 1005–1006. doi: 10.1097/01.smj.0000215641.58901.4c

Su, S., Wang, J., Lu, C., & Guo, H. (2006). Reducing urinary tract infections among female clean room workers. *Journal of Women's Health, 15*, 870–876. doi: 10.1089/jwh.2006.15.870

Wagenlehner, M. E., Weidner, W., & Naber, K. G. (2009). An update on uncomplicated urinary tract infections in women. *Current Opinion in Urology, 19*, 368–374. doi: 10.1097/MOU.0b013e32832ae18c

23

Urinary Incontinence

Sandra H. Hines
Janis M. Miller

The International Continence Society defines urinary incontinence (UI) as "the complaint of any involuntary leakage of urine" (Abrams et al., 2002, p. 168). Other experts define UI as the involuntary leakage of urine, regardless of whether the patient reports symptoms (Wallner et al., 2009). Sampselle, Palmer, Boyington, O'Dell, and Wooldridge (2004) observed that the prevalence of UI is stable until age 50 but increases steadily with age: As many as 40% of women 70 years of age and older experience symptoms of UI. However, the prevalence rates may actually be underreported because of the belief that UI is not a socially acceptable health problem; as a consequence, some women may be too embarrassed to discuss their concerns with their clinician. Many women mistakenly view UI as a normal occurrence that accompanies increasing age or results from childbirth. The development of chronic UI may occur gradually over time, and this factor probably contributes to women normalizing it. This normalization may be supported by well-meaning comments from clinicians as well as friends and family.

The experience of UI may also be associated with feelings of anxiety and social withdrawal. It is important for clinicians to routinely inquire about UI in women of all ages because women may not initiate this discussion unless prompted. Early identification may help thwart the negative effects UI has on women's lives. It is important for the clinician to elucidate which type of leakage is of greatest concern to the woman, such as urgency symptoms versus the occasional leakage with a sneeze, as well as her desire for treatment. UI might be accurately viewed as a concern or symptom rather than a specific pathophysiology.

Anatomy

Understanding UI requires an understanding of the pelvic structures and their relationship to one another. Bladder pressure must be lower than urethral pressure to maintain continence. In simple terms, the bladder is a reservoir, functioning as a low-pressure holding tank nearly 24 hours per day, with reversal to high-pressure emptying during only a few minutes of each day. The urethra forms a tight seal of high pressure against the urine-filled reservoir; this seal relaxes during voiding. There is also a reinforcing gate system: the levator ani muscle, which adds additional holding pressure against the outflow of urine by supporting the urethra and bladder neck from below. When conditions of high load or intra-abdominal pressure occur, the levator ani forms a resistive plate onto which the urethra compresses, thereby closing in response to downward forces. The interrelationship among these structures is represented in the continence equation presented in **Figure 23-1** and detailed in the anatomic sketch in **Figure 23-2**.

The Urinary Bladder: The Reservoir

The female urinary bladder is a muscular reservoir located within the pelvic cavity that is situated posterior to the symphysis pubis and anterior to the uterus and vagina. As the bladder fills, it expands toward the surrounding organs, taking on the shape created by the pressure of surrounding structures. Therefore, an enlarged uterus (as during pregnancy) and feces in the rectum both affect the shape of and pressure on the urinary bladder.

The wall of the urinary bladder contains the detrusor muscle, which is composed of smooth muscle fibers. When contracted, this muscle increases pressure within the bladder, reduces the size of the bladder, and forces urine into the urethra preparatory to expelling it from the body.

The urinary bladder floor contains a funnel-shaped opening called the bladder neck, which opens into the urethra (Shier, Butler, & Lewis, 2004). The neck of the bladder is sometimes referred to as the urethral sphincter or proximal sphincteric mechanism because it is the site where the funnel narrows to become the urethra. It is a common misperception that there is a circular ring of muscle at the bladder neck. In reality, the narrowing depends on adequate proximal distribution of circumferential urethral striated muscle (Perucchini, DeLancey, Ashton-Miller, Peschers, & Kataria, 2002).

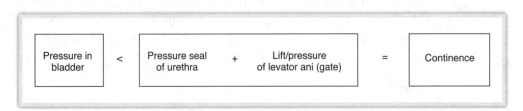

FIGURE 23-1 Continence equation.

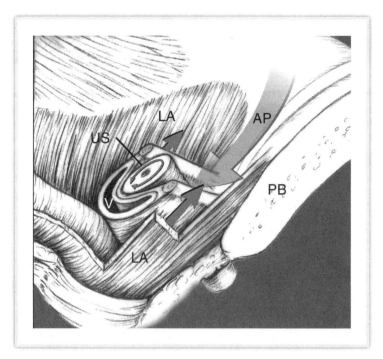

FIGURE 23-2 Interrelationship of pelvic structures to achieve continence. LA = levator ani, US = urethral sphincter, V = vagina, PB = pubic bone, AP = abdominal pressure

Source: © DeLancey, 2004. Used with permission.

The Urethra: The Seal

The urethra is a small tube beginning at the urinary bladder and ending at the urinary meatus. In adult women, the urethra is approximately 3.0 to 3.6 cm in length (Krantz, 1950). The most proximal 20% of the urethra is made up of smooth, involuntary muscles that transition with the smooth muscle of the bladder wall. The next 60% of the urethra includes both smooth muscle and circumferential, striated muscles called the urethrovaginal sphincter and compressor urethra muscles. The latter striated muscle structures are under voluntary control (Miller, Umek, DeLancey, & Ashton-Miller, 2004). The most distal 20% of the urethra, ending at the urinary meatus, has minimal impact on continence. For adequate resistant urethral closure pressure to occur, there must be coaptation ability (stickiness) of the mucosal inner lining, adequate tissue fullness from intravascular pressure, and both smooth and striated functional muscle structures. Adequate support from fibrous attachment and underlying muscle is also required.

The Pelvic Floor Structure: The Support Gate

The urethra rests on the anterior vaginal wall. This wall is supported by the levator ani muscle (Ashton-Miller, Howard, & DeLancey, 2001; DeLancey, 1990; Sampselle & DeLancey, 1998), which is commonly referred to as the pelvic floor or Kegel muscle. The levator ani actually consists of a group of muscles that, when contracted, stabilize and lift the rectum, vagina, and urethra in an anterior direction. The key band of support for the urethra is the most anterior portion of the levator ani, which is connected to the superior aspect of the pubic bone (Lien, Mooney, DeLancey, & Ashton-Miller, 2004). The arcus tendineus—a fibrous band extending from the pubic bone ventrally to the ischial spines dorsally—is a source of attachment for muscles making up the levator ani. With firm attachment, this group of muscles provides a shelf of support preventing prolapse of the pelvic organs.

The most superficial structural layer of tissue affecting continence is made up of the perineal membrane. This triangular fibrous complex attaches the perineal body to the pubic symphysis anteriorly and serves to support the pelvic organs during defecation, urination, and birth, when the levator ani muscle must relax.

To achieve urinary continence, the body must both maintain support of the vesicle neck and use the closure pressure of the urethral sphincteric mechanisms and the support of the levator gate mechanism. The closure pressure within the urethra must exceed the intra-abdominal pressure to avoid leakage of urine. Maintaining the high position of the bladder neck is important during a cough or sneeze because the increase in intra-abdominal pressure exerted during this action actually helps compress the urethra and maintain continence when a firm support exists beneath it. In contrast, when the bladder is allowed to descend, the internal sphincter is pulled open and closure pressure to the urethra during a cough or sneeze is compromised. When the detrusor muscle contraction overcomes the urethral pressure, voiding or leakage occurs.

Another component of the continence mechanism involves the innervation of the muscles. Without adequate innervation, the detrusor muscle is triggered when it should not be, or the strength and speed of the contraction in the urethral and levator muscles may be inadequate so that unwanted urine loss results. Although healthy components of the continence mechanism may compensate for injured or weaker ones, the continence mechanism is most effective when all components effectively function together.

Contributing Factors in Urinary Incontinence

Urinary incontinence occurs for a number of reasons and is classified according to the precipitating event or mechanism. The International Continence Society emphasizes the importance of fully assessing UI relative to "type, frequency, severity, precipitating factors, social impact, effect on hygiene and quality of life, the measures used to contain the leakage, and whether or not the individual seeks or desires help" (Abrams et al., 2002, p. 168). The following sections identify factors that are important to consider when caring for women with UI.

Fluid Intake

Fluid intake—both amount and type—may contribute to UI. Some women will limit fluids when UI is a concern; however, this practice may cause bladder irritation from overly concentrated urine, which increases the urge to urinate and raises the risk for UI. Drinking large amounts of fluids also is provocative, as it places an unnecessary overload on the bladder that results in either frequency or leakage.

High intake of particular types of fluids, such as caffeinated beverages, may worsen symptoms of UI, although data are inconclusive regarding this proposed mechanism. It is possible that volume is the key contributor. Women who experience UI are advised to eliminate caffeine intake to determine its effect on their symptoms (Gray, 2000). Similarly, alcoholic beverages, decaffeinated coffee or tea, carbonated beverages, and artificial sweeteners may play a role in urgency and frequency symptoms either because volume is high or because an unidentified ingredient may cause detrusor triggering.

Constipation

The accumulation of stool in the rectum may alter the position of the pelvic organs and press on the bladder, thereby reducing its capacity to hold urine. Severe limitation of fluids may contribute to constipation. Fiber in the diet helps prevent constipation and decreases symptoms of UI caused by constipation. In a systematic review of the literature, researchers found that the relationship between constipation and UI is inconclusive and warrants further investigation (Ostaszkiewicz, Ski, & Hornby, 2005)

Habitual Preventive Emptying

Habitual preventive emptying of the bladder may result in training the bladder to hold only small amounts of urine. Some women empty their bladders on initial urge or whenever a toilet is available. This practice can lead to urge sensations at increasingly lower bladder volumes. A recommended interval target between urinations is three to four hours (Sampselle et al., 1997). Women who drink very large amounts of fluid may need to reduce their fluid intake to achieve this interval. Women who have habitually emptied more frequently may have to gradually retrain their bladders to achieve normative capacity. Bladder retraining is covered in more detail later in this chapter.

Familial or Racial Incidence

Women reporting UI have a greater likelihood of having at least one immediate family member who also has UI (Giovanni, Bergman, & Dye, 2002). Racial and ethnic differences have been identified in incidence and types of UI in middle-aged and older women. For example, Sze, Jones, Ferguson, Barker, and Dolezal (2002) found Euro-American women reported UI at a significantly higher rate than African American or Hispanic women (41% compared to 31% and 30%, respectively). In contrast, Thom et al. (2006) found the highest rates of both stress and urge UI among Hispanic women. Fenner et al. (2008) compared African American and Euro-Caucasian women in an epidemiology study of women living in lower Michigan. By race, urinary incontinence prevalence was 14.6% for African American women and 33.1% for white women. Both Thom et al. (2006) and Fenner et al. (2008) found that a larger proportion of Euro-Caucasian women with incontinence reported symptoms of pure stress incontinence compared to African American women (25.0%), whereas a larger proportion of African American women reported symptoms of pure urge incontinence compared to Euro-Caucasian women.

Age

Age-related anatomic changes may be a factor in the development of UI. Striated muscle takes longer to develop force and attains a lower maximum force as an individual ages (Ashton-Miller et al., 2001). In addition, a significant decline in the number and density of urethral striated muscle fibers is observed with increasing age (Perucchini et al., 2002).

Urge UI has been identified as a significant independent risk factor for falls in women aged 75 to 86 years. In one study, urge UI increased the odds of a fall by 1.75. The exact mechanism underlying this relationship is unclear; however, a focus on trying to prevent urine leakage may distract a woman's attention from obstacles that might lead to a fall (Teo, Briffa, Devine, Dhaliwal, & Prince, 2006).

Pregnancy and Childbirth

Pregnancy, childbirth, and increased parity have long been associated with UI. Studies demonstrate the prevalence of UI in nulliparous women is lower than the prevalence in parous women (Fenner et al., 2008; Hunskaar et al., 2000; Jolleys, 1988; Sampselle, Harlow, Skurnick, Brubaker, & Bondarenko, 2002). The tendency toward urinary incontinence during pregnancy increases as the fetal size increases; following birth, however, most women experience resolution of UI symptoms over the first year postpartum (Chaliha, Kalia, Stanton, Monga, & Sultan, 1999; Sampselle et al., 1998).

The role of childbirth as a predisposing factor to UI may be related to loss of support to pelvic structures or damage to structures during the birthing process, although the data are not conclusive and prospective trials are needed to confirm this hypothesis (DeLancey, Kearney, Chou, Speights, & Binno, 2003; DeLancey et al., 2007). Some evidence indicates that strength of the pelvic muscle contraction decreases following a vaginal birth (Sampselle, 1990; Sampselle et al., 1998). Childbirth classes frequently emphasize the importance of practicing pelvic muscle exercises during pregnancy. In their study, Sampselle et al. (1998) report that primiparous women who practiced pelvic muscle exercises during pregnancy and on a postpartum basis experienced earlier recovery from symptoms of UI compared to those in the control group.

Body Mass Index

Women's risk of developing UI of all types increases with increasing body mass index (BMI) (Townsend et al., 2007; Waetjen et al., 2008). Townsend et al. (2007) found that women with a BMI of 35 or greater were more than twice as likely to experience at least monthly UI compared with women whose BMI was in the range of 21 to 22.9 kg/m². The development of UI also increased with adult weight gain. Women who gained approximately 5.1 to 10 kg after early adulthood were 1.44 times more likely to experience at least weekly UI compared to women who maintained their weight within 2 kg. Women who gained 30 kg after early adulthood were 4.04 times more likely to experience at least weekly UI (Townsend et al.). One study found a 5% to 10% weight loss in women with a BMI in the range of 25 to 45 to be as effective as other nonsurgical treatments for UI (Subak et al., 2005).

Comorbidities

Risk for UI development increases with comorbid conditions. For example, childhood enuresis, fecal incontinence, and other bowel problems are all associated with UI. Women who smoke cigarettes, whether currently or in the past, have a higher risk of experiencing UI. Additionally, many medications are associated with UI, such as diuretics, estrogen, benzodiazepines, tranquilizers, antidepressants, hypnotics, laxatives, and antibiotics. Specific health conditions associated with UI include diabetes, stroke, hypertension, cognitive impairment, Parkinson's disease, arthritis, back problems, and hearing and visual impairments. Functional impairment is also associated with UI (Holroyd-Leduc & Straus, 2004).

Female UI has been associated with major depressive disorders, which suggests that women with UI should be screened for depression and offered treatment (Fitzgerald, Link, Litman, Travison, & McKinaly, 2007; Melville, Delancy, Newton, & Katon, 2005; Vigod & Stewart, 2006). Some authors have suggested this convergence of symptoms directs clinicians to find medical treatment to address both conditions concurrently (Thor, Kirby, & Viktrup, 2007).

Assessment

Because of the comorbid nature of UI, full assessment and therapeutic plans for UI may require collaboration with numerous healthcare professionals. Scope and standards of practice for nurses and other clinicians working with patients diagnosed with UI have been defined by the Society of Urologic Nurses and Associates (SUNA, 1997).

The first step in assessment is helping women to identify and discuss their UI. A long-standing screening questionnaire has just two questions: "How often do you experience urinary leakage?" and "How much urine do you lose each time?" (Sandvik et al., 1993). Answers indicating UI concerns can be followed up by using the eight-item Leakage Index Questionnaire developed by Antonakos, Miller, and Sampselle (2003) to specify and quantify the subjective experience of UI (**Figure 23-3**). In addition to the presence of symptoms, assessment of "bother" to the woman should be determined. A simple question about bother used in one study asked a question such as "On a scale of 1 to 5, with 1 being 'very little bother' and 5 being 'very much bother,' how much does this leakage bother you?" (Sampselle et al., 2000). An

Leakage Index Questionnaire

Other than the few drops right after urinating, have you involuntarily lost or leaked any amount of urine or been unable to hold your water and wet yourself?

	YES	NO
	1	0

Next is a list of things that some people say can cause them to leak urine and wet themselves. Tell me whether each one has caused you to lose urine since we last saw you [date of last visit].

	YES	NO
Coughing hard	1	0
Laughing...	1	0
Sneezing..	1	0
Not being able to wait at least 5 minutes until it is convenient to go to the toilet.................	1	0
Arriving at your door or putting your key in the lock	1	0
Suddenly finding that you are losing or about to lose urine with very little warning.................	1	0

Imagine that you are standing in the check-out line at the grocery store with a full bladder that you would like to empty as soon as possible. Now imagine that you have to sneeze or cough several times very hard. What is most likely to happen about urine leakage?

Check One

0   Stay dry

1   Leak a few drops, *or*
           Wet underpants but not soak through, *or*
           Possibly drip onto the floor

TOTAL SCORE
(Sum All Items)

FIGURE 23-3 Leakage Index Questionnaire.
Source: Antonakos, Miller, & Sampselle, 2003.

alternative assessment is the International Consultation on Incontinence Questionnaire, which contains four items to assess both UI and its effect on quality of life (Avery et al., 2004).

The assessment process for UI also involves targeting the specific problem underlying an individual woman's symptoms. The most common types of UI (**Table 23-1**) in women

TABLE 23-1 Classification of Urinary Incontinence

Type of Incontinence	Definition	Description	Associated Conditions or Findings
Stress urinary incontinence	Involuntary leakage with effort or exertion, sneezing, or coughing	Involuntary leakage with effort or exertion, sneezing, or coughing	Hypermobility of bladder neck or insufficient urethral closure pressure
Urge urinary incontinence	A strong desire to urinate that is difficult to postpone	Involuntary leakage accompanied by or immediately preceded by urgency	Uninhibited contractions of the detrusor muscle, frequency
Mixed urinary incontinence	Involuntary urine leakage associated with symptoms of both stress and urge urinary incontinence	Involuntary leakage with symptoms of both stress and urge incontinence	
Continuous urinary incontinence	Continuous urine leakage	Continuous urine leakage	Extremely low urethral closure pressure
Extra-urethral urinary incontinence	Leakage of urine from areas other than the urethral meatus	Leakage of urine from areas other than the urethral meatus	Fistula
Functional urinary incontinence	Urine loss related to physical conditions outside of the urinary tract or cognitive impairment	Involuntary urine leakage related to physical conditions outside the urinary tract or by cognitive impairment	Immobility, often diagnosis of exclusion
Uncategorized urinary incontinence	Involuntary urine leakage that cannot be classified by signs and symptoms	Involuntary urine leakage that cannot be classified by signs and symptoms	

Sources: Adapted from Abrams et al., 2002; Fantl et al., 1996.

are stress UI, urge UI, and mixed UI. Less common forms are continuous UI, extraurethral UI, uncategorized UI, and functional UI (Abrams et al., 2002).

Once the etiology is identified, treatment follows logically in the direction of correcting the causative pathology. The equation for continence (Figure 23-1) can be used as a diagnostic guideline. The variables that contribute to the continence equation are multifactorial, with each factor potentially altering the delicate balance between bladder pressure and urethral pressure.

Assessing the Urinary Bladder

Pressure on the Bladder Many situations can result in high intra-abdominal pressure, which transfers downward onto the bladder and affects the continence equation. Women who are overweight have elevated intra-abdominal pressure, as do women who experience frequent episodes of coughing because of asthma, bronchitis, a history of heavy smoking, or use of angiotensin-converting enzyme (ACE) inhibitors. Occupations involving operatic singing, lifting heavy loads, aerobic exercise, and other high-impact activities are also associated with increased intra-abdominal pressure. Women with otherwise healthy bladders may experience leakage of urine because of their inability to compensate for such exceptionally high abdominal loads. Ultimately, there is a threshold of load beyond which all women will leak urine.

Assessment to determine the underlying cause of UI includes identifying situations of high intra-abdominal pressure as potential causative factors. For this purpose, the primary assessment tool is the targeted history, which includes inquiry about occupation, physical activity, smoking, or other respiratory factors, and a physical assessment indicating both BMI and body habitus proportions.

The leak point pressure test is administered by placing a catheter, specially equipped with a pressure transducer, into the bladder. It measures intra-abdominal pressure indirectly (transferred to the bladder) and determines how large the pressure increase must be to produce leakage in an individual woman—for instance, during coughing. It is important for the woman to validate the finding as consistent with her experience of symptoms. For example, following a cough test with leakage, the clinician asks, "Do you routinely cough this hard outside the clinic setting, or undertake activities that would impose an equal level of pressure?" and "Is this the type of leakage that you experience and that you find bothersome?" If not, further assessment should be undertaken to determine whether additional causative factors might account for the problematic leakage or bother. The goal is to mimic a natural situation that instigates leakage, with treatment prioritized according to the symptom of highest concern to the woman.

Pressure Within the Bladder Several situations can account for increased pressures within the bladder that act to change the balance of the continence equation. For some women, situations such as occupational restrictions beyond their control can lead to habitual over-filling of the bladder. This situation is so common that in certain occupations the bladder problem is known by the occupation itself, such as "teacher's bladder," "nurse's bladder," or "factory worker's bladder." Women who are restricted in their access to toilets can, over long intervals, train their bladders to be unresponsive to normal urge sensations. Instead of receiving mild and then progressively stronger urge sensations as the bladder fills, these women receive only a late and very strong urge sensation without adequate warning to make it to the bathroom in time. These women complain they are unable to delay urination despite having what they perceive to be a "strong" bladder, when actually the detrusor muscle is weakened and overstretched.

A similar scenario occurs in women who drink excessive amounts of fluid. Typically, these women are acting on inappropriate information by which they believe pushing fluids is good for them and without adverse consequences. In reality, women who drink excessive amounts of fluids will also need excessive numbers of voids per day or risk suffering the consequences of UI from an overly full bladder.

Paradoxically, women can also suffer consequences from habitually emptying the bladder before it fills to normative capacity (approximately 240 cc). These are women with voiding intervals of every hour, who "map the bathrooms" across the city and live in fear of being unable to reach one in time. These women with low bladder capacity demonstrate an imbalance in the continence equation because their bladders are trained toward detrusor activation at low volumes. Known as detrusor instability, this overtriggering of the detrusor muscle results in high within-bladder pressure at lower than normal capacity volumes, sometimes with accompanying leakage.

A 3-day voiding diary (**Figure 23-4**) is a simple and valuable tool in illuminating situations that might be responsible for increased pressure within the bladder. Although a diary can be inconvenient for women to fill out, willingness is typically improved when women understand the value of the tool in providing a picture to the clinician of the daily struggles caused by bladder problems. A clinic visit devoted entirely to a review of the diary helps reinforce the message from the clinician that the diary data are truly needed and drive treatment. Four types of data are critical to record:

1. Frequency and amount of voiding
2. Frequency and time of day of UI
3. Description of UI episodes and associated events
4. Type and amount of fluid intake

The diary, although certainly an assessment tool, can be viewed equally as an intervention in and of itself. A woman may not be fully aware of her own patterns and can find the self-monitoring experience to be illuminating. "I had no idea I was drinking this much coffee in a day," represents the type of comment frequently heard from first-time diary keepers. The diary also serves to monitor progress over time when a repeat diary is recorded later in treatment.

Assessing the Urethra

The factor that is perhaps most critical in maintaining a high margin of continence (i.e., urethral pressure greater than bladder pressure) is the urethra itself. This small structure is responsible for holding back a load in the bladder that reaches 300 to 400 mL several times daily, and can occasionally reach 600 to 700 mL of urine.

A weak urethra is highly suspected if a woman describes leakage not only with coughing, but also with bending or reaching, or says, "I just find myself wet." Although these symptoms are often associated with women aged 60 years or older (Perucchini et al., 2002), younger

Instructions: Please record each time you drink fluids, you empty your bladder, you lose urine accidentally, and you perform pelvic muscle contractions for 3 consecutive days.

- "Time" columns: Be sure to write AM or PM.
- "Type" column: Write caffeinated or decaf for beverages such as coffee, tea, and cola. Other examples of beverage types include milk, juice, water, alcohol, milkshakes, etc.
- "Amount" column: Write one of the following numbers to indicate the amount of accidental urine loss:
  - 1 – leak a few drops
  - 2 – wet underpants, but not soak through
  - 3 – soak all the way through to outer clothes
  - 4 – possibly drip onto the floor
- "Urge" column: Write 'yes' if you had a sudden urge and couldn't get to the bathroom in time.
- "Activity" column: Please describe what you were doing when you accidentally lost urine (i.e., coughing, sneezing, laughing, reaching, jumping, lifting a heavy object, rising from chair, heard running water, etc.).

DATE BEGUN

_____/_____/_____

Day 1   Awakening Time: _____   Bedtime: _____

Fluids I Drank Today:		
Time (AM/PM)	Type	Amount oz or ml

Urinated in Toilet:			
Time (AM/PM)	Time (AM/PM)	Time (AM/PM)	Time (AM/PM)

Accidental Leakage of Urine:			
Time (AM/PM)	Amount	Urge (yes/no)	Activity

FIGURE 23-4 Voiding diary example.

women may also present with a weak urethra, particularly those of Asian or Euro-American descent.

Quantification of urethral closure pressures can be obtained by performing a urethral pressure profilometry. Unfortunately, the expensive equipment involved is not readily accessible in general practice environments. An estimate of urethral pressure adequacy can be made by using a paper towel to quantify urine loss during a full bladder standing stress test (Miller, Ashton-Miller, & DeLancey, 1998a). With the woman in a standing position and with a full bladder (150–450 cc), she is asked to hold a trifold brown paper towel lightly against the perineum while coughing hard. The resulting wetted area (from a few drops to saturation) of the paper towel provides an indicator of relative functional urethral closure pressure (**Figure 23-5**). A weak urethra is particularly suspected if the wetted area of the paper towel

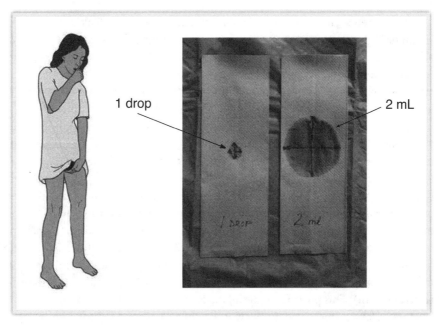

FIGURE 23-5 Use of a paper towel to quantify volume of urine loss upon coughing.

test cannot be reduced through intentional contraction of the pelvic floor muscles during coughing. Volitional contraction of the urethral striated muscle is possible, as it is with other striated muscles of the body. Thus an increase in circular contractile force should occur, and does when adequate functional striated urethral muscle is available. If not, a weak urethra—sometimes called "intrinsic sphincter deficiency"—likely underlies the UI.

Assessing the Pelvic Floor Support

Two muscles increase urethral closure pressure when women volitionally contract their pelvic floor muscles: the striated portion of the urethral muscles and the striated levator ani support muscles. In a healthy state, the levator ani muscle shortens under volitional contraction effort, compressing and closing the rectal, vaginal, and urethral orifices. When the levator ani is fully relaxed, the orifices open, allowing urine, feces, and birthing babies to pass through.

Babies, by nature of their size, impose a great deal of stretching and compression force onto the levators during vaginal birth. Approximately 1 in 10 women sustain injury to the levators during childbirth that persists over time (DeLancey et al., 2003). With injury, the muscles lose their ability to dynamically alter their stiffness in response to varying loads, which results in poor support and hypermobility of the urethra and bladder. The result is loss of compression on the urethra during increased intra-abdominal pressure—the very moment the urethral seal is most essential to preventing UI.

An injured levator ani muscle is suspected in women who leak urine only during a hard cough or high-impact exercise activities. Hypermobility of the urethra can be documented on ultrasound, although the availability and cost of imaging equipment sometimes limit the feasibility of this diagnostic technique.

Upon palpation, additional evidence that hypermobility may be the causative factor in UI can be detected in a weak, thin, or absent pubococcygeus portion of the levator ani muscle. The levator muscle is readily palpated by placing the index finger laterally in the lower one-third of the vagina, so that the middle of the distal phalanx is hooked to the right or the left, 2 to 3 cm beyond the hymen. Upon asking a woman to contract, a gross assessment of function can be obtained by estimating the response of the muscle beneath the palpating finger. A strong muscle bulks palpably beneath the finger. A weak, thinned, or missing band of muscle will offer imperceptible bulking, or the woman may instead elicit a straining down maneuver in response to instruction to contract. A second method of assessing a weak or injured levator ani muscle is accomplished by measuring the genital hiatus or introitus while the woman strains down. The genital hiatus is measured from the middle of the external urethral meatus to the posterior midline hymen border (or perineal body if the hymen is not clearly evident). This portion of the vagina is typically less than 4 cm in women with healthy levators. A larger measurement likely indicates a weakened levator support system.

A weak or injured levator muscle in combination with high intra-abdominal pressure is an indication of leakage consistent with hypermobility. Such leakage might be of smaller volume; again, it is important to ask the question, "Is this the type of leakage that you find most bothersome?" For some women, leakage that is of smaller volume, perhaps transient or with predictable exacerbations (for instance, during a cold), and that can readily be contained by a pad, may be of less consequence than the unpredictable, larger-volume leakage associated with detrusor instability.

Pelvic organ prolapse may also create a condition of UI and, therefore, should be assessed. The woman should be asked to strain down fully so that the clinician can observe the presence or absence of prolapse. The type of prolapse is not always immediately evident, but a pink bulge will indicate the need of further assessment. A speculum, split in half and used only to suppress the posterior vaginal wall, will help lend visual clarity to determine if the bulge represents anterior wall descent. If so, it is important to determine that leakage is not resulting from a cystocele that is causing inadequate emptying. A postvoid residual should be obtained to rule out large residuals (greater than 100 cc) that may be indicative of overflow-related leakage. In some women, prolapse of the bladder may actually support continence because the urethra is kinked, comparable to bending a garden hose to reduce flow. In such a case, correcting the cystocele (surgically or with a pessary) unkinks the urethra and may worsen UI in these women. If a rectocele or uterine prolapse is evident, then the anatomic misalignment may get in the way of the levators' active support to the urethra.

Sometimes the feeling of wetness has an origin other than urine—for instance, sweating or vaginal discharge. If there is doubt, a phenazopyridine (Pyridium) test can be performed. After taking phenazopyridine (available without prescription), urine becomes orange or red. The woman is instructed to wear an absorbent pad and note if the wetness is red or orange, which indicates the leakage is urine. If the leakage is urine, then appropriate laboratory testing (such as urinalysis or fasting blood glucose), neurologic assessment, diagnostic testing, or referral for specialized evaluation will assist in ruling out underlying factors.

In summary, adequate treatment of UI relies on careful elucidation of the underlying factors that are causing an imbalance in the continence equation. Treatment is aimed at education about normal anatomy and correction of the underlying causative factors. The woman's indication of which situation of leakage is most bothersome is critically important in the prioritization of treatment.

Differential Diagnosis

Urinary incontinence may sometimes be a symptom of broader system pathology. Bacterial urinary tract infection, diabetes mellitus, neurologic disorders (e.g., multiple sclerosis, dementia or Alzheimer's disease, stroke), and traumatic injury (e.g., back injury, pelvic trauma, surgical trauma) can all initially present as UI. Moreover, studies have demonstrated an association between depression and UI, with a possible common underlying physiologic mechanism (Melville, 2004; Nygaard, Turvey, Burns, Crischilles, & Wallace, 2003).

Management of Urinary Incontinence

Management of UI is aimed at reducing the factors that allow bladder pressure to exceed urethral pressure, resulting in urine leakage. Interventions related to lifestyle, diet, fluid habits, toilet habits, constipation, medications, and coexisting diseases form the basis for initial treatment.

Behavioral Interventions

Women living with UI experience a sense of powerlessness that may be addressed through supervised behavioral treatments (Hagglund & Ahlstrom, 2007). Behavioral interventions for UI are effective alone or in combination with pharmaceuticals. Behavioral interventions are recommended as a first consideration for treatment of UI because these interventions are less invasive and lower in risk than other treatments. "Pelvic muscle training, along with education on good bladder habits in general, provides … women with the needed wellness intervention for a lifelong sense of control" (Miller, 2002, p. 307).

The Knack Maneuver Application The Knack is a pelvic muscle contraction (incorporating the levator ani and urethral striated muscle) that is strategically timed to increase intraurethral pressure just before and during an event that causes leakage. This maneuver is taught to women as a self-help technique to intentionally increase the margin of continence enough to decrease urine leakage during a woman's day-to-day routine (Miller, Ashton-Miller, &

DeLancey, 1998b; Miller, Sampselle, Ashton-Miller, Son, & DeLancey, 2008). Steps for teaching the Knack are described in **Box 23-1**.

Women can practice the Knack during planned maneuvers such as blowing the nose, voluntary coughs, prior to turning on the water faucet, or upon arriving home to suppress latchkey urgency. As skill with this technique develops, women will be ready to handle the surprise cough, sneeze, or urge sensation. An additional Knack habit is to contract the pelvic floor muscles after voiding, thereby resetting the continence mechanism into holding mode. Women who are unable to achieve a voluntary pelvic muscle contraction or who have pelvic organ prolapse below the hymenal ring will probably be unable to effectively perform the Knack maneuver (Miller et al., 1998b).

Pelvic Floor Muscle Exercise Pelvic muscle exercise, commonly known as Kegel exercises, is accomplished by putting the pelvic floor muscles through a repetitive contraction regimen. The goal is to increase muscle mass and strength. Kegel exercises offer rehabilitation for women whose muscles have been weakened.

Assessment of a woman's ability to contract the levator ani muscle must be completed prior to recommending either pelvic muscle training or the Knack for UI. Recommending either will likely be ineffective and frustrating if a woman is unable to voluntarily contract her

---

BOX 23-1 *Steps in Teaching the Knack*

1. Confirm voluntary control: Palpate the body of the muscle bilaterally through the vaginal wall while the woman attempts a pelvic muscle contraction. You should feel a bulking up of the muscle. If not, or if she bears down (Valsalva maneuver), instruct her in an easy flick of the muscles, the same maneuver she would use to hold back gas, to see if this elicits correct isolation.

2. Maximize the contraction: The woman should be taught to contract the pelvic muscles as deeply into the vagina as she is able. In some women, this is most easily accomplished by learning a stacking contraction. Start with a small flick-and-release maneuver, then build into stacking two to three small flicks. This is commonly known as the "elevator" technique (imagined as moving from one floor to the next).

3. Begin to coordinate: Teach her to maintain a steady hold of the pelvic muscle contraction while inhaling and exhaling. Remind her to avoid the tendency to incorrectly hold her breath during the pelvic muscle contraction. The coordination maneuver eventually required is to be able to hold a contraction steadily throughout a secondary activity, such as diaphragm movement. She can practice by talking while holding, or blowing her nose while holding. As soon as she is ready, she is taught to hold the contraction during a voluntary cough, or other activity that she expects to cause leakage.

4. The final goal is habit establishment. With practice she should nearly reflexively contract the pelvic muscles just prior to any event known to increase intra-abdominal pressure or cause an unwanted urge sensation. The contraction should be held until the abdominal wall relaxes or upon completion of the event.

levator ani muscle. It is important to assess that women are not bearing down (i.e., Valsalva maneuver) during an attempt to contract the muscles.

Sampselle et al. (1997) recommend 30 contractions of moderate to near maximum intensity each day; each contraction should be followed by at least 10 seconds of rest. An alternative individualized protocol prescribes one of five levels of training matched to a particular woman's muscle ability (Miller, 2002). Most women will notice improvement in strength and control within one month, although three months or more may be needed to see full results.

Biofeedback is sometimes added to pelvic muscle training to facilitate skill development, particularly in the early stages. Although studies demonstrate no statistically significant difference in reduction of urine leakage between groups undertaking pelvic muscle training with or without biofeedback (Morkved, Bo, & Fjortoft, 2002), some women find the visual feedback motivating and reassuring. Numerous physical therapists are now trained in supervising pelvic muscle training.

Bladder Training Bladder training (also known as retraining) is recommended for women experiencing urge UI (also known as overactive bladder or detrusor instability). This intervention is designed to reduce urgency and frequency of urination. A voiding diary should be kept and evaluated prior to recommending bladder training. It is important to consider the type and amount of fluid intake as part of this effort, because simply scaling back on overconsumption of fluids may reduce urinary frequency.

Simple bladder retraining involves educating the woman to delay the first urge sensation and reassuring her that it is healthy to do so when known low-volume filling underlies her bladder issues. She should be taught to contract the pelvic floor muscles as an urge suppression technique (Knack) and to use distraction strategies (such as counting backward) to ignore the urge.

Women who do not respond to simple bladder retraining can advance to strict bladder retraining. The latter intervention is thought to work by reducing frequent urges to urinate by emptying the bladder before an urge occurs. The voiding diary helps determine baseline voiding frequency. The initial bladder retraining interval should start 15 minutes earlier than the normal voiding time to preempt urge sensation. For instance, if baseline voids occur hourly, begin strict bladder retraining at voids every 45 minutes. If the urge to urinate occurs prior to the scheduled time, the woman should attempt to delay emptying until the scheduled time (or at least delay 5 minutes past the initial urge). Each week (or longer if necessary to become comfortable with the new interval), she should try to increase the interval by 15 to 30 minutes until the interval is, on average, three to four hours between voiding. For most women, an average interval of three to four hours between voids means two to three hours in the morning, four to five hours in the afternoon, and three to four hours in the evening, assuming normal fluid intake. The scheduled voiding is followed only during waking hours. The purpose of this training is to regain control over the bladder so voiding can occur on the individual woman's schedule.

Women who take diuretics or have a high fluid intake may have to adjust their voiding to a realistic level that accommodates an increased voiding frequency. As a rule of thumb, women should aim for approximately one cup of urine every three to four hours with a yellow color to the urine, neither dark nor nearly colorless. Providing women with a container that fits into their toilet for urine collection to monitor color and amount of output is a valuable tool. This guideline helps monitor both intake and voiding intervals, adjusting for healthy levels.

Reverse Bladder Retraining For selected women with urge UI experienced as late signaling (no urge sensation until the bladder is excessively full and signals a strong and uncontrollable urge), reverse bladder retraining is appropriate. These women routinely report high volumes per void (greater than 350 cc) and describe themselves as having no early warning of bladder filling. Bladder training for these women involves voiding by the clock until normalized urge sensations can be relied upon. The time interval to begin reverse bladder retraining is again established by the baseline diary. The woman should reduce her interval void time to the level that will produce no more than 300 cc per void (the first morning void may be larger).

Electrical Stimulation for Urinary Incontinence

Electrical stimulation is an additional nonsurgical treatment that has demonstrated efficacy in patients with stress UI and detrusor instability. The electrical stimulation treatments contract the same muscles as do pelvic muscle exercises and can be administered in the clinician's office or at home, using a home unit. These units should not be used on women who are pregnant, nor should they be used in individuals who have a heart pacemaker. An investigation of home-managed electrical stimulation found this management routine to be both practical and well accepted (Indrekvam & Hunskaar, 2002). A wide range of side effects, including pain, psychological distress, and local irritation, were reported, but none were deemed serious. In a randomized trial comparing intravaginal stimulation to standard therapy for stress UI and detrusor instability, electrical stimulation was found to be safe and as effective as standard therapy, though not statistically better (Smith, 1996).

Other treatments similar to electrical stimulation are available. A surgically implanted sacral nerve stimulator is available for select individuals experiencing urge UI. Satisfaction measured by a quality of life survey revealed 60.5% of patients who received such an implant reported satisfaction with urinary symptoms on follow-up at a mean length of 22 months (range, 3–162 months) (Sutherland et al., 2006).

Barrier Devices for Urinary Incontinence Vaginal pessaries are designed to support the pelvic organs as a space-filling device, replacing normal pressure on the vaginal walls when levator ani support is unreliable. Pessaries come in many forms, and fitting may require a number of visits to find the correct size and type.

Some women with mild stress UI may obtain satisfactory relief with the use of tampons, based on the same principle of a space-filling supportive device. Tampons should be worn for short periods of time to decrease the risk of infection; they can be quite effective for exercise-related UI (Nygaard, 1995).

Pharmacologic Treatment

Pharmacologic treatment for UI varies according to underlying etiology. Currently, the most effective pharmacologic treatments are available for urge UI. The main limitation in their efficacy relates to these agents' lack of selectivity for the tissues in the urinary tract.

Urge Urinary Incontinence   The drugs prescribed for urge UI (also referred to as overactive bladder) belong to the class known as anticholinergic antimuscarinic agents. They target the parasympathetic muscarinic cholinergic receptor sites of smooth muscle in the bladder. The action of these drugs reduces the involuntary contractions of the detrusor muscle of the urinary bladder and increases the bladder capacity. They do not reliably increase the time between urge and emptying or the ability to suppress the urge, however, so they are most effective when combined with behavioral therapies. The most common side effects of the antimuscarinic agents include dry mouth, blurred vision, constipation, nausea, dizziness, and headaches.

The drugs approved for treatment of urge UI are oxybutynin (Ditropan), tolterodine (Detrol) in various forms including extended-release oral and patch products (Oxytrol), fesoterodin (Tovias), darifenacin (Eablex), and solifenacin (Vesicare). Propantheline bromide (Probanthine) is an anticholinergic prescribed for UI on an off-label basis (Wein & Rovner, 2002). Immediate-release oxybutynin is considered the gold standard of treatment based on its long-time use, but newer formulations are reported to be as effective with a lower incidence of dry mouth, which is the most frequently reported side effect with these agents (Appell, 2002). Tricyclic antidepressants, usually imipramine (Tofranil), have been used on an off-label basis for UI, but not as first-line pharmacologic agents for this indication.

Stress Urinary Incontinence   There are no drugs approved specifically for stress UI, although off-label use of some agents occurs. Drugs used on an off-label basis to treat stress UI are selected for their ability to increase outlet resistance (i.e., urethral pressure). Alpha-adrenergic agonists act on the $alpha_1$-receptor sites in the bladder neck and proximal urethra; ephedrine and pseudoephedrine (Sudafed) are the most often prescribed of these agents. Potential side effects include elevated blood pressure, headaches, dry mouth, insomnia, anxiety, nervousness, tachycardia, and palpitations (Wein & Rovner, 2002). Duloxetine is a dual serotonin and norepinephrine reuptake inhibitor that is also known be used on an off-label basis for stress incontinence (Thor et al., 2007).

Surgical Interventions for Urinary Incontinence

Implanted sacral nerve stimulator (discussed previously) is the only surgery for urge UI. Other forms of surgery are contraindicated for urge UI and can actually exacerbate symptoms. There are, however, a number of good surgical treatments for stress UI.

Injection of bulking agents is one surgical procedure used for this indication, particularly when stress UI is primarily caused by poor urethral closure pressure and without hypermobility. Bulking agents are injected under local anesthesia by direct vision into the proximal urethra. Although the means by which bulking agents improve UI is not fully understood, they are believed to reduce UI by adding bulk to the periurethral tissue, which increases urethral closure pressure and improves resistance to urine outflow (Kershen, Dmochowski, & Appell, 2002). Bovine collagen is an approved injectable agent, although studies demonstrate variable results with its use. Carbon-coated zirconium beads suspended in a water-based carrier gel are also approved as a bulking agent, similar in efficacy to collagen (Dmochowski & Appell, 2003). There has been some concern about migration of bulking agents after injection. The efficacy of bulking agents may be transient, but the procedure is repeatable.

Surgical treatment for stress UI includes a number of variations on surgical suspensions and slings. The aim of these procedures is to support and stabilize the urethra. The tension-free vaginal tape (TVT) sling procedure is the least invasive and is typically performed on an outpatient basis. The current trend is to perform a TVT, pubovaginal sling, or retropubic urethropexy. More traditional surgeries including the Marshall-Marchetti-Krantz or Burch procedure and transvaginal bladder neck suspensions such as the Stamey-Raz or Gittes surgical approach are also still being performed.

Referral

Many women will respond to behavioral instruction, pharmacologic treatments, or pessary use; some may be satisfied with education about UI, even if their symptoms persist. If management is ineffective, if it does not meet expectations for improvement, or if complicating factors are suspected, women should be referred to a UI specialist or specialty clinic. Some women find it difficult to identify and contract the targeted pelvic muscles and should be referred for physical therapy when the muscles are functional but very weak. Referral for electrical stimulation might be appropriate for some individuals in this population. If the muscles have clearly been injured beyond functional capacity, and stress UI is the dominant symptom of bother, then referral for surgical evaluation should be considered.

If possible, referral to a urogynecologist or a urologist with specialty practice in correcting female UI should be the priority. Education about the full scope of treatment modalities is important in the evaluation of UI. Some women will choose an intervention because the results are more immediate and require less personal involvement; others prefer to exhaust the full complement of behavioral approaches before considering pharmaceutical or surgical options. It is important to recognize each individual's self-knowledge in her choice of treatment modalities.

Evidence for Practice

Urinary incontinence receives much attention from the research community, probably because it affects a large number of women. Evidence for treatment, diagnosis, and prevention continues to evolve.

Prevention of Urinary Incontinence

Behavioral practices have been recommended to prevent UI, but evidence supporting this advice is scant. Diokno et al. (2004) reported results related to a behavioral modification program using pelvic muscle training, bladder training, and education about UI. In their sample of postmenopausal women who reported zero to five days of UI in the year prior to entering the study, the women in the treatment group were twice as likely not to have experienced UI in the year of the study as the women in the control group. The women in the behavior modification program were instructed in a group setting. In addition to demonstrating the efficacy of this program in preventing UI, these findings suggest that the information can be effectively disseminated in a group setting.

Emerging Knowledge

New instrumentation—particularly the imaging technologies of ultrasound and magnetic resonance—along with histologic and anatomic studies, are rapidly advancing understanding about the continence mechanism, pathologic factors involved, predictive variables for dysfunction, and hopes for developing improved prevention and treatment modalities. Given that these research findings are accumulating on a nearly daily basis, the literature should be reviewed routinely to keep abreast of the rapidly unfolding advancements. Along with the advancing knowledge about the physiologic and mechanical factors, new understandings of women's lived experiences of UI are informing practice in this area. Further development of a language and public knowledge of UI and continence-mechanism understanding is still needed. Currently, clinicians have only limited knowledge with which to answer the postpartum woman's question: "Why do I feel different down there, is this degree of change normal, and must I live with it?" There is even less certainty in answering another key question: "Why does my bladder trigger unexpectedly, and will this ever completely go away?" New advances are bringing new hope and a larger body of knowledge to draw from to reduce or cure UI.

Special Considerations

Adolescents

Women of all ages should receive information about healthy bladder practices. Learning pelvic muscle exercises and the Knack will provide adolescents with tools that can allow those participating in high-impact sports to concentrate on their performance rather than potential urine leakage. Of course, they can also use these tools over the course of their entire adult lives.

Culture

In certain religious groups, it is required that women perform ritual cleansing before prayer. An episode of UI renders a woman who has cleansed to be unclean; thus she must cleanse again before she can resume prayer rituals (Wilkinson, 2001). Women in this situation may hesitate to discuss incontinence outside of their family for concern they may be perceived as unclean. In one study, Jewish and Muslim women experienced the greatest restrictions as a result of UI (Chaliha & Stanton, 1999).

Conclusion

Urinary incontinence detracts from a woman's quality of life and may unduly direct her concentration to how well her body is behaving. Women who experience UI become vigilant about hiding evidence on clothes and odors, and they may experience a sense of losing control. Clinicians, through assessment and education, can provide the opportunity for women to discuss UI, weigh options for treatment, and make informed judgments about caring for this basic bodily function of urine storage and emptying.

Internet Resources

American Urogynecologic Society (Information for Women)
http://www.augs.org or http://www.mypelvichealth.org
Cochrane Consumers Network
http://www.cochrane.org/consumers/reviewgrp.htm
National Association for Continence
http://www.nafc.org
National Institute of Diabetes & Digestive & Kidney Diseases
http://kidney.niddk.nih.gov/kudiseases/pubs/uiwomen
Simon Foundation for Continence
http://www.simonfoundation.org
Women's Health Foundation—Total Control
http://www.womenshealthfoundation.org/default.php

References

Abrams, P., Cardozo, L., Fall, M., Griffiths, D., Rosier, P., Ulf, U., et al. (2002). The standardization of terminology of lower urinary tract function: Report from the standardization sub-committee of the International Continence Society. *Neurourology and Urodynamics, 21*, 167–178.

Antonakos, C. L., Miller, J. M., & Sampselle, C. M. (2003). Indices for studying urinary incontinence and levator ani function in primiparous women. *Journal of Clinical Nursing, 12*, 554–561.

Appell, R. A. (2002). The newer antimuscarinic drugs: Bladder control with less dry mouth. *Cleveland Clinic Journal of Medicine, 69*(10), 761–769.

Ashton-Miller, J. A., Howard, D., & DeLancey, J. O. L. (2001). The functional anatomy of the female pelvic floor and stress continence control system. *Scandinavian Journal of Urological Nephrology, 207*(suppl), 1–7.

Avery, K., Donovan, J., Peters, T. J., Shaw, C., Gotoh, M., & Abrams, P. (2004). ICIQ: A brief and robust measure for evaluating the symptoms and impact of urinary incontinence. *Neurourology and Urodynamics, 23*, 322–330.

Chaliha, C., Kalia, V., Stanton, S. L., Monga, A., & Sultan, A. H. (1999). Antenatal prediction of postpartum urinary and fecal incontinence. *Obstetrics and Gynecology, 94*, 689–694.

Chaliha, C., & Stanton, S. L. (1999). The ethnic cultural and social aspects of incontinence: A pilot study. *International Urogynecology Journal, 10*, 166–170.

DeLancey, J. O. L. (1990). Anatomy and physiology of urinary continence. *Clinical Obstetrics and Gynecology, 33*(2), 298–307.

DeLancey, J. O., Kearney, R., Chou, Q., Speights, S., & Binno, S. (2003). The appearance of levator ani muscle abnormalities in magnetic resonance images after vaginal delivery. *Obstetrics & Gynecology, 101*(1), 46–53.

DeLancey, J. O., Miller, J., Kearney, R., Howard, D., Reddy, P., Umek, W., et al. (2007). Vaginal birth and de novo stress incontinence: Relative contributions of urethral dysfunction and support loss. *Obstetrics and Gynecology, 110*(2 Pt 1), 354–362.

Diokno, A. C., Sampselle, C. M., Herzog, A. R., Raghunathan, T. E., Hines, S., Messer, K. L., et al. (2004). Prevention of urinary incontinence by behavioral modification program: A randomized, controlled trial among older women in the community. *Journal of Urology, 171*, 1165–1171.

Dmochowski, R., & Appell, R. A. (2003). Advancements in minimally invasive treatments for female stress urinary incontinence: Radio frequency and bulking agents. *Current Urology Reports, 4*, 350–355.

Fantl, J. A., Newman, D. K., Colling, J., DeLancey, J. O. L., Keeys, C., Loughery, R., … Whitmore, K. (1996). *Urinary incontinence in adults: Acute and chronic management* (AHCPR Publication No. 96-0682). Rockville, MD: U.S. Department of Health and Human Services, Public Health Service, Agency for Health Care Policy and Research.

Fenner, D., Trowbridge, E., Patel, P., Fultz, N., Miller, J., Howard, D., & DeLancey, J. (2008). Establishing the Prevalence of Incontinence (EPI) Study: Racial differences in women's patterns of urinary incontinence. *Journal of Urology, 179*, 1455–1460.

Fitzgerald, S., Link, M., Litman, H., Travison, T., & McKinaly, J. (2007). Beyond the lower urinary tract: The association of urologic and sexual symptoms with common illnesses. *European Urology, 52*(2), 407–415.

Giovanni, E., Bergman, J., & Dye, T. D. (2002). Familial incidence of urinary incontinence. *American Journal of Obstetrics and Gynecology, 187*, 53–55.

Gray, M. (2000). Caffeine and urinary continence. *Journal of Wound, Ostomy, and Continence Nursing, 28*(2), 66–69.

Hagglund, D., & Ahlstrom, G. (2007). The meaning of women's experience of living with long-term urinary incontinence is powerlessness. *Journal of Clinical Nursing, 16*, 1946–1954.

Holroyd-Leduc, J. M., & Straus, S. E. (2004). Management of urinary incontinence in women: Scientific review. *Journal of the American Medical Association, 291*(8), 986–995.

Hunskaar, S., Arnold, E. P., Burgio, K., Diokno, A. C., Herzog, A. R., & Mallett, V. T. (2000). Epidemiology and natural history of urinary incontinence. *International Urogynecological Journal, 11*, 301–319.

Indrekvam, S., & Hunskaar, S. (2002). Side effects, feasibility, and adherence to treatment during home-managed electrical stimulation for urinary incontinence: A Norwegian national cohort of 3,198 women. *Neurourology and Urodynamics, 21*, 546–552.

Jolleys, J. V. (1988). Reported prevalence of urinary incontinence in women in a general practice. *British Medical Journal, 296*, 1300–1302.

Kershen, R. T., Dmochowski, R. R., & Appell, R A. (2002). Beyond collagen: Injectable therapies for the treatment of female stress urinary incontinence in the new millennium. *Urologic Clinics of North America, 29*(3), 559–574.

Krantz, K. E. (1950). The anatomy of the urethra and anterior vaginal wall. *American Journal of Obstetrics and Gynecology, 62*(2), 374–386.

Lien, K. C., Mooney, B., DeLancey, J. O., & Ashton-Miller, J. A. (2004, January). Levator ani muscle stretch induced by simulated vaginal birth. *Obstetrics and Gynecology, 103*(1), 31–40.

Melville, J. (2004, August). *Urinary incontinence in U.S. women: A population-based study*. Paper presented at the International Continence Society Annual Meeting, Paris, France.

Melville, J. L., Delancy, K., Newton, K., & Katon, W. (2005). Incontinence severity and major depression in incontinent women. *Obstetrics and Gynecology, 106*(3), 585–592.

Miller, J. M. (2002). Criteria for the therapeutic use of pelvic floor muscle training in women. *Journal of Wound, Ostomy, and Continence Nursing, 29*(6), 301–311.

Miller, J. M., Ashton-Miller, J. A., & DeLancey, J. O. L. (1998a). Quantification of cough-related urine loss using the paper towel test. *Obstetrics and Gynecology, 91*, 705–709.

Miller, J. M., Ashton-Miller, J. A., & DeLancey, J. O. L. (1998b). A pelvic muscle precontraction can reduce cough-related urine loss in selected women with mild SUI. *Journal of the American Geriatrics Society, 46*(7), 870–874.

Miller, J., Sampselle, C., Ashton-Miller, J., Son, G., & DeLancey, J. (2008). Clarification and confirmation of the effect of volitional pelvic floor muscle contraction to preempt urine loss (the knack maneuver) in stress incontinent women. *International Urogynecology Journal and Pelvic Floor Dysfunction, 19*(6), 773–782.

Miller, J. M., Umek, W. H., DeLancey, J. O., & Ashton-Miller, J. A. (2004). Can women increase urethral closure pressures without their pubococcygeus muscles? *American Journal of Obstetrics and Gynecology, 191*(1), 171–175.

Morkved, S., Bo, K., & Fjortoft, T. (2002). Effect of adding biofeedback to pelvic floor muscle training to treat urodynamic stress incontinence. *Obstetrics and Gynecology, 100*(4), 730–739.

Nygaard, I. (1995). Prevention of exercise incontinence with mechanical devices. *Journal of Reproductive Medicine, 40*(2), 89–94.

Nygaard, I., Turvey, C., Burns, T. L., Crischilles, E., & Wallace, R. (2003). Urinary incontinence and depression in middle-aged United States women. *Obstetrics and Gynecology, 101*, 149–156.

Ostaszkiewicz, J., Ski, C., & Hornby, L. (2005). Does successful treatment of constipation or faecal impaction resolve lower urinary tract symptoms? A structured review of the literature. *Australian and New Zealand Continence Journal, 11*(3), 70–80.

Perucchini, D., DeLancey, J. O. L., Ashton-Miller, J. A., Peschers, U., & Kataria, T. (2002). Age effects on urethral striated muscle. *American Journal of Obstetrics and Gynecology, 186*, 351–355.

Sampselle, C. M. (1990). Changes in pelvic muscle strength and stress urinary incontinence associated with childbirth. *Journal of Obstetric, Gynecologic and Neonatal Nursing, 19*(5), 371–377.

Sampselle, C. M., Burns, P. A., Dougherty, M. C., Newman, D. K., Thomas, K. K., & Wyman, J. F. (1997). Continence for women: Evidence-based practice. *Journal of Obstetric, Gynecologic and Neonatal Nursing, 26*, 375–385.

Sampselle, C. M., & DeLancey, J. O. L. (1998). Anatomy of female continence. *Journal of Wound, Ostomy, and Continence Nursing, 25*, 63–74.

Sampselle, C. M., Harlow, S. D., Skurnick, J., Brubaker, L., & Bondarenko, I. (2002). Urinary incontinence predictors and life impact in ethnically diverse perimenopausal women. *Obstetrics and Gynecology, 100*(6), 1230–1238.

Sampselle, C. M., Miller, J. M., Mims, B. L., DeLancey, J. O. L, Ashton-Miller, J. A., & Antonakos, C. L. (1998). Effect of pelvic muscle exercise on transient incontinence during pregnancy and after birth. *Obstetrics and Gynecology, 91*, 406–412.

Sampselle, C. M., Palmer, M., Boyington, A., O'Dell, K., & Wooldridge, L. (2004). Prevention of incontinence in adults: Population-based strategies. *Nursing Research, 53*(6S), S61–S67.

Sampselle, C. M., Wyman, J. F., Thomas, K. K., Newman, D. K., Gray, M., Dougherty, M., & Burns, P. A. (2000). Continence for women: A test of AWHONN's evidence-based protocol in clinical practice. *Journal of Obstetric, Gynecologic, and Neonatal Nursing, 29*(1), 18–26.

Sandvik, H., Junskaar, S., Seim, A., Hermstad, R., Vanvik, A., & Bratt, H. (1993). Validation of a severity index in female urinary incontinence and its implementation in an epidemiological survey. *Journal of Epidemiology and Community Health, 47*(6), 497–499.

Shier, D., Butler, J., & Lewis, R. (2004). *Hole's human anatomy and physiology* (10th ed.). Boston: McGraw-Hill.

Smith, J. J., III. (1996). Intravaginal stimulation randomized trial. *Journal of Urology, 155*(1), 127–130.

Society of Urologic Nurses and Associates (SUNA). (1997). *Scope and standards of urologic nursing practice.* Pitman, NJ: Author.

Subak, L. L., Witcomb, E., Shen, H., Saxton, J., Vittinghoff, E., & Brown, J. S. (2005). Weight loss: A novel and effective treatment for urinary incontinence. *Journal of Urology, 174*(1), 190–195.

Sutherland, E. S., Lavers, A., Carlson, A., Holtz, C., Kesha, J., & Siegel, S. W. (2006). Sacral nerve stimulation for voiding dysfunction: One institution's 11-year experience. *Neurourology and Urodynamics, 26*, 19–28.

Sze, E. H., Jones, W. P., Ferguson, J. L., Barker, C. D., & Dolezal, J. M. (2002). Prevalence of urinary incontinence symptoms among black, white, and Hispanic women. *Obstetrics and Gynecology, 99*, 572–575.

Teo, J., Briffa, K., Devine, A., Dhaliwal, S. S., & Prince, R. L. (2006). Do sleep problems or urinary incontinence predict falls in elderly women? *Australian Journal of Physiotherapy, 52*, 19–24.

Thom, D. H., van den Eeden, S. K., Ragins, A. I., Wassel-Fyr, C., Vittinghof, E., Subak, L. L., & Brown, J. S. (2006). Differences in prevalence of urinary incontinence by race/ethnicity. *Journal of Urology, 175*(1), 259–264.

Thor, K. B., Kirby, M., & Viktrup, L. (2007). Serotonin and noradrenaline involvement in urinary incontinence, depression and pain: Scientific basis for overlapping clinical efficacy from a single drug, duloxetine. *International Journal of Clinical Practice, 61*(8), 1349–1355.

Townsend, M. K., Danforth, K. N., Rosner, B., Curhan, G. C., Resnick, N. M., & Grodstein, F. (2007). Body mass index, weight gain, and incident urinary incontinence in middle-aged women. *Obstetrics and Gynecology, 110*(2 Pt 1), 346–353.

Vigod, S. N., & Stewart, D. E. (2006). Major depression in female urinary incontinence. *Psychosomatics, 47*(2), 147–151.

Waetjen, L. E., Feng, W. Y., Ye, J., Johnson, W. O., Greendale, G. A., Sampselle, C. M., … Gold, E. B. (2008, March). Factors associated with worsening and improving urinary incontinence across the menopausal transition. *Obstetrics and Gynecology, 111*(3), 667–677.

Wallner, L., Porten, S., Meenan, R., Rosetti, M., Calhoun, E., Sarma, A., & Clemens, J. (2009). Prevalence and severity of undiagnosed urinary incontinence in women. *American Journal of Medicine, 122*, 1037–1042.

Wein, A. J., & Rovner, E. S. (2002). Pharmacologic management of urinary incontinence in women. *Urologic Clinics of North America, 29*(3), 537–550.

Wilkinson, K. (2001). Pakistani women's perceptions and experiences of incontinence. *Nursing Standard, 16*(5), 33–39.

CHAPTER 24

Menstrual Cycle Pain and Discomforts

Diana Taylor
Kerri Durnell Schuiling
Beth A. Collins Sharp

Overview

Most women, at some time during their childbearing years, experience cyclic pelvic pain (CPP) and other discomforts associated with the menstrual cycle (Clayton, 2008; Collins Sharp, Taylor, Kelly-Thomas, Killeen, & Dawood, 2002).

Historically, paternalistic views of menstrual-related experiences prevailed and biomedical language predominated, with little attention being paid to alternative perspectives from other disciplines or, more importantly, from a woman's perspective. In the mid-1980s, professional medical organizations in the United States and the United Kingdom met to define premenstrual syndrome (PMS), and the published proceedings established the medical basis for the presentation and clinical existence of PMS as a disease classification (Dawood, McGuire, & Demers, 1985; Halbreich, 1997). From that point forward, paternalistic labeling shifted to medical diagnosis.

Recognized in the *International Classification of Diseases* manual developed by the World Health Organization (WHO, 1992), the popular and quasi-medical term PMS describes the cyclical recurrence of symptoms that impair a woman's health, relationships, and occupational functioning. Although its decision met with much controversy, the American Psychiatric Association (APA) recognized the diagnostic term *premenstrual dysphoric disorder* (PMDD) in the third, fourth, and fifth editions of its *Diagnostic and Statistical Manual* (APA, 1987, 1994, 2000). PMDD is a diagnostic label that applies to a much smaller number of menstruating women experiencing severe PMS with predominantly negative affect symptoms.

Development of Evidence-Based Clinical Practice Guidelines

In 2003, an interdisciplinary group of scientists and clinicians sponsored by the Association of Women's Health, Obstetric and Neonatal Nurses (AWHONN) developed clinical practice guidelines based on a broad range of clinical, empirical, and theoretical evidence (Collins Sharp et al., 2002). The goal was to provide a comprehensive description of a complex women's health problem that encompasses more than the individual concepts of dysmenorrhea, PMS, and PMDD. These guidelines recommend use of the term *cyclic pelvic pain and discomfort* (CPPD) to differentiate normal cyclic changes associated with menstruation from the severe, debilitating menstrual and premenstrual symptom experiences that require professional or pharmacologic intervention. *Perimenstrual* refers to the period from about 7 to 10 days before menstrual flow begins until the first or second day of menstrual flow (Collins Sharp et al.; Woods, Most, & Dery, 1982a). Although the term CPPD references the negative end of the perimenstrual experience spectrum, it reflects the woman's experience, rather than her personal attributes or a medically imposed diagnosis, and is based on a range of rigorously reviewed empirical studies conducted using both quantitative and qualitative methods.

The American College of Obstetricians and Gynecologists (2000, reaffirmed 2010) has also developed clinical management guidelines designed to aid clinicians in making decisions about appropriate PMS diagnosis and treatment. The diagnostic criteria for PMS are included in these guidelines, as are recommendations for therapeutic interventions that include both self-care strategies and pharmacologic approaches.

Scope and Prevalence of the Problem

The menstrual cycle is a normative process. Nevertheless, approximately 10% of women experience severe recurring symptoms associated with their menstrual cycle. In well-designed studies of community-based, nonclinical samples, the prevalence of perimenstrual symptoms was 30% to 50%, with pain, fatigue, mood swings, and physical discomforts being the most commonly reported symptoms (Woods, Most, & Dery, 1982b). Ballagh and Heyl (2008) and Clayton (2008) suggest that an even greater proportion of women—as many as 85%—will experience physical and emotional changes during the menstrual cycle. Ballagh and Heyl also note that as many as 40% of women experience menstrual-related conditions such as PMS and PMDD that can have a significant impact on a woman's daily life.

As the *Diagnostic and Statistical Manual*, Fourth Edition, Text Revision (DSM-IV-TR) definition of PMDD acknowledges, mild symptoms such as bloating and breast tenderness affect as many as 70% of menstruating women; thus these symptoms should not be considered "disordered" (APA, 1994, 2000). However, between 5% and 14% of women report perimenstrual symptoms so severe that they are considered disabling (Angst, Sellaro, Merikangas, & Endicott, 2001; Vigod, Ross, & Steiner, 2009), and another 30% to 40% of women have perimenstrual symptoms that are bothersome enough that they seek professional advice (Woods, Lentz, Mitchell, Heitkemper, & Shaver, 1997; Woods, Taylor, Mitchell, & Lentz, 1992). A review of several studies suggests that between 4% and 7% of women may qualify for a diagnosis of PMDD (Ross & Steiner, 2003). Based on these prevalence studies, an estimated 35 million women in the United States are believed to experience mild to moderate PMS and 5 to 7 million have severe PMS (Woods, Mitchell, Lentz, Taylor, & Lee, 1987; Woods et al., 1982b). **Table 24-1** compares the clinical labels and diagnostic classifications of the perimenstrual symptom experience.

Focusing on perimenstrual symptoms rather than a disease-oriented syndrome provides a model for understanding complex gender-specific conditions that include biologic, psychosocial, and cultural factors. This holistic model can also be applied to other women's health problems, such as stress-related conditions (e.g., heart disease, arthritis, and immune system disorders), psychiatric disorders, or normative menstrual cycle transitions (e.g., menarche, postpartum, and menopause).

Clinical Presentation

Research has identified several common patterns of perimenstrual symptoms (Collins Sharp et al., 2002; Moos, 1969; Taylor, 1986; Woods, Mitchell, & Lentz, 1999). In a factor and cluster analysis of data from a cross-sectional population-based sample, Woods, Mitchell, and Lentz (1999) identified four symptom clusters that accounted for much of the variance in women's experience of the premenstrual phase:

- Turmoil: hostility, depression, anger, feeling out of control, tension, guilt feelings, tearfulness, anxiety, rapid mood changes, nervousness, irritability, desire to be alone, loneliness, and impatience
- Fluid retention: weight gain, abdominal bloating or swelling, painful breasts, swelling of hands and feet, and skin disorders
- Somatic symptoms: nausea, lowered desire to move, decreased food intake, abdominal pain, headaches, decreased sexual desire, and aches and pains

TABLE 24-1 Perimenstrual Symptom Experience: Comparing Clinical Labels and Diagnostic Classifications

	Perimenstrual Symptom Experience		
Clinical Label and Diagnostic Classification	Cyclic Perimenstrual Pain and Discomforts (CPPD)	Premenstrual Syndrome (PMS)	
	Perimenstrual Symptoms–Primary Dysmenorrhea		Premenstrual Dysphoric Disorder (PMDD)
Intensity/Distress	Mild to moderate	Moderate	Severe
Pattern	Few hours to 5 days	6–9 days	10–14 days

- Arousal: bursts of energy or activity, increased sexual desire, impulsiveness, increased food intake, increased sense of well-being, and cravings for certain foods or tastes

Turmoil was the dominant symptom cluster in terms of explaining variance in premenstrual symptoms, and fluid retention was the most important cluster for distinguishing women with low-symptom severity from those with PMS or premenstrual magnification. Woods, Mitchell, and Lentz (1999) conclude that these symptom clusters are reliable indicators of premenstrual symptoms that are sensitive to cycle phase differences. Somatic symptoms and arousal symptoms appear to be highly stable across the menstrual cycle, and these clusters are poorly correlated with one another. The researchers speculate that somatic and arousal symptoms might be independent of menstrual cycle phases.

Cyclic Perimenstrual Pain and Discomfort

Cyclic perimenstrual pain and discomfort addresses symptom clusters that occur both before and after the menstrual flow begins (**Box 24-1**). The primary feature of CPPD is a cluster of cyclic symptoms that includes pain, discomfort, and mood symptoms (Collins Sharp et al., 2002), and that encompasses three nursing diagnoses, each representing a cluster of symptoms (AWHONN, 2003).

The recognition of CPPD as a diagnosis distinct from medical diagnoses relative to menstrual cycle pain and discomforts does not negate the importance of the biologic-based diag-

---

BOX 24-1 *CPPD Symptom Clusters*

Cyclic perimenstrual pain and discomforts (CPPD) includes dysmenorrhea and pelvic pain as well as other perimenstrual physical and mood symptoms. It is distinguished by three major symptom clusters: cyclic pelvic pain, perimenstrual physical discomforts, and perimenstrual mood discomforts. Perimenstrual refers to the span of time from approximately 7–10 days before menstrual flow (premenstrual phase) begins through the first 1 to 2 days of menstrual flow (menstrual phase).

Dysmenorrhea is subjectively identified acute discomfort that occurs in the abdominal area circumscribed by the pelvis and that recurs in a pattern associated with the menstrual cycle. Other pain symptoms related to CPP are abdominal cramps, backache, nausea, vomiting, diarrhea, and change in bowel frequency.

Perimenstrual physical discomforts are painful physical symptoms other than those commonly associated with CPP that escalate around the time of menstruation and subside after menses begins. Symptoms include fatigue, headaches, fluid retention, joint aches and pains, breast tenderness, leg/thigh discomforts, and change in energy and appetite.

Perimenstrual mood discomforts are psychological symptoms that escalate around the time of menstruation and subside after menses begins. Symptoms include depression, irritability, tension, impatience, anxiety, anger, mood swings, hostility, change in sexual desire, guilt, feeling out of control, and tearfulness.

Source: Adapted from AWHONN, 2003.

noses and therapies. Instead, a more inclusive diagnosis encourages an integrated approach to assessment and treatment. This approach is woman centered and relies on the woman as the expert knower. Her description of her symptoms, their severity, and their effect on her life assists in the diagnosis and management of the problem. Using an integrated approach to assess, diagnose, and treat perimenstrual symptoms encourages the use of complementary and pharmacologic treatment modalities. In addition, an integrated approach encourages women to participate in decision making and to take responsibility for those aspects of the treatment regimens within their control, such as nutrition and exercise.

Dysmenorrhea

Dysmenorrhea is categorized as primary or secondary based on the presence of known etiology or pelvic pathology. As medically defined, primary dysmenorrhea is diagnosed by exclusion when painful menstruation occurs in the absence of pathology. Primary dysmenorrhea tends to begin shortly after the establishment of menses (Hoffman, 2008), and increased endometrial prostaglandin production is believed to be the cause of the associated pain (Lentz, 2007). Secondary dysmenorrhea involves an underlying pathology acting directly or indirectly on the pelvic anatomy to cause pain symptoms during menstrual flow. It may be associated with dyspareunia, dysuria, abnormal uterine bleeding, or infertility (Hoffman, 2008). The pain associated with either primary or secondary dysmenorrhea is the same; thus the mere presence of pain does not indicate which type of dysmenorrhea the woman is experiencing.

Many women report experiencing dysmenorrhea that significantly diminishes their quality of life. Detrimental effects may include lost work or school time, expenses for self-care, over-the-counter (OTC) treatments, and visits to healthcare professionals (AWHONN, 2003). The incidence of dysmenorrhea is as high as 80% among women in their teens and early 20s, with one-half of these women experiencing loss of time from school or work as a result of this condition (Dawood, 1990). For 10% to 20% of women, the dysmenorrhea is so severe it is disabling (Harlow & Park, 1996; Smith, 1993).

Premenstrual Conditions

Premenstrual Syndrome

The term *premenstrual syndrome* is used to indicate the cyclic recurrence of distressing physical, mood, and behavioral experiences that often affect interpersonal relationships, personal health, and a woman's ability to function (Woods et al., 1999) (**Box 24-2**). The hallmark of PMS has been defined as the repeated occurrence of behavioral, somatic, and mood symptoms severe enough to impair a woman's social and work-related functioning during the perimenstrual phase of the menstrual cycle (Mitchell, Woods, Lentz, & Taylor, 1991). PMS has a distinct symptom pattern: no or low severity of symptoms after menses, followed by an escalation in symptom frequency and severity premenses, that subsides again at the onset (or

---

BOX 24-2 *Menstrual Diagnoses*

Dysmenorrhea is difficult or painful menses. The medical literature differentiates primary and secondary dysmenorrhea. Primary dysmenorrhea is associated with multiple symptoms including: abdominal cramps, headache, backache, general body aches, continuous abdominal pain, and other somatic discomforts (Dawood & Ramos, 1990) and is more common than secondary dysmenorrhea. There is no evidence of organic pathophysiology in the uterus, fallopian tubes, or ovaries with primary dysmenorrhea (Kinch & Robinson, 1985). Secondary dysmenorrhea involves underlying pathology that causes pain during menses.

Premenstrual syndrome (PMS) is a diagnostic term used to indicate cyclical recurrence of distressing physical, mood, and behavioral experiences that often affect interpersonal relationships and personal health and function (Woods, Mitchell, & Taylor, 1999). A PMS symptom pattern can be discerned by the absence of symptoms or low severity symptoms after menses (post-menses, defined as approximately days 6 through 10 of the cycle), followed by an escalation in symptoms premenses during the seven days preceding the next menses that subside again at the onset (or first few days) of menses.

Premenstrual dysphoric disorder (PMDD) is a diagnostic label now included in the *Diagnostic and Statistical Manual IV-TR* of the American Psychiatric Association (2000) and replaces the earlier label of late luteal phase dysphoric disorder. This diagnosis applies to a subset of women suffering from severe PMS with an emphasis on mood symptoms.

Premenstrual magnification (PMM) is a variant of the premenstrual syndrome pattern in which women experience moderately severe symptoms postmenses, and more severe symptoms premenses (Mitchell, Woods, & Lentz, 1994). This variant may represent an exacerbation of an ongoing mental health problem or physical disorder (Harrison, 1985). Women with conditions such as eating disorders, bipolar disorder, substance abuse disorder, major depression, anxiety, or personality disorders will experience symptoms of their disorder throughout the menstrual cycle, but the symptoms are more severe during the premenstrual phase.

---

first few days) of menses (Mitchell, Woods, & Lentz, 1994). Changes in other perceptions are also evident, such as emotional and physical feelings of stress, including anticipatory stress in advance of symptoms (Hamilton, Alagna, & Sharpe, 1985; Rubinow, Schmidt, & Roca, 1998a; Taylor, Woods, Lentz, Mitchell, & Lee, 1991; Woods, Lentz, Mitchell, Taylor, & Lee, 1992). Behavioral patterns, such as angry outbursts or low impulse control that precipitate interpersonal conflict, may also occur (Woods, Mitchell, & Lentz).

Successful management of PMS begins with the assessment of symptom clusters, symptom severity patterns, and their degree of impact on a woman's functional status. The diagnosis of PMS should include review of a symptom diary that clearly suggests the symptoms are related to the luteal phase of the menstrual cycle (American College of Obstetricians and Gynecologists, 2000, reaffirmed 2010). Typically the clinician should look for a pattern of symptoms that are present 3 days prior to the onset of the menses, that end within 4 days after the menstrual flow ceases, and that occur for at least 3 consecutive menstrual cycles. The symptoms should be severe enough that they interfere with some of the woman's normal activities (American College of Obstetricians and Gynecologists, 2010; Panay, 2008).

Premenstrual Magnification

Premenstrual magnification (PMM) is another syndrome distinct from PMS (Box 24-2). This term refers to the exacerbation of somatic or mood symptoms in the late luteal or menstrual phase of the cycle (Harrison, 1985). Conditions that may worsen during the premenstrual or menstrual phase include depressive disorders, panic or anxiety disorders, migraines, seizure disorders, irritable bowel syndrome (IBS), asthma, chronic fatigue syndrome, and allergies (Mitchell et al., 1994). Premenstrual symptoms may coexist with other conditions such as mood disorders, asthma, migraines, thyroid disorders, seizure disorders, or arthritis. This is considered a dual diagnosis. Women who have PMM of an illness or who feel sick before or during menstruation may also have some characteristics of PMS.

Premenstrual Dysphoric Disorder

PMDD is a separate diagnostic label that applies to a much smaller number of menstruating women and requires at least one affective symptom (Box 24-2). The APA first included the diagnostic term *late luteal phase dysphoric disorder* (LLPDD) in the third revised edition of its *Diagnostic and Statistical Manual* (DSM-III-R), published in 1987 (APA, 1987). Although this term was listed in the research appendix as a condition "requiring further study," it was given a diagnostic code, list of symptoms, and cutoff points—exactly like the diagnostic labels in the main text of the DSM-III-R that were considered to be supported by scientific evidence. After an extensive literature review, an LLPDD subcommittee of the APA concluded in 1994 that very little research supported the existence of premenstrual mental illness (in contrast to PMS). Nevertheless, the term LLPDD was revised to PMDD and is included in the DSM-IVTR in the research appendix and also in the main text under the heading "Depressive Disorders" (APA, 2000).

There is no question that some women experience a more severe form of PMS, but the legitimization of PMDD or severe PMS as a psychiatric disorder troubles many feminist and medical scholars. In spite of the U.S. Food and Drug Administration (FDA) approval of the antidepressant fluoxetine (Prozac/Sarafem) as a treatment for PMDD in 1999, a European drug regulator required the drug's manufacturer (Lilly) to delete PMDD as an indicated disorder for fluoxetine treatment (Moynihan, 2004). The European Committee for Proprietary Medicinal Products found that PMDD was "not a well-established disease entity across Europe," was not listed in the International Classification of Diseases (ICD), and was listed only as a research diagnosis in the DSM-IV-TR (Moynihan, 2004).

Etiology

Biologic

A strong body of knowledge supports a biologic etiology for cyclic menstrual pain or dysmenorrhea. Dawood and associates (1985) established that an increase or imbalance in the quantity of prostaglandins present in menstrual fluid occurs in women with dysmenorrhea.

The excessive amounts of prostaglandins cause the uterus to contract abnormally and reduce uterine blood flow and oxygenation, thereby giving rise to pain. However, almost any process that can affect the pelvic viscera and cause acute or intermittent recurring pain might be a source of cyclic perimenstrual pain, including urinary tract infection, endometriosis, pelvic inflammatory disease, uterine fibroids, interstitial cystitis, hernia, IBS, and pelvic relaxation (Dawood, 1990; Smith, 1993). Identifying the cause of perimenstrual cyclic pelvic pain can be difficult, because the clinician must distinguish dysmenorrhea from other pelvic pain that occurs in a cyclic manner outside the time of the menstrual flow (American College of Obstetricians and Gynecologists, 2004, reaffirmed 2010; Rapkin & Howe, 2007; Smith).

The etiologic mechanisms for cyclic perimenstrual physical and mood discomforts, PMS, or PMDD are even less clear. Although a number of biologic and neuroendocrine etiologies have been proposed, they have comprised mostly simple, direct, unsubstantiated pathophysiologic models such as hormonal imbalances, sodium retention, nutritional deficiencies, or abnormal hypothalamic–pituitary–adrenal axis function (Backstrom et al., 1983; Keye, 1989; O'Brien, 1987; Reid & Yen, 1981). A number of investigators have hypothesized that ovarian hormones have neuroregulatory effects on humans' central serotonin systems, as inferred from (mostly animal) studies demonstrating the impact of gender, estrus cycle, or hormone manipulation (Rubinow, Schmidt, & Roca, 1998b). This menstrual cycle hormone–serotonin hypothesis remains unconfirmed as yet, and is based primarily on indirect tests using selective serotonin reuptake inhibitor (SSRI) antidepressants (Freeman, 1997).

In the end, the cause of these disorders is complex. When working with a patient, the clinician must consider both factors that may be correlates and useful as identifiers of the pathophysiology and those that may contribute to the disorder (Vigod et al., 2009).

Integration of Biologic, Genetic, and Environmental Factors

Empirical and theory testing research points to an integrative etiology that links genetics, environmental stressors, and hormonal processes with individual vulnerabilities (Endicott, 2001; Halbreich, 1997, 1999; Kendler, Karkowski, Corey, & Neale, 1998; Rubinow & Schmidt, 1995; Schmidt, Nieman, Danaceau, Adams, & Rubinow, 1998; Taylor et al., 1991). Perimenstrual symptoms and syndromes may act as modulators of other disorders, or they may be an abnormal response to normal biologic rhythms (e.g., the menstrual cycle, circadian rhythms, adrenocortical pulses) (Cahill, 1998; Lewis, Greenblatt, Rittenhouse, Veldhuis, & Jaffe, 1995; Reame et al., 1996; Reame, Marshall, & Kelch, 1992; Ross, Sellers, Gilbert-Evans, & Romach, 2004; Taylor et al., 1991; Thys-Jacobs, 2000; Ussher, 2002). PMS is most likely a psychoneuroendocrine disorder in which psychosocial variables exert their influence by lowering the individual's threshold to experience perimenstrual symptoms in response to normal or abnormal biologic changes of the menstrual cycle in the context of a multifaceted interaction between the central nervous system (CNS), hormones, and other modulators.

A few well-designed studies have empirically tested the hypothesis that biologic and psychosocial variables interact to result in vulnerability to mood and behavioral changes across the menstrual cycle (Taylor et al., 1991). In these studies, the effect of stressors and stress response was not only direct, but also operated through generalized distress mediated by poor health behaviors. Multiple well-crafted laboratory studies from the National Institutes of Mental Health's Behavioral Endocrinology Branch have tested the putative roles of pituitary, ovarian, and adrenal steroids in the etiology of PMS. The results of these investigations do not support a primary endocrine abnormality in PMS patients, but rather indicate that the understanding of these disorders lies in contextual factors instead of in hormonal excesses or deficiencies (Bloch, Schmidt, Su, Tobin, & Rubinow, 1998; Rubinow et al., 1998a; Schmidt et al., 1998).

In a study of 1312 menstruating twins, lifetime major depression, premenstrual tiredness, sadness, and irritability were retrospectively assessed twice over 6 years. Premenstrual depression and anxiety remained moderately stable over time, with the investigators estimating that the heritability of this stable component of premenstrual symptoms was 56%. Moreover, the results of this investigation suggest that there is no close etiologic relationship between PMS and major depression. Although premenstrual symptoms and major depression were found to share genetic and environmental risk factors, 88% of the genetic variance for premenstrual symptoms and 88% of the environmental variance were not shared with major depression (Kendler et al., 1998). PMDD may have a different pattern of heritability, as suggested by a report on the relationship between a polymorphism in the serotonin transporter gene and the severity of PMDD symptoms (Praschak-Rieder et al., 2002).

Psychosocial Stressors and Sociocultural Factors

A number of studies have suggested that the manifestation of PMS, particularly perimenstrual mood discomforts, may result from a combination of multiple stressors, a heightened stress response, few supports, and a vulnerable period of biologic reactivity. Stress perception and stressful experiences appear to influence the reporting of premenstrual symptoms, and biopsychosocial factors (altered stress hormones, low self-esteem, negative life changes, increased stress response) increase the severity of PMS (Gallant, 1991; Taylor et al., 1991; Woods et al., 1999). Notably, women with PMS report more stressors and experience them as more distressing than women without PMS (Freeman, Sondheimer, & Rickels, 1988; Gise, Lebovits, Paddison, & Strain, 1990). Women with premenstrual symptoms may use relatively ineffective methods of coping with stress, such as avoidance or wishful thinking, rather than effective strategies such as problem-solving, communication, or direct action (Ross, 2004; Taylor, 1996).

A history of sexual abuse, particularly in childhood, seems to be common among women seeking treatment for severe PMS. Among 42 women with severe PMS who agreed to be interviewed about their sexual abuse history, 95% reported at least one attempted or completed sexual abuse event, with 81% reporting rape with penetration (Golding, Taylor, Menard, & King, 2000). A more recent study of 568 women with and without PMS ages 18 to 45 years revealed that the severity of PMS patterns were significantly correlated with whether the woman had been abused as an adolescent (Koci & Strickland, 2006).

Sociocultural factors appear to influence which symptoms women notice and which symptoms they consider to be problematic. Two of the largest cross-cultural studies suggest that the reported incidence of various premenstrual changes is high in many different countries and that a large number of women throughout the world report physical discomfort and mood changes associated with menstruation (Janiger, Riffenburgh, & Kersh, 1972; WHO, 1981). Perimenstrual symptom experiences appear to differ by geographic location, marital status, parity, education, and occupation (Futterman, Jones, Miccio-Fonseca, & Quigley, 1992; Huerta-Franco & Malacara, 1993; Woods, Dery, & Most, 1982). Some analyses of cross-cultural differences suggest that women in Western societies have been socialized to have negative expectations about menstruation. In one study, Mexican women who viewed a videotape describing the negative consequences of PMS later reported more severe premenstrual symptoms compared with women in a control group who watched a neutral video (Marvan, Diaz-Erosa, & Montesinos, 1998).

The onset of PMS or severe perimenstrual symptoms seems to occur across the reproductive life span, although women who report experiencing the most severe symptoms tend to be in their late 30s. Perhaps more severe symptoms are experienced during this period of life because they coincide with increasing stress in a woman's life (Lee & Rittenhouse, 1992; Taylor, 1996). The menopausal transition has also been associated with the onset of perimenstrual mood discomforts or PMS (Woods et al., 1997). One hypothesis suggests that as women age, their brain receptors become less resilient to hormonal fluctuations than they were in earlier years (Rubinow et al., 1998b). In general, studies reveal that older women report more symptoms prior to menses, whereas younger women report more symptoms during menstruation. There is evidence that two-thirds of adolescent females have some degree of dysmenorrhea, with rates being higher for adolescents than for adults (Freeman, Rickels, & Sondheimer, 1993; Sundell, Milsom, & Andersch, 1990).

Young girls learn about symptoms from observing their mothers, sisters, and peers, including their expectations regarding menstrual experiences and the effects of menstruation on feelings and behavior (Woods, Mitchell, & Lentz, 1999). Mothers' experiences with premenstrual symptoms appear linked to daughters' subsequent symptom experiences and illness behavior. Indeed, exposure to a mother with premenstrual symptoms and teachings about negative effects of menstruation have been associated with negative affect symptomatology during premenses and menses for adult women (Taylor et al., 1991). Women who have perimenstrual symptoms may come to anticipate having them, which in turn prompts them to perceive events around the time of menstruation as more stressful.

It is unlikely that any single general theory can explain the flare-up of premenstrual symptoms for all women. Although PMS and PMDD have been predominantly regarded as biologically based illnesses, strong evidence suggests that variables such as life stress, stress response, history of sexual abuse, and cultural socialization are important determinants of perimenstrual symptoms. The prevailing view is that women with PMS are more sensitive to what are essentially normal hormonal shifts, and as a result they develop symptoms that do not affect other menstruating women. Some of these physiologic changes may make more of a difference for some women who experience PMS than for others. For example, one woman may be particularly sensitive to premenstrually induced low blood sugar, whereas another might be hypersensitive to changes in serotonin levels. Perhaps changes in the levels of gonadal steroids that are released by the pituitary gland trigger a change in some women's moods, or otherwise predispose them to mood instability. For some women, response to stress may be the key factor. Moreover, women with PMS might potentially have trouble coping with physiologic shifts as well as with other stressful aspects of their lives, which in turn exacerbates the intensity of their premenstrual symptoms.

Translating Research into Practice

Cyclic perimenstrual pain and discomfort represent a family of symptom clusters that require the clinician to balance several seemingly dichotomous views: normative versus pathologic, one-dimensional versus multidimensional, acute versus chronic, and protocol versus individualized care. The goal for practice related to the menstrual cycle and perimenstrual experiences is to normalize these experiences for women, and to help women understand them in the context of their life transitions, personal characteristics, and environmental stressors.

A few of the assumptions that underpin the assessment and therapeutic strategies for women experiencing perimenstrual pain and discomforts include the following:

- Personal and social changes have health effects that are as important as, if not more important than, the biologic changes of the menstrual cycle.
- Biologic changes should not be ignored, but rather viewed in the context of biobehavioral relationships, including, but not restricted to, the levels of hormones.
- Multiple factors both promote and prevent women from caring for their own health.

Clinicians can have a significant impact on the care of women with cyclic perimenstrual pain, discomforts, and PMS by using the evidence-based approach to assessing, diagnosing, and managing cyclic perimenstrual pain and discomfort (Collins Sharp et al., 2002).

Assessment

The conventional medical approach to assessment and diagnosis focuses on ruling out pathology. Data for assessment and diagnosis are collected during the medical history, physical examination, laboratory assessments, and differential diagnoses. The challenge for women's health clinicians is to integrate the strengths of a feminist approach to clinical practice with biomedical knowledge and skills. A feminist model of intervention focuses on women-centered care, advocacy, health promotion, and self-care.

The goal for assessment is to understand each individual woman's perimenstrual experience and to help her define and manage distressing symptoms and their concomitant problems. Much of the assessment process can be assumed by the woman herself with the help of self-assessment tools (Taylor & Colino, 2002) and professional guidance (AWHONN, 2003). Prospective assessment of individual symptoms or symptom clusters—the recommended method—can be accomplished by the use of a calendar or symptom checklist kept for two to three consecutive cycles (Mitchell, 1991; Panay, 2008; Shaver & Woods, 1985).

In addition to a focused health history and physical examination, distinguishing perimenstrual symptoms and discomfort patterns across at least three menstrual cycle phases is optimal: the premenstrual phase (up to 14 days prior to the onset of menses), the menstrual phase (the days during menses), and the postmenstrual phase (after menses and before ovulation) (AWHONN, 2003; Mitchell, 1991; Mitchell et al., 1991; Panay, 2008).

According to the American College of Obstetricians and Gynecologists (2000, reaffirmed 2010), the key criteria for a diagnosis of PMS are as follows:

- Symptoms consistent with PMS
- Consistent occurrence of the symptoms only during the luteal phase of the menstrual cycle
- Negative impact of the symptoms on some facet of the woman's life
- Exclusion of other diagnoses that may better explain the symptoms

For a diagnosis of PMDD, the APA (2000) requirements are as follows:

- Five or more symptoms, including affective and physical symptoms, are present during the week before menses and are absent in the follicular phase.
- One of the symptoms is irritability, depressed mood, anxiety, or affective lability.
- The symptoms markedly interfere with occupational or social functioning.
- The symptoms are not due to an exacerbation of another disorder.
- The preceding criteria have been confirmed by prospective daily ratings over at least two menstrual cycles.

However, evidence suggests there is not enough support to establish PMDD as a separate classification from severe PMS or CPPD (Moynihan, 2004).

Symptom Assessment

Based on research and professional recommendations, CPPD and PMS appear to be individualized experiences requiring a dynamic and personalized assessment and diagnosis, which includes self-monitoring of symptoms, rating of symptom severity, and the identification of patient-specific symptom clusters and patterns. Screening should assess for pelvic pain at or around the time of menstruation, other related discomforts, and the effectiveness of currently used therapies. AWHONN (2003) suggests completing a focused nursing assessment that includes screening questions, a health history, and a focused physical examination (**Figure 24-1**).

Symptom Monitoring

Symptom monitoring essentially consists of educating women in self-diagnosis. Getting in touch with their symptoms includes simply listing and rating feelings, symptoms, and behavioral changes, as well as focusing on social and physical environmental factors. Careful

Focused Nursing Assessment

SCREENING QUESTIONS

- Do you ever have pelvic pain or cramps during or around the time of your period?
- Are you able to treat this pain so it doesn't bother you?
- Do you ever have other physical or mood discomforts during or around the time of your period?
- Are you able to treat these discomforts so they don't bother you?

FOCUSED HEALTH HISTORY

- **Investigation of presenting problem/chief complaint**
  - Identify the individual woman's pattern of CPPD. The cycle may be divided into three phases: premenstrual, early menstrual (days 1–3 or days of heavy flow) and late menstrual (day 4 and onward or days of lighter flow).
    - Pattern of severity of CPP across pre- and early menstrual phases
    - Rating of overall distress caused by CPP
    - Pattern of severity of other cyclic discomforts across pre- and early menstrual phases
    - Rating of overall distress caused by cyclic discomforts
    - Influences on the cyclic symptoms — e.g., work stress, diet or exercise
  - A symptom checklist and calendar are useful for collecting these data (Figure 19–2).
- **Medical history**
  - Medical problems
  - Depression, anxiety, eating disorders
  - Surgeries
- **Focused family history**
  - Maternal and sibling CPPD experience and beliefs
  - Family response to CPPD
  - Cultural remedies
- **Menstrual history**
  - Age at menarche
  - First day of last menstrual period
  - Description of usual cycle (length, flow, regularity)
  - Any changes in usual cycle
- **Present health status**
  - Health perception
  - Current medications, complementary therapies
  - Drug allergies

- **Identification of the individual woman's pattern of symptom management**
  - Interventions, including self-care strategies
  - Pattern of use across pre- and early menstrual phases
  - Rating of relief obtained from intervention
  - Rating of satisfaction with pain and symptom control
  - Rating of adherence (consistent use of treatment)
- **Sexual history**
  - Sexual orientation and current sexual activity
  - Number of partners
  - Satisfaction with current sexual practices
  - Protection from sexually transmitted infections
  - Contraception
  - Physical or sexual assault or abuse
  - Risk-taking behaviors (alcohol, drugs, age of partners)
- **Obstetric history**
  - Gravity, parity, abortions
  - Living children
  - Complications related to pregnancy and birth
- **Health behaviors/functional status**
  - Nutrition
  - Exercise
  - Sleep/rest
  - Self-perception/concept
  - Roles and relationships
  - Family, social and occupational stressors
  - Coping skills
    - Health promoting
    - Health damaging

FOCUSED PHYSICAL EXAMINATION

- Abdominal examination: inspection, auscultation, percussion, palpation
  - Assess rebound tenderness (peritoneal inflammation)
  - Iliopsoas and obturator muscle tests (appendicitis)
- Percussion for costovertebral angle tenderness and palpation for suprapubic tenderness (pyelonephritis, urinary tract infection)
- External examination: inspection, palpation
- Internal examination: inspection, palpation, assessment cervical motion and tenderness
- Laboratory evaluation as indicated by history and examination

FIGURE 24-1 Focused health history and physical examination.

symptom assessment through daily monitoring and use of a diary of daily experiences can be therapeutic (Taylor, 1996). Women can see their own patterns of symptoms and identify the relationship between these symptoms and the circumstances of their lives as well as the menstrual cycle. Not only will daily monitoring of these factors help women determine the severity and pattern of their symptoms, but it will also provide them with a basis for making healthy changes all month long.

Although prospective assessment is the recommended method of assessing symptom severity, distress, and pattern, retrospective assessment can be an initial first step in determining symptom distress. Retrospective symptom severity reports are likely to overestimate severity and do not provide data about symptom patterns. Prospective ratings are critical to precise diagnosis and to rule out other chronic illnesses. Retrospective assessment can include the following questions:

- In your own words, describe the pain and discomforts that are the most severe and distressing to you.
- What is the pattern of pain and discomforts during a typical menstrual cycle? How many days before, during, or after your period do you notice symptoms? Do the symptoms occur around ovulation?
- Does anything in particular—such as work stress, dietary influences, or exercise—worsen or alleviate symptoms?

Identifying and Rating Symptom Cluster Severity and Distress

Once a woman has identified her most distressing or bothersome discomforts by symptom cluster, she can then rate the severity and degree of distress prospectively over one to two menstrual cycles. Prospective assessment of cyclic pain and discomforts can be accomplished through the use of a calendar or symptom checklist. A menstrual or symptom calendar is useful for women who are able to describe their unique symptoms and symptom clusters, as well as to visualize symptom severity patterns. Women fill in their most distressing symptoms beginning on the first day of their last menstrual period, using a five-point rating scale:

    0: no severity
    1: minimal severity
    2: mild severity
    3: moderate severity
    4: extreme severity

Examples of a calendar method of symptom assessment can be found in **Figure 24-2** (AWHONN, 2003; Taylor & Colino, 2002) and in the American College of Obstetricians and Gynecologists' *Education Pamphlet AP057: Premenstrual Syndrome* (2010), which is available on the College's website. Women who have difficulty describing their symptoms or who have many symptoms may find it easier to use a symptom-severity checklist to identify symptoms and symptom clusters (Mitchell et al., 1991; Mitchell, Woods, Lentz, Taylor, & Lee, 1992; Taylor & Colino, 2002).

CPPD Symptom Calendar

INSTRUCTIONS

Menstrual cycle day:	Begin with the first day of menstrual flow and end with the last day of your menstrual cycle. If you are only experiencing symptoms during your menstrual flow (and not before), you may stop your calendar when your flow stops.
Month and date:	Write the month and the corresponding date in the box under each menstrual cycle day.
Bleeding/menstrual flow:	Record your menstrual flow or vaginal bleeding as heavy (H), moderate (M), light (L), spotting (S) or, if no bleeding, leave the box blank. Note the last day of your menstrual flow with an asterisk (*).
Symptoms:	Rate these symptoms or behavior changes daily as mild (1), moderate (2), severe (3) or extreme (4) throughout the cycle.

Menstrual cycle day	1	2	3	4	5	6	7	8	9	10	11	12	13	14	15	16	17	18	19	20	21	22	23	24	25	26	27	28	29	30	31
Month/date																															
Bleeding/menstrual flow																															
Cyclic pelvic pain																															
• Abdominal cramps																															
• Nausea, vomiting																															
• Backache																															
• Change in bowel frequency																															
Physical discomforts																															
• Fatigue																															
• Headaches																															
• Fluid retention																															
• Joint aches and pain																															
• Breast tenderness																															
• Leg/thigh discomfort																															
• Change in energy and appetite																															
Mood discomforts																															
• Depression																															
• Irritability																															
• Tension																															
• Impatience																															
• Anxiety																															
• Anger																															
• Mood swings																															
• Hostility																															
• Change in sexual desire																															
• Guilt																															
• Feeling out of control																															
• Tearfulness																															

Note: From *Taking Back the Month: A Personalized Solution for Managing PMS and Enhancing Your Health* (p. 285), by D. Taylor and Stacey Colino, 2002, New York: Berkley Publishing. Copyright 2002 by Diana Taylor and Stacey Colino. Adapted with permission. This form may be duplicated for use in clinical practice only. Permission for use in any other form must be obtained from AWHONN.

FIGURE 24-2 Calendar method for perimenstrual symptom assessment.

Source: Copyright © 2003 by the Association of Women's Health, Obstetric and Neonatal Nurses. All rights reserved.

Determining Symptom Cluster Severity and Distress Patterns

It is important to clearly delineate symptoms, their patterns, and the ways that they are related (or not) to the menstrual cycle, because PMS and perimenstrual symptom clusters have no clearly defined cause. A number of investigators have found that many women who believed they had PMS were later found to have another problem, such as endometriosis, that worsened around the time of menstruation. In other instances, a woman's mood or behavior changes—which may have been heightened during the premenstrual phase—were attributed to PMS when, in fact, they were a result of external problems such as work-related stress, relationship difficulties, problems with children, on-the-job harassment, violence, and other legitimate sources of anxiety, fear, and frustration. Alternatively, when examining a completed chart, women may discover that certain symptom clusters—pain and fatigue, for example—continue all month long but just worsen premenstrually. This exercise helps a woman to gain a sense of self-awareness and become more attuned to how her perimenstrual experiences manifest themselves as symptoms, feelings, or behaviors, as well as the degree to which they affect her life.

Once symptom clusters have been identified and tracked for one or two menstrual cycles, symptom patterns can be classified. Three or four classifications of cyclic pain and discomfort patterns are typically employed:

- When women have a low severity of perimenstrual pain and discomforts, they experience few bothersome symptoms of low to mild severity in the menstrual or premenstrual phases, or they may have one or two symptoms that are rated as moderate to severe but last only for 1 or 2 days.
- The classic dysmenorrhea pattern includes multiple pain symptoms that are rated as moderate or severe for 1 day premenstrually and 3 to 5 menstrual days. Symptoms completely subside after menses but might also include cyclic headaches and physical discomforts such as bloating.
- The classic PMS pattern or cyclic perimenstrual mood and physical discomforts include symptoms that are rated as moderate to extremely severe for up to 2 weeks before the onset of menses, and symptoms that subsequently disappear or become much milder within 1 to 4 days of the onset of bleeding.
- With PMM, women have symptoms that are cyclic in the sense that they are present during the postmenstrual (follicular) and early premenstrual (luteal) phases, but often increase in severity during the premenstrual phase. Many women who demonstrate this pattern deserve careful evaluation to determine whether they are experiencing a premenstrual exacerbation of another disorder such as depression, anxiety, substance abuse, headaches, allergies, asthma, IBS, or chronic pelvic pain.

Laboratory Assessments

There are no specific tests for CPPD, PMS, or PMM, although some laboratory tests can be helpful in ruling out underlying problems. Simple blood tests can identify conditions such as anemia, thyroid disorders, diabetes, or hypoglycemia. Ovarian hormone testing is unnecessary unless premature menopause (before the age of 40 years) is suspected.

Differential Diagnoses

The patterns and severity of symptoms are the best guide for sorting out whether a woman has cyclic or chronic perimenstrual pain, mild or severe perimenstrual physical or mood discomforts, PMM, severe PMS, or a dual diagnosis. Symptom-tracking charts and calendars along with menstrual and health history data will provide essential clues for making a diagnosis.

PMS and CPPD need to be distinguished from endocrine abnormalities and from conditions that are subject to PMM (discussed previously). Furthermore, the transition to menopause may be a vulnerable period when women experience the onset or a worsening of CPPD or PMS, especially mood disturbances and fatigue (Woods et al., 1997).

Although the underlying cause of this phenomenon is unknown, a considerable body of evidence indicates there are many possible manifestations of PMM. Many medical and psychiatric conditions may be exacerbated in the premenstrual or menstrual phase of the cycle, leading a woman to believe that she must be experiencing PMS. In particular, thyroid disease is frequently overlooked because of the many symptoms associated with hypothyroid or hyperthyroid disease syndromes (Girdler, Pedersen, & Light, 1995). Mood disorders—primarily depression—are twice as common as anxiety disorders, and both may become exacerbated premenstrually (Rubinow & Schmidt, 1995; Yonkers & White, 1992). Other psychiatric disorders, such as substance abuse and bulimia, can be exacerbated during the luteal phase of the menstrual cycle. Many women with epilepsy experience changes in seizure frequency and severity with changes in reproductive cycles, including at puberty, over the menstrual cycle, with pregnancy, and at menopause.

Musculoskeletal pain syndromes, such as arthralgias, arthritis, and fibromyalgia, can cause symptoms that overlap with PMS (e.g., generalized pain, fatigue, sleep disturbances, or cognitive impairment) and may go undiagnosed in women with moderate to severe PMS (Shaver et al., 1997). Cyclic perimenstrual pain that is severe and begins at mid-cycle or worsens premenstrually may indicate an underlying gynecologic condition such as endometriosis, pelvic inflammatory disease, or chronic pelvic pain (see Chapters 21, 27, and 29, respectively). Clinical management guidelines for the diagnosis of chronic pelvic pain have been published by the American College of Obstetricians and Gynecologists (2004, reaffirmed 2010) that differentiate pathophysiology between acute and chronic pelvic pain. In addition, migraine-type headaches appear to increase during the premenstrual and menstrual phases. Menstrual migraines tend to occur 1 to 3 days before menstruation begins or during the first day or two of menstruation when hormone levels drop considerably.

All menstruating women report that gastrointestinal (GI) symptoms, such as stomach pain, nausea, and loose stools, are highest during menses, and almost 50% of women with IBS report a perimenstrual increase in their symptoms. Women with Crohn's disease report more premenstrual and menstrual GI symptoms (e.g., diarrhea, abdominal pain, and constipation) than other women with bowel disease. Women with functional bowel disease (FBD)—that is, bowel disease not yet classified as a GI disorder—report more stomach pain, nausea, and diarrhea at menses than women without FBD.

Infections seem to increase or worsen during the premenstrual phase of the menstrual cycle. Vaginal infections, especially yeast infections, often occur right before or during menstruation and have been found to be related to alterations in the normal vaginal pH level. The incidence of urinary cystitis increases both premenstrually and during menstruation for the same reason. Viral infections, such as herpes, seem to flare up during this time as well. Some women report sinus congestion and symptoms of colds or other upper respiratory infection premenstrually, which then disappear after the onset of their menses.

Beginning the Therapeutic Process

Setting Goals

Sometimes the process of assessment is therapeutic in itself—raising self-awareness and validating women's symptom experience. Setting goals and outcome criteria formalizes the therapeutic process while continuing an interactive process that includes and encourages the woman's participation in her self-care. For example, outcomes identified may include comfort level, type of treatment, pain and discomfort relief, role performance change, or economic costs. Setting goals should include both health-related outcomes and other outcomes, such as functional status and economic impact. In terms of functional status, the detrimental effects of inadequately treated cyclic perimenstrual pain range from missed life opportunities, such as work, school, or other activities, to increased costs for women seeking relief from pain (Dawood et al., 1985; Harlow, 1986; Harlow & Park, 1996; Smith, 1993).

The clinician—in collaboration with the woman—facilitates the therapeutic process, which is dependent on the following elements:

1. Desired patient outcome
2. Characteristics of the diagnosis
3. Research base associated with the intervention
4. Feasibility of successfully implementing the intervention
5. Acceptability of the intervention to the client
6. Capability of the clinician (Bulecheck & McCloskey, 1999)

Therapeutic Options

Most women use OTC remedies to manage their pelvic pain. Drugs such as acetaminophen (Tylenol), naproxen (Aleve), and ibuprofen (Advil, Motrin) have proved effective in managing pain (Jarrett, Heitkemper, & Shaver, 1995). Nonetheless, it appears that many women—particularly adolescents—do not always use OTC medications effectively and would benefit from additional information on pain management and evidence-based self-care strategies (Campbell & McGrath, 1997). **Table 24-2** identifies interventions for the treatment of CPPD and PMS.

Treatments for perimenstrual symptoms and PMS range from dangerous options (ovarian radiation) to those treatments that obviously are ineffective (hiding in one's room). For many years, the focus on singular (usually pharmacologic) therapy has dominated treatments for perimenstrual symptoms and PMS. However, clinical research has suggested that a combination of treatments may prove more satisfactory than a single treatment (Taylor, 1988, 1996; Taylor & Woods, 1991). Moreover, outcomes from symptom-management programs suggest that when symptoms are comprehensively managed, women are more likely to remain in treatment and show improved outcomes. New models of symptom management that combine self-care, social support, medical therapies, and psychosocial strategies applied to specific conditions have shown promising results. In a clinical trial of multimodal symptom-management strategies for women experiencing severe PMS, Taylor (1999) found

TABLE 24-2 CPPD and PMS Interventions

CPPD and PMS Interventions: Interventions are organized within a conceptual framework of symptom management in the left column. Interventions for which there is an evidence base are identified under each symptom cluster. Specific details about implementation of the intervention are presented in this chapter, the AWHONN evidence-based guideline (Collins Sharp et al., 2002), or Taylor and Colino (2002).

	Cyclic Pelvic Pain	Physical Discomforts	Mood Discomforts	Severe PMS
1. Fundamental Symptom Management				
• Collaborative Symptom Assessment & Self-Monitoring	X Symptom cluster, severity, pattern assessment	X	X	X
• Mutual Goal-Setting	X	X	X	X
• Coping Enhancement	X	X	X	X
2. Symptom-Regulation				
a. Pharmacologic				
• Over-the-Counter Medication	X NSAIDs, analgesics	X NSAIDs, analgesics		
• Prescription Medication	X NSAIDs, analgesics	X	X	X Antidepressants
• Hormones	X Oral contraceptives, progestin IUD	X Oral contraceptives		X Micronized progesterone (inconsistent evidence)
• Nutraceuticals	X Calcium, magnesium, essential fatty acids, vitamin E, vitamin B1	X	X	X

(continues)

TABLE 24-2 CPPD and PMS Interventions *(Continued)*

	Cyclic Pelvic Pain	Physical Discomforts	Mood Discomforts	Severe PMS
b. Topical-Cutaneous				
• Heat Application	X	X		
• Therapeutic Massage	X	X	X	
• Acupressure	X	X		
• Transcutaneous Nerve Stimulation	X			
c. Behavioral-Cognitive				
• Behavioral Relaxation	X Breathing, stretching, PMR	X	X Breathing, stretching, PMR, AT	
• Cognitive Relaxation			X Cognitive exercises, imagery, meditation, biofeedback	X
• Environmental Modification			X Time management, healthy communication, problem solving	X
3. Self-Modification				
• Nutritional Counseling: General Dietary Modification	X Multivitamin-mineral supplement, lowfat and vegetarian diet, increase fluid premenstrually	X	X Decrease caffeine, alcohol, simple sugars, salt premenstrually, increase fluids, meal frequency	X

• Health Risk Reduction: Smoking Cessation	X		
• Exercise Promotion	X Aerobic exercise postmenstrually; premenstrual or menstrual activity modification	X	X

4. Referral and/or Co-management

• Acupuncture	X	X	
• Traditional Chinese Medicine	X	X	X
• Homeopathy	X	X	
• Botanical/Herbal Therapy		X	X Vitex, SAM-e
• Chiropractic Therapy	X		
• Surgical Evaluation	X		
• Mental Health Evaluation		X	X
• Emerging Therapies		X	X Light therapy, SAM-e,

that women prefer to select multiple strategies for symptom management, that perimenstrual symptom severity declined markedly within the first few months with this approach, and that this effect could be maintained over the long term.

These strategies, although focused on perimenstrual symptom relief, are generally health promoting. Establishing healthy dietary and exercise habits along with managing personal and environmental stress during early adulthood may lead to lifelong healthy behaviors that result in chronic disease prevention in later adult life. Symptom management interventions can also be considered as complementary to pharmacologic therapy in women with a dual diagnosis or a depressive disorder that regularly worsens during a specific menstrual cycle phase. **Table 24-3** identifies science-based self-management of the symptoms of PMS.

TABLE 24-3 Translating Research into Practice: Science-Based PMS Self-Management

Putting the science back into self-care has been a significant extension of menstrual cycle research, resulting in consumer education about this research. Taylor and Colino (2002) have published one of the first science-based self-help books for women that describes step-by-step strategies for self-assessment and self-management of perimenstrual symptoms, PMS, and stress. This book can be used in combination with the American College of Obsteticians and Gynecologists or AWHONN guidelines in ways such as the following:

- Tracking symptoms and stress—Empowered self-diagnosis strategies
- The anti-PMS diet—How food increases and decreases stress and PMS
- Nutritional supplements for PMS and stress management
- Reducing body stress—Breathing, physical activity, and relaxation strategies
  - Behavioral relaxation strategies include breathing and stretching exercises that can be accomplished in a few minutes twice daily, along with how to choose between progressive muscle relaxation and autogenic training relaxation.
- Adding the mind to the body—Breaking the cycle of mental bad habits, dealing with thoughts that won't stop, changing thinking to change mood, retraining the mind, and thinking up better realities.
  - As body relaxation is effective for only 50% of women (Taylor, 1996), cognitive relaxation strategies have been found to be helpful in relaxing the mind. For example, meditation, guided imagery, prayer, and biofeedback are ways to reduce mental stress. Instructions for thought stopping and reducing toxic self-talk have been found to be effective in reducing both mind and body tension.
- Managing stress from the "outside," such as making and taking time, learning to communicate effectively, developing an everyday talk therapy, and other effective ways to manage work, home, and relationship stress that increase perimenstrual negative moods and stress responses.
  - Managing time vs. letting time take over—Assessing time problems, managing time, and reclaiming time
  - Controlling relationship stress at home and work—Everyday talk therapy, revamping communication styles, developing a "can do" process for dealing with relationship stress, overcoming resistance from others, and starting a support group.
- Putting the pieces together—Developing a personalized prescription
- Solve new symptoms as they arise, such as common stress-related headaches, fatigue, insomnia, or menstrual pain and bloating.

Management of Severe PMS

Evidence-Based Recommendations

Some women experience severe PMS or have a dual diagnosis that includes noncyclic mood disorders, seasonal depression, or intense menstrual pain that may benefit from medication in combination with various aspects of a symptom-management program. Others may be so acutely sensitive to hormonal fluctuations that it may make sense to suppress the ovarian cycle to help obtain symptom relief.

Certain psychotropic medications, hormonal therapies, and diuretics have been found to be helpful in dealing with noncyclic moods, PMM, or severe mood and physical discomforts. Although the SSRI drugs appear to lessen the cyclic agitated–depressive symptoms, micronized progesterone has been found to act as an antianxiety agent, which means it may be better suited for relieving the perimenstrual mood discomfort cluster of symptoms (tension, irritability, anger, feeling out of control, or mood swings). Women who are experiencing both CPPD and perimenopausal menstrual irregularities may be more responsive to micronized progesterone. If a woman is not sensitive to exogenous hormones and needs contraception, ovarian suppression using a combined contraceptive (i.e., pill, patch, or vaginal ring; see Chapter 12) may help decrease the mood, pain, and other physical symptoms that have not been completely relieved by nonpharmacologic symptom-management strategies.

General caveats for all the pharmacologic therapies include avoidance during pregnancy or pregnancy planning. In addition, it is recommended that these medications be tried for at least two or three menstrual cycles to gauge their effects on symptoms and to overcome any side effects.

Pharmacologic Symptom Management

Antidepressants For patients with severe PMS and for those who do not respond to fundamental symptom management, the American College of Obstetricians and Gynecologists' (2000, reaffirmed 2010) practice guidelines recommend that SSRIs—particularly fluoxetine (Prozac) and sertraline (Zoloft)—be taken daily or intermittently during the premenstrual phase of the menstrual cycle. Level I evidence supported by a meta-analysis and three placebo-controlled trials (Steiner, Korzekwa, Lamont, & Wilkins, 1997; Steiner et al., 2001; Steiner et al., 1995) shows that SSRIs resulted in a 40% to 55% decrease in PMDD (especially negative mood symptoms) but had a high rate of side effects (especially at the 60 mg level of fluoxetine), even when used cyclically. Level II evidence suggests that SSRIs can be used for a shorter duration when combined with multimodal symptom-management strategies (Taylor, 2000). To date, a considerable body of evidence demonstrating the benefits of using SSRIs in the successful treatment of PMS has been published (Dimmock, Wyatt, Jones, & O'Brien, 2000).

Serotonergic-activating agents, including the SSRIs fluoxetine, sertraline, paroxetine (Paxil), and citalopram (Celexa), have all been shown to mediate severe premenstrual symptoms. A relabeled form of fluoxetine has been approved by the FDA for the treatment of

PMDD or severe PMS under the brand name Sarafem. Notably, the European counterpart to the FDA has not approved these drugs for treatment of PMDD, claiming lack of evidence to establish PMDD as a treatable disorder (Moynihan, 2004).

The most common side effects of SSRIs are headaches, sleep disturbances, dizziness, weight gain, dry mouth, and decreased libido. Other, less often reported side effects include decreased appetite, weight loss, drowsiness, impaired concentration, altered taste, nausea, diarrhea, and nervousness. If these problems occur, they can usually be lessened by prescribing lower dosages of the medications. Notably, a substantial amount of evidence indicates that SSRIs do not increase the risk of spontaneous abortion, major malformation, decreased birth weight, prematurity, or postnatal complications following in utero exposure, nor is there evidence that SSRIs are teratogenic.

Anxiolytic Drugs The most commonly prescribed antianxiety medication for noncyclic anxiety or panic disorders is alprazolam (Xanax). Other agents in this class include diazepam (Valium), lorazepam (Ativan), and buspirone (BuSpar). Research on the use of antianxiety medications to relieve PMS symptoms has shown mixed results. In the only two randomized, crossover, placebo-controlled clinical trials of alprazolam for use during the premenstrual phase, women taking the drug experienced less anxiety, depression, and headaches (Freeman, Rickels, Sondheimer, & Polansky, 1995; Schmidt, Grover, & Rubinow, 1993). However, alprazolam has also been shown to stimulate increased appetite premenstrually, which could make it difficult to control food cravings or binges. Furthermore, alprazolam has the potential to produce addiction, tolerance, and bothersome sedation, and it is not recommended as a first-line treatment by the American College of Obstetricians and Gynecologists' (2000, reaffirmed 2010) PMS Practice Guidelines.

These medications are for short-term use only, and continued use should not exceed 8 weeks without medical or psychiatric evaluation, because physical and psychological dependencies can occur quickly with anxiolytic drugs. Physical tolerance develops quickly, and relying on pills supersedes the development of nonpharmacologic stress-management strategies. Side effects of anxiolytic agents may include visual problems, mood swings, and joint stiffness. Other, less frequently reported side effects include drowsiness, headaches, dizziness, blurred vision, dry mouth, weakness, confusion, nausea, constipation, agitation, and depression. Oral contraceptives can increase the potency of antianxiety drugs, which in turn may increase the risk of side effects. By contrast, alcohol, if consumed while taking an antianxiety drug, increases depression of the CNS.

Hormonal Therapy A progesterone deficiency has not been proven as a causal mechanism for PMS, and results of research using progestogens as a treatment for PMS are inconsistent. A systematic review of 14 trials with progestogens given orally, vaginally, or rectally did not support the use of progestogen therapy for this indication (Wyatt, Dimmock, Jones, Obhrai, & O'Brien, 2001). Although the FDA has not approved progestogen therapy for PMS, micronized progesterone is an FDA-recognized hormone therapy for perimenopausal symptoms, especially when a woman is still menstruating and estrogen supplementation is contraindicated (Martorano, Ahlgrimm, & Colbert, 1998). Cyclic physical and mood discomforts that are experienced by women in the menopausal transition combined with menstrual irregularities have been successfully treated with 300 mg of micronized progesterone at bedtime or medroxyprogesterone (Provera) in a dose of 10 mg per day for 16 days of the menstrual cycle (Prior, 2002). Micronized progesterone appears to play a role in bone formation, whereas the synthetic progestins are implicated in bone loss (Prior et al., 2001). Micronized progesterone has been recognized as a treatment for PMS in the United Kingdom since the 1970s and few side effects have been reported beyond mild sedation or drowsiness, nor has the drug been linked with fetal abnormalities if it is used during pregnancy. Current contraindications to the use of oral progestogens, such as medroxyprogesterone, include liver dysfunction, known or suspected cancer, genital bleeding of unknown cause, and blood clotting disorders.

A number of investigators have found that temporarily suppressing ovulation can reduce cyclic perimenstrual pain as well as cyclic perimenstrual physical and mood discomforts in some women (Bjorn et al., 2002; Bjorn, Bixo, Nojd, Nyberg, & Backstrom, 2000; Freeman et al., 2001; Sanders, Graham, Bass, & Bancroft, 2001). Level III evidence indicates that combined oral contraceptives (COCs) can reduce perimenstrual negative mood symptom severity and variability (Oinonen & Mazmanian, 2002). Nevertheless, in a controlled trial of a COC that contains the newer progestin drospirenone (Yasmin), the results showed an insignificant decrease in mood symptoms (10% decrease in premenstrual mood symptoms and PMDD) and a 10% to 20% rate of side effects such as nausea, headaches, and depression, which are similar to side effects reported for all COCs (Freeman et al., 2001). According to the American College of Obstetricians and Gynecologists (2000, reaffirmed 2010), oral contraceptives should be considered only if symptoms are primarily physical.

There is limited and inconsistent evidence supporting the utility of hormonal ovulation suppression with gonadotropin-releasing hormone (GnRH) agonists or surgical oophorectomy in treating PMS and related disorders. Although some women have benefited from these therapies, GnRH agonists are associated with significant side effects, and surgical oophorectomy is an irreversible therapeutic option.

Diuretics Diuretics have been widely prescribed for severe premenstrual bloating and fluid retention. However, no evidence exists to show that thiazide diuretics are of benefit, and they can actually make symptoms worse via potassium depletion, which results in stimulation of the autonomic nervous system. An aldosterone antagonist with antiandrogenic properties, spironolactone, is the only diuretic that has demonstrated evidence in reducing severe premenstrual bloating and headaches. According to the American College of Obstetricians and Gynecologists (2000, reaffirmed 2010), there is Level I evidence to support the use of spironolactone, although not all reports evaluating spironolactone have shown a benefit from this therapy.

Emerging Therapies

Several promising alternative or complementary therapies for perimenstrual pain and discomforts have emerged in recent years. These approaches differ from those used by conventional, Western medical practitioners, and although the science behind these nonmedicinal remedies is often sparse, many of them have some research data that support their use. They are included in the discussion here because alternative or complementary treatments, such as herbal remedies, homeopathy, massage, and nutritional supplements, are popular among women who have perimenstrual discomforts.

Although the use of light therapy sprang from high-tech research interventions, many of the therapies included here, such as acupuncture, are based on centuries-old practices and ancient healing systems. Often these techniques are based on Eastern philosophies that do not separate the body from the mind, or health from lifestyle. Instead, the Eastern view perceives a woman's body as an integrated whole, with body and mind working in concert. The aim behind these disciplines is to create balance and harmony in the body; to produce subtle, positive effects over time; or to bolster the body's own healing abilities rather than relying on a potent drug that would intervene in a more aggressive way. Because of the complexity of these approaches, this section can merely provide an overview of how they could help relieve various premenstrual symptoms. To err on the side of caution, herbal or nutritional remedies are included in this section only if they are considered safe and have well-documented efficacy studies to support them.

Alternative Healing Systems: Traditional Chinese Medicine and Homeopathy

In traditional Chinese medicine (TCM), both herbs and acupuncture are used separately or in combination to treat health conditions that result from disruptions to the flow of the body's vital energy (qi or chi), which represents an imbalance between the eternal opposites of yin and yang. The National Institutes of Health has found acupuncture—the ancient Chinese art of needle placement—to be helpful in the treatment of menstrual cramps, low back pain, joint pain, headaches, and severe PMS. Acupuncture treatment manipulates the vital energy sources of the body by introducing ultrathin needles into specific points along the *meridians*, or energy pathways, of the body. Most TCM practitioners use a combination of acupuncture and herbs in the treatment of severe PMS.

Homeopathy is a holistic treatment system based on the principle that giving a person the right dose of a natural substance that might disturb the body in the wrong amounts can actually trigger healing. In a meta-analysis of 105 clinical trials of homeopathic treatments, researchers found that 75% of interpretable trials showed a positive result (Chapman, Angelica, Spitalny, & Strauss, 1994). More recently, a randomized, controlled, double-blind clinical trial at the Hebrew University, Hadassah Medical School, in Israel found that 90% of the women participating in the study experienced an improvement of more than 30% in their premenstrual symptoms after an oral dose of a homeopathic medication (Yakir et al., 2001). Although homeopathic remedies have no side effects and are available without a prescription, it is wise to consult a professional homeopath who can help choose the most appropriate treatments.

Dietary Supplements: Calcium and Vitamin D

Research suggests that supplemental calcium may be beneficial in the treatment of PMS (Canning, Waterman, & Dye, 2006; Bertone-Johnson, Hankinson, Johnson, & Manson, 2007). Canning et al.'s (2006) systematic review of dietary and herbal treatments used by women with PMS revealed that the evidence supports the use of calcium and continuous vitamin B_6 in treating the symptoms of PMS. Vitamin B_6 doses in the range of 50 to 150 mg/day may be beneficial, whereas intermittent usage was not shown to improve symptoms (Wyatt, Dimmock, & O'Brien, 1999).

Botanic, Herbal, and Alternative Therapies

Several herbs seem to have beneficial effects on both PMS and menstrual cramps, including Vitex (chaste tree berry), cramp bark, and evening primrose oil, among others. All of these herbs are available without a prescription at pharmacies and health food stores. Not all herbs have enough clinical or research evidence to document their safety or efficacy, however. Only those herbs that have been recommended by the German Commission E (which was established more than 20 years ago and has reviewed all the available literature on more than 300 herbs) or by the late Varro Tyler, a professor of pharmacognosy at Purdue University and author of *Tyler's Honest Herbal* (Foster & Tyler, 2000), are included here. To learn about safe, therapeutic dosages, the reader may want to consult *The American Pharmaceutical Association Practical Guide to Natural Medicines* (Pierce, 1999), the American Botanical Council's (2003) *The ABC Guide to Herbal Medicine*, or the National Center for Complementary and Alternative Medicine (http://nccam.nih.gov).

Vitex Agnus-Castus (Chaste Tree Berry) The only botanical treatment with Level I evidence to support its use in PMS is chaste tree berry. Native to the Mediterranean and central Asia, chaste tree (also called Vitex) is a shrub that produces dark brown to black fruit the size of a peppercorn. Preparations of the fruit as an extract or in powdered form have been approved by German health authorities for the treatment of menstrual irregularities, such as PMS and breast pain associated with a woman's menstrual period. This herb appears to have a dopamine-like activity and effect on the pituitary gland, helping to reinstate the normal balance between estrogen and progesterone during the luteal phase of the menstrual cycle. Clinical trials have shown that chaste tree berry extract keeps the overproduction of progesterone in check and effectively reduces breast pain associated with a woman's menses (Schellenberg, 2001). In the first placebo-controlled trial to clearly demonstrate the herb's effectiveness in treating PMS, German scientists found that women taking 20 mg of Vitex reported a 52% overall reduction in PMS symptoms compared with only 24% for those taking placebo (Berger, Schaffner, Schrader, Meier, & Brattstrom, 2000; Schellenberg, 2001). Reports of side effects were rare, with only 5% of the women experiencing mild symptoms, such as acne, skin rash, and bleeding between their periods. None of these symptoms caused women to drop out of the study.

Although chaste tree berry extracts do not contain hormones, they should not be used with combined contraceptives or other hormone therapies without the guidance of a clinician. Chaste tree berry extract also should not be used during pregnancy, as it can stimulate premature lactation.

Evening Primrose Oil The seed oil of the evening primrose, a weed that is native to North America, contains high concentrations of the essential fatty acid gamma linolenic acid, which is a precursor to prostaglandin. More than 120 studies in 15 countries have reported on the potential benefits of evening primrose oil, and the studies of its use for PMS suggest that it helps to regulate hormones (American Botanical Council, 2003). Two well-controlled studies failed to show any beneficial effects for evening primrose oil, although because the trials were relatively small, modest effects cannot be excluded. Although the results of research have been mixed, some scientists have found that consuming evening primrose oil supplements decreases premenstrual mood symptoms, breast pain, and fluid retention (Budeiri, Li Wan Po, & Dornan, 1996), whereas other researchers state there is no clear evidence of clinical benefit (Bayles & Usatine, 2009). The safety of the herb seems well established, but approximately 2% of those persons who take evening primrose oil experience stomach discomfort, nausea, or headaches.

SAM-e S-Adenosylmethionine, or SAM-e, is neither a drug nor an herb. Rather, SAM-e is a molecule manufactured in the body from the amino acid methionine during metabolism, which has been discovered to be related to metabolic disturbances found in patients with psychiatric and neurologic disorders. Available by prescription for years in Europe, SAM-e has been shown to be both safe and effective in treating depression and comparable to standard tricyclic antidepressants for this indication, according to a 1994 meta-analysis (Bressa, 1994). A double-blind, placebo-controlled trial found no difference between the antidepressive efficacy of 1600 mg of Sam-e and 400 mg of imipramine, except that Sam-e was more easily tolerated (Delle Chiaie, Pancheri, & Scapicchio, 2002).

A neuropharmacologist at Baylor University Medical Center Institute of Metabolic Disease in Dallas, Texas, has been studying SAM-e for more than 15 years and considers it to be safe and effective for mild to moderate depressive symptoms (Bottiglieri, 2002). This agent has also been found to be helpful in reducing joint pain associated with osteoarthritis and may be used as an alternative therapy for people who experience adverse effects when taking NSAIDs. SAM-e has been reported to cause mild and transient insomnia, nervousness, lack of appetite, constipation, headaches, heart palpitations, nausea, dry mouth, sweating, and dizziness.

Because SAM-e is converted into homocysteine (a protein associated with heart disease) in the body, it is unclear whether rising levels of homocysteine secondary to SAM-e metabolism will increase the risk of heart disease. SAM-e must be taken with a daily multivitamin along with a diet high in fruits and vegetables. Three of the B vitamins (folic acid [B_3], B_6, and B_{12}) can lower the homocysteine levels that SAM-e elevates.

Unfortunately, there is no way to find a standardized dose of SAM-e, because raw SAM-e degrades quickly unless stored at proper temperatures, and there is no guarantee that the pills available for sale have been properly handled. SAM-e is also very expensive. A daily dose can vary in price from $2.50 to $18.00 and needs to be taken over a few weeks to see results.

Light Therapy

Research suggests a link exists between PMS and seasonal affective disorder (SAD), a type of depression that typically occurs in the fall and winter months when levels of natural light decline in countries north of the equator (Brown & Robinson, 2002; Parry et al., 1997). Exposure to full-spectrum light, including ultraviolet light, in women who are highly sensitive to light has been found to decrease the moodiness and depressive symptoms of PMS. One study found that women with severe PMS who were treated with 30 minutes of evening light therapy for 2 weeks during the luteal phase of their menstrual cycles experienced a significant reduction in depression and premenstrual tension (Parry et al.). It is theorized that bright light corrects disturbances in the body's internal sleep–wake cycle that are linked with PMS or, alternatively, that the light promotes the effects of the feel-good brain chemical serotonin.

Light therapy may be considered a viable option for women who feel depressed all month long during the fall and winter months and experience an increased severity of premenstrual mood symptoms during these seasons. Formal light therapy should be initiated with the consultation of a psychotherapist or mental health counselor. Informally, women can brighten their world by increasing their light exposure, especially to morning light. Science-based self-help books offer additional recommendations (Brown & Robinson, 2002; Taylor & Colino, 2002).

Conclusion

Although CPPD is a term that describes the actual experiences of women and encompasses the medical diagnoses of dysmenorrhea and PMS, the definition of PMS has become a popularized entity as well as a recognized ICD classification. Biomedically, PMS has been defined as an illness experience or syndrome characterized by the repeated occurrence of behavioral, somatic, and mood symptoms severe enough to impair a woman's social and work-related functioning during the premenstrual and luteal phases of the menstrual cycle. PMDD, a severe form of PMS, is a controversial label now defined as a psychiatric diagnosis, and PMM refers to the premenstrual magnification of an underlying medical or psychiatric condition.

CPPD encompasses three diagnoses, each representing a cluster of symptoms supported by empirical research. Identifying the severity and patterns of these symptom clusters provides an evidence-based guide for sorting out whether a woman has cyclic or chronic perimenstrual pain, mild or severe perimenstrual physical or mood discomforts, premenstrual magnification, severe PMS, or a dual diagnosis. Prospective symptom self-monitoring using tracking charts or calendars combined with menstrual and health history data will provide additional diagnostic clues and is supported by good-quality evidence.

Under the evidence-based guidelines developed by the American College of Obstetricians and Gynecologists and AWHONN, multimodal symptom management is recommended as a first-line treatment for cyclic perimenstrual physical and mood discomforts or for mild to moderately severe PMS, to include the following components:

- Symptom monitoring
- Dietary counseling
- Nutritional supplements
- Personal and environmental stress management
- Exercise promotion

There is also fair to good evidence to support the use of selective pharmacologic therapies, such as SSRI antidepressants, for severe PMS that does not respond to nonpharmacologic symptom management. Inconsistent evidence exists for other pharmacologic therapies such as hormonal or singular therapies. More effective than a singular therapy is a multimodal package of symptom-management strategies as outlined in the AWHONN clinical practice guidelines, including the following elements:

- Exercise and dietary changes with self-monitoring
- Behavioral therapies
- Cognitive exercises
- Training in time management, role redefinition, communicating, and problem solving

Note

Beth A. Collins Sharp was an employee of the U.S. federal government when this work was conducted and prepared for publication. The views expressed in this chapter are those of the authors and do not necessarily reflect those of the Agency for Healthcare Research and Quality or the U.S. Department of Health and Human Services.

References

American Botanical Council. (2003). *The ABC guide to herbal medicines*. Austin, TX: Author.

American College of Obstetricians and Gynecologists. (2000, reaffirmed 2010). *ACOG Practice Bulletin (No. 15): Premenstrual syndrome*. Washington, DC: Author.

American College of Obstetricians and Gynecologists. (2004, reaffirmed 2010). *ACOG Practice Bulletin (No. 51): Chronic pelvic pain*. Washington, DC: Author.

American College of Obstetricians and Gynecologists. (2010). *ACOG educational pamphlet AP057: Pre-menstrual syndrome*. Retrieved from http://www.acog.org

American Psychiatric Association (APA). (1987). *Diagnostic and statistical manual of mental disorders (DSM-III-R)*. Washington, DC: Author.

American Psychiatric Association (APA). (1994). *Diagnostic and statistical manual of mental disorders (DSM-IV-R)*. Washington, DC: Author.

American Psychiatric Association (APA). (2000). *Diagnostic and statistical manual of mental disorders (DSM-IV-TR)*. Washington, DC: Author.

Angst, J., Sellaro, R., Merikangas, K., & Endicott, J. (2001). The epidemiology of perimenstrual psychological symptoms. *Acta Psychiatrica Scandinavica, 104*, 110–116.

Association of Women's Health, Nurses and Neonatal Nursing (AWHONN). (2003). *Evidence-based clinical practice guideline: Nursing management for cyclic perimenstrual pain and discomfort.* Washington, DC: Author.

Backstrom, T., Sanders, G., Leask, R., Davidson, D., Warner, P., & Bancroft, J. (1983). Mood, sexuality, hormones, and the menstrual cycle: II. Hormone levels and their relationship to premenstrual syndrome. *Psychosomatic Medicine, 45*, 503–507.

Ballagh, S., & Heyl, A. (2008). Communicating with women about menstrual cycle symptoms. *Journal of Reproductive Medicine, 53*, 837–846.

Bayles, B., & Usatine, R. (2009). Evening primrose oil. *American Family Physician, 80*, 1405–1408.

Berger, D., Schaffner, W., Schrader, E., Meier, B., & Brattstrom, A. (2000). Efficacy of Vitex agnus castus L. extract Ze 440 in patients with pre-menstrual syndrome (PMS). *Archives of Gynecology & Obstetrics, 264*(3), 150–153.

Bertone-Johnson, E., Hankinson, S., Johnson, S., & Manson, J. (2007). Assessing premenstrual syndrome in large prospective studies. *Journal of Reproductive Medicine, 52*(9), 779–786.

Bjorn, I., Bixo, M., Nojd, K., Collberg, P., Nyberg, S., Sundstrom-Poromaa, I., et al. (2002). The impact of different doses of medroxyprogesterone acetate on mood symptoms in sequential hormonal therapy. *Gynecology and Endocrinology, 16*(1), 1–8.

Bjorn, I., Bixo, M., Nojd, K., Nyberg, S., & Backstrom, T. (2000). Negative mood changes during hormone replacement therapy: A comparison between two progestogens. *American Journal of Obstetrics and Gynecology, 183*(6), 1419–1426.

Bloch, M., Schmidt, P., Su, T., Tobin, M., & Rubinow, D. (1998). Pituitary–adrenal hormones and testosterone across the menstrual cycle in women with premenstrual syndrome and controls. *Biological Psychiatry, 43*(12), 897–903.

Bottiglieri, T. (2002). S-Adenosyl-L-methionine (SAMe): From the bench to the bedside: Molecular basis of a pleiotrophic molecule. *American Journal of Clinical Nutrition, 76*(5), 1151S–1157S.

Bressa, G. (1994). S-Adenosyl-l-methionine (SAMe) as antidepressant: Meta-analysis of clinical studies. *Acta Neurologica Scandinavica, 154*(suppl), 7–14.

Brown, M. A., & Robinson, J. (2002). *When the body gets the blues.* New York: Rodale.

Budeiri, D., Li Wan Po, A., & Dornan, J. (1996). Is evening primrose oil of value in the treatment of premenstrual syndrome? *Controlled Clinical Trials, 17*(1), 60–68.

Bulecheck, G., & McCloskey, J. (1999). *Nursing interventions: Effective nursing treatments.* Philadelphia: Saunders.

Cahill, C. A. (1998). Differences in cortisol, a stress hormone, in women with turmoil-type premenstrual symptoms. *Nursing Research, 47*, 278–284.

Campbell, M. A., & McGrath, P. J. (1997). Use of medication by adolescents for the management of menstrual discomfort. *Archives of Pediatrics and Adolescent Medicine, 151*, 905–913.

Canning, S., Waterman, M., & Dye, L. (2006). Dietary supplements and herbal remedies for premenstrual syndrome (PMS): A systematic research review of the evidence for their efficacy. *Journal of Reproductive and Infant Psychology, 24*(4), 363–378.

Chapman, E., Angelica, J., Spitalny, G., & Strauss, M. (1994). Results of a study of the homeopathic treatment of PMS. *Journal of the American Institute of Homeopathy, 87*, 14–21.

Clayton, A. (2008). Symptoms related to the menstrual cycle: Diagnosis, prevalence, and treatment. *Journal of Psychiatric Practice, 14*, 13–21.

Collins Sharp, B., Taylor, D., Kelly-Thomas, K., Killeen, M. B., & Dawood, M. Y. (2002). Cyclic perimenstrual pain and discomfort: The scientific basis for practice. *Journal of Obstetric, Gynecological, and Neonatal Nursing, 31*, 637–649.

Dawood, M. Y. (1990). Dysmenorrhea. *Clinical Obstetrics & Gynecology, 33*(1), 168–178.

Dawood, M. Y., McGuire, J. L., & Demers, L. M. (1985). *Premenstrual syndrome and dysmenorrhea.* Baltimore/Munich: Urban & Schwarzenberg.

Dawood & Ramos (1990). Transcutaneous electrical nerve stimulation (TENS) for the treatment of primary dysmenorrhea: A randomized, crossover comparison with placebo TENS and ibuprofen. *Obstetrics & Gynecology, 75*, 656–660.

Delle Chiaie, R., Pancheri, P., & Scapicchio, P. (2002). Efficacy and tolerability of oral and intramuscular S-adenosyl-L-methionine 1,4-butanedisulfonate (SAMe) in the treatment of major depression: Comparison with imipramine in 2 multicenter studies. *American Journal of Clinical Nutrition, 76*(5), 1172S–1176S.

Dimmock, P., Wyatt, K., Jones, P., & O'Brien, P. (2000). Efficacy of selective serotonin-reuptake inhibitors in premenstrual syndrome: A systematic review. *Lancet, 30*, 1131–1136.

Endicott, J. (2001). The epidemiology of perimenstrual psychological symptoms. *Acta Psychiatrica Scandinavica, 104*, 110–116.

Foster, S., & Tyler, V. (2000). *Tyler's honest herbal: A sensible guide to the use of herbs and related remedies.* Binghamton, NY: Haworth Press.

Freeman, E. W. (1997). Premenstrual syndrome: Current perspective on treatment and etiology. *Current Opinions in Obstetrics and Gynecology, 9*, 147–153.

Freeman, E., Kroll, R., Rapkin, A., Pearlstein, T., Brown, C., Parsey, K., et al. (2001). Evaluation of a unique oral contraceptive in the treatment of premenstrual dysphoric disorder. *Journal of Women's Health & Gender Based Medicine, 10*(6), 561–569.

Freeman, E., Rickels, K., & Sondheimer, S. (1993). Premenstrual symptoms and dysmenorrhea in relation to emotional distress factors in adolescents. *Journal of Psychosomatic Obstetrics & Gynecology, 14*, 41–50.

Freeman, E., Rickels, K., Sondheimer, S., & Polansky, M. (1995). A double-blind trial of oral progesterone, alprazolam, and placebo in treatment of severe premenstrual syndrome. *Journal of the American Medical Association, 274*(1), 51–57.

Freeman, E., Sondheimer, S., & Rickels, K. (1988). Effects of medical history factors on symptom severity in women meeting criteria for premenstrual syndrome. *Obstetrics & Gynecology, 72*, 236–239.

Futterman, L. A., Jones, J. E., Miccio-Fonseca, L. C., & Quigley, M. E. (1992). Severity of premenstrual symptoms in relation to medical/psychiatric problems and life experiences. *Perceptual and Motor Skills, 74*, 787–799.

Gallant, S. J. (1991). The role of psychological factors in the experience of premenstrual symptoms. *Proceedings of the 9th Conference of the Society for Menstrual Cycle Research*, 139–152.

Girdler, S., Pedersen, C., & Light, K. (1995). Thyroid axis function during the menstrual cycle in women with premenstrual syndrome. *Psychoneuroendocrinology, 20*(4), 395–403.

Gise, L., Lebovits, A., Paddison, P. L., & Strain, J. J. (1990). Issues in the identification of premenstrual syndromes. *Journal of Nervous & Mental Diseases, 178*(4), 228–234.

Golding, J. M., Taylor, D. L., Menard, L., & King, M. J. (2000). Prevalence of sexual abuse history in a sample of women seeking treatment for premenstrual syndrome. *Journal of Psychosomatic Obstetrics and Gynaecology, 21*(2), 69–80.

Halbreich, U. (1997). Menstrually related disorders: Towards interdisciplinary international diagnostic criteria. *Cephalalgia, 17*, 1–4.

Halbreich, U. (1999). Premenstrual syndromes: Closing the 20th century chapters. *Current Opinions in Obstetrics and Gynecology, 9*, 147–153.

Hamilton, J., Alagna, S., & Sharpe, A. (1985). Cognitive approaches to understanding and treating premenstrual depression. In H. Ofofsky (Ed.), *Premenstrual syndrome* (pp. 69–84). Washington, DC: American Psychiatric Press.

Harlow, S. (1986). Function and dysfunction: A historical critique of the literature on menstruation and work. *Health Care for Women International, 7*(1–2), 39–50.

Harlow, S., & Park, M. (1996). A longitudinal study of risk factors for the occurrence, duration and severity of menstrual cramps in a cohort of college women. *British Journal of Obstetrics and Gynecology, 103*, 1134–1142.

Harrison, M. M. (1985). *Self-help for premenstrual syndrome* (2nd ed.). New York: Random House.

Hoffman, B. (2008). Pelvic pain. In J. Schorge, J. Schaffer, L. Halvorsen, B. Hoffman, K. Bradshaw & F. Cunningham (Eds.), *Williams gynecology* (pp. 244–268). New York: McGraw-Hill.

Huerta-Franco, M. R., & Malacara, J. M. (1993). Association of physical and emotional symptoms with the menstrual cycle and life-style. *Journal of Reproductive Medicine, 38*, 448–454.

Janiger, O., Riffenburgh, M., & Kersh, M. (1972). A cross-cultural study of premenstrual symptoms. *Psychosomatics, 13*, 226–235.

Jarrett, M., Heitkemper, M., & Shaver, J. (1995). Symptoms and self-care strategies in women with and without dysmenorrhea. *Health Care for Women International, 16*, 167–178.

Kendler, K., Karkowski, L., Corey, L., & Neale, M. (1998). Longitudinal population-based twin study of retrospectively reported premenstrual symptoms and lifetime major depression. *American Journal of Psychiatry, 155*, 1234–1240.

Keye, W. R., Jr. (1989). The biomedical model of premenstrual syndrome: Past, present and future. In A. Voda & R. Conover (Eds.), *Proceedings of the 8th Conference of the Society for Menstrual Cycle Research* (pp.

589–600). Salt Lake City, UT: Society for Menstrual Cycle Research.

Kinch, R., & Robinson, G. (1985). Premenstrual syndrome—current knowledge and new directions. *Canadian Journal of Psychiatry, 30*(7):467–468.

Koci, A., & Strickland, O. (2006). Relationship of adolescent physical and sexual abuse to perimenstrual symptoms (PMS) in adulthood. *Issues in Mental Health Nursing, 28,* 75–87.

Lee, K., & Rittenhouse, C. A. (1992). Prevalence of perimenstrual symptoms in employed women. *Women & Health, 17*(3), 17–32.

Lentz, G. (2007). Primary and secondary dysmenorrheal, premenstrual syndrome, and premenstrual dysphoric disorder. In V. Katz, G. Lentz, R. Lobo, & D. Gershenson (Eds.), *Comprehensive gynecology* (pp. 901–914). Maryland Heights, MO: Mosby Elsevier.

Lewis, L. L., Greenblatt, E. M., Rittenhouse, C. A., Veldhuis, J. D., & Jaffe, R. B. (1995). Pulsatile release patterns of luteinizing hormone and progesterone in relation to symptom onset in women with premenstrual syndrome. *Fertility and Sterility, 64,* 288–292.

Martorano, J., Ahlgrimm, M., & Colbert, T. (1998). Differentiating between natural progesterone and synthetic progestins: Clinical implications for premenstrual syndrome and perimenopause management. *Comprehensive Therapeutics, 24*(6–7), 336–339.

Marvan, M. L., Diaz-Erosa, M., & Montesinos, A. (1998). Premenstrual symptoms in Mexican women with different educational levels. *Journal of Psychology, 132,* 517–526.

Mitchell, E. S. (1991). Identification of recurrent symptom severity patterns across multiple menstrual cycles. In *Proceedings of the 9th Conference of the Society for Menstrual Research* (pp. 73–82). Seattle, WA: Society for Menstrual Cycle Research.

Mitchell, E. S., Woods, N. F., & Lentz, M. J. (1994). Differentiation of women with three premenstrual symptom patterns. *Nursing Research, 43*(1), 25–30.

Mitchell, E., Woods, N., Lentz, M., & Taylor, D. (1991). Recognizing PMS when you see it: Criteria for PMS sample selection. In D. L. Taylor & N. F. Woods (Eds.), *Menstruation, health and illness* (pp. 89–102). New York: Hemisphere.

Mitchell, E. S., Woods, N. F., Lentz, M. J., Taylor, D., & Lee, K. (1992). Methodological issues in the definition of perimenstrual symptoms. In A. Dan & L. Lewis (Eds.), *Menstrual health in women's lives* (pp. 7–14). Urbana, IL: University of Illinois Press.

Moos, R. (1969). Typology of menstrual cycle symptoms. *American Journal of Obstetrics & Gynecology, 103,* 390–402.

Moynihan, R. (2004). Controversial disease dropped from Prozac product information. *British Medical Journal, 328,* 365.

O'Brien, P. M. S. (1987). Controversies in premenstrual syndrome: Etiology and treatment. In B. E. Ginsburg & B. F. Carter (Eds.), *Premenstrual syndrome: Ethical and legal implications in a biomedical perspective* (pp. 3177–3328). New York: Plenum.

Oinonen, K. A., & Mazmanian, D. (2002). To what extent do oral contraceptives influence mood and affect? *Journal of Affective Disorders, 70,* 229–240.

Panay, N. (2008). Understanding the pain: Managing severe PMS. *The Practising Midwife, 11,* 26–29.

Parry, B. L., Udell, C., Elliott, J. A., Berga, S. L., Klauber, M. R., Mostofi, N., et al. (1997). Blunted phase-shift responses to morning bright light in premenstrual dysphoric disorder. *Journal of Biological Rhythms, 12*(5), 443–456.

Pierce, A. (1999). *The American Pharmaceutical Association practical guide to natural medicines.* New York: William Morrow.

Praschak-Rieder, N., Willeit, M., Winkler, D., Neumeister, A., Hilger, E., Zill, P., et al. (2002). Role of family history and 5-HTTLPR polymorphism in female seasonal affective disorder patients with and without premenstrual dysphoric disorder. *European Neuropsychopharmacology, 12*(2), 129–134.

Prior, J. (2002). The ageing female reproductive axis II: Ovulatory changes with perimenopause. *Novartis Foundation Symposium, 242,* 172–192.

Prior, J., Hitchcock, C., Kingwell, E., Vigna, Y., Bishop, C., & Pride, S. (2001). Perimenopausal bone loss: More than estrogen depletion. *Journal of Bone Mineral Research, 16*(12), 2365–2366.

Rapkin, A. & Howe, C. (2007). Pelvic pain and dysmenorrhea. In J. Berek (Ed.), *Berek and Novak's gynecology* (14th ed., pp. 505–540). Philadelphia: Lippincott Williams & Wilkins.

Reame, N., Kelch, R., Beitins, I., Yu, M., Zawacki, C., & Padmanabhan, V. (1996). Age effects of FSH and pulsatile LH secretion across the menstrual cycle of premenopausal women. *Journal of Clinical Endocrinology and Metabolism, 81,* 1512–1518.

Reame, N., Marshall, J., & Kelch, R. (1992). Pulsatile LH secretion in women with premenstrual syndrome (PMS): Evidence for normal neuroregulation of the menstrual cycle. *Psychoneuroendocrinology, 17*, 205–213.

Reid, R. L., & Yen, S. S. C. (1981). Premenstrual syndrome. *American Journal of Obstetrics & Gynecology, 139*, 85.

Ross, L. (2004). Rethinking mental health and disorder: Feminist perspectives. *Archives of Women & Mental Health, 7*(2), 151–152.

Ross, L., Sellers, E., Gilbert-Evans, S., & Romach, M. (2004). Mood changes during pregnancy and the postpartum period: Development of a biopsychosocial model. *Acta Psychiatrica Scandinavica, 109*(6), 457–466.

Ross, L., & Steiner, M. (2003). A biopsychosocial approach to premenstrual dysphoric disorder. *Psychiatric Clinics of North America, 26*, 529–546.

Rubinow, D. R., & Schmidt, P. J. (1995). The neuroendocrinology of menstrual cycle mood disorders. *Annals of the New York Academy of Sciences, 771*, 648–659.

Rubinow, D. R., Schmidt, P. J., & Roca, C. A. (1998a). Hormone measures in reproductive endocrine-related mood disorders: Diagnostic issues. *Psychopharmacology Bulletin, 34*, 289–290.

Rubinow, D. R., Schmidt, P. J., & Roca, C. A. (1998b). Estrogen–serotonin interactions: Implications for affective regulation. *Biological Psychiatry, 44*, 839–850.

Sanders, S., Graham, C., Bass, J., &, Bancroft, J. (2001). A prospective study of the effects of oral contraceptives on sexuality and well-being and their relationship to discontinuation. *Contraception, 64*(1), 51–58.

Schellenberg, R. (2001). Treatment for the premenstrual syndrome with agnus castus fruit extract: Prospective, randomised, placebo-controlled study. *British Medical Journal, 322*(7279), 134–137.

Schmidt, P., Grover, G., & Rubinow, D. (1993). Alprazolam in the treatment of premenstrual syndrome: A double-blind, placebo-controlled trial. *Archives of General Psychiatry, 50*(6), 467–473.

Schmidt, P. J., Nieman, L. K., Danaceau, M. A., Adams, L. F., & Rubinow, D. R. (1998). Differential behavioral effects of gonadal steroids in women with and in those without premenstrual syndrome. *New England Journal of Medicine, 338*, 209–216.

Shaver, J. F., & Woods, N. F. (1985). Concordance of perimenstrual symptoms across two cycles. *Research in Nursing and Health, 8*, 313–319.

Shaver, J. L., Lentz, M., Cho, S. K., Cirelli, R. A., Pollice, M., Hastie, A. T., et al. (1997). Sleep, psychological distress, and stress arousal in women with fibromyalgia. *Research in Nursing & Health, 20*, 247–257.

Smith, R. (1993). Cyclic pelvic pain and dysmenorrhea. *Obstetrics and Gynecologic Clinics of North America, 20*(4), 753–764.

Steiner, M., Korzekwa, M., Lamont, J., & Wilkins, A. (1997). Intermittent fluoxetine dosing in the treatment of women with premenstrual dysphoria. *Psychopharmacology Bulletin, 33*(4), 771–774.

Steiner, M., Romano, S., Babcock, S., Dillon, J., Shuler, C., Berger, C., et al. (2001). The efficacy of fluoxetine in improving physical symptoms associated with premenstrual dysphoric disorder. *British Journal of Obstetrics and Gynecology, 108*(5), 462–468.

Steiner, M., Steinberg, S., Stewart, D., Carter, D., Berger, C., Reid, R., et al. (1995). Fluoxetine in the treatment of premenstrual dysphoria. *New England Journal of Medicine, 332*, 1529–1534.

Sundell, G., Milsom, I., & Andersch, B. (1990). Factors influencing the prevalence and severity of dysmenorrhea in young women. *British Journal of Obstetrics and Gynaecology, 97*(7), 588–594.

Taylor, D. (1986). Development of perimenstrual symptom typologies. *Communicating Nursing Research, 19*, 168.

Taylor, D. (1988). *Nursing interventions for premenstrual syndrome: A longitudinal therapeutic trial*. Seattle: University of Washington.

Taylor, D. (1996). The perimenstrual symptom management program: Elements of effective treatment. *Capsules & Comments in Perinatal/Women's Health Nursing, 2*, 140–151.

Taylor, D. (1999). Effectiveness of professional-peer group treatment: Symptom management for women with PMS. *Research in Nursing & Health, 22*(6), 496–511.

Taylor, D. (2000). More than personal change: Effective elements of symptom management. *Nurse Practitioner Forum, 11*, 79–86.

Taylor, D., & Colino, S. (2002). *Taking back the month: A personalized solution to managing PMS and enhancing your health*. New York: Perigee/Putnam-Penguin.

Taylor, D., & Woods, N. F. (Eds.). (1991). *Menstruation, health and illness*. New York: Taylor & Francis.

Taylor, D., Woods, N., Lentz, M., Mitchell, E., & Lee, K. (1991). Premenstrual negative affect: Development and testing of an explanatory model. In D. Taylor & N. Woods (Eds.), *Menstruation, health and illness* (pp. 103–109). New York: Hemisphere.

Thys-Jacobs, S. (2000). Micronutrients and the premenstrual syndrome: The case for calcium. *Journal of the American College of Nutrition, 19*, 220–227.

Ussher, J. M. (2002). Processes of appraisal and coping in the development and maintenance of premenstrual dysphoric disorder. *Journal of Community & Applied Social Psychology, 12*, 309–322.

Vigod, S., Ross, L., & Steiner, M., (2009). Understanding and treating premenstrual dysphoric disorder: An update for the women's health practitioner. *Obstetric Gynecologic Clinics of N. America, 36*, 907–924. doi: 10.1016/j.ogc.2009, 10.010

Woods, N., Dery, G., & Most, A. (1982). Stressful life events and perimenstrual symptoms. *Journal of Human Stress, 8*, 23–31.

Woods, N., Lentz, M., Mitchell, E., Heitkemper, M., & Shaver, J. (1997). PMS after 40: Persistence of a stress-related symptom pattern. *Research in Nursing & Health, 20*, 329–340.

Woods, N. F., Lentz, M. J., Mitchell, E. S., Taylor, D., & Lee, K. (1992). Perimenstrual symptoms and the health-seeking process. In A. Dan & L. Lewis (Eds.), *Menstrual health in women's lives* (pp. 155–167). Urbana, IL: University of Illinois Press.

Woods, N. F., Mitchell, E. S., & Lentz, M. (1999). Premenstrual symptoms: Delineating symptom clusters. *Journal of Women's Health and Gender-Based Medicine, 8*, 1053–1062.

Woods, N. F., Mitchell, E. S., Lentz, M. J., Taylor, D., & Lee, K. (1987, July–August). Premenstrual symptoms: Another look. *Public Health Reports* (suppl), 106–112.

Woods, N., Mitchell, E., & Taylor, D. (1999). From menarche to menopause: Contributions from nursing research and recommendations for practice. In I. Hinshaw, S. Feetham, & J. L. Shaver (Eds.), *Clinical Nursing Research* (Vol. 1, pp. 485–507). New York: Saunders.

Woods, N., Most, A., & Dery, G. (1982a). Estimating perimenstrual distress: A comparison of two methods. *Research in Nursing & Health, 5*, 81–91.

Woods, N., Most, A., & Dery, G. (1982b). Estimating the prevalence of perimenstrual symptoms. *American Journal of Public Health, 72*, 1257–1264.

Woods, N. F., Taylor, D., Mitchell, E. S., & Lentz, M. J. (1992). Premenstrual symptoms and health-seeking behavior. *Western Journal of Nursing Research, 14*(4), 418–443.

World Health Organization (WHO). (1981). A cross-cultural study of menstruation: Implications for contraceptive development and use. *Studies in Family Planning, 12*, 3–16.

World Health Organization (WHO). (1992). *International statistical classification of diseases and related health problems* (Vol. 10). Geneva, Switzerland: Author.

Wyatt, K., Dimmock, P., Jones, P., Obhrai, M., & O'Brien, S. (2001). Efficacy of progesterone and progestogens in management of premenstrual syndrome: Systematic review. *British Medical Journal, 323*(7316), 776–780.

Wyatt, K., Dimmock, P., & O'Brien, P. (1999). Efficacy of vitamin B-6 in the treatment of premenstrual syndrome: Systematic review. *British Medical Journal, 318*, 1375–1381.

Yakir, M., Kreitler, S., Brzezinski, A., Vithoulkas, G., Oberbaum, M., & Bentwich, Z. (2001). Effects of homeopathic treatment in women with premenstrual syndrome: A pilot study. *British Homeopathic Journal, 90*, 148–153.

Yonkers, K., & White, K. (1992). Premenstrual exacerbation of depression: One process or two? *Journal of Clinical Psychiatry, 53*, 289–292.

25

Normal and Abnormal Uterine Bleeding

Mary Ann Faucher
Kerri Durnell Schuiling

A feminist model of health care keeps the woman whole with her body and avoids medicalizing symptoms that are, in fact, representations of normal. For example, the term *dysfunctional uterine bleeding* suggests pathology and the need to fix a "problem." It is important to appreciate that some of the knowledge about women's cyclicity has been medicalized, socially constructed, or both. Some cases of "abnormal" or "dysfunctional" bleeding actually represent a variation of normal and signify the physiologic passage of women's bodies into the next stage of development—for example, menarche or menopause. For this reason, it is important to look beyond the biomedical model when providing health care. A medical model inscripts the disorder on the body, necessitating symptom interpretation from the clinician's expertise alone (Bordo, 1993).

Medical intervention, particularly surgical, should be the last resort in many cases of abnormal uterine bleeding. When the uterine bleeding diagnosed as irregular or abnormal is actually a variation of normal, treatment with exercise, diet, relaxation, and stress reduction may sometimes be more appropriate. As more clinicians embrace the normalcy of menstrual variations, there will be less temptation to "cure" normal female processes (Tavris, 1992). The expert clinician is one who actively listens, values input provided by the woman, and then carefully evaluates all available information before determining whether the bleeding is truly abnormal or just a variation of normal.

A feminist approach to women's health care using a health-oriented, normalizing model allows normalcy to be validated. This paradigm enables assessment, diagnosis, and treatment that is woman centered and that values her standpoint, background, ethnicity, and culture.

Abnormal and Dysfunctional Uterine Bleeding

Abnormal uterine bleeding (AUB) is one of the more common reasons why women seek health care. It accounts for as much as one-third of all annual gynecologic visits and affects as many as 50% of women worldwide (American College of Obstetricians and Gynecologists, 2006a). AUB has a significant impact on the quality of life for the women it affects. Bleeding patterns range from amenorrhea (no menses) to menorrhagia (abnormally long or heavy menses). An estimated 30% of women of reproductive age experience menorrhagia, and menorrhagia and uterine fibroids are believed to account for as many as 75% of all hysterectomies performed worldwide (Vilos, Lefebvre, & Graves, 2001). Clearly, AUB imposes a heavy economic burden. A recent study conservatively estimated the annual direct costs of AUB to be approximately $1 billion, with the annual indirect costs totaling $12 billion (Liu, Doan, Blumenthal, & Dubois, 2007). These estimates do not include intangible costs or productivity losses, such as time lost from work.

AUB is an all-encompassing diagnosis referring to any uterine bleeding that is irregular in amount, frequency, duration, or timing (i.e., cycle irregularity). It may or may not be related to a woman's menstrual cycle. AUB can occur as a normal physiologic event, such as the irregular bleeding that often accompanies menarche or perimenopause. However, it can also signal pathologic, life-threatening conditions such as an ectopic pregnancy or endometrial cancer.

Terms commonly used to describe patterns of AUB are defined in **Table 25-1**. Although these terms continue to be used, a group of experts recognized that globally there was no consensus on the meaning of the terms. In 2007, an international group of clinicians and scientists came together with the goal of developing an international clinical standardized terminology (Ducholm, 2008; Fritz & Speroff, 2011). **Table 25-2** provides the recommendations from this meeting. If adopted, the new terminology would provide a clear meaning of the terms for both clinicians and patients.

Dysfunctional uterine bleeding (DUB) is the term traditionally used to describe abnormal bleeding for which no pelvic pathology or underlying medical cause is found (Hillard, 2007). In the past few years, this term has begun to fall out of favor, however, with fewer clinicians using DUB and more using the term anovulatory uterine bleeding (American College of Obstetricians and Gynecologists, 2006a). Although the authors of this chapter agree that the term DUB should be retired, DUB is referred to in this chapter because many clinicians still use it. DUB is irregular and unrelated to organic pathology, medications, pregnancy-related disorders, systemic conditions, iatrogenic causes, or genital tract pathology (Albers, Hull, & Wesley, 2004; Bradley, 2010; Fritz & Speroff, 2011). DUB is a diagnosis of exclusion. It is important to emphasize that clinicians should be consistent in the definition they use in practice because this definition often guides assessment. It is equally important to clarify the meaning of the term for the woman so she has a full understanding of the meaning of her diagnosis. For the purposes of this chapter, all DUB is considered anovulatory uterine bleeding.

TABLE 25-1 Abnormal Bleeding Terminology and Patterns

Term	Definition	Interval
Amenorrhea	Absence of menses	
Primary amenorrhea	Absence of menses by age 14 with delay in maturation of secondary sexual characteristics or absence of menses by age 16 with evidence of secondary sexual characteristics	
Secondary amenorrhea	Absence of periods for a length of time equivalent to a total of at least three of the previous cycle intervals or 6 months of amenorrhea	
Intermenstrual bleeding	Bleeding or spotting between normal menses; flow is usually light	Between normal menses
Menorrhagia	Excessive amount or prolonged duration of bleeding; in excess of 80 ml	Regular
Menometrorrhagia	Heavy, prolonged menstrual bleeding	Irregular
Metrorrhagia	Uterine bleeding that is excessive in flow or duration or both	Irregular
Oligomenorrhea	Decreased, scanty flow	> 35 days
Polymenorrhea	Regular, frequent menstruation	< 24 days

Source: Adapted from Fritz & Speroff, 2011.

Physiology and Patterns of Normal Menses

The physiology of normal menstrual processes and the anatomic and functional structure of the genital tract provide a foundation for understanding AUB (see Chapter 5). Normal menses results from a functional hypothalamic–pituitary–ovarian axis (HPOA) and a precise sequence of hormonal events that lead to ovulation. If conception does not occur and if the outflow tract is patent, menses ensues. Normal menses may vary in length, duration, and amount of flow from woman to woman; reflecting this fact, normal parameters are provided as ranges (**Table 25-3**). It is always wise to ask women who present with a concern about abnormal bleeding, "What is a normal pattern for you?"; the woman is always the best authority in describing her cycles.

Menses resulting from ovulatory cycles tend to demonstrate the same interval, amount, and duration from cycle to cycle unless significant health changes occur that negatively affect the HPOA. Menses in individual women tend to have consistent patterns once ovulation is established. Women who have regular, ovulatory menstrual cycles often experience premenstrual symptoms such as bloating, fatigue, constipation, and mood changes. These symptoms (collectively called *molimina*) are a result of higher levels of progesterone in the body. The

TABLE 25-2 Uniform Descriptions of Terms Used to Describe AUB

Frequency			Regularity			Duration of Flow			Volume of Monthly Blood Loss		
Old Term	New Term	Days	Old Term	New Term	Variation	Old Term	New Term	Days	Old Term	New Term	mL
Polymenorrhea	Frequent	< 24	Amenorrhea	Absent	Not applicable	Hypermenorrhea	Prolonged	> 8.0	Menorrhagia	Heavy	> 80
Normal	Normal	24–38	Regular	Regular	± 2–20 days	Normal	Normal	4.5–8.0	Normal	Normal	5–80
Oligomenorrhea	Infrequent	> 38	Metrorrhagia	Irregular	> 20 days	Hypomenorrhea	Shortened	< 4.5	Hypomenorrhea	Light	< 5

Source: Data from Ducholm, 2008; Fritz & Speroff, 2011.

TABLE 25-3 Ranges of Normal Menstrual Cycles

Parameter	Range of Normal
Cycle interval	21–34 days
Duration of flow	3–8 days
Amount of flow	30–80 mL

progesterone surge in the luteal phase sustains the corpus luteum for a finite period of time. When conception does not occur, the corpus luteum atrophies, with resultant progesterone withdrawal bleeding. The withdrawal of progesterone also causes the production of arachidonic acid, which in turn stimulates the production of PGF_2 alpha. Although the pathology of dysmenorrhea is not well understood, it is believed that dysmenorrhea associated with ovulatory bleeding results from the effects of PGF_2 alpha that cause vasoconstriction and contraction of smooth muscle (Greydanus, Omar, Tsitsika, & Patel, 2009; Lentz, 2007).

Etiology and Pathophysiology of Abnormal Uterine Bleeding

The causes of abnormal bleeding can be physiologic, pathologic, or pharmacologic (**Table 25-4**). Disruption of endocrine function at any level of the HPOA can disrupt normal menstrual physiology and disturb menstrual cycle regularity, frequency, duration, or volume. In women of reproductive age, the most common cause of a bleeding pattern that is suddenly different from a woman's established menstrual pattern is a complication of pregnancy, including threatened or incomplete abortion, ectopic pregnancy, retained products of conception, and gestational trophoblastic disease (Fritz & Speroff, 2011). The latter two conditions are less likely but still need to be considered in the differential diagnosis (Fritz

TABLE 25-4 Causes of Abnormal Uterine Bleeding

Pregnancy

- Ectopic
- Spontaneous abortion (threatened, inevitable, missed, incomplete)

Endocrine

- Adrenal hyperplasia
- Cushing's syndrome
- Diabetes
- Pituitary
- Polycystic ovary syndrome (PCOS)
- Thyroid disease

(continues)

TABLE 25-4 Causes of Abnormal Uterine Bleeding *(Continued)*

Medications—substances—herbs

- Amphetamines
- Anticoagulants
- Antipsychotics
- Benzodiazepines
- Corticosteroids
- Herbs (ginkgo, ginseng, soy)
- Hormone therapy
- Isoniazid
- Selective serotonin reuptake inhibitor (SSRI) antidepressants

Problems with the hypothalamic–pituitary–ovarian axis

- Systemic illness (e.g., PCOS, pituitary, thyroid)
- Premature ovarian failure
- Postmenarche
- Perimenopause
- Stress
- Eating disorders
- Severe dieting and/or weight loss
- Excessive exercise

Genital tract disease/dysfunction

- Atrophy
- Cancer
- Endometrial hyperplasia
- Endometriosis
- Infections
- Fibroids (leiomyomas, leiomyomatas, myomas)
- Outflow tract obstruction
- Ovarian tumors
- Polyps
- Trauma

Systemic disease

- Thyroid dysfunction
- Coagulation defects
- Von Willebrand disease
- Leukemia
- Idiopathic thrombocytopenia

& Speroff). As a consequence, clinicians treating women of childbearing age—especially adolescents who may not be forthcoming about their sexual activity—who present with AUB should always first exclude pregnancy or a complication of pregnancy as a cause of the bleeding.

Anovulatory Uterine Bleeding/Dysfunctional Uterine Bleeding

The diagnosis of anovulatory uterine bleeding or DUB is made after excluding all other causes of the abnormal bleeding. When all other causes of bleeding are firmly ruled out, then and only then can the diagnosis of DUB be made.

Evidence from histologic and molecular studies suggests that anovulatory bleeding is a result of an increased density of abnormal vessels that have a fragile structure prone to focal rupture that is followed by the release of lysosomes (proteolytic enzymes) from surrounding epithelial and stromal cells and migratory leukocytes and macrophages (Fritz & Speroff, 2011). This condition is generally caused by one of three hormonal imbalances: estrogen withdrawal, estrogen breakthrough, or progesterone breakthrough (American College of Obstetricians and Gynecologists, 2006a).

Estrogen withdrawal bleeding is attributable to a decrease in estrogen levels, with the cause often being iatrogenic, such as cessation of estrogen therapy (American College of Obstetricians and Gynecologists, 2006a). Women with high sustained levels of estrogen tend to experience the heaviest bleeding. They often include women who have polycystic ovary syndrome (PCOS), are obese, or are perimenopausal (Fritz & Speroff, 2011).

Estrogen breakthrough bleeding occurs as a result of the endometrium being stimulated by long-term chronic unopposed estrogen, such as that observed in women experiencing chronic anovulation. For example, women with PCOS often have estrogen breakthrough bleeding because of chronic anovulation (Fritz & Speroff, 2011). See Chapter 26 for additional information about PCOS.

Progesterone breakthrough bleeding occurs when the progesterone–estrogen ratio becomes elevated (American College of Obstetricians and Gynecologists, 2006a). This type of abnormal bleeding is sometimes seen in women using progestin-only pills or other forms of progestin-only contraception (Fritz & Speroff, 2011).

Anovulatory cycles characterized by a lack of progesterone in the luteal phase lead to an unstable, excessively vascular endometrium. Heavy and irregular bleeding results from an imbalance in the vasoconstricting and vasodilating properties of prostaglandins and an imbalance in platelet aggregation and inhibition (Hoffman, 2008). The abnormal microvasculature is most probably the cause of the abnormal bleeding that results from this phenomenon (Fritz & Speroff, 2011). **Table 25-5** identifies physiologic and pathologic causes of anovulation.

Anovulatory bleeding, in contrast to the regular, predictable, and often painful bleeding experienced with ovulatory cycles, frequently leads to abnormal cycle intervals (e.g., polymenorrhea or metrorrhagia) or abnormal amounts of bleeding (e.g., oligomenorrhea,

TABLE 25-5 Physiologic and Pathologic Causes of Anovulation

Physiologic causes

- Pregnancy
- Lactation
- Perimenarche
- Perimenopause

Pathologic causes

- Hypoandrogenic disorders/syndromes (e.g., PCOS)
- Hypothyroidism
- Hyperprolactinemia
- Iatrogenic
- Extreme stress (physical and psychological)

menorrhagia, or menometrorrhagia). Anovulatory bleeding also tends to be heavy secondary to the high and sustained levels of unopposed estrogen that can result in endometrial hyperplasia. Endometrial hyperplasia, in turn, can result in episodes of amenorrhea, menorrhagia, and intermenstrual bleeding. Fritz and Speroff (2011) provide a clear description of anovulation and its effect on a woman's cycle:

> By definition, the anovulatory woman is always in the follicular phase of the ovarian cycle and in the proliferative phase of the endometrial cycle. There is no luteal or secretory phase because there is no ovulation or cycle. The only ovarian steroid signal the endometrium receives is estrogen, levels of which constantly fluctuate, rising and falling as each new cohort of follicles begins to grow but ultimately loses its developmental momentum and, sooner or later, lapses into atresia. Although the amplitude of the signal may vary, the message, growth, stays the same. (p. 599)

It is important for the clinician to consider a variety of causes including other organic (i.e., systemic, genital tract, or iatrogenic) causes before concluding that anovulation is the cause of the abnormal bleeding.

The most common times for a woman to experience irregular menstrual cycles are at the beginning and the end of her reproductive life cycle: postmenarche and perimenopause. The HPOA is most affected by the normal life-cycle transitions that occur during the first 2 years after menarche and 3 years prior to menopause (Fritz & Speroff, 2011); thus irregular bleeding during this time may be a reflection of normal functioning. The least variation in menses occurs during the childbearing years, which generally encompass ages 20 to 40, although most women will experience some variation from their established normal pattern from time to time. Even though bleeding patterns may fall within the range of normal, it is important to listen to the woman's description prior to making a diagnosis, because for her, the bleeding may be abnormal and require follow-up.

Ovulatory Abnormal Uterine Bleeding

Ovulatory AUB occurs significantly less often than abnormal bleeding due to anovulation. It occurs most often in the postadolescent years and during the premenopausal years. Ovulatory abnormal bleeding cycles are regular and tend to be cyclic, although the bleeding patterns are often abnormal and may include polymenorrhea, oligomenorrhea, midcycle spotting, and menorrhagia. Menorrhagia is the pattern most frequently observed with ovulatory abnormal bleeding and is commonly associated with pelvic pathology such as uterine fibroids, adenomyosis, or endometrial polyps (Livingstone & Fraser, 2002). Therefore, women with ovulatory abnormal bleeding need an evaluation to rule out endometrial lesions and other pathology. Menorrhagia is also frequently associated with bleeding dyscrasias, and as many as 20% of adolescents who present with menorrhagia have a bleeding disorder (Bevan et al., 2001; Claessens & Cowell, 1981; Fritz & Speroff, 2011).

Systemic Causes of AUB

AUB can be a sign of significant systemic disease, especially if findings from the pelvic examination are normal. Systemic diseases cause AUB by altering the HPOA or the uterine endometrium, which is the target tissue of the HPOA. Abnormal bleeding patterns with systemic etiologies typically include amenorrhea, oligomenorrhea, and menorrhagia.

Common systemic causes of AUB include renal disease, liver disease, thyroid disease, coagulopathies, thrombocytopenia, von Willebrand disease (VWD), and coagulation factor deficiencies (Hoffman, 2008). Liver and renal diseases result in an inability to adequately clear estrogen, which allows levels of biologically active, free-floating estrogen to increase; this buildup then negatively impacts the HPOA, with resultant anovulation (Mohan, Page, & Higham, 2007). VWD—one of the most common genetically inherited bleeding disorders—is frequently the cause of lifelong abnormal bleeding patterns in women (American College of Obstetricians and Gynecologists, 2009b; James, 2005, 2006; Lobo, 2007). One of the hallmarks of VWD is menorrhagia (American College of Obstetricians and Gynecologists, 2009b). Women presenting with a history of easy bruising, prolonged bleeding following dental work or surgery, menorrhagia, or metrorrhagia warrant further follow-up, particularly if other treatment has failed (American College of Obstetricians and Gynecologists, 2009b).

Thyroid dysfunction may cause bleeding abnormalities; consequently, endocrine pathology should always be considered when evaluating a woman for AUB. Graves' disease, which occurs four to five times more often in women than in men, is one of the most common causes of hyperthyroidism (Hillard, 2007). Hyperthyroidism can result in oligomenorrhea or amenorrhea. Hypothyroidism can cause either amenorrhea (particularly if the hypothyroidism is chronic) or menorrhagia (if the hypothyroidism is recent) (Mohan et al., 2007). Pituitary disease and some pituitary tumors may result in elevated levels of prolactin. Amenorrhea associated with elevated prolactin levels is due to prolactin inhibition of the pulsatile secretion of gonadotropin-releasing hormone (GnRH) (Fritz & Speroff, 2011). Prolactin-secreting pituitary adenomas are the most common type of pituitary tumor (Fritz & Speroff). Approximately one-third of women with elevated prolactin levels will also have galactorrhea. Nevertheless, many individuals (10%) have silent pituitary masses that are not endocrinologically active and have no adverse impact on health and well-being. If there is no evidence of hormonal disturbance, no immediate action is probably necessary, although long-term surveillance is appropriate (Fritz & Speroff).

Diseases or syndromes causing insulin resistance, such as PCOS, increase circulating levels of insulin, which in turn leads to an elevation in androgen production and concomitant anovulation (Hoffman, 2008). The relationship between insulin and androgens is believed to be an underlying cause of PCOS (see Chapter 26 for further discussion of PCOS).

Genital Tract Etiologies of AUB

All women of childbearing age who present with AUB should be considered pregnant until proven otherwise. Reproductive disorders that may result in AUB include pregnancy complications such as ectopic pregnancy; threatened, missed, or incomplete abortion; subinvolution of the placental site; and trophoblastic disease (Hoffman, 2008).

Signs of gynecologic malignancies such as endometrial and cervical cancer may present as AUB, often in the form of metrorrhagia. For this reason, gynocologic cancers should be ruled out whenever a woman presents with AUB. Additionally, uterine bleeding that occurs in women who are postmenopausal is always considered abnormal and endometrial cancer needs to be ruled out.

Infections such as chlamydia, gonorrhea, and endometritis may cause irregular spotting due to irritation and inflammation of the tissues of the cervix or endometrium. A thorough history and physical examination (including pelvic examination) will assist in ruling out infection as a cause of the abnormal bleeding.

Fibroids, adenomyosis, and cervical polyps can cause irregular or heavy abnormal uterine bleeding (see Chapter 27 for further discussion of these conditions). Leiofibroids are a frequent cause of abnormal bleeding during the reproductive years and frequently cause menorrhagia or menometrorrhagia (Fritz & Speroff, 2011; Hoffman, 2008). Polyps are commonly encountered, benign growths on the cervix. They are easily visualized with a speculum, appearing as smooth, deep to bright red growths that are fragile and bleed with little encouragement during examination. Women with cervical polyps may present with a concern about postcoital bleeding.

Trauma to the genital tract can also cause AUB. Tampons can irritate the cervix and cause spotting. Women who have been sexually assaulted may experience abnormal bleeding from lacerations and other injuries affecting the internal organs and genitals.

Outflow Tract Causes of AUB

Normal menses depends on a normally functioning outflow tract (among other factors). Anatomic abnormalities at any level of the outflow tract can interfere with normal menstrual flow, and generally problems associated with the outflow tract result in amenorrhea. For example, uterine or cervical congenital or structural abnormalities can cause AUB. When the uterus or vagina has congenital structural abnormalities, it may be impossible for menses to flow properly. Rarely, segments of the Müllerian tube fail to develop, resulting in abnormalities such as imperforate hymen, lack of a vaginal orifice, lapses in the continuity of the vaginal canal, an absent uterus or cervix, an absent uterine cavity, or an absence of endometrium. Obstruction of menses may lead to painful distention due to hematometra, hematocolpos, or hemoperitoneum. Affected women are genotypically and phenotypically normal females with functioning ovaries. Such abnormalities are uncommon, however (Fritz & Speroff, 2011). If a patient presents with amenorrhea, and her pelvic examination and bimanual examination are normal and there is no history of infection or trauma, then an abnormality of the outflow tract is not likely.

Iatrogenic Causes of AUB

Many medications predispose women to AUB, including glucocorticoids, tamoxifen, and anticoagulants (Fritz & Speroff, 2011). Ginseng, ginkgo, and soy products have been associated with alterations in estrogen levels and affecting clotting parameters (American College of Obstetricians and Gynecologists, 2001, reaffirmed 2010). A thorough history should reveal whether a patient is taking any medication that might cause AUB. It is important to clarify the regimen followed in taking the medication, because sometimes taking a medication incorrectly will result in AUB. In particular, this effect is frequently observed in women taking oral contraceptives for the first time.

Lifestyle Causes of AUB

Athletic women, particularly long-distance runners, gymnasts, and professional ballet dancers, are at risk for oligomenorrhea and amenorrhea, as are women who have anorexia and other eating disorders (Fritz & Speroff, 2011; Polotsky, 2010). Typically, the amenorrhea occurs as secondary amenorrhea that follows the start of an intensive training regimen, although some reports indicate that when intensive training begins prior to menarche, menarche can be delayed by as much as 3 years (Fritz & Speroff). It is extremely important to understand that it is not the fact of exercise itself that causes the amenorrhea, but rather the specific type of exercise (Fritz & Speroff). For example, swimming is less likely to cause amenorrhea than long-distance running. In particular, the combination of low body weight and lean body mass with the physical activity is more often associated with amenorrhea (Fritz & Speroff). According to Fritz and Speroff, "The potential adverse effects of exercise and body weight on menstrual function are synergistic" (p. 490).

The pathophysiology of exercise-induced amenorrhea is complex and is probably due to the combination of low body fat and diminished secretion of GnRH. Decreased GnRH results in fewer luteinizing hormone (LH) and follicle-stimulating hormone (FSH) pulses, which in turn decreases the amount of estrogen produced by the ovaries. The critical weight theory hypothesizes that there is a critical weight and amount of body fat that must be maintained for women to experience regular menstrual cycles (Fritz & Speroff, 2011). Interestingly, opponents of the critical weight theory have suggested that the newly discovered protein hormone leptin and the leptin receptors in the hypothalamus, which provide a feedback mechanism for central regulation of body fat content, have more to do with weight than does the existence of a critical weight point (Fritz & Speroff). If body weight is maintained by this feedback mechanism, then this relationship refutes the theory that a critical body weight is necessary for normal menses.

Illicit drugs have been shown to inhibit ovulation due to hyperprolactinemia, which results in amenorrhea. A descriptive study focusing on the endocrine profiles of women who were admitted to a substance-abuse unit found that hyperprolactinemia and macrocytosis (increased mean corpuscular volume [MCV]) was evident in as many as 60% of women who were of reproductive age and who abused alcohol, tranquilizers, and opiates or used illicit drugs including marijuana and cocaine (Teoh, Lex, Mendelson, Mello, & Cochin, 1992). More than 80% of the women in the study who were postmenopausal and had an alcohol dependency also had hyperprolactinemia, increased MCV, or both (Teoh et al.).

Assessment

History

A detailed menstrual history provides the most useful information in differentiating anovulatory bleeding from other causes and may be enough to confidently make a diagnosis and proceed with treatment without further testing. It is critical to remember that if the woman is of reproductive age and presents with abnormal uterine bleeding, pregnancy should be ruled out prior to any other testing. Only 2% of endometrial carcinomas occur before the age of 40. However, approximately 6% of cancers occur in women with heavy regular bleeding, and endometrial carcinoma increases in prevalence in women in their late 40s (Pitkin, 2007). In women with postmenopausal bleeding, the absolute risk for endometrial cancer ranges from 5.7% to 11.5% (Sadoon, Salman, Smith, Henson, & McCullough, 2007).

For example, the diagnosis of DUB can be confidently made in women with irregular, unpredictable bleeding in the absence of molimina or other associated symptoms. However, in women with regular, heavy bleeding that is prolonged, menstrual history alone is likely to be inadequate in obtaining an accurate diagnosis (Fritz & Speroff, 2011).

Start the interview by asking the woman to describe in detail what brought her in for the visit and then obtain a detailed menstrual history. Questions should include her current age as well as her age at menarche and menopause (if appropriate); cycle length, duration, and estimated amount of flow; and when the menstrual pattern changed. When questioning women about cycle length, duration, and flow, it is important to understand how the woman calculates each of these factors. Some women do not include the first day of spotting or may not include the days when the flow is light when determining cycle length. Teaching the woman the parameters of what is considered normal may also provide her with a useful guide for describing her cycles. Her observation about how the bleeding deviates from her established pattern is a valuable tool to use in the assessment. Studies have repeatedly demonstrated that estimation of the amount of blood loss can be highly imprecise (Chimera, Anderson, & Turnball, 1980; Halberg, Hogdahl, Nillson, & Rybo, 1966). Counting pads or tampons has not been shown to be helpful in establishing the amount of bleeding, because the brands vary widely in absorption rates (Grimes, 1979; Jannsen, Scholten, & Heintz, 1995). A reliable indicator of heavy bleeding is the passage of clots accompanied by heavy bleeding (Warner et al., 2004).

It is particularly helpful to determine whether the bleeding occurs at regular or irregular intervals, as the pattern of bleeding provides clues to its etiology. For example, a woman who is postmenopausal and reports that she experienced spontaneous, painless, and irregular bleeding indicates to the clinician that endometrial hyperplasia should be part of the differential diagnosis. A woman who reports she is having regular cycles that have now become heavy and are accompanied by the passage of clots, and who says she has noticed a sensation of pelvic fullness, suggests to the clinician that her menorrhagia may be secondary to uterine fibroids. Whenever a woman reports that the duration of flow has changed—for example, from 3 to 6 days—it must be considered abnormal (Katz, Lentz, Lobo, & Gershenson, 2007).

Ask the patient about the dates of her last three menstrual periods and the date of her last normal menses. Often a calendar will assist her in answering these questions accurately. Inquire about the color and character of her flow and related signs and symptoms such as pain, odor, and postcoital spotting. Inquire whether hot flushes or the sensation of a racing heartbeat are present—these signs accompanied by abnormal bleeding may indicate menopause is approaching, particularly if the woman is in the perimenopausal years. Inquiring about other associated symptoms is important. For example, the presence of premenstrual molimina may indicate ovulation along with the presence of dysmenorrhea, whereas reports of dyspareunia or intermenstrual bleeding lead to a different set of differential diagnoses.

The gynecologic history may reveal other episodes of abnormal bleeding. Question the woman about previous treatment for abnormal bleeding. Inquire about Papanicolaou (PAP) test history, gynecologic surgeries, sexually transmitted infections, or other infections of the genital tract or organs.

If the woman is currently using or has used contraception in the past, obtain information about the type, the length of use, and any side effects encountered. Contraceptive history may reveal that her abnormal bleeding is mechanically caused by an intrauterine device (IUD) or is related to the use of hormonal contraception, such as oral contraceptives or injectable depot medroxyprogesterone acetate (Depo-Provera). In addition, inquire about hormone therapy in postmenopausal women to rule out a history of taking unopposed estrogen that can lead to endometrial hyperplasia.

Obtain a complete medication history. Glucocorticoids, tamoxifen, and anticoagulants may predispose women to abnormal uterine bleeding. Ask about over-the-counter and herbal medications. Notably, the herb bromelain may increase the risk of bleeding.

A medical history or general health history, including family history, provides information that may reveal underlying medical conditions that might be the cause of the abnormal bleeding. Ask about symptoms of thyroid disorders (e.g., cold intolerance, fatigue, hyperactivity, weight gain or loss) and hormone-secreting tumors (e.g., hair loss, changes in breast size, hirsutism, headache, breast discharge). Findings in the health history may suggest the presence of a systemic disease; therefore, pay particular attention to signs and symptoms such as easy bruising, presence of petechiae, weight or appetite changes, or changes in elimination patterns. Given that bleeding and endocrine disorders can be inherited, it is important to look for familial patterns. Including questions about lifestyle is also important to obtain information about drug use or abuse, exercise patterns, and nutrition.

Physical Examination

The physical examination provides additional information about possibilities of systemic disease, particularly organic pathology. Height, weight, body mass index (BMI), vital signs, hair, and body fat distribution are important parameters to include. Note signs of possible androgen excess, including hirsutism, acne, and alopecia (see Chapter 26). Tanner staging (see Chapter 2) is helpful when examining adolescents because it can validate information from the history and may help to determine ovulatory status. Observe for signs that are indicative of anemia, such as pale skin tone and delayed capillary refill. Palpating the thyroid may identify enlargement or tumors related to either hypothyroidism or hyperthyroidism. A breast examination can rule out the presence of galactorrhea, which may indicate an elevated prolactin level.

A pelvic examination is essential for a woman of any age who is (or has been) sexually active or has abdominal pain, anemia, irregular bleeding, or bleeding that is so heavy her hemodynamic stability is compromised. In contrast, if the patient is a young adolescent who is not sexually active and only recently began menstruating, and who has a normal hematocrit, a pelvic examination is most likely unnecessary. The pelvic examination should include a general assessment of the genitalia. Observe for bruising, lacerations, lesions, or evidence of infection. Clitoromegaly suggests the possibility of an endocrine disorder.

A speculum examination enables observation of the vagina and cervix for evidence of infection, trauma, or foreign objects. Cervical cultures to rule out infection and a Pap test should be obtained at this time. Clinicians who have young clients who are not sexually active but who require a pelvic examination to rule out the cause of the abnormal bleeding should use a pediatric speculum, inserting it with great care and gentleness. At times, a pelvic examination in these instances may need to be done under anesthesia to provide physical comfort.

A bimanual examination provides the opportunity to assess for the presence of tumors, cervical polyps, ovarian cysts, uterine tenderness or enlargement, and adnexal pain or masses. If the bimanual examination is performed on a young adolescent, the clinician should use only one digit and, again, proceed with great care and gentleness.

Laboratory and Diagnostic Testing

Laboratory tests used to diagnose AUB can be invasive and expensive. Decisions regarding which tests to perform should be based on the differential diagnosis and directed by the information collected during the history and physical, including the woman's age and her reproductive status (**Table 25-6**).

TABLE 25-6 Laboratory Testing for AUB		
Test	**Differential Diagnosis**	**Abnormal Results**
Qualitative urine: human chorionic gonadotropin (hCG)	Pregnancy; threatened, missed, or incomplete spontaneous abortion	May be positive or negative
Quantitative serum hCG	Ectopic pregnancy or impending spontaneous abortion	Level lower than expected for gestational age and/or lack of doubling in 48 hours
Complete blood count (CBC) with platelets	Anemia	Hemoglobin less than 10 mg/dl
	Clotting abnormalities	Platelets less than 150,000
Prothrombin time (PT), activated partial thromboplastin time (aPTT), bleeding time	Von Willebrand disease, leukemia, prothrombin deficiency	Bleeding time increased
Serum iron/ferritin	Iron deficiency anemia secondary to bleeding	Decreased levels
Follicle-stimulating hormone (FSH)	Amenorrhea due to menopause; premature ovarian failure	Levels greater than 30 mIU/ml, some texts cite 40 mIU/ml
Progesterone	Anovulatory	Levels less than 10 ng/ml
Thyroid-stimulating hormone (TSH)	Hypothyroidism or hyperthyroidism	Levels less than 0.8 or greater than 4.0
Pap test	Dysplasia; carcinoma	Atypical cells suggestive of dysplasia and/or carcinoma
Prolactin	Pituitary adenoma	Levels greater than 100 ng/mL
Cultures and/or microscopic examination of vaginal secretions	Vaginal infection (e.g., gonorrhea, chlamydia, trichomoniasis, vulvovaginal candidiasis)	Positive test or microscopy (see Chapters 20 and 21)

General tests to consider obtaining for all types of AUB include the following:

1. A pregnancy test (if the patient is of childbearing age):
   • Qualitative urine human chorionic gonadotropin (hCG).
   • Serial serum quantitative b-hCG may help to diagnose specific pregnancy disorders.
2. Complete blood count:
   • Order only if indicated or anemia is suspected.
3. Thyroid-stimulating hormone (TSH):
   • Order especially if hypothyroidism or hyperthyroidism or other thyroid abnormality is suspected.
4. Prolactin level:
   • Order if the woman reports headaches and has galactorrhea and/or peripheral vision changes.
5. Pap test (unless the patient is an adolescent who is not sexually active).
6. Nucleic acid amplification test (NAAT) for gonorrhea and chlamydia if the woman is sexually active.
7. Microscopic examination of vaginal secretions with normal saline and potassium hydroxide.
8. Coagulation studies if there is suspicious history of bleeding or easy bruising; unexplained menorrhagia.
   • Include both a prothrombin time (PT) and an activated partial thromboplastin time (aPTT).
9. A serum progesterone if the menstrual history does not indicate whether the woman is ovulating. Obtain between cycle days 22 and 24.

Additional tests should be ordered only for specific indications (**Table 25-7**). For example, if the patient says she is experiencing heavy bleeding and is passing clots greater than 1 inch in diameter and has to change her pads or tampons frequently, particularly during the night, a serum ferritin test should be considered. Warner et al. (2004) found that if the aforementioned clinical signs are accompanied by a low serum ferritin, it is highly likely the woman is experiencing menorrhagia.

Although menstrual history alone is often sufficient to make the diagnosis of DUB, after organic, systemic, and iatrogenic causes for the AUB are ruled out, other diagnostic tests may be required for definitive diagnosis of endometrial pathology. If a woman is experiencing ovulatory menorrhagia, then endocervical curettage and pelvic sonography have been recommended (Katz et al., 2007). Transvaginal ultrasonography (TVS) of the pelvis is often one of the first-line diagnostic tools used because it is convenient and reliable for detecting polyps and submucosal fibroids, measuring endometrial thickness, evaluating pregnancy complications, and assessing ovarian masses (Abou-Salem, Elmazny, & El-Sherbiny, 2010; Vilos et al., 2001). TVS can reliably measure endometrial thickness in postmenopausal women and rule out endometrial carcinoma in women with a thin endometrium, defined as 5 mm or less. Studies have investigated different thresholds of endometrial thickness as

TABLE 25-7 Differential Diagnosis and Laboratory Assessment of AUB

To rule out:	Laboratory tests to order:
Endocrine causes of AUB	General labs + prolactin, FSH & LH levels
Adrenal causes (see Chapter 26)	General labs + adrenal studies, testosterone levels Adjunct: CT scan of abdomen, cortisol levels
Hormone-producing tumor	General labs + MRI, CT scan, cortisol levels
Structural abnormalities	General labs + ultrasound
Infection	General labs + gonorrhea and chlamydia tests + wet mount; consider need for WBC
Cervical or uterine pathology	General labs + colposcopy with biopsy; endometrial biopsy; hysteroscopy
Amenorrhea	General labs + FSH, LH, prolactin levels, TSH, T_3, and T_4
Von Willebrand disease (VWD)	Ristocetin cofactor assay
Liver disease	Liver function tests
Renal disease	Renal function tests
Coagulation disorders other than VWD	PTT, PT, assessment of platelet function

Note: CT = computed tomography; FSH = follicle-stimulating hormone; LH = luteinizing hormone; MRI = magnetic resonance imaging; PT = prothrombin time; PTT = partial thromboplastin time; T_3 = triiodothyronine; T_4 = thyroxine; TSH = thyroid-stimulating hormone; WBC = white blood cell count.

Source: Data from Fritz & Speroff, 2011.

cutoff points in the assessment for endometrial hyperplasia. Although no threshold completely eliminates the possibility of endometrial hyperplasia, lowering the threshold to less than 5 mm does not increase the diagnostic accuracy of TVS (Batzer, 2007; Sadoon, Salman, Smith, Henson, & McCullough, 2007). If the result of TVS is abnormal, it might be prudent for the clinician to consult with a physician or refer the woman for medical management.

An endometrial biopsy is easily accomplished in the office setting and can be performed by clinicians who have had the education and training required for carrying out the test accurately. Endometrial biopsy can be useful in the diagnosis of both ovulatory and anovulatory AUB. With the former condition, the results will report a secretory endometrium or reveal a uterine lesion such as polyps, submucous fibroids, or carcinoma (Katz et al., 2007; Telner & Jakubovicz, 2007). The sensitivity of endometrial biopsy for the detection of endometrial cancer ranges from 83% to 96%, but this technique may miss as many as 18% of local lesions, including fibroids and polyps, because only a small part of the endometrium is sampled at any one time (Clark et al., 2002; Mahajan, Mahajan, & Soni, 2007). In their study, Svirksy and colleagues (2008) evaluated 639 women for focal intrauterine pathology. Two experienced clinicians performed both an in-office hysteroscopy and an endometrial biopsy with a Novak curette on each of the participants. The results were compared with hysteroscopic findings in 558 cases in which complete findings were available for both procedures, with hysteroscopy being used as the reference. The findings suggest that hysteroscopy and endometrial biopsy should be used as complementary tools in women undergoing evaluation for endometrial pathology.

Hysteroscopy remains the most popular—albeit the most invasive—method for evaluating the endometrium (van Dongen, de Kroon, Jacobi, Trimbos, & Jansen, 2007); however, some evidence suggests that saline-infusion sonohysterography (SIS) with endometrial biopsy offers the most complete evaluation of the endometrium with the least risk to the patient (Brooks, 2007; Espindola, Kennedy, & Fischer, 2007). A comparison study of the diagnostic accuracy of TVS and SIS in the evaluation of the endometrial cavity in women who were premenopausal ($n = 100$) and women who were postmenopausal ($n = 33$) found that the sensitivity and specificity of TVS in diagnosing endometrial pathologies were 83% and 70.6%, respectively, whereas the sensitivity and specificity of SIS in the diagnosis were 97.7% and 82.4%, respectively (Erdem, Bilgin, Bozkurt, & Erdem, 2007). The sensitivity and specificity of SIS in the diagnosis of endometrial polyps were 100% and 91.8%, respectively, and in the diagnosis of polyps were 95% and 100% (Erdem et al.). These findings suggest that SIS is more accurate than TVS alone when used to evaluate the endometrial cavity of women with AUB. Both SIS and hysteroscopy are indicated when endometrial biopsy or transvaginal ultrasonography results are normal but the woman continues to be symptomatic (Bradley, 2004).

Magnetic resonance imaging (MRI) and computed tomography (CT) scan may be used to diagnose adnexal masses, adenomyosis, uterine fibroids, and pituitary adenomas. The costs of these technologies may be considered excessive, however, if other types of evaluation methods would provide the same information (Fritz & Speroff, 2011).

As mentioned earlier, none of these diagnostic tests is generally necessary for evaluation of a woman with anovulatory AUB, because often the menstrual history is sufficient for making a diagnosis. Nevertheless, an endometrial biopsy or hysteroscopy should always be included in the assessment of abnormal bleeding in women who are perimenopausal or postmenopausal, adolescents who are obese and have had long-term (3 or more years) of unexplained abnormal bleeding, or any woman whose endometrium has been exposed to unopposed estrogen.

Management

Management goals for treating AUB are to (1) normalize the bleeding, (2) correct any anemia, (3) prevent cancer, and (4) restore quality of life. Concomitant therapy may be necessary to achieve these goals, particularly if the bleeding is severe and threatens hemodynamic stability. For example, a woman who presents with severe bleeding from a raw and denuded endometrium may require high-dose estrogen to stop the bleeding. Estrogen therapy will provide rapid growth of a denuded endometrium. However, the administration of estrogen to stop the acute bleeding will not address the cause of the bleeding; thus additional treatment, such as endometrial ablation (e.g., laser ablation, roller-ball electrocoagulation, thermal balloon ablation) or hysterectomy, may be required (Bayer & DeCherney, 1993; Chapple, 1999; Choung & Brenner, 1996; Espindola et al., 2007). Additionally, if the woman is anemic because of the bleeding, she will need iron therapy.

Age, desire for future fertility, and patient preference all need to be considered when determining treatment options for women with AUB. Treatment falls into two categories: treatment of acute bleeding and treatment of chronic bleeding. Women who present with excessive heavy bleeding and who have a dangerously low hematocrit require physician consultation. All episodes of acute hemorrhagic bleeding should be managed by a physician.

Acute Life-Threatening Hemorrhage

Acute hemorrhage always necessitates physician referral and medical management in the hospital setting.

Acute Non-Life-Threatening Menorrhagia Due to Anovulation

A variety of pharmacologic choices are available for women with heavy uterine bleeding due to anovulation, including combined oral contraceptives (COCs), progestogen-only therapy, and the levonorgestrel-releasing intrauterine system (LNG-IUS; Mirena) (Schuiling & Brucker, 2011). If bleeding is nonemergent and hospitalization is not required, and a significantly denuded endometrium is suspected as the cause of the heavy bleeding, then administration of high-dose estrogen usually will stop the bleeding and allow for further evaluation. In contrast, if the patient is hemodynamically unstable, hospitalization is required and a physician needs to be consulted.

Estrogen therapy stimulates rapid endometrial proliferation and resolves the bleeding from a denuded endometrium (Casablanca, 2008; Fritz & Speroff, 2011). Concomitant use of antiemetics (e.g., meclizine) is indicated when high-dose estrogen is used because of the nausea that often accompanies its use. The clinician needs to be mindful that estrogens—particularly high-dose estrogens—may precipitate thromboembolism and, therefore, are contraindicated in women with a history of thrombosis or family history of idiopathic venous thromboembolism. A usual dosage regimen of high-dose estrogen in these instances is 1.25 mg conjugated estrogen or 2.0 mg micronized estradiol every 4 to 6 hours for 24 hours. The amount of estrogen may be tapered then to once daily for 7 to 10 days after the bleeding is under control (Casablanca).

As noted earlier, heavy bleeding resulting in hemodynamic instability requires hospitalization. Usually intravenous estrogen therapy is instituted in such cases. Following intravenous administration of estrogen, high-dose estrogen therapy should be continued orally, tapering to once daily when bleeding is under control and adding a progestogen such as medroxyprogesterone acetate (Fritz & Speroff, 2011). This same treatment is effective for the woman whose bleeding is acute but not yet considered an emergency.

A monophasic COC given twice daily should also result in the reduction of bleeding within 24 hours. If the flow does not stop with 48 hours, further evaluation is indicated. The COC is typically tapered to once daily after 5 to 7 days and continued with 21 days of active pills, followed by 7 days of placebo pills or no pills. An alternative to the 21/7-day cycle is an extended regimen of 84 days of monophasic COCs followed by a 7-day pill-free interval (Kaunitz, Westhoff, & Leonhardt, 2002; Schuiling & Brucker, 2011).When the bleeding stops, 2.5 mg of conjugated equine estrogens (CEE; Premarin) can be given daily, followed by the addition of 10 mg of medroxyprogesterone acetate (MPA; Provera), given during the last 10 days of therapy to initiate withdrawal bleeding. **Table 25-8** describes medical therapies for menorrhagia.

TABLE 25-8 Medical Therapies for Menorrhagia

Acute bleeding—estrogen therapy

(Note: High-dose estrogen often causes nausea; therefore, concurrent treatment with an antiemetic is recommended.)

- Replete intravascular volume
- CEE 25 mg IV q 4–6 hrs PRN then CEE 2.5 mg–5 mg po 4×/day for 2–3 days then add MPA 10 mg for 10–14 days (continue CEE)
- COCs 2×–3×/day then taper

Acute bleeding—progestin therapy

(Use only if endometrium is normal or increased in thickness. Treatment should continue for 3 weeks decreasing to once daily treatment after 7–10 days).

- Medroxyprogesterone acetate 10–20 mg 2×/day or
- Megestrol 20–40 mg 2×/day or
- Norethindrone 5 mg 2×/day

Acute prolonged bleeding—estrogen–progestin therapy

- Any monophasic COC beginning with 1 pill 2×/day decreasing to 1 pill daily. Continue treatment for a minimum of 2 weeks.

Long-term/chronic management

- Cyclic MPA 10 mg/day for 10–14 days, every 30–40 days
- Combined contraceptives (oral, patch, ring)
- Oral micronized progesterone 300 mg for 10–14 days, every 30–40 days
- Depot medroxyprogesterone acetate (Depo-Provera) 150 mg IM every 3 months
- Levonorgestrel intrauterine system (LNG-IUS, Mirena)
- NSAIDs

Note: High doses of estrogen may precipitate a thrombotic event and therefore are contraindicated in women with a history of thrombosis or a family history of idiopathic venous thromboembolism. Also, warn the woman using progestin therapy that withdrawal of progestin will result in heavy menses. In women who desire contraception, treatment with an estrogen–progestin contraceptive is a better choice (Fritz & Speroff, 2011).

CEE = conjugated equine estrogen; COC = combined oral contraceptive; IM = intramuscular; IV = intravenous; MPA = medroxyprogesterone acetate; NSAIDs = nonsteroidal anti-inflammatory drugs; OCP = oral contraceptive pill; PRN = as needed

Progestogen Therapy

Progestogens can be used to treat chronic heavy bleeding that is due to anovulation (**Table 25-9**). After the withdrawal bleeding ends, several therapeutic medical options are available for the woman to consider, but a definitive diagnosis should be made by reviewing endometrial histology (Katz et al., 2007). Other authorities suggest that 3 months of CEE/MPA or COC therapy should be provided; if there is no significant improvement with this regimen, then the woman should be reevaluated (Society of Obstetricians and Gynaecologists of Canada [SOGC], 2001). Women with chronic menorrhagia can be offered cyclic MPA at doses of 10 mg a day for 10 to 14 days, with the therapy being repeated every 30 to 40 days. Progestogens are not as effective as estrogen in stopping acute bleeding but are effective for long-term treatment once the acute bleeding episode has been resolved. Additionally, progestogens may be the management regimen of choice if the woman has contraindications to taking estrogen. To induce normal bleeding, a progestogen is given for 7 to 12 days each month. Withdrawal bleeding should occur within 2 to 7 days of discontinuing the progestogen. If bleeding fails to occur or if irregular bleeding persists, diagnostic reevaluation is necessary and physician consultation is recommended. Do not use progestogen therapy if the woman thinks she might be pregnant, even if her pregnancy test is negative.

The LNG-IUS (see Chapter 12) is a particularly effective therapy for menorrhagia caused by fibroids. The reduction in mean blood loss with this treatment has been reported to be as high as 80% (Katz et al., 2007; Lethaby, Cooke, & Rees, 2003; Mansour, 2007). Women with fibroids are candidates for the LNG-IUS if the fibroid does not distort the uterine cavity and the uterus is less than 12 weeks in size. A small study demonstrated resolution of anemia in 95% of woman who used the LNG-IUS for bleeding and a 40% prevalence of amenorrhea after 12 months of use (Grigorieva, Chen-Mok, Tarasova, & Mikhailov, 2003).

The LNG-IUS also has been compared with endometrial ablation in the treatment of menorrhagia. In this study, women were referred from their primary care provider for lack of efficacy with medical therapy. One group received thermal ablation and the other group received the LNG-IUS. Both therapies were found to be equally efficacious by measurement with a pre- and post-pictorial blood-loss assessment chart (Barrington, Arunkalaivannan, & Abdel-Fattah, 2003).

In addition, the LNG-IUS has been compared with hysterectomy in women with leiofibroids but not the subserosal type. At follow-up, 20% of the women with the LNG-IUS had undergone a hysterectomy, and 68% of the women were still using the LNG-IUS. Both

---

TABLE 25-9 Progestogen Therapy for Chronic Anovulation

- Medroxyprogesterone acetate (Provera) 10 mg × 10 days
- Norethindrone 5 mg 2x/day × 10 days
- Oral micronized progesterone (Prometrium) 200 mg/day × 10 days
- Depot medroxyprogesterone acetate (Depo-Provera) 150 mg IM every 12 weeks
- Levonorgestrel-releasing intrauterine system (LNG-IUS, Mirena)

groups reported improvement in quality of life (Hurskainen et al., 2004). Another multi-center trial in which women were treated with either the LNG-IUS or hysterectomy found no difference between the two groups with regard to symptom improvement. Although 42% of women in the LNG-IUS group had a hysterectomy, the LNG-IUS was found to be much less expensive (Hurskainen et al.).

Gonadotropin-Releasing Hormone Agonists

Gonadotropin-releasing hormone agonists (GnRHa) such as leuprolide acetate (Lupron), nafarelin acetate (Synarel), and goserelin acetate (Zoladex) may be used for a short period of time while a woman is awaiting surgical treatment for her heavy bleeding. GnRHa are not recommended for long-term use because of their many side effects related to estrogen deficiency, such as negative impact on bone density, hot flashes, and night sweats (Casablanca, 2008). Women taking a GnRHa should be forewarned about the estradiol "flare" that occurs around day 5 and lasts until day 14 and that is accompanied by heavy uterine bleeding (Munro, 2008). For this reason, GnRHa use in women who are anemic needs to be carefully considered.

GnRHa therapy is also quite expensive—another reason for using it on only a short-term basis. Nevertheless, these agents are very effective in stemming the bleeding with resultant amenorrhea. In the interim, the woman's hemoglobin has time to rise, thereby making her a better candidate for surgery.

Nonhormonal Medications to Treat Acute Heavy Bleeding

Nonsteroidal anti-inflammatory drugs (NSAIDs) are useful for ovulatory–idiopathic menorrhagia. The heavier the bleeding, the better the effect, although the mechanism of action for NSAIDs used for menorrhagia remains poorly understood. Theoretically, the NSAIDs interfere with the transformation of arachidonic acid to cyclic endoperoxidases and, therefore, block the production of prostaglandins. This effect on the prostaglandin cascade results in a 12% to 50% increase in platelet aggregation (Lethaby, Augood, & Duckitt, 2003; Smith, Abel, Kelly, & Baird, 1982). Optimally, an NSAID should be initiated 3 days prior to the start of menses, although some experts suggest starting the drug with the onset of menses (Schuiling & Brucker, 2011). All NSAIDs are contraindicated in women with ulcers or bronchospastic lung disease. **Table 25-10** identifies NSAIDs that are commonly used to manage heavy bleeding.

In 2009, tranexamic acid (cyklokapron), an antifibrinolytic agent that reduces menstrual bleeding by 45% to 60%, was approved in the United States for the treatment of heavy bleeding (Farrell, 2004; Fritz & Speroff, 2011). Tranexamic acid is particularly useful as a second-line option for women who cannot or do not wish to use hormonal options ("New Option," 2010; "Pharmacological Treatment," 2008) and is considered a first-line treatment for ovulatory AUB (Farrell, 2004). It is also effective in managing the severe bleeding that accompanies von Willebrand disease. In a recent multicenter, double-blind, parallel-group study of 196 women

TABLE 25-10 NSAID Therapy for Menorrhagia

- Mefanamic acid 500 mg 3×/day*
- Ibuprofen 600 mg 3×/day
- Naproxen sodium 550 mg loading dose then 275 mg every 6 hours

*FDA approved

that compared women who received tranexamic acid (n = 123) with women who received a placebo (n = 73), the researchers found that women who were treated with tranexamic acid achieved a statistically significant reduction (P < .001) in their mean menstrual blood loss (Lukes et al., 2010). A concern with use of this therapy is venous thromboembolism (VTE); however, to date no increase in VTE incidence with tranexamic acid use has been observed ("Pharmacological Treatment"). Use of the drug is generally contraindicated in women with a history or who are at risk of thrombosis. The prescribed dose is 1 gm taken 3 to 4 times daily (Farrell). Side effects are rare but include nausea and leg cramps.

Surgical Treatment of Menorrhagia

When medical therapy fails, surgical management options for menorrhagia include dilatation and curettage (D & C), endometrial ablation, uterine artery embolization, and hysterectomy. In the presence of a thin endometrium, medical therapy for excessive uterine bleeding is reasonable. When ultrasound is available and the endometrial stripe is greater than 10 mm in the presence of acute excessive uterine bleeding, D &C should be considered (Katz et al., 2007). Additionally, D & C is the quickest way to stop acute bleeding and should be considered in a woman 35 years or older with symptoms of hypovolemia because pathology is more likely in this age group (Katz et al.).

Endometrial ablation was introduced in the 1990s as an alternative to hysterectomy. A less invasive operative procedure, it results in destruction of the endometrium using heated fluid either contained within a balloon or circulating freely within the uterine cavity, tissue freezing, microwaves, or radiofrequency electricity (American College of Obstetricians and Gynecologists, 2007a, reaffirmed 2009). Endometrial ablation should not be performed on a woman who desires to maintain her fertility.

Several devices can be used to perform uterine ablation. The most commonly employed is a modified urological resectoscope that uses radiofrequency current (American College of Obstetricians and Gynecologists, 2007a, reaffirmed 2009). The types of electrodes used range from loop electrodes to grooved or spiked electrodes, all of which serve to destroy the endometrium and cause coagulation of adjacent tissues (American College of Obstetricians and Gynecologists).

Nonresectoscopic systems destroy the endometrium using various devices and techniques. Cryotherapy essentially freezes the endometrial tissues. The use of heated free fluid (as is used in the Hydro ThermAblator) achieves endometrial ablation with heated normal saline (American College of Obstetricians and Gynecologists, 2007a, reaffirmed 2009) and results in tissue necrosis. Hysteroscopic monitoring enables the clinician to visualize the progress during the procedure.

Two approved ablation devices employ microwaves; one is disposable, while the other is reusable. The probe used in this technique transmits information about the temperature of the surrounding tissues back to the control module.

The NovaSure system uses radiofrequency electricity; its probe also provides a feedback system to monitor the endometrial cavity. The NovaSure system results in electrosurgical vaporization and desiccation of endometrial tissues in approximately 90 seconds (American College of Obstetricians and Gynecologists, 2007a, reaffirmed 2009).

The thermal balloon is a probe with a balloon tip; this tip is extended with heated fluid, which then results in destruction of the endometrium. At this time, the only device approved by the U.S. Food and Drug Administration is the ThermaChoice (American College of Obstetricians and Gynecologists, 2007a, reaffirmed 2009).

Endometrial ablation has been best studied in women who are premenopausal and have fibroids less than 2 cm in size. Endometrial ablation has fewer complications, costs less, and has the same postoperative satisfaction as hysterectomy (Marjoribanks, Lethaby, & Farquhar, 2003; Pinion et al., 1994; Zupi et al., 2003). However, 30% to 40% of ablations require subsequent surgical intervention (i.e., re-ablation or hysterectomy), although the number of overall hysterectomies is decreased when ablation is used (Marjoribanks et al.).

A number of complications have been associated with resectoscopic ablation devices, including distention media fluid overload, with the excess fluid being absorbed into the systemic circulation and causing hyponatremia, hyposmolality, brain edema, permanent neurologic damage, and death (American College of Obstetricians and Gynecologists, 2007a, reaffirmed 2009). Other potential complications include uterine trauma due to cervical injury or perforation of the uterus during the procedure, burns to the vagina and vulva, postablation tubal ligation syndrome, and pregnancy complications. Although pregnancy after ablation is rare, it does occur; women who elect to continue the pregnancy have a high rate of malpresentation, prematurity, placenta accreta, and perinatal mortality (American College of Obstetricians and Gynecologists).

Complications associated with nonresectoscopic devices are rarer than those with resectoscopic devices. They include distention fluid overload, cervical laceration, uterine corpus perforation, and postprocedural hematometra (Lethaby, Hickey, & Garry, 2005).

Some authorities do not recommend ablation in women 50 years of age or older because of the increased risk of endometrial cancer in this age group. However, this guideline is a subject of debate and to date a consensus of opinion on this topic has not been achieved. Women with abnormal bleeding who are considering ablation should undergo hysteroscopy before ablation to confidently rule out the presence of endometrial disease. Limitations of use include very specific candidate criteria (**Table 25-11**).

Because 20% to 50% of women have fibroids and many of these women are young, uterine artery embolization was introduced as a surgical intervention that provides relief from the effects of this condition but maintains the possibility of future fecundity. In one well-designed

TABLE 25-11 Candidates and Contraindications for Endometrial Ablation

Candidates	Contraindications
• Cancer has been ruled out	• Known or suspected uterine cancer
• No previous myomectomy	• Uterine hyperplasia
• Nondistorted uterine cavity	• Thin myometrium
• Past childbearing	• Intrauterine device
• Refractory to medical therapy	• Pregnancy
	• Previous classical cesarean birth
	• Pelvic, uterine, cervical, or vaginal infection
	• Uterus sounds to < 4 cm or uterus sounds outside of the device parameter
	• Disorders of Müllerian fusion or absorption

Source: Adapted from American College of Obstetricians and Gynecologists, 2007a, reaffirmed 2009; Barrington et al., 2003; Pinion et al., 1994.

study, 200 women with a mean age of 43 years underwent uterine artery embolization. An 85% to 95% improvement in bleeding and a 93% improvement in overall symptoms were reported. Uterine size decreased 38% and fibroid size decreased 58%. A minor complication rate of 6.3% also was reported, with the occurrence of one pulmonary embolism that resolved successfully (Spies et al., 2001). Uterine artery embolization is a safe and effective option for women who desire to retain their fertility (American College of Obstetricians and Gynecologists, 2007a, reaffirmed 2009). All candidates for this procedure need to be evaluated by an obstetrician–gynecologist prior to the procedure and provide informed consent, indicating an understanding about the rare but possibly deadly complications of this procedure.

Each year, more than 500,000 women in the United States have a hysterectomy (Gambone, Reiter, & Gluck, 2007). This procedure is reserved as the last resort for women who experience ongoing menorrhagia that has not resolved with other treatments. Generally speaking, hysterectomy as treatment for menorrhagia should be limited to women who have other indications for the surgery, such as fibroids or uterine prolapse (Lobo, 2007). Many advantages of hysterectomy have been reported, including improved quality of life, but postoperative morbidity and mortality, including postsurgical fatigue, weight change, and changes in sexual satisfaction, are widespread. The debate about posthysterectomy sexuality is complex due to the presence of many confounding variables, although most studies do not confirm a negative impact on sexual satisfaction (Dragisic & Milad, 2004; Maas, Weijenborg, & ter Kuile, 2003; Roussis, Waltrous, Kerr, Robertazzi, & Cabbad, 2004).

Studies have shown that women facing the decision about hysterectomy want their clinician to provide them with information about the physical effects of the procedure, the body parts involved, issues concerning sexuality and femininity, and the availability of support groups for dealing with some of these postoperative issues (Wade, Pletsch, Morgan, & Menting, 2000). Research demonstrates that when patients are provided with written and video information preoperatively and have an opportunity to discuss the advantages, disadvantages, and alternatives to hysterectomy, fewer women will choose hysterectomy compared with women who only receive information but do not have the opportunity to have an interview with their clinician (Kennedy et al., 2002).

Alternative Treatments for Heavy Bleeding

A systematic review of Chinese herbal medicine (CHM) as compared to conventional Western medicine was performed to determine the efficacy and safety of using CHM for DUB. Four randomized clinical trials (RCTs) involving 452 patients were reviewed. The conclusion was that all but one of the RCTs had methodological problems that rendered their findings unsuitable for use as evidence for practice (Tu, Huang, & Tan, 2009). No adverse effects with the use of CHM were identified, however, and findings in one of the trials that used an appropriate methodology suggest that CHM may be effective. More research is needed in this area.

A pilot clinical trial ($n = 10$) was conducted to determine whether *Portulaca oleracea L.* (purslane) is effective in treating AUB (Shobeiri, Sharei, Heidari, & Kianbakht, 2009). It is common for women in Iran to use purslane to treat symptoms of AUB. Purslane seeds are obtained from the purslane plant. These seeds are washed, dried, and ground into a powder, which is then distributed in 5-gm bags. The powder is mixed in hot water (sugar is often added) and taken orally every 4 hours, beginning 48 hours after the start of the menses and continuing for 3 days. Women in the study had a diagnosis of AUB and had not responded to standard medications, making them candidates for hysterectomy. The women self-reported on the volume, duration, and pattern of their bleeding following the use of purslane seeds. All women completed the study (3 months' duration), and 8 of the women reported significant improvement of their symptoms; 2 women continued to have AUB symptoms. No adverse effects were reported. The results of this study suggest a need for larger clinical trials on the effect of purslane seeds and AUB (Shobeiri et al.).

Nonemergent Anovulatory AUB

Treatment of nonemergent AUB due to anovulation can be managed by administration of COCs (Fritz & Speroff, 2011), although this therapy will be ineffective if the endometrium is raw and denuded. Any formulation is acceptable. Therapy consists of one pill taken twice daily for 5 to 7 days, then one pill daily. The flow may cease within 24 hours, but the therapy continues as prescribed. The therapy is continued for 3 months, at which time the endometrium should be of normal height, and unopposed endogenous estrogen should stimulate a withdrawal bleed of normal amount and duration. If the woman desires contraception, the COCs can be continued. If the flow does not stop, further evaluation is necessary. The combined contraceptive patch or ring may also be used. For further discussion of COCs and other types of contraception, see Chapter 12.

Chronic anovulatory AUB can also be managed with cyclic progestogen therapy, given during the last 10 days of the menstrual cycle (Table 25-9). In women with secondary amenorrhea due to anovulation, the progestational challenge should be administered. Bleeding should commence within 2 to 7 days after completion of the progestogen. Any amount of bleeding after the progestational challenge confirms adequate levels of endogenous estrogen and outflow tract patency. Generally, progestogens will not induce bleeding when the woman has hypopituitarism caused by a tumor or has profound hypothalamic suppression (Fritz & Speroff, 2011). Women who do not bleed after a progestational challenge merit further evaluation. Typically cyclic progestogen therapy is reserved for women who do not need contraception. In adolescents with anovulatory AUB, however, progestogen therapy for 10 days each month will result in regular cyclic withdrawal bleeding, and this therapy can continue until maturation of the HPOA and without interfering with HPOA maturation.

Amenorrhea

Amenorrhea simply means absence of menses. Fritz and Speroff (2011, p. 436) state patients meeting any of the following criteria should be evaluated for amenorrhea:

- No menses by age 14 in the absence of growth or development of secondary sexual characteristics
- No menses by age 16 regardless of the presence of normal growth and development of secondary sexual characteristics
- In women who have menstruated previously, no menses for an interval of time equivalent to a total of at least three previous cycles, or 6 months

Amenorrhea typically is categorized as either primary or secondary. Primary amenorrhea is the failure to begin menses by the age of 16, whereas secondary amenorrhea is the cessation of established, regular menstruation for 6 months or longer (Dickerson, Raghunath, & Atkin, 2009). Because primary and secondary amenorrhea can have the same causes, the initial investigation for both is similar.

Physiologic causes of amenorrhea include anatomic defects, ovarian failure, chronic anovulation, anterior pituitary disorders, and central nervous system disorders. Age is an important criterion in making the differential diagnosis of primary versus secondary amenorrhea, and is relevant in determining the types of questions to ask when taking the medical history. Primary amenorrhea in a young woman may be indicative of HPOA disorder or anatomic factors, such as outflow tract obstruction. With primary amenorrhea, the physical examination needs to focus on identifying the maturation of secondary sex characteristics (e.g., Tanner staging for breast development and pubic hair pattern; see Chapter 2) and establishing outflow tract patency. The clinician should ask, "Has any vaginal bleeding occurred?" Other important interview questions to consider relate to lifestyle patterns (e.g., exercise, medication, and drug use) and eating habits (e.g., possible eating disorders). A family history of anatomic or genetic abnormalities should be explored as well.

Normal menstrual function requires that four anatomic and structural components are in working order: the uterus, ovary, pituitary, and hypothalamus (Fritz & Speroff, 2011). This understanding enables the clinician to categorize the amenorrhea according to the site or level of disturbance (Fritz & Speroff, p. 438):

- Disorders of the genital outflow tract
- Disorders of the ovary
- Disorders of the anterior pituitary
- Disorders of the hypothalamus or central nervous system

The differential diagnosis for nonpregnant women presenting with amenorrhea is either primary amenorrhea or secondary amenorrhea, although Fritz and Speroff (2011) warn that premature categorization of amenorrhea can lead to diagnostic omissions and, frequently, unnecessary and expensive diagnostic testing. The most common causes of amenorrhea are pregnancy, hypothalamic amenorrhea, and PCOS (Golden & Carlson, 2008).

Assessment

Evaluation begins with obtaining a medical history and then proceeding with a careful physical examination (see Chapter 6). The first step is always to rule out pregnancy if the woman is of childbearing age.

During the history the clinician should explore the woman's general overall health, her lifestyle, and any chronic diseases, history of trauma, or stress factors in her life. Factors such as being an adolescent, having a family history of eating disorders, and participating in competitive athletics are risks for lifestyle stress that can interrupt the function of the HPOA and lead to amenorrhea (Dickerson et al., 2009). A contraceptive history may reveal that the woman is a long-term user of hormonal contraceptives and, therefore, is more likely to experience amenorrhea due to endometrial atrophy (Fritz & Speroff, 2011). Changes in body weight or body distribution (e.g., large waist circumference) suggest PCOS and chronic anovulation, whereas weight gain and temperature intolerance suggest thyroid disorders. A history of headaches and galactorrhea may be related to a prolactin-secreting tumor or hypothyroidism. A history of hot flushes, cessation of menses, or vaginal dryness suggests menopause as a possible etiology for amenorrhea. A history of multiple D & C procedures, significant endometrial infections, or cervical treatments (e.g., cryotherapy) indicates that cervical stenosis may be the cause of the amenorrhea.

The physical examination should include an overall body assessment noting general habitus, weight, body fat distribution, and hair patterns. The thyroid should be assessed for size, presence of nodules, and tenderness. Vital signs, particularly the pulse rate and skin changes, may be helpful in diagnosing thyroid disease. Include a breast examination and note Tanner staging when doing a work-up for primary amenorrhea. The extent of breast development is an indicator of estrogen production or exposure to exogenous estrogen (Fritz & Speroff, 2011). Assessing for the presence of galactorrhea (whose presence often indicates high prolactin levels) and performing a visual field evaluation are important when women present with headaches or galactorrhea, both of which are suggestive of pituitary disease.

Prior to the pelvic examination, visually assess the external genitalia and the presence of pubic hair, which indicates androgen production or exposure (Fritz & Speroff, 2011). Visual inspection of the external genitalia may also reveal clitoral hypertrophy and the possibility of virilization (Reid, 2000).

The pelvic examination is helpful in identifying if genital anatomy is normal, if the outflow tract is patent, and if there are signs of estrogen depletion.

Diagnosis and Management

Outflow tract abnormalities are due to abnormal development of the Müllerian duct. Although these abnormalities are not common, they should be considered if the cervix is not visible or if the vagina is not patent. Obstruction of the vagina in the presence of a bulging, bluish-colored membrane indicates imperforate hymen. An obstructed bimanual examination needs referral and follow-up for possible presence of a vaginal septum or a blind pouch at the end of the vagina. Both physical findings suggest the possibility of uterovaginal agenesis and should prompt a medical referral (Reid, 2000). **Table 25-12** lists the causes of primary and secondary amenorrhea.

TABLE 25-12 Causes of Primary and Secondary Amenorrhea

Primary Amenorrhea	Secondary Amenorrhea

• Pregnancy
• Upper genital tract causes
  • Müllerian agenesis (absence of uterus and vagina, normal secondary sex characteristics)
  • Testicular feminization (absence of uterus, blind ending vaginal pouch, normal breast development, scant pubic and axillary hair)
• Lower genital tract causes
  • Labial agglutination
  • Imperforate hymen
  • Transverse vaginal septae
• Hypergonadotropic-hypogonadism
  • Follicle-stimulating hormone (FSH) > 40 mIU/L
  • Gonadal dysgenesis
  • Ovarian enzyme disorder
  • Resistant ovarian syndrome
	• Pregnancy
	• Asherman's syndrome
	• Cervical stenosis
	• Hormonal contraception
	• Hyperthyroidism/hypothyroidism
	• Polycystic ovary syndrome (PCOS)
	• Pituitary tumor
	• Premature ovarian failure
	• Menopause
	• Hypothalamic/central nervous system (CNS) disorders (e.g., lifestyle stress, eating disorder, extreme athleticism)

Ovarian function abnormalities are the most common cause of amenorrhea, and estrogen production is the most reliable measure of ovarian function (Fritz & Speroff, 2011). Laboratory tests to assess estrogen production include serum estradiol levels, progestogen challenge test, measurement of endometrial thickness, and serum FSH concentration.

A random serum estradiol level that is greater than 40 pg/mL indicates functioning ovaries. If the level is low, the woman may be amenorrheic because of ovarian failure or have hypothalamic amenorrhea.

A progestogen challenge test that produces withdrawal bleeding is indicative of functioning ovaries because bleeding will occur only if enough circulating estrogen is present. A progestogen challenge can be accomplished by administering micronized progesterone (Prometrium) 300 mg daily or medroxyprogesterone acetate (Provera) 10 mg daily for 5 days. Withdrawal bleeding should occur within 7 to 10 days after the progestogen is discontinued if the level of endogenous estrogen is appropriate to produce a withdrawal bleed and the outflow tract is patent. If the patient chooses to use micronized progesterone, it is suggested that she take this medication at bedtime, because it is known to cause drowsiness in some women. If the response to the progestogen challenge is positive (withdrawal bleeding occurs), the patient does not have galactorrhea, and her prolactin level is normal, the possibility of a pituitary tumor is effectively ruled out (Fritz & Speroff, 2011). In this case, the diagnosis is anovulation, and the treatment is a progestogen for the first 10 days of each month or a combined contraceptive (pill, patch, or vaginal ring). The patient should also be evaluated for PCOS. If the patient does not have a positive progestational challenge, then a physician consult is warranted for further evaluation and management options.

The endometrial thickness measurement should correlate with the findings of both the serum estradiol level and the progestogen challenge test.

A serum FSH indirectly measures ovarian function. A low result suggests normal functioning ovaries. In contrast, an elevated result may indicate serious disease, and the woman needs to be evaluated further. If the aforementioned tests reveal that the ovaries are producing estrogen and the FSH level is normal, the diagnosis is chronic anovulation (Fritz & Speroff, 2011). Other than pregnancy, the most common causes of chronic anovulation are thyroid disease and hyperprolactinemia (Heiman, 2009). A TSH level will detect either hypothyroidism (TSH is elevated) or hyperthyroidism (TSH is low), both of which can cause amenorrhea. Menstrual cycles almost always return to normal once the thyroid level is normalized.

Hyperprolactinemia can be diagnosed by obtaining a serum prolactin level. Galactorrhea does not always accompany hyperprolactinemia, however, so ordering a serum prolactin test is reasonable for women with amenorrhea. Hyperprolactinemia has many causes (see Chapter 16) but if it and the accompanying amenorrhea cannot be attributed to medication or another condition, then further evaluation to rule out pituitary tumors and hypothalamic mass lesions is necessary (Fritz & Speroff, 2011). Some medications, including antidepressants, opiates, calcium-channel blockers, and estrogens, can cause an elevated prolactin level; therefore, it is important to ask about medications when obtaining the health history. A dopamine agonist is the treatment of choice in the treatment of hyperprolactinemia (Fritz & Speroff).

All women with anovulation require management of this condition: If left untreated, endometrial cancer can occur, regardless of the woman's age. Typically treatment consists of inducing menses using a progestogen such as medroxyprogesterone acetate 5 to 10 mg daily for the first 12 to 14 days of the cycle. It is important for the woman to know she is not protected against pregnancy during this treatment. If she does not have her menses, she should have a pregnancy test if she has engaged in intercourse during the treatment period.

Ovarian failure is diagnosed when low estrogen production is identified while the serum FSH is high. Premature ovarian failure can be due to many causes, including genetic conditions. For this reason, Fritz and Speroff (2011) recommend a karyotype test for all patients younger than the age of 30 years who have a diagnosis of ovarian failure. Ovarian failure may also be due to autoimmune diseases, particularly Addison's disease. Consequently, it is reasonable to test for anti-adrenal antibodies in women who have premature ovarian failure (Fritz & Speroff).

MRI assessment is suggested in those instances where there is no clear explanation for either the hypogonadism or the hyperprolactinemia (Fritz & Speroff, 2011). If no lesions are found, there is no need to perform further pituitary testing, and the diagnosis is functional hypothalamic amenorrhea (Fritz & Speroff).

Functional hypothalamic amenorrhea is characterized by "the absence of menses due to the suppression of HPOA in which no anatomic organic disease is identified" (Gordon, 2010, p. 365). The typical picture of a woman diagnosed with functional amenorrhea is the adolescent who is underweight, overexercises, and is experiencing a great deal of stress. In this setting, an energy deficit occurs, and there is a resultant negative impact on the HPOA (Gordon). Treatment generally focuses on weight gain and exercise reduction, though psychological counseling may also be helpful. A goal of treatment is to offset the bone loss that occurs during the estrogen-deficient periods of time (Gordon). The underlying pathophysiology of functional hypothalamic amenorrhea is not well understood, however, and more research about this condition is needed.

Evidence for Practice

Level I evidence consistently demonstrates that the treatment of choice for anovulatory uterine bleeding is pharmacologic treatment with combined contraceptives. Cyclic progestogens also work well (American College of Obstetricians and Gynecologists, 2000, reaffirmed 2009). Recommendations that are based primarily on consensus and expert opinion (Level III) are as follows:

- Underlying coagulopathies should be considered in all patients (particularly adolescents) with abnormal bleeding if the bleeding does not respond to treatment and is not able to be explained.
- The efficacy of using CEE therapy in anovulatory bleeding is based on limited evidence, but it is effective in controlling the abnormal bleeding (American College of Obstetricians and Gynecologists, 2000, reaffirmed 2009).

Special Considerations

Adolescents

The American College of Obstetricians and Gynecologists Committee on Adolescent Health and the American Academy of Pediatrics encourage using the menstrual cycle as a vital sign because of the important information it provides about overall health (American College of Obstetricians and Gynecologists, 2006b, reaffirmed 2009).

Nutrition has a considerable impact on the gynecologic health of adolescents. Adolescent females with eating disorders such as anorexia, bulimia nervosa, or obesity frequently have menstrual abnormalities (Seidenfeld & Rickert, 2001) and, therefore, history and physical assessment are important diagnostic tools in these patients.

It is also important for clinicians to make no assumptions about an adolescent's sexual activity. It is essential to question teens about their sexual and gynecologic histories. Confidentiality is an important part of therapeutic interactions with all teens.

Once a thorough history is obtained, decide if a pelvic examination is necessary. The new cervical cytology guidelines (see Chapter 8) do not recommend a Pap test for an adolescent who is not having sex. Therefore, a pelvic examination should be done only if there is an indication such as infection.

Most adolescents with anovulatory bleeding can be treated with medical therapy (American College of Obstetricians and Gynecologists, 2000, reaffirmed 2009) and nutritional counseling. Teaching patients with significant anemia about consumption of a diet rich in iron and folic acid is important, and often a short course of iron supplementation is appropriate (Benjamin, 2009).

Women with Disabilities

Women with physical or mental disabilities and their caregivers may be particularly challenged by menstruation. It is important for the clinician to assess the level of knowledge the adolescent or adult has about her body and about menstruation. Communication should be directed to the adolescent or adult, not to the caregiver (American College of Obstetricians and Gynecologists, 2009a). It is important to ascertain if specific concerns need to be addressed. It is also important to use developmentally appropriate education to teach the patient about hygiene, contraception, sexually transmitted infections, and abuse prevention (American College of Obstetricians and Gynecologists).

When the evaluation is complete, communicating with the patient and her parents or caregiver is important. There may be a need to treat dysmenorrhea, or contraception may be desired. If contraception is desired, the level of cognitive disability will help to determine which method might work best. Some contraceptives may not be suggested if the woman is immobile (e.g., those contraceptives that have VTE risks associated with their use); therefore, the clinician should assess the risk–benefit profile prior to prescribing any option (American College of Obstetricians and Gynecologists, 2009a).

If the family or caregiver is requesting a hysterectomy or sterilization procedure for the adolescent, it is important to find out the specific reason for the request. States have different laws about surgical procedures resulting in sterilization of minors (American College of Obstetricians and Gynecologists, 2007b, reaffirmed 2009; 2009a). The American College of Obstetricians and Gynecologists' slide program Reproductive Health Care for Women with Disabilities (http://www.acog.org/departments/dept_notice.cfm?recno=38&bulletin=4526) is a helpful resource for clinicians who provide care to this population.

Perimenopause

The incidence of AUB increases as women approach the menopause. The onset of anovulatory cycles actually represents a continuation of declining ovarian function. Women should be educated early about health-promoting activities that offset risks associated with menopause, such as osteoporosis. They should be encouraged to exercise regularly and modify their diets to include foods rich in iron and calcium; in addition, if they smoke, they should be counseled about quitting (American College of Obstetricians and Gynecologists, 2000, reaffirmed 2009).

Older Women

One of the most important goals in the assessment of AUB is to rule out endometrial cancer, particularly in older women. The risk of developing endometrial cancer increases with age. The overall incidence is 10.2 cases per 100,000 in women aged 19 to 39 years, increasing to 36.5 cases per 100,000 in women aged 40 to 49 years (Albers et al., 2004). The American College of Obstetricians and Gynecologists (2000, reaffirmed 2009) recommends endometrial evaluation in women aged 35 years and older who present with abnormal bleeding.

Estrogen stimulation resulting in endometrial hyperplasia increases a woman's risk for developing endometrial cancer. Symptoms of endometrial cancer include postmenopausal bleeding; thus all uterine bleeding in a woman who is postmenopausal should be considered cancer until proven otherwise.

Table 25-13 lists the risk factors for endometrial cancer. Chapter 28 provides further discussion about endometrial cancer.

Cultural Factors

Culturally, the need for regular menses seems to be an essential part of their health for many women, such that deviations from established regular patterns are often perceived as pathologic (Livingstone & Fraser, 2002). Previous studies have demonstrated that some women will reject modes of contraception that do not

TABLE 25-13 Risk Factors for Endometrial Cancer

- Age 40 years or older
- Anovulation
- Polycystic ovary syndrome (PCOS)
- Family history of endometrial cancer
- New onset of heavy irregular bleeding, particularly after menopause
- Nulliparity
- Overweight
- Unopposed estrogen stimulation of endometrium
- Tamoxifen therapy

produce a regular bleeding cycle (Thomas & Ellerton, 2000), although more recent studies indicate women are interested in avoiding bleeding (Andrist et al., 2004; Hardy, Hebling, deSousa, Kneuper, & Snow, 2009). Interestingly, however, a qualitative study of 9 women who had been deployed to U.S. military operations recognized that menstrual suppression would help alleviate issues they experience around their menstrual cycles while deployed, but were reluctant to try it (Trego, 2007). It is important for clinicians to listen to the woman who presents with a concern about abnormal bleeding and to ascertain her perception of the bleeding, to learn how her individual culture defines abnormal bleeding, and to learn what for her might be acceptable modes of management and treatment.

Conclusion

The clinical management of AUB is complex and requires the clinician to consider not only the physical etiology but also the individual, emotional, and economic aspects of management. Age, history, and physical examination are reliable tools that suggest etiologic factors. For the clinician, it is essential to always rule out pregnancy first, and to never assume the cause of the bleeding. Be thorough and consider cancer in the algorithm. If bleeding persists even in the face of negative or reassuring tests, re-instigate the investigation and consider consultation and referral. Order laboratory tests selectively, and always involve the woman actively in the decision-making process and management plan.

References

Abou-Salem, N., Elmazny, A., & El-Sherbiny, W. (2010). Value of 3-dimensional sonohysterography for detection of intrauterine lesions in women with abnormal uterine bleeding. *Journal of Minimally Invasive Gynecology, 17*, 200–204. doi: 10:1016/j.jmig.2009.12.010

Albers, J., Hull, S., & Wesley, R. (2004). Abnormal uterine bleeding. *American Family Physician, 69*, 1915–1926.

American College of Obstetricians and Gynecologists. (2000, reaffirmed 2009). Management of anovulatory bleeding. *ACOG Practice Bulletin, 14*, 1–12. Retrieved from http://www.acog.com/ publications/educational_bulletins/pb014.cfm

American College of Obstetricians and Gynecologists. (2001, reaffirmed 2010). Use of botanicals for management of menopausal symptoms. *ACOG Practice Bulletin, 28*. Retrieved from http://www.acog/from_home/publications/misc/pb028.htm

American College of Obstetricians and Gynecologists. (2006a). *Management of abnormal uterine bleeding* [PowerPoint slides]. Retrieved from http://www.acog.org

American College of Obstetricians and Gynecologists. (2006b, reaffirmed 2009). Menstruation in girls and adolescents: Using the menstrual cycle as a vital sign. (ACOG Committee Opinion No. 349). *Obstetrics & Gynecology, 108*, 1323–1328.

American College of Obstetricians and Gynecologists. (2007a, reaffirmed 2009). ACOG Practice Bulletin No. 81: Endometrial ablation. *Obstetrics & Gynecology, 109*, 1233–1248.

American College of Obstetricians and Gynecologists. (2007b, reaffirmed 2009). Sterilization of women, including those with mental abilities (ACOG Committee Opinion No. 371). *Obstetrics & Gynecology, 110*, 217–220.

American College of Obstetricians and Gynecologists. (2009a). Menstrual manipulation for adolescents with disabilities (ACOG Committee Opinion No. 448). *Obstetrics & Gynecology, 114*, 1428–1431.

American College of Obstetricians and Gynecologists. (2009b). Von Willebrand disease in women (ACOG Committee Opinion No. 451). *Obstetrics & Gynecology, 114*, 1439–1443.

Andrist, L., Arias, R., Nucatola, D., Kaunitz, A., Musselman, B., Reiter, S., et al. (2004). Women's and providers' attitudes toward menstrual suppression with extended use of oral contraceptives. *Contraception, 70,* 359–363.

Barrington, J., Arunkalaivannan, A., & Abdel-Fattah, M. (2003). Comparison between the levonorgestrel intrauterine system (LNG-IUS) and thermal balloon ablation in treatment of menorrhagia. *European Journal of Obstetrics & Gynecology and Reproductive Biology, 108,* 72–74.

Batzer, F. R. (2007). Abnormal uterine bleeding: Imaging techniques for evaluation of the uterine cavity and endometrium before minimally invasive surgery: The case for transvaginal ultrasound. *Journal of Minimally Invasive Gynecology, 14,* 9–11.

Bayer, S., & DeCherney, A. (1993). Clinical manifestations and treatment of dysfunctional uterine bleeding. *Journal of the American Medical Association, 269,* 1823–1828.

Benjamin, L. J. (2009). Practice guideline: Evaluation and management of abnormal uterine bleeding in adolescents. *Journal of Pediatric Health, 23,* 189–193.

Bevan, J., Maloney, K., Hillary, C., Gill, J., Montgomery, R., & Scott, J. (2001). Bleeding disorders: A common cause of menorrhagia in adolescents. *Journal of Pediatrics, 13,* 856–861.

Bordo, S. (1993). *Unbearable weight: Feminism, Western culture, and the body.* Berkeley, CA: University of California Press.

Bradley, L. (2004). Assessment of abnormal uterine bleeding: 3 office-based tools. *OBG Management Online.* Retrieved August 30, 2004, from http://www.obmanagement.com/content/obg_featurexml.asp?file=2003/05/obg_0504_00

Bradley, L. (2010). *Menstrual dysfunction.* Retrieved from http://www.clevelandclinicmeded.com/medicalpubs/diseasemanagement/womens-health

Brooks, P. G. (2007). In the management of abnormal uterine bleeding, is office hysteroscopy preferable to sonography? The case for hysteroscopy. *Journal of Minimally Invasive Gynecology, 14,* 12–14.

Casablanca, Y. (2008). Management of dysfunctional uterine bleeding. *Obstetric Gynecologic Clinics of North America, 35,* 219–234.

Chapple, A. (1999). Menorrhagia: Women's perception of this condition and its treatment. *Journal of Advanced Nursing, 29,* 1500–1506.

Chimera, T., Anderson, A., & Turnball, A. (1980). Relation between measured menstrual blood and patient's subjective assessment of loss during bleeding, number of sanitary towels used, uterine weight, and endometrial surface area. *British Journal of Obstetrics & Gynecology, 87,* 603–609.

Choung, C., & Brenner, P. (1996). Management of abnormal uterine bleeding. *American Journal of Obstetrics & Gynecology, 175,* 787–792.

Claessens, E., & Cowell, C. (1981). Acute adolescent menorrhagia. *American Journal of Obstetrics & Gynecology, 139,* 227–280.

Clark, T., Mann, C., Shah, N., Kahn, K., Song, F., & Gupta, J. (2002). Accuracy of outpatient endometrial biopsy in the diagnosis of endometrial cancer: A systemic quantitative review. *British Journal of Obstetrics & Gynecology, 109,* 313–321.

Dickerson, E. H., Raghunath, A. S., & Atkin, S. L. (2009). Initial investigation of amenorrhea. *British Medical Journal, 339,* b2184. doi: 10.1136/bmj.b2184

Dragisic, K., & Milad, M. (2004). Sexual functioning and patient expectations of sexual functioning after hysterectomy. *American Journal of Obstetrics & Gynecology, 190,* 1416–1418.

Ducholm, M. (2008). Perspectives on "Abnormal uterine bleeding: An international agreement on terminologies and definitions." *Gynecologic Surgery, 5,* 81–84. doi: 10.1007/s10397-007-0359-5

Erdem, M., Bilgin, U., Bozkurt, N., & Erdem, A. (2007). Comparison of transvaginal ultrasonography and saline infusion sonohysterography in evaluating the endometrial cavity in pre- and postmenopausal women with abnormal uterine bleeding. *Menopause, 14,* 846–852.

Espindola, D., Kennedy, K., & Fischer, E. (2007). Management of abnormal uterine bleeding and the pathology of endometrial hyperplasia. *Obstetric and Gynecology Clinics of North America, 34,* 717–737.

Farrell, E. (2004). Dysfunctional uterine bleeding. *Australian Family Physician, 33,* 906–908.

Fritz, M., & Speroff, L. (2011). *Clinical gynecologic endocrinology and infertility.* Philadelphia: Wolters Kluwer Lippincott Williams & Wilkins.

Gambone, J., Reiter, R., & Gluck, P. (2007). Quality assessment, performance improvement and patient safety. In J. Berek (Ed.), *Berek and Novak's gynecology* (pp. 39–54). Philadelphia: Lippincott Williams & Wilkins.

Golden, N., & Carlson, J., (2008). The pathophysiology of amenorrhea in the adolescent. *Annals of the New York Academy of Science, 1135,* 163–178.

Gordon, C. (2010). Functional hypothalamic amenorrhea. *New England Journal of Medicine, 363*, 365–371.

Greydanus, D., Omar, H., Tsitska, A., & Patel, D. (2009). Menstrual disorders in adolescent females: Current concepts. *Disease-a-Month, 55*:45–113. doi: 10.1016/j.disamonth.2008.10.004

Grigorieva, V., Chen-Mok, M., Tarasova, M., & Mikhailov, A. (2003). Use of a levonorgestrel-releasing intrauterine system to treat bleeding related to uterine leiofibroids. *Fertility and Sterility, 79*, 1194–1198.

Grimes, D. (1979). Estimating vaginal blood loss. *Journal of Reproductive Medicine, 22*, 190–192.

Halberg, L., Hogdahl, A., Nillson, L., & Rybo, G. (1966). Menstrual blood loss: A population study. *Acta Obstetrics Gynecology Scandinavia, 44*, 347–351.

Hardy, E., Hebling, E. M., deSousa, M. H., Kneuper, E., & Snow, R. (2009). Association between characteristics of current menses and preference for induced amenorrhea. *Contraception, 80*, 266–269.

Heiman, D. L. (2009). Amenorrhea. *Primary Care Clinics in Office Practice, 36*(1), 130–131.

Hillard, P. J. (2007). Benign diseases of the female reproductive tract. In J. Berek (Ed.), *Berek and Novak's gynecology* (pp. 431–504). Philadelphia: Lippincott Williams & Wilkins.

Hoffman, B. L. (2008). Abnormal uterine bleeding. In J. Schorge, J. Schaffer, L. Halvorson, B. Hoffman, K. Bradshaw, & F. G. Cunningham (Eds.), *Williams gynecology* (pp. 174–196). New York: McGraw-Hill Medical.

Hurskainen, R., Teperi, J., Rissanen, P., Aalto, A., Grenman, S., Kivela, A., et al. (2004). Clinical outcomes and costs with the levonorgestrel-releasing intrauterine system or hysterectomy for treatment of menorrhagia: A randomized trial 5-year follow-up. *Journal of the American Medical Association, 29*, 1503–1504.

James, A. (2005). More than menorrhagia: A review of the obstetric and gynaecological manifestations of bleeding disorders. *Haemophilia, 11*, 295–307.

James, A. (2006). Von Willebrand disease. *Obstetrics & Gynecology Survey, 61*, 136–145.

Jannsen, C., Scholten, P., & Heintz, A. (1995). A preliminary study of factors influencing perception of menstrual blood loss volume. *American Journal of Obstetrics & Gynecology, 85*, 977–982.

Katz, V., Lentz, G., Lobo, R., & Gershenson, D. (2007). *Comprehensive gynecology*. Philadelphia: Mosby Elsevier.

Kaunitz, A., Westhoff, C., & Leonhardt, K. (2002, April). Therapeutic options to reduce or halt menstruation. *Female Patient* (suppl), 12–16.

Kennedy, A., Sculpher, M., Coulter, A., Dwyer, N., Rees, M., Abrams, K., et al. (2002). Effects of decision aids for menorrhagia on treatment choices, health outcomes, and costs: A randomized controlled trial. *Journal of the American Medical Association, 288*, 2701–2708.

Lentz, G. (2007). Primary and secondary dysmenorrheal, premenstrual syndrome, and premenstrual dysphoric disorder. In V. Katz, G. Lentz, R. Lobo, & D. Gershenson (Eds.), *Comprehensive gynecology* (pp. 901–914). Philadelphia: Mosby Elsevier.

Lethaby, A., Augood, C., & Duckitt, K. (2003). Nonsteroidal anti-inflammatory drugs for heavy menstrual bleeding. *Cochrane Database Systematic Reviews*, CD000400.

Lethaby, A., Cooke, I., & Rees, M. (2003). Progesterone/progestogen releasing intrauterine systems versus either placebo or any other medication for heavy menstrual bleeding. *Cochrane Database Systematic Reviews*, CD002126.

Lethaby, A., Hickey, M., & Garry, R. (2005). Endometrial destruction techniques for heavy menstrual bleeding. *Cochrane Database of Systematic Reviews, 4*, CD000329. doi: 10.1002/14651858.CD001501.pub2

Liu, Z., Doan, Q., Blumenthal, P., & Dubois, R. (2007). A systematic review evaluating health-related quality of life, work impairment, and health-care costs and utilization in abnormal uterine bleeding. *International Society for Pharmacoeconomics & Outcomes Research, 10*, 183–194. doi: 10.1111/j.1524-4733.2007.00168x

Livingstone, M., & Fraser, I. (2002). Mechanisms of abnormal uterine bleeding. *Human Reproduction Update, 8*(1), 60–67.

Lobo, R. (2007). Abnormal uterine bleeding. In V. Katz, G. Lentz, R. Lobo, & D. Gershenson (Eds.), *Comprehensive gynecology* (pp. 915–932). Philadelphia: Mosby Elsevier.

Lukes, A. S., Moore, K. A., Muse, K. N., Gersten, J. K., Hecht, B. R., Edlund, M., et al. (2010). Tranexamic acid treatment for heavy menstrual bleeding. *Obstetrics & Gynecology, 116*, 865–875.

Maas, C., Weijenborg, P., & ter Kuile, M. (2003). The effect of hysterectomy on sexual functioning. *Annual Review of Sex Research, 14*, 83–113.

Mahajan, N. N., Mahajan, K., & Soni, R. (2007). Endometrial thickness screening in premenopausal women with abnormal uterine bleeding. *Journal of Obstetrics and Gynaecologic Research, 33*(6), 886.

Mansour, D. (2007). Modern management of abnormal uterine bleeding: The levonorgestrel intra-uterine system. *Best Practice & Research Clinical Obstetrics & Gynecology, 21*(6), 1007–1021. doi: 10.1016/j.bpobgyn.2007.03.023

Marjoribanks, J., Lethaby, A., & Farquhar, C. (2003). *Surgery versus medical therapy for heavy menstrual bleeding* (Issue 3). Oxford, UK: Update Software.

Mohan, S., Page, L., & Higham, J. (2007). Diagnosis of abnormal uterine bleeding. *Best Practice & Research Clinical Obstetrics and Gynaecology, 6,* 891–903. doi: 10.1016/j.bpobgyn.2007.03.013

Munro, M. G. (2008, January). New concepts in non-gestational acute uterine bleeding. *Contemporary OBGYN.net.* Retrieved from http://www.modernmedicine.com/modernmedicine/*CME++ACCREDITED+ARTICLES/Grand-Rounds-New-concepts-in-nongestational-acute-/ArticleStandard/Article/detail/483468

New option available for heavy menstrual bleeding. (2010, March). *Contraceptive Technology,* 30.

Pharmacological treatment of heavy menstrual bleeding varies according to the need for contraception and the presence of haemostatic impairment. (2008). *Drugs & Therapy Perspectives, 24,* 13–16.

Pinion, S., Parkin, D., Abramovich, D., Naji, A., Alexander, D., Russell, I., et al. (1994). Randomized trial of hysterectomy, endometrial laser ablation, and transcervical endometrial resection for dysfunctional uterine bleeding. *British Medical Journal, 309,* 979–983.

Pitkin, J. (2007). Dysfunctional uterine bleeding. *British Medical Journal, 334,* 1110–1111.

Polotsky, A. (2010). Amenorrhea caused by extremes of body mass: Pathophysiology and sequelae. *ContemporaryOBGYN.net.* Retrieved from http://www.modernmedicine.com/modernmedicine/Modern+Medicine+Now/Amenorrhea-caused-by-extremes-of-body-mass-pathoph/ArticleStandard/Article/detail/682086

Reid, R. (2000). Amenorrhea. In L. Copeland (Ed.), *Textbook of gynecology* (pp. 365–390). Philadelphia: Saunders.

Roussis, N., Waltrous, L., Kerr, A., Robertazzi, R., & Cabbad, M. (2004). Sexual response in the patient after hysterectomy: Total abdominal versus supracervical versus vaginal procedure. *American Journal of Obstetrics & Gynecology, 65,* 2073–2083.

Sadoon, S., Salman, G., Smith, G., Henson, C., & McCullough, W. (2007). Ultrasonographic endometrial thickness for diagnosing endometrial pathology in postmenopausal bleeding. *Journal of Obstetrics and Gynaecology, 27*(4), 406–408.

Schuiling, K., & Brucker, M. (2011). Pelvic and menstrual disorders. In T. King & M. Brucker (Eds.), *Pharmacology for women's health* (pp. 916–949). Sudbury, MA: Jones and Bartlett.

Seidenfeld, M., & Rickert, V. (2001). Impact of anorexia, bulimia and obesity on the gynecologic health of adolescents. *American Family Physician, 64,* 445–450.

Shobeiri, S. F., Sharei, S., Heidari, A., & Kianbakht, S. (2009). *Portulaca oleracea L.* in the treatment of patients with abnormal uterine bleeding: A clinical trial. *Phytotherapy Research, 23,* 1411–1414.

Smith, S., Abel, M., Kelly, R., & Baird, D. (1982). The synthesis of prostaglandins from persistent proliferative endometrium. *Journal of Clinical Endocrinology and Metabolism, 55,* 284–289.

Society of Obstetricians and Gynaecologists of Canada (SOGC). (2001, August). Guidelines for the management of abnormal uterine bleeding. *SOGC Clinical Practice Guidelines, 106,* 1–6.

Spies, J., Ascher, S., Roth, A., Kim, J., Levy, E., & Gomez-Jorge, J. (2001). Uterine artery embolization for leiofibroidta. *Obstetrics & Gynecology, 98,* 29–34.

Svirsky, R., Smorgick, N., Rozowski, U., Sagiv, R., Feingold, M., Halperin, R., & Pansky, M. (2008). Can we rely on blind endometrial biopsy for detection of focal intrauterine pathology? *American Journal of Obstetrics & Gynecology, 199,* 115e–115.e.3. doi: 10.1016/j.ajog.2008.02.015

Tavris, C. (1992). *The mismeasure of woman.* New York: Simon & Schuster.

Telner, D. E., & Jakubovicz, D. (2007). Approach to diagnosis and management of abnormal uterine bleeding. *Canadian Family Physician, 53*(1), 58–64.

Teoh, S., Lex, B., Mendelson, J., Mello, N., & Cochin, J. (1992). Hyperprolactinemia and macrocytosis in women with alcohol and polysubstance abuse. *Journal of Studies on Alcohol, 53,* 176–182.

Thomas, S., & Ellerton, C. (2000). Nuisance or natural and healthy: Should monthly menstruation be optional for women? *Lancet, 355,* 922–924.

Trego, L. L. (2007). Military women's menstrual experiences and interest in menstrual suppression during deployment. *Journal of Obstetric Gynecology and Neonatal Nursing, 36*, 342–347.

Tu, X., Huang, G., & Tan, S. (2009). Chinese herbal medicine for dysfunctional uterine bleeding: A meta-analysis. *eCAM, 6*, 99–105. doi: 10.1093/ecam/nem063

van Dongen, H., de Kroon, C. D., Jacobi, C. E., Trimbos, J. B., & Jansen, F. W. (2007, January). Diagnostic hysteroscopy in abnormal uterine bleeding: A systematic review and meta-analysis. *British Journal of Obstetrics & Gynaecology*, 664–675.

Vilos, G., Lefebvre, G., & Graves, G. (2001). Guidelines for the management of abnormal uterine bleeding. *Journal of Obstetrics & Gynaecology Canada, 106*, 1–6.

Wade, J., Pletsch, P., Morgan, S., & Menting, S. (2000). Hysterectomy: What do women need and want to know? *Journal of Obstetric, Gynecologic, and Neonatal Nursing, 29*, 33–42.

Warner, P. E., Critchley, H., Lumsden, M., Campbell-Brown, M., Douglas, A., & Murray, G. C. (2004). Menorrhagia I: Measured blood loss, clinical features, and outcome in women with heavy periods: A survey with follow-up data. *Obstetrics and Gynecology, 190*(5), 1216–1223.

Zupi, E., Zullo, F., Marconi, D., Sbracia, M., Pellicano, P., Solima, E., et al. (2003). Hysteroscopic endometrial resection versus laparoscopic supracervical hysterectomy for menorrhagia: A prospective randomized trial. *American Journal of Obstetrics & Gynecology, 188*, 7–12.

26

Hyperandrogenic Disorders

Christine L. Anderson

In the past, clinicians often regarded women with hirsutism, acne, alopecia, irregular menses, and other symptoms of hyperandrogenism as suffering from a mainly cosmetic disorder or a menstrual annoyance requiring only symptomatic treatment. The health implications of hyperandrogenism, such as hyperinsulinemia and psychological distress, were either unknown or ignored. Fortunately, there have been many advances in the understanding and management of hyperandrogenic disorders. Clinicians now have an opportunity to positively affect the quality and duration of life experienced by women with these conditions by providing screening, treatment, and education related to hyperandrogenic disorders. It is important for clinicians to approach a woman who has symptoms of hyperandrogenism in a sympathetic and concerned manner. Hyperandrogenism is both an endocrine disorder and a cosmetic problem. The affected woman may have concerns on many levels regarding her health, sexuality, fertility, and social acceptance. This chapter reviews the pathophysiology, clinical presentation, diagnostic evaluation, and therapy for hyperandrogenism, while focusing on the most common hyperandrogenic disorder, polycystic ovary syndrome, and its sequelae.

Description of Hyperandrogenic Disorders

Scope of the Problem

Hyperandrogenism in reproductive-aged women is most frequently associated with polycystic ovary syndrome (PCOS), an extremely common endocrinopathy. PCOS occurs in 6% to 8% of all women, and in more than 70% of women presenting with hirsutism, acne, or androgenic alopecia (Azziz et al., 2009; Carmina, Rosato, Jannì, Rizzo, & Longo, 2006).

Patients with PCOS may experience a variety of symptoms, including clinical hyperandrogenism (e.g., hirsutism, acne, or androgenic alopecia), menstrual irregularity, or infertility. Women with PCOS also have an increased risk for adverse health outcomes such as endometrial cancer and type 2 diabetes (Teede, Deeks, & Moran, 2010). Women with PCOS need to have regular, comprehensive, preventive health care and education to decrease the long-term sequelae associated with the syndrome. Other causes of hyperandrogenism, such as nonclassical adrenal hyperplasia and androgen-producing tumors, are rarely seen but must be included in the diagnostic evaluation of women with hyperandrogenism.

Etiology

Androgen production occurs in the ovaries and adrenal glands (**Figure 26-1**). The major circulating androgens in women are dehydroepiandrosterone sulfate (DHEA-S), dehydroepiandrosterone (DHEA), androstenedione, testosterone, and dihydrotestosterone (DHT). DHEA-S, DHEA, and androstenedione must be converted to testosterone to cause androgenic effects. Women normally produce testosterone in the range of 0.2 to 0.3 mg/day, 50% of which is derived from the peripheral conversion of androstenedione. The ovaries are the most common source of increased testosterone and androstenedione. Adrenal causes of excess production of these hormones are rare (Fritz & Speroff, 2011).

Circulating testosterone is bound to sex hormone-binding globulin (SHBG), which is produced in the liver. It is normal for approximately 80% of circulating testosterone to be bound to SHBG, 19% loosely bound to albumin, and the remaining 1% left unbound. The level of SHBG is suppressed by elevated production of androgens and insulin, and increased by estrogens and thyroid hormone. Therefore, more testosterone is bound making less biologically available with high levels of thyroid hormone and estrogen. It is mainly the unbound portion of testosterone that is responsible for androgenicity, although the fraction associated with albumin makes some contribution. If SHBG is suppressed, or if androgen production increases, the amount of free (unbound) testosterone will increase without necessarily increasing the total testosterone level and the woman may develop symptoms of hyperandrogenism. Thus, because of the interplay between SHBG, insulin, thyroid hormone, estrogen, and androgen production, the total testosterone concentration may remain in the normal range, with symptoms reflecting only the decreased binding capacity of the SHBG and the increased percentage of unbound testosterone (Fritz & Speroff, 2011).

Although testosterone is the major circulating androgen, DHT is the hormone responsible for the clinical expression of androgen stimulation in many androgen-sensitive tissues, such as the skin, the pilosebaceous unit, and the hair follicles (see **Color Plate 26**). Conversion of testosterone to DHT is accomplished by 5α-reductase, an enzyme that is present in these target tissues. Racial and ethnic differences have been noted in the number of hair follicles present on the body and in the degree of 5α-reductase activity present in the hair follicles. The sensitivity of the hair follicle to the effect of androgens depends on the degree of 5α-reductase activity and is genetically predetermined. In women who are

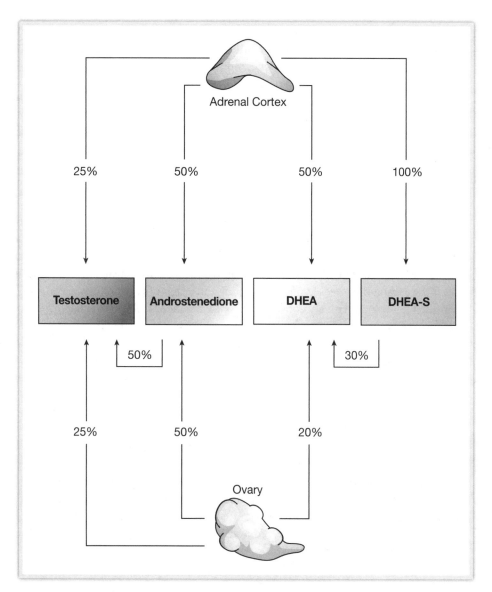

FIGURE 26-1 Sources of androgen production.

Source: Reprinted with permission from Fritz, M. A., & Speroff, L. (2011). *Clinical gynecologic endocrinology and infertility* (8th ed.). Baltimore: Lippincott Williams & Wilkins.

genetically predisposed to excessive 5α-reductase activity, normal levels of androgen can stimulate hair growth, leading to idiopathic hirsutism (Fritz & Speroff, 2011).

The symptoms of hirsutism, acne, alopecia, and, frequently, anovulation can all be traced to increased androgen levels, to decreased production of SHBG, or to increased 5α-reductase activity in the skin and hair follicles that has caused an initial stimulus to androgen-sensitive areas and then acts to sustain continued sensitivity (Fritz & Speroff, 2011). The source of the increased androgen production is the key to determining the cause of hyperandrogenism.

Biochemical Features of PCOS

Women with PCOS are predominantly anovulatory, and they typically maintain relatively steady levels of gonadotropins and sex steroids instead of experiencing the fluctuations in these levels characteristic of the normal menstrual cycle. Serum concentrations of luteinizing hormone (LH) are higher than those found in women who ovulate normally. The elevated LH levels are a result of increased pulse frequency and amplitude, but mainly frequency. Women with PCOS have a relatively constant LH pulse frequency of approximately one pulse per hour, whereas women who are ovulatory have cyclic variation in LH frequency. The increased LH pulse frequency is caused by increased gonadotropin-releasing hormone (GnRH) pulse frequency, which also causes follicle-stimulating hormone (FSH) levels to be at the low end of the normal range. FSH levels are also decreased because of increased estrone levels resulting from peripheral conversion of increased androstenedione (Fritz & Speroff, 2011).

Most of the increased androgen production seen with PCOS occurs in the ovaries as a result of increased LH stimulation. Many women with PCOS also have some increased androgen production in the adrenal glands. Insulin resistance, which results in compensatory hyperinsulinemia, is common in women with PCOS and can further contribute to hyperandrogenism. Increased insulin levels stimulate androgen production in the ovaries, both in isolation and by potentiating LH, and suppress SHBG production in the liver. A vicious cycle is created in which the elevated androgens and insulin suppress SHBG synthesis, resulting in an increase in free testosterone, which in turn exacerbates the insulin resistance (Fritz & Speroff, 2011).

Clinical Presentation

Hirsutism

Hirsutism is defined as excessive terminal hair growth in women, occurring in anatomic areas where the hair follicles are most androgen sensitive. Androgens cause transformation of fine, soft, unpigmented vellus hair to coarse, dark, terminal hair in androgen-dependent areas of hair growth (Brodell & Mercurio, 2010). Common sites for involvement include the face and chin, upper lip, areolae, lower abdomen, inner thighs, and perineum. The presence of significant amounts of terminal hair in these areas is considered abnormal. The degree and extent of hirsutism is commonly evaluated using a modified version of the Ferriman–Gallwey scale (Ferriman & Gallwey, 1961; Hatch, Rosenfield, Kim, & Tredway, 1981) (see **Color Plate 27**). Use of this scale can be limited by the fact that many women who present with hirsutism are already removing excess hair. Assessment of the type(s) and frequency of hair removal methods can be more useful for assessment and follow-up of the response to therapy (Fritz & Speroff, 2011).

Nevertheless, not all women with PCOS have hirsutism. PCOS can be present in women with minimal unwanted hair growth and a low score (5 or lower) on the modified Ferriman–Gallwey scale (Souter, Sanchez, Perez, Bartolucci, & Azziz, 2004).

Alopecia

In contrast to hirsutism, prolonged exposure to circulating androgens may paradoxically cause hair loss. Elevated androgen levels are found in 15% of reproductive-aged women who have alopecia without other manifestations of hyperandrogenism (Goodman et al., 2001). Androgen-related hair loss generally occurs at the frontal region and the crown, with the frontal hairline being left intact.

Acne

Androgen stimulation of the pilosebaceous unit (PSU) can cause enlargement of the sebaceous glands and increased secretion of sebum. The extent of correlation between the severity of acne and plasma androgen levels is inconsistent (Lee & Zane, 2007). Acne is a common finding in adolescents that usually regresses by the time affected individuals reach their mid-20s. In contrast, acne that persists beyond this time or presents in the 20s should alert the clinician to the possibility of hyperandrogenism, especially if the acne is resistant to the usual dermatologic treatment strategies and is associated with hirsutism or menstrual dysfunction (Goodman et al., 2001).

Virilization

Virilization is characterized by clitoral hypertrophy, severe hirsutism, deepening of the voice, increased muscle mass, breast atrophy, and male pattern baldness. It may also be associated with severe hyperinsulinemia. Virilization, particularly if it progresses rapidly and is associated with pronounced oligomenorrhea or amenorrhea, can indicate the presence of one of the less common causes of hyperandrogenism, such as adrenal or ovarian tumors, congenital adrenal hyperplasia, or hyperthecosis (Goodman et al., 2001).

Menstrual Dysfunction and Infertility

Women with hyperandrogenism may have various degrees of ovulatory dysfunction. Indeed, menstrual irregularity is a hallmark feature of PCOS. Oligomenorrhea is the most common presentation of overt menstrual dysfunction, but women with PCOS can have amenorrhea or, more rarely, polymenorrhea (Azziz et al., 2009). Bleeding is generally irregular and unpredictable, and can be heavy as a result of continuous estrogenic stimulation of the endometrium and resultant endometrial hyperplasia. Typically, menstrual irregularity begins at menarche, but it can occur after regular cycles (Fritz & Speroff, 2011).

Regular menses do not rule out the possibility of oligo-anovulation. Subclinical menstrual dysfunction, in which women have regularly occurring menses but chronic anovulation, is common in individuals with PCOS (Azziz et al., 2009). With either type of menstrual function, an awareness of the impending arrival of menses before bleeding begins is usually absent due to the lack of premenstrual symptoms, which is a clinical indicator of anovulation.

Many patients with hyperandrogenism experience infertility as a result of anovulation. Women with PCOS can ovulate intermittently. More than half of women with PCOS are fertile (i.e., they will become pregnant within 12 months of trying), although it may take them longer to conceive (Teede at al., 2010).

Polycystic Ovaries

Since Stein and Leventhal originally described the thickened, glistening, white, enlarged multicystic ovary in 1935, it has been clear that PCOS is associated with a classic ovarian morphology. In women with PCOS, polycystic ovaries are a result of chronic anovulation (Fritz & Speroff, 2011). In 2003, a consensus definition of the polycystic ovary syndrome was developed at a joint European Society for Human Reproduction and Embryology (ESHRE) and American Society for Reproductive Medicine (ASRM) meeting; this new definition represented a revision of the consensus statement on PCOS sponsored by the National Institutes of Health (NIH) in 1990. At the 2003 meeting, the following description of the morphology of the polycystic ovary was agreed upon: one or both ovaries with 12 or more follicles measuring 2 to 9 mm in diameter and/or increased ovarian volume of more than 10 mL (Balen, Laven, Tan, & Dewailly, 2003). Some evidence indicates that normal ovarian size is 7.5 cm or smaller; if true, this information may warrant establishing a lower threshold for increased ovarian size. While the majority of women with PCOS have polycystic ovaries, the presence of polycystic ovaries is not required if other diagnostic criteria are met (Azziz et al., 2009). The definition of polycystic ovaries does not apply to women who take combined oral contraceptives (COCs) because COCs modify ovarian morphology. In addition, women who do not meet the diagnostic criteria for PCOS can have polycystic-appearing ovaries on ultrasound (Balen et al., 2003; Lobo, 2003).

Obesity

Approximately half of patients with PCOS are obese, and obesity increases the risk for developing PCOS. Typically the obesity occurs in the abdominal region (android obesity or apple shape), with an increase in the waist–hip ratio (WHR), as opposed to the lower body (gynoid obesity or pear shape). Obesity is associated with the three following alterations that interfere with normal ovulation:

- Increased peripheral aromatization of androgens, resulting in chronically elevated estrogen concentrations
- Decreased levels of hepatic SHBG, resulting in increased circulating concentrations of free estradiol and testosterone
- Insulin resistance, leading to a compensatory increase in insulin levels that stimulates androgen production in the ovarian stroma, resulting in high local androgen concentrations that impair follicular development (Fritz & Speroff, 2011, p. 500)

As a result, obesity increases the likelihood of menstrual dysfunction and infertility (Fritz & Speroff, 2011). Patients with PCOS who are obese are more likely to develop impaired glucose tolerance, hypertension, dyslipidemias, and estrogen-dependent tumors than women with PCOS who are of normal or low weight (Goodman et al., 2001).

Insulin Resistance

Between 50% and 70% of women with PCOS are insulin resistant—a condition that often results in compensatory hyperinsulinemia (Azziz et al., 2009). Hyperinsulinemia plays a pathogenic role in the etiology of PCOS by stimulating ovarian androgen production and decreasing serum SHBG concentrations. Obesity further complicates the condition by increasing insulin resistance due to excess adiposity (Goodarzi & Korenman, 2003). Although insulin resistance is more likely to arise with obesity, it also occurs in women whose weight is in normal ranges and who have PCOS. Insulin resistance increases the risk for impaired glucose tolerance and type 2 diabetes. A recent systematic review and meta-analysis found that women with PCOS have more than twice the odds of impaired glucose tolerance (odds ratio 2.48; 95% confidence interval, 1.63–3.77) and more than four times the odds of type 2 diabetes mellitus (odds ratio 4.43; 95% confidence interval, 4.06–4.82) compared to women without PCOS (Moran, Misso, Wild, & Norman, 2010).

Dyslipidemia

Most women with PCOS (70%) have at least one lipid level that is borderline or high (Azziz et al., 2009). Dyslipidemias commonly found in women with PCOS include decreased high-density lipoprotein (HDL) cholesterol and increased triglycerides, low-density lipoprotein (LDL) cholesterol, and non-HDL cholesterol. While dyslipidemias are typically more severe in women with PCOS who have a higher body mass index (BMI), prevalence of dyslipidemias is higher in women with PCOS regardless of BMI than in women without PCOS (Wild, Rizzo, Clifton, & Carmina, 2011).

Metabolic Syndrome

Obesity, insulin resistance, and dyslipidemia are part of the metabolic syndrome, which is a cluster of risk factors for cardiovascular disease and diabetes (Alberti et al., 2009). Criteria for diagnosing this condition are found in **Table 26-1**. One-third to one-half of women with PCOS have the metabolic syndrome (Essah, Wickham, & Nestler, 2007). A recent systematic review and meta-analysis found women with PCOS have nearly three times the odds of developing metabolic syndrome (odds ratio 2.88; 95% confidence interval, 2.40–3.45) compared to women without PCOS (Moran et al., 2010).

Psychological Impact

The expression of hyperandrogenism (hirsutism, alopecia, and acne), the annoyance and unpredictability of irregular menstrual bleeding, and the pain of infertility can have significant negative impacts on a woman's psychological health and well-being. Additionally, the frequent occurrence of obesity with hyperandrogenism can have a further negative effect on self-esteem and self-image. Despite these known psychological implications of PCOS, research on the effect of PCOS on mental health is lacking (Himelein & Thatcher, 2006). Rates of depressive disorders, anxiety disorders, and binge eating are higher in women with PCOS than those without the condition (Hollinrake, Abreu, Maifeld, Van Voorhis, & Dokras, 2007). Moreover, it appears PCOS is associated with decreased sexual satisfaction and lowered health-related quality of life (Himelein & Thatcher).

Cancer Risks

Women with PCOS are at a threefold increased risk of developing endometrial cancer because of chronic, unopposed estrogen stimulation of the endometrium (Chittenden, Fullerton, Maheshwari, & Bhattacharya, 2009). Women who are obese are thought to be at the greatest risk of developing endometrial cancer because of the peripheral conversion of androgens to estrogen in adipose tissue (Rotterdam ESHRE/ASRM-Sponsored PCOS Consensus Workshop Group [Rotterdam PCOS Consensus Group], 2004). The risk of developing ovarian cancer appears to be increased twofold in women with PCOS. The etiology for the increased risk of ovarian cancer is unclear, and data on this relationship are limited. It does not appear women with PCOS have an increased risk of breast cancer (Chittenden et al.).

TABLE 26-1 Diagnostic Criteria for the Metabolic Syndrome in Women

Three or more of the following:

1. Waist circumference ≥ 88 cm (35 in.)
2. Triglycerides ≥ 150 mg/dL or drug treatment for elevated triglycerides
3. High-density lipoprotein cholesterol (HDL-C) < 50 mg/dL or drug treatment for reduced HDL-C
4. Systolic blood pressure ≥ 130 mm Hg and/or diastolic blood pressure of ≥ 85 mm Hg or drug treatment for hypertension
5. Fasting glucose ≥ 100 mg/dL or drug treatment for elevated glucose

Source: Adapted from Alberti et al., 2009.

Assessment

Women with hyperandrogenism can have a range of clinical manifestations and associated problems. Therefore, appropriate diagnosis, therapeutic management, and follow-up are essential. A thorough history and physical examination will give clues to the etiology of hyperandrogenism.

History

Ask the patient's age at thelarche (onset of breast development), adrenarche (onset of pubic hair), and menarche, and the menstrual pattern since menarche. Obtain a complete pregnancy history, including time to conceive and history of miscarriages. Note the age of onset and progression of obesity, hirsutism, seborrhea, acne, and alopecia, along with the any treatments for these conditions and their success or failure. If alopecia is present, assess for other causes of hair loss, such as nutritional deficiencies, recent surgery, rapid weight loss, anemia, thyroid dysfunction, or major illness (Shapiro, 2007).

A complete medication history is important to seek a pharmacologic cause of the symptoms. Medications that have been associated with hyperandrogenism include testosterone, anabolic steroids, danazol, certain progestins, glucocorticoids, and valproic acid (Brodell & Mercurio, 2010; Somani, Harrison, & Bergfeld, 2008).

Especially important in the history is the rapid development of symptoms of hirsutism and any rapid progression to virilization over the course of several months. Ask the patient if she has experienced increased libido, increased muscle bulk, voice deepening, breast atrophy, or clitoromegaly. Although rare, this phenomenon should raise the suspicion of an androgen-producing tumor (Fritz & Speroff, 2011).

In addition, assess the patient for polydipsia or polyuria, which suggest glucose intolerance; galactorrhea, visual disturbance, or headache, which are associated with hyperprolactinemia and pituitary tumor; hot or cold intolerance and weight loss or gain, which suggest thyroid dysfunction; and striae, mood changes, easy bruisability, or weight gain, which suggest Cushing syndrome (Somani et al., 2008). Identify cardiovascular risk factors including cigarette smoking and history of hypertension, dyslipidemia, or diabetes mellitus (Wild et al., 2010). Ask about family history of hirsutism, acne, infertility, diabetes mellitus, cardiovascular disease (especially first-degree relatives with premature cardiovascular disease, occurring before age 55 in men and before age 65 in women), dyslipidemia, or obesity (American College of Obstetricians and Gynecologists, 2009; Wild et al., 2010).

Physical Examination

The physical examination should be geared toward establishing the degree of severity of hyperandrogenism and its related symptoms. In addition to assessing height and weight, measurement of the waist circumference and BMI (see Chapter 6) are important in assessing the degree of obesity in women with hyperandrogenism. It is also important to measure blood pressure, as abnormalities may indicate an increased risk for morbidity and mortality related to the metabolic syndrome (Wilson, 2011).

Conduct a thorough skin examination, paying particular attention to the presence of hirsutism, acne, and alopecia. The pattern of body hair distribution and degree of hirsutism may be evaluated using a grading tool such as the modified Ferriman–Gallwey scale (**Color Plate 27**). Racial, familial, genetic, and hormonal influences that affect body hair distribution and amount should be considered, however. Northern Europeans, natives of North and South America, and African Americans generally have less hair than persons of Mediterranean descent. East Asians tend to have less hair than Euro-Americans, albeit with no difference in testosterone levels (Goodman et al., 2001). Acanthosis nigricans (skin that is velvety, warty, and hyperpigmented), which is associated with insulin resistance, may be present in the neck area or axillae or under the breasts.

Perform a thyroid examination and breast examination to evaluate for thyroid conditions or evidence of galactorrhea. Observe for signs of Cushing syndrome such as moon facies, dorsocervical fat pad (buffalo hump), and abdominal striae. Perform a complete pelvic examination including evaluation of the clitoris for hypertrophy and bimanual examination to determine the size of the uterus and ovaries, and the presence of masses (American College of Obstetricians and Gynecologists, 2009; Somani et al., 2008)

Diagnostic Testing

Laboratory Studies Laboratory tests for patients with evidence of hyperandrogenism should be selected based on the individual patient's history and physical examination. There is some disagreement in the literature regarding which tests are essential and which are superfluous. The following recommendations for laboratory studies to be completed during the initial assessment of hyperandrogenism are based on guidance from the American College of Obstetricians and Gynecologists (2009), the Androgen Excess and PCOS Society (Azziz et al., 2009), and Fritz and Speroff (2011).

All women who have hyperandrogenism with ovulatory dysfunction should have a serum prolactin, serum thyroid-stimulating hormone (TSH), fasting lipid profile, and 2-hour oral glucose tolerance test (American College of Obstetricians and Gynecologists, 2009; Fritz & Speroff, 2011). The prolactin and TSH levels are used to exclude hyperprolactinemia and thyroid disorders, both of which can cause ovulatory dysfunction. The prevalence of dyslipidemias in women with PCOS warrants baseline assessment of a fasting lipid profile. The 2-hour oral glucose tolerance test is used to identify impaired glucose tolerance (2-hour glucose test result in the range of 140–200 mg/dL) and diabetes mellitus (2-hour glucose test result of 200 mg/dL or greater). Routine screening for insulin resistance is not recommended due to the lack of a uniformly accepted test (Fritz & Speroff).

Women who have clinical signs of hyperandrogenism with regular menstrual cycles should be evaluated for ovulatory dysfunction by obtaining a serum progesterone level between days 20 and 24 of the menstrual cycle (Azziz et al., 2009). If this luteal-phase progesterone level is less than 3 to 4 ng/mL, the cycle is oligo-anovulatory. Repeating the progesterone level during a second cycle can confirm the diagnosis of chronic oligo-anovulation and PCOS.

Routine measurement of androgen levels in women with clinical signs of hyperandrogenism is controversial because of the limitations in accuracy and sensitivity of testosterone assay methods. Given that there is no standardized assay, clinicians must be aware of the type and quality of assay being used as well as the laboratory's reference ranges (Rosner, Auchus, Azziz, Sluss, & Raff, 2007). The American College of Obstetricians and Gynecologists (2009) recommends routine free testosterone measurement either directly by equilibrium dialysis or calculated from high-quality measurements of total testosterone and SHBG. According to Fritz and Speroff (2011), routine testosterone measurement is unnecessary when clinical signs of hyperandrogenism are present. These authors recommend reserving testosterone testing for women who have moderate or severe hirsutism, sudden onset or rapid progression of hirsutism, or signs of virilization, as these findings suggest that an androgen-producing tumor is present. Women in whom a tumor is suspected should have a serum total testosterone, ideally performed after extraction and chromatography by mass spectrometry or immunoassay rather than on whole serum (Fritz and Speroff; Rosner et al.). Women with a serum total testosterone level of 150 ng/dL or greater (100 ng/dL or greater in postmenopausal women) need evaluation for an androgen-producing tumor (see the next section on imaging studies). Neither the American College of Obstetricians and Gynecologists nor Fritz and Speroff recommend routine DHEA-S testing.

Measurement of 17-hydroxyprogesterone (17-OHP) is performed to assess for nonclassical or "late-onset" congenital adrenal hyperplasia, which is characterized by excessive adrenal androgen production and can present very similarly to PCOS. The American College of Obstetricians and Gynecologists (2009) recommends routine 17-OHP testing. Fritz and Speroff (2011) state that routine testing is reasonable but note that it is safe to reserve 17-OHP testing for women who have pre- or peri-menarcheal onset of hirsutism, have a family history of nonclassical congenital adrenal hyperplasia, or are members of a high-risk ethnic group (Hispanic, Mediterranean, Slavic, Ashkenazi Jew, or Yupik Eskimo). 17-OHP testing is performed in the morning during the follicular phase. Values less than 200 ng/dL exclude the condition, whereas values greater than 800 ng/dL establish the diagnosis. Values from 200 to 800 ng/dL warrant referral to an endocrinologist for an adrenocorticotropic hormone (ACTH) stimulation test (Fritz & Speroff).

Testing for Cushing syndrome, which results from excess adrenal cortisol secretion, should be reserved for women with symptoms of this condition (American College of Obstetricians and Gynecologists, 2009; Fritz & Speroff, 2011). Screening for Cushing syndrome consists of the overnight dexamethasone suppression test, which is performed by giving 1 mg of dexamethasone orally between 11 p.m. and 12 a.m., and then drawing a serum cortisol at 8 a.m. the next morning. Values less than 1.8 mcg/dL are considered normal (Fritz & Speroff).

Imaging Studies and Endometrial Biopsy Pelvic ultrasonography can be used to assess for polycystic ovaries and identify endometrial hyperplasia in women who are oligomenorrheic or amenorrheic (American College of Obstetricians and Gynecologists, 2009; Fritz & Speroff, 2011). An endometrial biopsy is recommended for any patient who has long-standing anovulation because of the risk for endometrial carcinoma. The decision to perform an endometrial biopsy should not be based on a woman's age, as endometrial cancer can be encountered in young women who are anovulatory. Thus it is the duration of exposure to unopposed estrogen that is critical, rather than the patient's age (Fritz & Speroff).

If a virilizing tumor is suspected but an adnexal mass is not palpable, transvaginal ultrasound of the ovaries is indicated. If no ovarian tumor is identified on ultrasound, adrenal computed tomography (CT) imaging should be performed. Routine adrenal imaging should be avoided because it can lead to unnecessary evaluation of nonfunctioning adrenal masses (incidentalomas) (Fritz & Speroff, 2011).

Making the Diagnosis of PCOS

If history, physical examination, and laboratory testing rule out all other possible causes of hyperandrogenism, the most likely diagnosis is PCOS. It is important to remember that PCOS is a syndrome; thus no single diagnostic criterion is sufficient for clinical diagnosis. Two sets of diagnostic criteria are commonly used today: those developed by the Rotterdam PCOS Consensus Group (2004) and those developed by the Androgen Excess and Polycystic Ovary Syndrome Society (Azziz et al., 2009).

According to the Rotterdam PCOS Consensus Group (2004), the exclusion of other etiologies and two out of three of the following criteria must be present to make the diagnosis of PCOS:

1. Oligo- or anovulation
2. Clinical and/or biochemical signs of hyperandrogenism
3. Polycystic ovaries

The Androgen Excess and Polycystic Ovary Syndrome Society criteria for the diagnosis of PCOS (Azziz et al., 2009) are as follows:

1. Hyperandrogenism: hirsutism and/or hyperandrogenemia
2. Ovarian dysfunction: oligo-anovulation and/or polycystic ovaries
3. Exclusion of other androgen excess or related disorders

The primary difference between these diagnostic criteria is that the Androgen Excess and Polycystic Ovary Syndrome Society criteria require hyperandrogenism for diagnosis of PCOS. Clinicians should be aware which diagnostic criteria were used when reviewing research studies (Fritz & Speroff, 2011).

Differential Diagnoses

Differential diagnoses for hyperandrogenism include PCOS; congenital adrenal hyperplasia; hyperandrogenism, insulin resistance, and acanthosis nigrans (HAIR-AN) syndrome; androgen-producing ovarian or adrenal tumors; idiopathic hirsutism; Cushing syndrome; thyroid disorders; androgenic medications; conditions associated with pregnancy; and hyperprolactinemia. The most likely of these is PCOS. Key points for differential diagnoses can be found in **Table 26-2**.

TABLE 26-2 Differential Diagnoses for Hyperandrogenism

Polycystic ovary syndrome (PCOS)	• Most common cause of hyperandrogenism, occurs in approximately 80% of women with androgen excess • Clinical and/or biochemical evidence of hyperandrogenism • Oligo-anovulation • Polycystic ovaries • Exclusion of other etiologies
Nonclassical congenital adrenal hyperplasia	• Occurs in approximately 2% of women with androgen excess • Clinically indistinguishable from PCOS • Elevated 17-hydroxyprogesterone (17-OHP), greater than 800 ng/dL
Hyperandrogenism, insulin resistance, and acanthosis nigrans (HAIR-AN) syndrome	• Occurs in approximately 4% of women with androgen excess • Severe hyperandrogenism, possible virilization • Acanthosis nigricans • Severe hyperinsulinemia/insulin resistance
Androgen-producing tumors (ovarian or adrenal)	• Rare • Acute, rapid course of virilizing symptoms • Testosterone usually elevated to more than 150 ng/dL in premenopausal women or 100 ng/dL in postmenopausal women • Palpable adnexal mass or mass on imaging of ovaries or adrenal glands
Idiopathic hirsutism	• Occurs in approximately 5% of women with androgen excess • Normal serum androgen levels • Normal ovulation by basal body temperature charting or luteal-phase progesterone measurements
Cushing syndrome	• Frequent referral diagnosis, one of the least common final diagnoses • Evidence of striae over abdomen, central weight distribution, muscle weakness, altered mood, easy bruisability • Failure of cortisol suppression after overnight dexamethasone suppression test
Thyroid disorders	• Palpable thyroid enlargement or mass • Suspect with presence of alopecia • Elevated thyroid-stimulating hormone
Androgenic medication use	• May be systemic or topical • Hirsutism is common
Pregnancy	• Rapid virilization occurs during pregnancy • Common causes are pregnancy luteoma or theca-lutein cysts (hyperreactio luteinalis)
Hyperprolactinemia	• Galactorrhea • Elevated prolactin level

Sources: Adapted from Azziz et al., 2004; Fritz & Speroff, 2011; Goodman et al., 2001; Kanova & Bicikova, 2011; Rotterdam ESHRE/ASRM-Sponsored PCOS Consensus Workshop Group, 2004; Somani et al., 2008.

Management

This section focuses on management of PCOS. Management goals are to treat current clinical manifestations and ameliorate long-term sequelae. Management should address any cosmetic manifestations of hyperandrogenism that the patient finds distressing as well as the psychological stress associated with PCOS.

Nonpharmacologic Management

Lifestyle Modification All women with PCOS, regardless of their weight, must be aware of the importance of a healthy diet, regular exercise, and weight management in controlling symptoms of PCOS and preventing sequelae. Weight loss is the first-line treatment for women who are obese. Weight loss, even in relatively small amounts (2% to 5%), decreases androgen levels and increases SHBG. Additional benefits include decreased hirsutism, resumption of ovulation, improved menstrual function, increased pregnancy rates, and reduced risk of miscarriage. Weight loss also improves fasting insulin, glucose, glucose tolerance, and lipid levels, which are important for preventing and treating diabetes and cardiovascular disease (Fritz & Speroff, 2011; Moran, Pasquali, Teede, Hoeger, & Norman, 2009).

The most important dietary strategy for weight loss is decreased caloric consumption, entailing a reduction of 500 to 1000 kcal/day. A fat intake that constitutes fewer than 30% of total calories, with fewer than 10% of calories coming from saturated fat, and an increase in consumption of fiber, whole grains, fruits, and vegetables are recommended. Specific macronutrient composition of the diet, such as high protein or very low carbohydrate consumption, has been studied, but there is not yet clear evidence to recommend any specific approach as superior to the others (American College of Obstetricians and Gynecologists, 2009; Fritz & Speroff, 2011; Moran et al., 2009).

The weight management program should include at least 30 minutes of structured exercise per day. It appears that exercise offers benefits even if significant weight loss does not occur (Farrell & Antoni, 2010).

Structure and support for any weight management program are important, and the clinician must provide close follow-up and monitoring (Moran et al., 2009). Evidence supporting the use of antiobesity medications (e.g., phentermine, sibutramine, and orlistat) and bariatric surgery in women with PCOS is limited, and further research is needed to assess their use when other weight management options prove unsuccessful (Moran et al.; Wild et al., 2010).

Mechanical Hair Removal Contrary to popular belief, mechanically removing hair by shaving, plucking, waxing, or depilatory creams does not stimulate further hair growth. These methods may be used in conjunction with pharmacologic therapy to remove hair as needed. Electrolysis and photoepilation with laser or intense pulsed light (IPL) can be used for permanent hair reduction. Both strategies require several sessions of treatment and can cause pigment changes and scarring. The Endocrine Society recommends laser over electrolysis because laser is faster and less painful than electrolysis; however, electrolysis is less expensive than laser therapy (Martin et al., 2008).

Pharmacologic Management

This section focuses on pharmacologic treatment for women who are not trying to conceive. When selecting a medication, it is important to consider the specific treatment goals for the patient, such as improving clinical signs of hyperandrogenism (e.g., hirsutism, acne, and alopecia), regulating menstrual cycles, protecting the endometrium, and preventing long-term sequelae of PCOS. Most patients have multiple treatment goals, and some individual medications (e.g., combined oral contraceptives and insulin sensitizing agents) address more than one treatment goal.

Combined Oral Contraceptives Combined oral contraceptives (COCs) are recommended as a first-line pharmacologic treatment for women with PCOS (American College of Obstetricians and Gynecologists, 2009; Fritz & Speroff, 2011; Martin et al., 2008; Wilson, 2011). COCs treat hyperandrogenism by inhibiting LH secretion and subsequently LH-dependent ovarian androgen production, and by raising the concentration of SHBG, which binds free testosterone. As a result, COCs provide cosmetic relief of acne and hirsutism. These medications also regulate menstrual cycles and provide protection against endometrial cancer by interrupting the steady state of estrogen stimulation on the uterus and inducing a monthly withdrawal bleed. Some concerns have been raised about COCs' safety in women with PCOS, given that COCs may decrease insulin resistance or glucose tolerance. There is no evidence that these risks are substantially higher in women with PCOS, however (Fritz & Speroff).

A COC with a low dose of estrogen (less than 50 mcg) and a nonandrogenic progestin component is recommended. Formulations containing desogestrel, norgestimate, or drospirenone are commonly used because of their low androgenic effects (Radosh, 2009). Drospirenone functions as an androgen receptor agonist. The drospirenone dose in COCs (3 mg) is equivalent to approximately 25 mg of spironolactone, which may not be enough for hirsutism treatment but should be considered if additional spironolactone is given because hyperkalemia can occur with such therapy (Martin et al., 2008). The maximal effect of COCs on acne is usually observed within 2 months. In contrast, the maximal effect on hair growth may take as long as 9 to 12 months for its realization because of the length of the hair growth cycle (Ehrmann & Rychlik, 2003). The nonoral combined contraceptives—that is, the transdermal patch and the vaginal ring—are also likely to be beneficial for women with PCOS, but evidence and literature on their use in this population is limited. More detailed information about combined contraceptives can be found in Chapter 12.

Progestogens Women who have contraindications to COCs or do not wish to take these agents can use progestogens to prevent endometrial hyperplasia and cancer. Women who need contraception can use the levonorgestrel-releasing intrauterine system (LNG-IUS), progestin-only pills (POPs), the depot medroxyprogesterone acetate injection, or the subdermal implant. These contraceptive methods are discussed in Chapter 12. Women who do not need contraception can take a dose of 5 to 10 mg medroxyprogesterone acetate or 200 mg micronized progesterone daily for the first 14 days of each month. Progestational therapy alone will not treat hirsutism, however (American College of Obstetricians and Gynecologists, 2009; Fritz & Speroff, 2011).

Antiandrogens Antiandrogens are effective in the treatment of hirsutism. They should always be used in combination with effective contraception in a woman who is sexually active because of their potential for having teratogenic effects on a fetus. COCs are generally used as a first-line treatment for hirsutism, but for women whose hirsutism remains refractory after 6 months of COC use, the addition of an antiandrogen medication may be more effective than administration of either agent alone (Martin et al., 2008; Wilson, 2011). Antiandrogens can be used as first-line therapy in women who do not want or need to take COCs. These medications include spironolactone, finasteride, and flutamide.

Spironolactone is effective in the treatment of hirsutism and androgenic alopecia. It works by inhibiting testosterone from binding to its receptors, thereby inhibiting its action. The usual dose is 50 to 100 mg twice daily, with the effects being dose dependent. It can take 6 months or more to see the full clinical effect. Side effects may include lightheadedness, dizziness, fatigue, diuresis, and a risk of hyperkalemia. Spironolactone may also cause menstrual irregularity when used as monotherapy. Combination therapy with COCs reduces this side effect, and improves clinical response (American College of Obstetricians and Gynecologists, 2009; Fritz & Speroff, 2011; Martin et al., 2008).

Finasteride inhibits 5α-reductase activity, which blocks the conversion of testosterone to DHT in the skin. A dose of 5 to 7.5 mg/day is effective in decreasing hirsutism without engendering any adverse effects. In studies comparing finasteride to spironolactone, the former agent proved slightly less or equally efficacious than spironolactone in doses of 100 mg daily. The major benefit of finasteride is its lack of side effects. Women who are treated with finasteride should be aware that this medication can adversely affect the development of the genital tract in male fetuses, and must be counseled to use a highly effective contraceptive method. Pregnant women should not touch crushed or broken finasteride tablets due to their teratogenicity (American College of Obstetricians and Gynecologists, 2009; Fritz & Speroff, 2011; Martin et al., 2008).

Flutamide is a pure antiandrogen that has shown some benefit in treating hirsutism and hyperandrogenic alopecia (Carmina & Lobo, 2003). Unfortunately, flutamide is associated with hepatotoxicity that can cause liver failure and rarely death. The Endocrine Society does not recommend flutamide for hirsutism treatment (Martin et al., 2008).

Insulin Sensitizing Agents Metformin is an oral antihyperglycemic agent whose primary mechanisms of action are inhibition of hepatic glucose production and increases in peripheral insulin sensitivity. Metformin has been shown to increase ovulatory frequency, regulate cycles, reduce hirsutism, and decrease androgen levels in women with PCOS, but it has a minimal effect on weight loss. In women with PCOS and hyperinsulinemia, this agent decreases fasting insulin levels, blood pressure, and LDL cholesterol levels (American College of Obstetricians and Gynecologists, 2009; Mathur, Alexander, Yano, Trivax, & Azziz, 2008; Practice Committee of the ASRM, 2008).

While metformin can treat some clinical manifestations of PCOS and has the potential to prevent or delay the onset of diabetes mellitus, routine therapy with this medication in all women with PCOS is not recommended. Metformin should be considered for women with impaired glucose tolerance whose weight does not respond to diet and exercise or whose weight is normal such that weight loss is not appropriate (Practice Committee of the ASRM, 2008; Wild et al., 2010). Metformin is also used in infertility treatment for women with PCOS (Thessaloniki ESHRE/ASRM-Sponsored PCOS Consensus Workshop Group, 2008). Metformin should not be given solely to treat hirsutism or promote weight loss (Martin et al., 2008; Mathur et al., 2008).

The usual dose of metformin is 1500 to 2550 mg per day, with the dose being started low and then gradually increased over 4 to 6 weeks. Metformin is taken on an empty stomach unless the sustained-release formulation is used, in which case it is usually taken with the evening meal. It is contraindicated in cases of impaired renal function, congestive heart failure, hepatic dysfunction, sepsis, or history of alcohol abuse. The most serious side effect of metformin is the development of lactic acidosis, but this is rare. Vitamin B_{12} deficiency can also occur. Gastrointestinal side effects, which are more common, include nausea, abdominal discomfort, diarrhea, and anorexia (Mathur et al., 2008).

The thiazolidinediones (TZDs) or glitazones lower glucose levels by increasing the utilization in the skeletal muscles and decreasing hepatic glucose synthesis. Most studies on this class of drugs used troglitazone, which was withdrawn from the market because of its propensity to cause significant hepatocellular toxicity. Two related drugs, rosiglitazone and pioglitazone, have been investigated for use in PCOS. Both can cause or worsen congestive heart failure, and rosiglitazone has been associated with increased risk of myocardial infarction (Katsiki & Hatzitolios, 2010). Use of TZDs for PCOS is not recommended (Mathur et al., 2008).

Topical Preparations Eflornithine HCl 13.9% (Vaniqa) is a topical cream approved for the treatment of facial hirsutism. It is applied to affected areas twice daily, and improvement is noticeable in 6 to 8 weeks. This agent's primary mechanism of action is inhibition of the enzyme ornithine decarboxylase in human skin, which slows the rate of hair growth. It is not a depilatory, and hair growth returns after discontinuation of the cream. Its main side effects are itching and dry skin (Brodell & Mercurio, 2010; Martin et al., 2008).

Additional Medications Gonadotropin-releasing hormone (GnRH) analogs, such as leuprolide, have been used in the treatment of hirsutism. These medications work by inhibiting gonadotropin secretion and subsequent ovarian hormone secretion, which results in not only a slowing of hair growth, but also severe estrogen deficiency. GnRH treatment is expensive, requires injections and estrogen therapy, and may not be more effective than COCs and antiandrogens. For these reasons, the Endocrine Society recommends reserving use of GnRH analogs for women with severe hyperandrogenemia, such as ovarian hyperthecosis, that has not responded to COCs and antiandrogens (Martin et al., 2008). Glucocorticoids (prednisone, dexamethasone) are not indicated for treatment of hirsutism in women with PCOS, but are used in treating nonclassical congenital adrenal hyperplasia (Martin et al.).

Follow-Up

Patient education and comprehensive woman-centered care are crucial to the successful management of PCOS and reduction of negative long-term sequelae. Long-term follow-up with routine visits is appropriate to monitor response to treatment and development of complications. Screening for evidence of development of metabolic consequences must be undertaken at regular intervals. The clinician should assess the patient's BMI, waist circumference, and blood pressure at every visit (Wild et al., 2010). Encourage weight loss in women who are overweight or obese. If the baseline fasting lipid profile is normal, repeat this test every 2 years or sooner if the woman gains weight. If the baseline 2-hour oral glucose tolerance test is normal, repeat this test every 2 years or sooner if the woman develops additional risk factors. Screen women with impaired glucose tolerance annually for diabetes mellitus (Wild et al., 2010). Diabetes mellitus, hypertension, and dyslipidemia require prompt treatment (or referral for treatment) after diagnosis. Advise women that cigarette smoking further increases their risk for cardiovascular disease and provide smoking cessation interventions for women who smoke.

When to Refer Patients

Endocrinopathies If diagnostic testing reveals that the patient has congenital adrenal hyperplasia, HAIR-AN syndrome, Cushing syndrome, hyperprolactinemia, or androgen-producing tumors, she should be referred to an endocrinologist. An endocrinology consultation should also be considered for patients who are refractory to treatment for PCOS. Clinicians who are not experienced in the management of metabolic syndrome should seek consultation for treating women with PCOS who meet the criteria for metabolic syndrome.

Treatment of Infertility Treatment of infertility in women with PCOS can be challenging and is beyond the scope of this chapter. The consensus statement on infertility treatment in women with PCOS, which was developed by international experts at a workshop endorsed by the ESHRE and the ASRM, is recommended as an overview of this topic (Thessaloniki ESHRE/ASRM-Sponsored PCOS Consensus Workshop Group, 2008). Women with PCOS and infertility require care from a clinician experienced in treating these conditions concomitantly.

Special Considerations

Adolescents

Unfortunately, the symptoms of hyperandrogenism are not usually brought to the attention of clinicians until the patient is in her late teens, early twenties, or even older. The most common causes of hyperandrogenism, however, usually become active in early adolescence. Premature adrenarche may be a consequence of hyperinsulinemia. These adolescents go on to develop clinical signs of hyperandrogenism and/or irregular menses, for which they often are treated symptomatically without undergoing a thorough assessment of the causes of symptoms. Menstrual irregularity is common right after menarche but warrants investigation if it persists more than 2 years. Every attempt should be made to diagnose and treat hyperandrogenic conditions as early as possible because early treatment may help ameliorate symptoms and prevent the development of adverse sequelae and psychological dysfunction (Fritz & Speroff, 2011).

Pregnant Women

Virilization presenting in pregnancy should raise the suspicion for a luteoma—a condition that is an exaggerated reaction of the ovarian stroma to normal levels of chorionic gonadotropin and not a true tumor. The solid luteoma is associated with a normal pregnancy and is usually unilateral. Maternal virilization occurs in 25% to 35% of pregnancies affected by a luteoma. If the mother is virilized as a result of the luteoma, there is a 60% to 70% chance that her female fetus will show some signs of masculinization. The luteoma does not cause other maternal effects and regresses postpartum. Virilization may be recurrent in subsequent pregnancies (Kanova & Bicikova, 2011).

In contrast, a theca-lutein cyst or hyperreactio luteinalis is usually bilateral and is seen with trophoblastic disease or with the high human chorionic gonadotropin levels associated with a multiple gestation. Maternal virilization will occur in 30% of pregnancies affected with a theca-lutein cyst, but no risk of fetal masculinization is noted.

If a woman is experiencing virilization during pregnancy, a pelvic ultrasound can be very helpful in making the diagnosis. If a solid unilateral ovarian lesion is present, malignancy is likely (Fritz & Speroff, 2011; Kanova & Bicikova, 2011).

Women being treated for hyperandrogenism who become pregnant should be aware of the benefits and risks of any medications they are taking. Although metformin may prove beneficial during pregnancy by reducing the risk of gestational diabetes mellitus, evidence is insufficient to recommend its routine use during pregnancy. In fact, metformin should be discontinued when pregnancy is diagnosed (Mathur et al., 2008). Some medications, such as finasteride, flutamide, and spironolactone are contraindicated in pregnancy and should be discontinued immediately. A woman who becomes pregnant while taking anti-androgens needs counseling regarding these agents' potential effects on her fetus.

Talking with the Patient

Clinicians should provide informed consent to all women presenting for evaluation or treatment of hyperandrogenic disorders. The information required includes the risks and benefits of the proposed treatment, the alternative treatments available, these therapies' advantages and disadvantages, and the consequences of not receiving treatment at all. Clinicians should be careful to mention any important side effects of treatment or medication of which the patient should be aware. Consider giving the patient printed information about the condition or medication to supplement the amount of information that can be verbally communicated in the time constraints of typical clinical practice (Starr, 2004).

References

Alberti, K. G. M. M., Eckel, R. H., Grundy, S. M., Zimmet, P. Z., Cleeman, J. I., Donato, K., et al. (2009). Harmonizing the metabolic syndrome: A joint statement of the International Diabetes Federation Task Force on Epidemiology and Prevention; National Heart, Lung, and Blood Institute; American Heart Association; World Heart Federation; International Atherosclerosis Society; and International Association for the Study of Obesity. *Circulation, 120,* 1640–1645.

American College of Obstetricians and Gynecologists. (2009). Polycystic ovary syndrome. American College of Obstetricians and Gynecologists Practice Bulletin No. 108. *Obstetrics & Gynecology, 114,* 936–949.

Azziz, R., Carmina, E., Dewailly, D., Diamanti-Kandarakis, E., Escobar-Morreale, H. F., Futterweit, W., et al. (2009). The Androgen Excess and PCOS Society criteria for the polycystic ovary syndrome: The complete task force report. *Fertility and Sterility, 91,* 456–488.

Azziz, R., Sanchez, L. A., Knochenhauer, E. S., Moran, C., Lazenby, J., Stephens, K. C., et al. (2004). Androgen excess in women: Experience with over 1000 consecutive patients. *Journal of Clinical Endocrinology & Metabolism, 89,* 453–462.

Balen, A. H., Laven, J. S., Tan, S., & Dewailly, D. (2003). Ultrasound assessment of the polycystic ovary: International consensus definitions. *Human Reproduction Update, 9*(6), 505–514.

Brodell, L. A., & Mercurio, M. G. (2010). Hirsutism: Diagnosis and management. *Gender Medicine, 7,* 79–87.

Carmina, E., & Lobo, R. A. (2003). Treatment of hyperandrogenic alopecia in women. *Fertility and Sterility, 79*(1), 91–95.

Carmina, E., Rosatao, F., Jannì, A., Rizzo, M., & Longo, R. A. (2006). Relative prevalence of different androgen excess disorders in 950 women referred because of clinical hyperandrogenism. *Journal of Clinical Endocrinology & Metabolism, 91,* 2–6.

Chittenden, B. G., Fullerton, G., Maheshwari, A., & Bhattacharya, S. (2009). Polycystic ovary syndrome and the risk of gynaecological cancer: A systematic review. *Reproductive BioMedicine Online, 19,* 398–405.

Ehrmann, D. A., & Rychlik, D. (2003). Pharmacologic treatment of polycystic ovary syndrome. *Seminars in Reproductive Medicine, 21*(3), 277–283.

Essah, P. A., Wickham, E. P., & Nestler, J. E. (2007). The metabolic syndrome in polycystic ovary syndrome. *Clinical Obstetrics and Gynecology, 50,* 205–225.

Farrell, K., & Antoni, M. H. (2010). Insulin resistance, obesity, inflammation, and depression in polycystic ovary syndrome: Biobehavioral mechanisms and interventions. *Fertility and Sterility, 94,* 1565–1574.

Ferriman, D., & Gallwey, J. D. (1961). Clinical assessment of body hair growth in women. *Journal of Clinical Endocrinology and Metabolism, 21,* 1440–1447.

Fritz, M. A., & Speroff, L. (2011). *Clinical gynecologic endocrinology and infertility* (8th ed.). Baltimore: Lippincott Williams & Wilkins.

Goodarzi, M. O., & Korenman, S. G. (2003). The importance of insulin resistance in polycystic ovary syndrome. *Fertility and Sterility, 80*(2), 255–258.

Goodman, N. F., Bledsoe, M. B., Futterweit, W., Goldzieher, J. W., Petak, S. M., Smith, K. D., et al. (2001). American Association of Clinical Endocrinologists medical guidelines for clinical practice for the diagnosis and treatment of hyperandrogenic disorders. *Endocrine Practice, 7*(2), 120–134.

Hatch, R., Rosenfield, R. L., Kim, M. H., & Tredway, D. (1981). Hirsutism: Implications, etiology, and management. *American Journal of Obstetrics and Gynecology, 140,* 815–830.

Himelein, M. J., & Thatcher, S. S. (2006). Polycystic ovary syndrome and mental health: A review. *Obstetrical and Gynecological Survey, 61,* 723–732.

Hollinrake, E., Abreu, A., Maifeld, M., Van Voorhis, B. G., & Dokras, A. (2007). Increased risk of depressive disorders in women with polycystic ovary syndrome. *Fertility and Sterility, 87,* 1369–1376.

Kanova, N., & Bicikova, M. (2011). Hyperandrogenic states in pregnancy. *Physiological Research, 60,* 243–252.

Katsiki, N., & Hatzitolios, A. I. (2010). Insulin-sensitizing agents in the treatment of polycystic ovary syndrome: An update. *Current Opinion in Obstetrics and Gynecology, 22,* 466–476.

Lee, A. T., & Zane, L. T. (2007). Dermatologic manifestations of polycystic ovary syndrome. *American Journal of Clinical Dermatology, 8,* 201–219.

Lobo, R. A. (2003). What are the key features of importance in polycystic ovary syndrome? *Fertility and Sterility, 80*(2), 259–261.

Martin, K. A., Chang, J., Ehrmann, D. A., Ibanez, L., Lobo, R. A., Rosenfield, R. L., et al. (2008). Evaluation and treatment of hirsutism in premenopausal women: An Endocrine Society clinical practice guideline. *Journal of Clinical Endocrinology & Metabolism, 93,* 1105–1120.

Mathur, R., Alexander, C. J., Yano, J., Trivax, B., & Azziz, R. (2008). Use of metformin in polycystic ovary syndrome. *American Journal of Obstetrics and Gynecology, 199,* 596–609.

Moran, L. J., Misso, M. L., Wild, R. A., & Norman, R. J. (2010). Impaired glucose tolerance, type 2 diabetes and metabolic syndrome in polycystic ovary syndrome: A systematic review and meta-analysis. *Human Reproduction Update, 16,* 347–363.

Moran, L. J., Pasquali, R., Teede, H. J., Hoeger, K. M., & Norman, R. J. (2009). Treatment of obesity in polycystic ovary syndrome: A position statement of the Androgen Excess and Polycystic Ovary Syndrome Society. *Fertility and Sterility, 92,* 1966–1982.

Practice Committee of the American Society for Reproductive Medicine (ASRM). (2008). Use of insulin-sensitizing agents in the treatment of polycystic ovary syndrome. *Fertility and Sterility, 90,* S69–S73.

Radosh, L. (2009). Drug treatments for polycystic ovary syndrome. *American Family Physician, 79,* 671–676.

Rosner, W., Auchus, R. J., Azziz, R., Sluss, P. M., & Raff, H. (2007). Utility, limitations, and pitfalls in measuring testosterone: An Endocrine Society position statement. *Journal of Clinical Endocrinology & Metabolism, 92,* 405–413.

Rotterdam ESHRE/ASRM-Sponsored PCOS Consensus Workshop Group. (2004). Revised 2003 consensus on diagnostic criteria and long term health risks related to polycystic ovary syndrome (PCOS). *Human Reproduction, 19*(1), 41–47.

Shapiro, J. (2007). Hair loss in women. *New England Journal of Medicine, 357,* 1620–1630.

Somani, N., Harrison, S., & Bergfeld, W. F. (2008). The clinical evaluation of hirsutism. *Dermatologic Therapy, 21,* 376–391.

Souter, I., Sanchez, L. A., Perez, M., Bartolucci, A. A., & Azziz, R. (2004). The prevalence of androgen excess among patients with minimal unwanted hair growth. *American Journal of Obstetrics and Gynecology, 191,* 1914–1920.

Starr, D. S. (2004, April). The duties of informed consent. *The Clinical Advisor,* 83.

Teede, H., Deeks, A., & Moran, L. (2010). Polycystic ovary syndrome: A complex condition with psychological, reproductive and metabolic manifestations that impacts health across the lifespan. *BMC Medicine, 8,* 41.

Thessaloniki ESHRE/ASRM-Sponsored PCOS Consensus Workshop Group. (2008). Consensus on infertility treatment related to polycystic ovary syndrome. *Fertility and Sterility, 89,* 505–522.

Wild, R. A., Carmina, E., Diamanti-Kandarakis, E., Dokras, A., Escobar-Morreale, H. F., Futterweit, W., et al. (2010). Assessment of cardiovascular risk and prevention of cardiovascular disease in women with the polycystic ovary syndrome: A consensus statement by the Androgen Excess and Polycystic Ovary Syndrome (AE-PCOS) Society. *Journal of Clinical Endocrinology & Metabolism, 95,* 2038–2049.

Wild, R. A., Rizzo, M., Clifton, S., & Carmina, E. (2011). Lipid levels in polycystic ovary syndrome: Systematic review and meta-analysis. *Fertility and Sterility, 95,* 1073–1079.

Wilson, J. F. (2011). In the clinic: The polycystic ovary syndrome. *Annals of Internal Medicine, 154,* ITC2-2-ITC2-15.

27

Benign Gynecologic Conditions

Carol A. Verga

T his chapter addresses a variety of conditions commonly encountered in gynecologic care, including vulvar dermatoses, nabothian cysts, cervical polyps, uterine fibroids, adenomyosis, endometriosis, and ovarian cysts. These conditions, although usually not malignant (with exceptions as noted), are still significant to the women experiencing them. Some of these conditions are associated with physical symptoms that can be severe, and all of them have the potential to cause women distress and anxiety. Therefore, emotional support is an essential component of care. Many of the conditions described in this chapter are chronic and require ongoing, long-term care. Thorough patient education about the clinical course and treatment options is imperative, and the clinician should act in partnership with the woman to develop management plans that meet her individual needs.

Vulvar Dermatoses

The vulva is composed of skin and mucous membrane (see Chapter 5). Most dermatoses that affect either the skin or mucous membranes can appear on the vulva. This section describes the general assessment of vulvar dermatoses and the specific assessment and management of some of the more common benign vulvar dermatoses: primary irritant and allergic dermatitis, lichen sclerosus, lichen planus, squamous cell hyperplasia, and psoriasis. Vulvar cancer is addressed in Chapter 28. A list of vulvar dermatology resources is provided at the end of the chapter for the many conditions that are beyond the scope of this text. Most of these resources contain extensive color photographs; reviewing photographs can improve a clinician's ability to recognize the many lesions that can occur on the vulva.

Vulvar dermatoses cause physical symptoms and can have significant psychological consequences. A woman may have suffered for years with her condition and may present for care feeling frustrated and without hope. It is important for a clinician to convey realistic expectations for treatment and to explain to the woman that more than one therapy may be needed to effect resolution, or at least relief. At the same time, the clinician can express a commitment to helping the woman obtain relief of her symptoms. Women may have cosmetic concerns related to the physical changes caused by their dermatosis. These concerns, particularly in conjunction with physical symptoms, can interfere with sexual functioning and cause distress for the woman and her partner. Asking the woman about the psychological impact of her condition and providing emotional support are crucial components of care. In addition, women with chronic dermatoses may benefit from joining support groups, either locally or online.

Assessment of Vulvar Dermatoses

Many of the benign diseases of the vulva share similar appearances, symptoms, and even therapies. Having the precise diagnosis is essential for accurate client education, monitoring of therapy, and prevention of complications. In addition, malignancy must be ruled out. A systematic approach to assessment is essential for accurate diagnosis.

History The clinician needs to identify when the woman first became aware of the lesion. Ask about associated symptoms including pruritus, pain, burning, bleeding, and vaginal discharge, and determine whether there are aggravating or alleviating factors. Identify treatments that have already been tried, including whether they were successful. Ask if the woman has any history of dermatologic disease as well as any skin changes elsewhere on her body. Obtain a sexual history, paying specific attention to dyspareunia, changes in sexual activity related to the condition, and the presence or absence of symptoms in her partner. Note family history of dermatologic disease or malignancy. Complete gynecologic and general health histories should also be obtained (see Chapter 6).

Physical Examination Carefully examine the external genitalia using a good light source. A speculum examination should be performed because some vulvar conditions have vaginal manifestations. General inspection of the skin can be useful for detecting systemic dermatologic conditions. Any additional examination should be directed by the history and genital examination findings.

Diagnostic Testing Microscopic evaluation of vaginal discharge should be performed to rule out vaginitis. The definitive diagnostic technique for vulvar dermatoses is biopsy, which is relatively simple to perform (**Box 27-1**). Biopsy should be performed liberally when vulvar lesions are present to avoid delayed diagnosis of malignancy (American College of Obstetricians and Gynecologists, 2008b, reaffirmed 2010). Colposcopy may be warranted to more closely examine the vulva and to direct the biopsy. Additional evaluations, such as testing for sexually transmitted infections, may be appropriate depending on the history and physical examination findings (see Chapter 21).

BOX 27-1 *Technique for Vulvar Biopsy*

Begin by identifying the best location for the biopsy. This may be the entire lesion or a portion, depending on the size. Do not be reluctant to take more than one biopsy if needed to sample all the variations of the presenting lesion(s). Consider desensitizing the area by applying ice or a topical anesthetic before injecting the local anesthetic. Seldom is any medication stronger than 1% lidocaine with epinephrine needed, though 0.5% bupivacaine lasts longer after the procedure. Use the smallest dose needed for anesthesia to prevent skin distention and more discomfort. The usual needle size is 27 or 30 gauge, the length should fit the area to be anesthetized, and medication is injected with the bevel up. Only a small amount of medication is usually needed, but the size of the biopsy must be considered in determining how much to use.

Punch biopsy can be done with either a disposable or reusable unit; if the latter is used, be certain it has been sterilized and is still sharp. A sharp instrument assures the least pain, the least bleeding, and the most reliable specimen. Most of the vulva is soft tissue; therefore, be sure to provide support for the tissue as the sharp edge is gently twisted and pushed into the area being biopsied. Other tissue sampling devices include biopsy forceps used for colposcopy. Explain to the woman that the major portion of larger instruments is the handle, as their size can be intimidating.

Specimens of 3 mm or under often do not require suturing for closure. Drysol (20% aluminum chloride) or silver nitrate may be used to stop bleeding. The biopsy will heal readily and care after biopsy is simply good personal hygiene; most biopsies do not require topical or oral antibiotic therapy. When sutures are needed, small dissolvable suture material (e.g., 4–0 or 5–0 chromic) is used and usually only one or two sutures are required. If the woman has a known sensitivity to chromic, or if the sutures will need to be in for more than 5 to 7 days because of the site of biopsy, use inert suture material (e.g., Monopril, Dermalon, etc.). Sutures should be removed in 5 to 14 days depending on their site.

Differential Diagnosis

The differential diagnoses for vulvar lesions are identified in **Box 27-2**.

Contact Dermatitis

Irritant contact dermatitis (ICD) and allergic contact dermatitis (ACD) are often referred to collectively as contact dermatitis, although the two forms have some distinctions. The etiology is nonimmunologic in ICD and immunologic in ACD: ICD results from exposure to an irritant, whereas ACD is a delayed hypersensitivity reaction after sensitization to an allergen (Burrows, Shaw, & Goldstein, 2008). Typically symptoms of ICD appear quickly following exposure to the irritant, while ACD can take 48 to 72 hours to manifest after allergen exposure. ICD is more common and resolves more quickly than ACD (Schlosser, 2010). A detailed history to identify the irritant or allergen is necessary.

Irritant Contact Dermatitis Exposure of the vulva to an irritant can result in burning, pruritus, and pain. Potential irritants include perfumed soaps, feminine hygiene sprays

BOX 27-2 *Differential Diagnoses for Vulvar Lesions*

Acanthosis nigricans
Acrochordon (skin tags)
Allergic dermatitis
Aphthosis
Atrophic vaginitis
Basal cell carcinoma
Behçet's disease
Bullous pemphigoid
Candidiasis
Chancroid
Cicatricial pemphigoid
Condyloma acuminata (genital warts)
Crohn's disease
Desquamative inflammatory vaginitis
Eczema
Epidermal cysts
Erythema multiforme
Folliculitis
Granuloma inguinale
Hemangiomas
Herpes simplex virus
Herpes zoster
Hidradenitis suppurativa
Impetigo
Intertrigo
Lentigo

Lichen planus
Lichen sclerosus
Lichen simplex chronicus
Lupus
Lymphogranuloma venereum
Melanoma
Molloscum contagiosum
Nevi (moles)
Pityriasis versicolor
Paget's disease
Pemphigus vulgaris
Primary irritant dermatitis
Psoriasis
Pyoderma gangrenosum
Scabies
Seborrheic dermatitis
Squamous cell carcinoma
Squamous cell hyperplasia
Steroid-rebound dermatitis
Stevens-Johnson syndrome
Syphilis
Vitiligo
Vulvar intraepithelial neoplasia (VIN)
Vulvar vestibulitis
Vulvodynia

and deodorants, bath bubbles and oils, colored or scented toilet paper, laundry detergents, sanitary napkins, tampons, condoms, spermicides, tight clothing, adult wipes, topical medications, and body fluids. A detailed history of contact with potential irritants is crucial. Physical examination will typically reveal erythema of the involved skin (**Color Plate 28**). Edema, vesicles, and ulcerations are common with acute ICD, and there may be scale and excoriation with subacute or chronic ICD (American College of Obstetricians and Gynecologists, 2008b, reaffirmed 2010; Schlosser, 2010).

Allergic Contact Dermatitis   Known allergens that can cause vulvar dermatitis include medications (e.g., anesthetics, antibiotics, antifungals, and antiseptics, corticosteroids), douches, emollients, fragrances, nail polish, nickel, preservatives, rubber, sanitary napkins, and spermicides (Schlosser, 2010). Allergic dermatitis may also occur with generalized allergy symptoms in women who have a hereditary tendency to allergic reactions (atopic individual). The physical examination findings with acute ACD are similar to those noted with ICD. Women with subacute or chronic ACD may also develop plaques, scaling, and excoriations (**Color Plate 29**) (Schlosser).

Management Identification of the irritant or allergen and avoidance of further contact is essential to treatment. Topical corticosteroids are the mainstay of pharmacologic therapy. Depending on the severity of the dermatitis, a low-potency (e.g., hydrocortisone 2.5%), medium-potency (e.g., triamcinolone 0.1%), or very high-potency (e.g., clobetasol propionate 0.05% or halobetasol 0.05%) corticosteroid can be used; it is initially administered twice daily until lesions have healed (**Table 27-1**). Cool sitz baths and wet dressings with Burow's solution (Domeboro) can be used to reduce discomfort. Ice packs can be helpful for relieving pruritus. If symptoms are severe, systemic corticosteroids and/or oral antihistamines may be warranted (Burrows et al., 2008; Schlosser, 2010).

Lichen Sclerosus

Lichen sclerosus (LS) is a benign, chronic, progressive disease of the skin characterized by inflammation, epithelial thinning, and distinctive dermal changes. It can occur on the trunk, neck, forearms, axillae, and under the breasts, as well as on the vulva. LS is most common in postmenopausal women, but it can occur as early as childhood. Although the exact etiology of LS is unknown, it appears to be an autoimmune disorder (Burrows et al., 2008). An increased risk of vulvar cancer has been noted in women with LS (see Chapter 28).

TABLE 27-1 Topical Corticosteroid Ointments Used for Vulvar Dermatoses

Potency	Medication	Strength
Low	Alclometasone dipropionate (Aclovate)	0.05%
	Desonide (DesOwen)	0.05%
	Hydrocortisone (Hytone)	2.5%
Medium	Betamethasone valerate (Beta-Val, Valisone)	0.1%
	Fluticasone propionate (Cutivate)	0.005%
	Mometasone furoate (Elocon)	0.1%
	Triamcinolone (Aristocort, Kenalog)	0.1%
High	Betamethasone dipropionate (Diprosone, Maxivate)	0.05%
	Desoximetasone (Topicort)	0.05%, 0.25%
	Fluocinonide (Lidex)	0.05%
	Halcinonide (Halog)	0.1%
Very high Superpotent*	Betamethasone dipropionate (Diprolene)	0.05%
	Clobetasol propionate (Temovate)	0.05%
	Diflorasone diacetate (Psorcon)	0.05%
	Halobetasol propionate (Ultravate)	0.05%

*Avoid the use of occlusive dressings with superpotent agents.

Clinical Presentation Vulvar pruritus is the most common presenting symptom of LS—it may be so intense as to interrupt sleep. Anorectal symptoms, including pruritus ani, painful defecation, anal fissures, and rectal bleeding, may also occur. For some women, a dull, nonspecific vulvar discomfort is a prodrome to LS. Dyspareunia is a later symptom occurring from small lacerations or introital stenosis. Phimosis of the labia minora over the clitoris may lead to diminished sexual sensation. Dysuria may occur if there is fusion of the minora over the urethra. Some women may be asymptomatic, leading to a delay of diagnosis of LS until routine examination.

Physical Examination Findings Lichen sclerosus involves both the skin and mucosal surfaces of the vulva and perianal area (**Color Plate 30**). Initially lesions are macular, but later become macular–papular with a flat surface. Most often they eventually coalesce into plaques. A classic figure-eight formation surrounds the vulva and perianal area. Over time, the skin thins and takes on a wrinkled, "cigarette paper" appearance. The normal architecture of both the dermis and the mucosa are lost during this process. Eventually the labia minora atrophy and are subsumed into the labia majora completely or partially by a process called agglutination. Phimosis may occur over the clitoris and possibly the urethra. Introital stenosis is common in advanced disease but, unlike with the complete stenosis of the vagina itself seen in lichen planus, LS causes no reduction in the vaginal caliber (diameter).

Management The goals of LS treatment are relief of symptoms and discomfort, prevention of further architectural distortion, and theoretical reduction in the incidence of malignancy (Funaro, 2004). Treatment is recommended for women who have physical examination findings consistent with LS but are asymptomatic (Murphy, 2010). Prior to initiating therapy for LS, any concomitant vaginitis (particularly vulvovaginal candidiasis) should be treated. High-potency or very high-potency topical corticosteroids are recommended for women with LS, and clobetasol propionate is frequently prescribed. A common regimen is to apply the medication once daily for one month, then every other day for one month, then twice weekly for one month. Once-a-day application is adequate for initial therapy; twice-daily application is unnecessary. There is a lack of consensus on the need for maintenance therapy. Some clinicians recommend ongoing corticosteroid application once or twice weekly, whereas others recommend discontinuation of corticosteroids after a course of therapy with reinitiation if symptoms recur (American College of Obstetricians and Gynecologists, 2008b, reaffirmed 2010; Beecker, 2010; Murphy). Further information about corticosteroid therapy can be found in Table 27-1 and **Box 27-3**.

Women who do not respond to or are unable to use corticosteroid therapy can be treated with topical tacrolimus or pimecrolimus; both agents are immunomodulators (Assman, Becker-Wegerich, Grewe, Megahed, & Ruzicka, 2003; Goldstein, Creasey, Pfau, Phillips, & Burrows, 2011; Kunstfeld, Kirnbauer, Stingl, & Karlhofer, 2003). Persistent vulvar pain despite appropriate therapy and improvement in physical findings may indicate that vulval dysesthesia—a secondary vulval pain syndrome—is present. Treatment includes reassur-

BOX 27-3 *Guidelines for Topical Corticosteroid Therapy*

- Rule out or treat vulvovaginal infections, especially candidiasis, prior to initiating corticosteroid therapy, as steroids can worsen candidal infection.
- Corticosteroid use during pregnancy should be avoided or limited.
- Ointments should be used because creams contain alcohol, which is irritating to mucosal tissue.
- Potent or superpotent steroid therapy is often required for vulvar conditions because the modified mucous membranes of the vulva can be steroid resistant. Caution should be used when corticosteroids are applied to surrounding areas that are not steroid resistant (e.g., hair-bearing areas, perianal skin, and medial thighs) because atrophy can occur more easily in those areas.
- The taper protocol should be titrated to the amount of disease present and the extent of symptoms at the onset of therapy.
- A sample tapering protocol calls for twice-daily application of medication, then once-daily use, then use every other day, followed by twice-weekly use. The length of time for each frequency varies with the condition being treated.
- The woman should be reevaluated 8 to 12 weeks after beginning therapy to assess her response to the medication and to determine whether vulvar atrophy is developing.
- Once the desired response is achieved, the woman should be switched to a lower-potency corticosteroid for maintenance, if possible. Some women will require high-potency steroids for maintenance.
- Maintenance dosing is usually one to three times weekly.
- It is important to limit the quantity of medication prescribed and to have follow-up visits prior to providing refills.
- Ongoing assessment for vulvar atrophy should occur at least annually.
- Referral should be considered when symptoms are severe or unresponsive to therapy, or if management involves medications with which the clinician is unfamiliar.

ance and possibly pharmacologic therapy with amitriptyline or gabapentin. Increased use of topical corticosteroids is not indicated (Murphy, 2010).

Surgery is used only as treatment for release of phimosis, introital stenosis, or for the excision of malignancy. These procedures should not be performed until the disease is stable and the inflammation is well controlled by the use of corticosteroids.

All women being treated for LS should be examined at least yearly to be sure their symptoms are not returning, to evaluate the effect of any ongoing corticosteroid use, and to monitor for the appearance of vulvar dysplasia.

Lichen Planus

Lichen planus (LP) is an inflammatory condition of the scalp, skin, nails, and mucous membranes. Lesions may be isolated to the vulva, or they may be accompanied by other skin manifestations of LP. Women who present with LP are usually perimenopausal or postmenopausal (McPherson & Cooper, 2010).

Clinical Presentation Presenting symptoms of LP include vaginal discharge, vulvar pruritus (which may be intense), vulvar pain and burning, vaginal soreness, dyspareunia, and postcoital bleeding (Burrows et al., 2008). Papulosquamous LP may be asymptomatic. The onset of LP can be abrupt or gradual, and symptoms may return intermittently for years.

Physical Examination Findings Three major types of vulvar LP are classical/papulosquamous, hypertrophic, and erosive (**Color Plate 31**). Papulosquamous LP affects the vulva and presents as small, intensely pruritic papules with a violaceous hue that arise on keratinized and perianal skin. Milky striae may be visible on the inner aspects of the labia. Hypertrophic LP is associated with hyperkeratotic, rough lesions of the perineum and the perianal area (American College of Obstetricians and Gynecologists, 2008b, reaffirmed 2010; Burrows et al., 2008; McPherson & Cooper, 2010).

Erosive LP affects the vulva and vagina and is associated with brightly erythematous erosions with white striae or borders (Wickham's striae). The lesions of erosive LP are usually glassy or shiny in appearance. They can occur on the labia minora and vestibule as isolated lesions on otherwise normal-appearing tissue, or they can cause marked architectural distortion including loss of the labia minora. As many as 70% of women with erosive LP will have vaginal involvement. This high rate contrasts with the rate of vaginal involvement in LS, which is very rare (Burrows et al., 2008). The vaginal epithelium of women with LP bleeds easily with vaginal penetration by a speculum or during intercourse. The tissue appears denuded, and a serosanguineous vaginal discharge may occur. In severe cases, adhesions may develop, leading to stenosis or even obliteration of the vagina (McPherson & Cooper, 2010).

Vulvovaginal-gingival syndrome is a variant of erosive LP that involves all three of these areas. This form of LP responds poorly to treatment and warrants referral to a clinician experienced in its management. Ask women with LP about any oral symptoms and conduct an oral examination (McPherson & Cooper, 2010; Panagiotopoulou, Wong, & Winter-Roach, 2010).

Management Papulosquamous LP usually resolves spontaneously, and treatment is needed only if the woman is symptomatic. Treatment consists of a medium-potency topical corticosteroid and emollients. Betamethasone valerate 0.1% can be used twice daily for 4 to 6 weeks (McPherson & Cooper, 2010).

Hypertrophic LP is treated with a superpotent topical corticosteroid (e.g., clobetasol propionate 0.05% twice a day for 3 months). Vulvar biopsy should be performed for any hypertrophic lesions that do not respond well to treatment, as the appearance of LP and vulvar cancers is similar. Intralesional corticosteroid injection (e.g., 0.5 to 1.0 mL of triamcinolone acetonide 10 mg/mL repeated in 6 to 8 weeks if needed) can also be used as therapy for this variant (McPherson & Cooper, 2010).

Erosive LP is chronic, recurring, and challenging to treat. Super potent topical corticosteroid therapy (e.g., clobetasol propionate 0.05% once daily for 3 months) is the first-line therapy for vulvar disease. The frequency of application and potency of the corticosteroid can be decreased as lesions improve. Typically women with well-controlled disease will require once- or twice-weekly application of corticosteroids as maintenance therapy (McPherson & Cooper, 2010). Tacrolimus or pimecrolimus may be used for women who do not respond to corticosteroid therapy (Helgesen, Gjersvik, Jebsen, Kirschner, & Tanbo, 2010; Lonsdale-Eccles & Velangi, 2005); stinging or burning is more commonly reported with tacrolimus. Intralesional corticosteroid injection is another option. Systemic therapy with oral predniso-lone, antibiotics, or immunosuppressives (e.g., azathioprine, cyclosporine) may be used when topical treatments prove ineffective, but evidence for these treatments is limited and results with them have been inconsistent (Cooper & Wojnarowska, 2006). Vaginal disease is treated with intravaginal hydrocortisone (foam or suppositories) or prednisolone (foam) (Burrows et al., 2008; McPherson & Cooper). Systemic and intravaginal therapies are best prescribed by clinicians experienced in their use. Beta blockers and nonsteroidal anti-inflammatory drugs (NSAIDs) have been associated with LP (Clayton et al., 2010). Consider changing drug therapy in women taking these medications.

Therapy with progressively sized vaginal dilators may be needed if there is vaginal steno-sis or closure. The dilator can be coated with a steroid ointment and is retained in the vagina overnight by use of snug-fitting underwear. Begin with the smallest dilator that the woman can tolerate comfortably and gradually increase the size. The largest dilator may need to be used weekly for maintenance of vaginal patency. If labial or vaginal adhesions are severe, surgical excision may be needed (American College of Obstetricians and Gynecologists, 2008b, reaffirmed 2010).

Lichen Simplex Chronicus

Lichen simplex chronicus (LSC; formerly called squamous hyperplasia, hyperplastic dys-trophy, and leukoplakia) is a localized variant of atopic dermatitis (Stewart, 2010). LSC can arise spontaneously, typically in patients with a history of allergies or asthma, or result from any vulvar disorder that causes pruritus. As scratching and itching persist, epidermal thick-ening and hyperproliferation of the cells (lichenification) occur. As the tissue continues to thicken and blood flow is further compromised, itching becomes almost intractable and the itch–scratch–itch cycle progresses (Burrows et al., 2008; Stewart).

Clinical Presentation Many women present with a history of what they think are chronic yeast infections and describe recurrent pruritus that is relieved by topical therapies. However, the pruritus returns within days to weeks after treatment. This cycle may have been present for years. Scratching or rubbing the area is pleasurable as opposed to itching that does not resolve when scratched.

Physical Examination Findings Early in the disease process, LSC is characterized by local-ized edema with erythema and mild exaggeration of the skin architecture. Fissures and exco-riation may also be present. As the disease progresses, epidermal thickening and lichenified plaques become visible (**Color Plate 32**). Hyperpigmentation or unusual whiteness of the tissue (from scale) may also be evident. Pubic hair may be broken or lessened from chronic scratching (Stewart, 2010).

Management A superpotent topical corticosteroid ointment (e.g., clobetasol propionate 0.05%) is used for initial treatment of LSC (Table 27-1 and Box 27-3). Patients should be screened for secondary infections and treated with oral therapy to avoid further irritation to the vulva. Corticosteroids are not effective immediately, however; 2% lidocaine jelly can be used to relieve itching in the interim before the steroids take effect (Stewart, 2010). Tacrolimus or pimecrolimus can be used as second-line treatment if corticosteroid therapy proves ineffective (Goldstein, Thaci, & Luger, 2009). Itching and scratching are often worse at night, and medications that provide sedation can be helpful. The tricyclic antidepressants amitriptyline and doxepin (10 to 100 mg 2 hours before bedtime) provide better and longer sedation than antihistamines (e.g., hydroxyzine, diphenhydramine) and can improve anxiety and depression—both conditions that are common in women with LSC. Wearing gloves at night is also recommended (Stewart).

Psoriasis

Psoriasis is a chronic, immune-mediated, genetic disease that manifests in the skin and joints. Its peak incidence is observed in adolescence through the 20s, but it can develop at any age. The most common form of psoriasis is characterized by papules or plaques that are covered with silvery-white scales, and are most frequently found on the knees, elbows, and scalp. Vulvar psoriasis (**Color Plate 33**) can occur as an isolated manifestation of the disease or can coexist with psoriasis at other sites on the body. The major clinical variation noted in the vulvar form of psoriasis is that erythema is more common and scaling is finer, with thick plaques seldom seen in this variant. Topical corticosteroids are the mainstay of therapy for psoriasis (Table 27-1 and Box 27-3). Referral is indicated if vulvar psoriasis is unresponsive to corticosteroids.

Nabothian Cysts

Nabothian cysts of the cervix are a common finding. The exact incidence of such cysts is unknown because they are rarely symptomatic. They are usually an incidental finding on visual examination of the cervix, but occasionally a woman presents having felt one of the larger cysts during self-examination.

Nabothian cysts occur as a result of metaplasia. The endocervical columnar cells are always in the process of transformation to the pink, smooth, squamous cells that compose the ectocervix at the active transformation zone of the cervix. As the squamous tissue evolves toward the canal, occasionally a gland orifice becomes blocked. In this scenario, the glandular cells remain active and continue to secrete mucus while becoming trapped under the more dense squamous tissue. The secretions form a mucinous retention cyst (Casey, Long, & Marnach, 2011).

Nabothian cysts are smooth and often shiny (**Color Plate 34**). Usually the mucus is clear, but it can be cloudy and give a more opaque appearance to the cyst. Blood vessels parallel to the surface can frequently be seen in the overlying tissue. These vessels are long, usually curve over the surface of the cyst, and do not bleed on contact.

Assessment

Diagnosis of a nabothian cyst is made by physical examination. No laboratory testing is needed unless the cyst seems atypical. If the blood vessels seem short, comma-like, or corkscrew shaped, and if they bleed on contact, colposcopy should be performed because these findings may represent malignant or premalignant cervical changes.

Differential Diagnosis

Carcinoma of the cervix can appear somewhat similar to a nabothian cyst, but would have atypical findings, as noted in the discussion of assessment.

Management

A nabothian cyst will frequently resolve on its own with further evolution of the transformation zone; in such a case, no treatment is required. The evolution of the transformation zone may take as long as 12 weeks. Nabothian cysts may rupture or extrude their contents during labor or with deep penetration at intercourse. The cyst is rarely so large that obtaining a thorough Pap test is difficult. If the cyst is so large that it precludes access to the cervix, the clinician may puncture the cyst with a 21-gauge needle and extrude the mucinous material with pressure from a cotton-tipped swab. The cyst may then resolve or recur. Electrocautery ablation or excision can also be used to treat nabothian cysts but is rarely necessary (Casey et al., 2011). Referral is indicated if the clinician is unsure of the benign nature of the observed cyst or if the cyst seems atypical or bleeds on contact.

Cervical Polyps

Cervical polyps occur in 2% to 5% of women, but are very rarely (fewer than 2% of cases) malignant. The etiology of cervical polyps is unknown. Hormones, chronic inflammation, and cervical blood congestion have been proposed as playing a role in their development (Stamatellos, Stamatopoulos, & Bontis, 2007). Mucosal polyps are a result of benign hyperplasia of glandular tissue arising from the mucosa itself. Such polyps may arise anywhere on the body that has glandular mucosa, including the cervix. They often form on a pedicle or stalk. Cervical polyps are often asymptomatic and, therefore, are incidentally diagnosed during a speculum examination done for another purpose. If symptoms occur, they are most likely to consist of postcoital or intermenstrual spotting or bleeding.

Assessment

On speculum examination, cervical polyps appear moist, red, and glandular (**Color Plate 35**). They range in size from barely visible to greater than 5 cm, and arise from a stalk in the cervical canal. During the assessment, the clinician should note the size of the polyp, along with its location on the cervix, color, and friability, and determine whether the base arises from within the cervical canal. A Pap test should also be performed to rule out dysplasia or malignancy. Any polyp with an atypical appearance should be biopsied. Atypical findings would include necrosis, contact bleeding, or change in color; such findings could indicate dysplasia or malignancy. Histologic testing is the final confirmation of the benign or malignant nature of a cervical polyp.

Differential Diagnosis

Endometrial polyps appear very similar to those of cervical origin. If the base is not clearly seen or is too broad to allow visualization, biopsy should not be performed. Polyps that appear cervical may, in fact, be endometrial, and this origin could lead to significant bleeding if biopsy were performed in the office setting (Spiewankiewicz, Stelmachow, Sawicki, Cendrowski, & Kuzlik, 2003). Ultrasound to rule out endometrial origin should be performed if the base of the polyp cannot be clearly identified.

Management

Historically, all cervical polyps were removed whether they were symptomatic or not. Today, fewer clinicians remove benign, asymptomatic polyps because of the cost and potential discomfort to the patient for a harmless finding. When a polyp is not removed, the woman should be advised to report irregular bleeding or bleeding after intercourse.

Polyps that are bothersome or atypical should be removed. The technique for removal is to first clearly visualize the base of the stalk, then to cross-clamp the stalk with a curved instrument, such as a Kelly clamp or sponge-holding forceps. Moderately firm clamping pressure for one to three minutes should assure hemostasis but not tear the polyp. Using the same clamp, twist the polyp in the canal with gentle traction until the stalk is separated. The specimen is placed in a formalin laboratory jar and sent for histology. Bleeding from the base of the lesion can be treated using a silver nitrate stick, or the area can be covered with Monsel's paste if there is too much bleeding to be managed with silver nitrate alone. Atypical or broad-based polyps may need to be removed by operative hysteroscopy, which facilitates assessment and treatment of any concurrent intrauterine pathology (Spiewankiewicz et al., 2003; Stamatellos et al., 2007).

Special Considerations

Women who are pregnant have increased blood flow to the cervix, a factor that can cause significant bleeding with polyp biopsy or removal. Biopsy or removal of a cervical polyp should be performed during pregnancy only for indications that are too urgent to be postponed until after the woman gives birth, and referral for biopsies in pregnancy should be considered.

Uterine Fibroids

Uterine fibroids, also known as myomas or leiomyomatas, are benign growths that arise from the smooth muscle of the uterus. They are classified based on the uterine layer most involved in their location (see Chapter 5 for uterine anatomy); these growths can be located on the external surface of the uterus (subserosal), be found completely within the myometrium (intramural or myometrial), or have contact with the endometrial layer (submucosal) (**Color Plate 36A** and **B**). Fibroids may be pedunculated off the serosal surface and sometimes prolapse into the cervical canal. They range in size from microscopic to large tumors weighing several pounds. Multiple fibroids are common, but they also occur singularly.

Incidence

The exact incidence of fibroids is unknown because they are often asymptomatic. These growths may be clinically apparent in 25% to 40% of women and have been found in as many as 77% of surgical specimens (Cramer & Patel, 1990; Okolo, 2008). The incidence of fibroids increases with age. Fibroids are two to three times more prevalent in black women, who are younger at diagnosis and have larger, more numerous, more rapidly growing fibroids with worse symptoms compared to white women (Jacoby, Fujimoto, Giudice, Kuppermann, & Washington, 2010).

Etiology and Pathophysiology

Uterine fibroids develop when a normal myocyte becomes abnormal and grows into a tumor. This growth occurs by clonal expansion from a single cell (Okolo, 2008). Fibroids appear to have a genetic basis, and local growth factors contribute to their development (Practice Committee of the American Society for Reproductive Medicine [ASRM] in collaboration with Society of Reproductive Surgeons, 2008). Fewer than 1% of women with fibroids have uterine sarcoma (Parker, Fu, & Berek, 1994).

Presentation

The majority of fibroids do not cause symptoms; thus they are commonly identified as an incidental finding on examination, ultrasound, or surgery. Increased uterine bleeding at menses is the most frequent symptom of fibroids. Menses are typically heavier and longer, and intermenstrual or postcoital bleeding may occur as well. Other common symptoms include pelvic pressure or pain and dyspareunia (American College of Obstetricians and Gynecologists, 2008a, reaffirmed 2010; Gupta, Jose, & Manyonda, 2008). Pain related to a uterine fibroid may be chronic and mild in nature or severe and acute as occurs in the event of torsion or necrosis. Other symptoms may include increased abdominal girth, urinary symptoms, and rectal pain or pressure. Peritoneal signs will be present if there is bleeding into the abdominal cavity, necrosis, or infection.

Assessment

History When a woman presents with abnormal uterine bleeding, pelvic pain or pressure, or other symptoms that may be related to uterine fibroids, the clinician should obtain a detailed menstrual history. If alterations in the menstrual pattern have occurred, identify when these differences were first noted and what the specific changes have been. If the patient has intermenstrual bleeding, ask the woman if it is related to intercourse. If she is experiencing pain or pressure, ask about the onset, location, frequency, quality, intensity, and aggravating and alleviating factors. Obtain a detailed obstetric history, paying particular attention to complications of pregnancy and infertility. Ask if any female relatives have had fibroids, as there is a familial predisposition to this condition. Complete general health and gynecologic histories should also be obtained (see Chapter 6).

Physical Examination Perform abdominal and pelvic examinations. The uterus may be palpable abdominally if the fibroid is very large. Guarding or rebound tenderness can indicate irritation of the peritoneum. Whether or not fibroids are palpable depends on their location and size. The bimanual examination can be normal, for example, even though fibroids are present. Palpable subserosal fibroids most often feel like smooth cobbles on the uterine serosal surface. Pedunculated subserosal fibroids may be palpated as a firm mass in the adnexa, posterior or anterior to the uterus, or in the uterine ligaments. Intramural and submucosal fibroids may not be palpable but can be noted as generalized enlargement or asymmetry of the uterus on bimanual examination. Fibroids are typically nontender.

Diagnostic Testing Definitive diagnosis of fibroids is usually made by ultrasound. There are no specific laboratory tests for uterine fibroids. If a woman is experiencing frequent and heavy bleeding, a hematocrit or hemoglobin should be obtained to evaluate the extent of blood loss.

Differential Diagnosis

Numerous causes of abnormal uterine bleeding exist, and the most important to rule out is endometrial cancer (see Chapters 25 and 28). Symptoms of endometriosis and adenomyosis can be similar to those caused by uterine fibroids. Pelvic pressure symptoms can be caused by constipation, irritable bowel syndrome, and other gastrointestinal disorders; urinary tract disorders; ovarian masses; neoplasia of the abdomen or pelvis; and ascites.

Management

Asymptomatic uterine fibroids are managed expectantly. Treatment options for symptomatic fibroids include medical therapy, surgery, and uterine artery embolization. The timing and type of treatment depends on the number, size, and location of fibroids; the type and severity of symptoms; the woman's age and proximity to menopause; future childbearing plans; and preference regarding uterine preservation (Duhan & Sirohiwal, 2010). Treatment today is aimed more at sparing the uterus compared to the therapy undertaken in the past.

Medical Management Gonadotropin-releasing hormone (GnRH) agonists (**Table 27-2**) are used to reduce the size of the uterine fibroid prior to surgery or attempts at pregnancy. GnRH treatment not only reduces fibroid volume, but also increases the woman's blood volume, thereby lowering the risks associated with surgery by reducing fibroid size and decreasing surgical blood loss (Lethaby, Vollenhoven, & Sowter, 2002). Reduction of fibroid size by 35% to 65% occurs within 3 months of initiating therapy (American College of Obstetricians

TABLE 27-2 Gonadatropin-Releasing Hormone Agonists

Product Names	Approved Indication(s)	Route of Administration	Dosage
Leuprolide (Lupron)	Endometriosis and uterine fibroids	Intramuscular injection	3.75 mg monthly or 11.25 mg every 3 months
Nafarelin (Synarel)	Endometriosis	Nasal spray, 200 mcg per spray	400–800 mcg per day • 400 mcg: One spray in one nostril in the morning and one spray in the other nostril in the evening • 800 mcg: one spray in each nostril twice a day
Goserelin (Zoladex)	Endometriosis	Subcutaneous injection in the upper abdomen	3.6 mg monthly

Note: These medications are contraindicated in pregnancy and must be used in conjunction with contraception. See the specific prescribing reference for full information on doses, side effects, contraindications, and cautions.

and Gynecologists, 2008a, reaffirmed 2010). Vasomotor symptoms and decrease in bone density are the major concerns with the use of GnRH agonists. These side effects can be ameliorated by "add-back therapy" or giving estrogen and/or a progestogen in addition to the GnRH agonist. The disadvantage of GnRH agonists is that the effects are usually reversed within months of discontinuation, so surgery or pregnancy attempts must ensue shortly after therapy to maximize the benefits.

The levonorgestrel intrauterine system (LNG-IUS, Mirena) is a treatment option for women whose fibroids are relatively small (uterine size smaller than 12 cm is typically recommended) and do not distort the uterine cavity significantly. The LNG-IUS improves menorrhagia associated with fibroids. Reduced uterine volume or fibroid size with the LNG-IUS has not been reported consistently across studies (Rodriguez, Warden, & Darney, 2010). Further information about the LNG-IUS can be found in Chapter 12.

The antiprogesterone agent mifepristone, also known as a progesterone modulator, decreases fibroid volume at a rate comparable to that achieved with GnRH agonists. Amenorrhea is common when mifepristone is administered, and endometrial hyperplasia without atypia can occur. Use of this agent is limited by the fact that the dosages used for fibroid treatment are not currently available in the United States, so the services of a compounding pharmacy are needed (American College of Obstetricians and Gynecologists, 2008a, reaffirmed 2010; Steinauer, Pritts, Jackson, & Jacoby, 2004).

Other medical therapies used in the management of fibroids include progestogens, combined estrogen and progestin contraceptives, and NSAIDs. These therapies appear to provide symptom relief rather than actually altering the fibroids.

Surgical Management Surgical options for the treatment of fibroids include myomectomy and hysterectomy.

Myomectomy preserves the uterus and can be performed laparoscopically, abdominally, or hysteroscopically depending on fibroid quantity, size, and location. This procedure can also be performed in conjunction with a cesarean birth. Myomectomy will not prevent growth of new lesions, and women may require a second procedure if fibroids recur.

Hysterectomy is the definitive therapy for symptomatic fibroids; indeed, fibroid removal is the most frequent indication for hysterectomy. Laparoscopically assisted vaginal hysterectomy, which reduces postoperative recovery time, is possible for many women with fibroids. Hysterectomy is the final resort when other therapies have failed. Treatment with GnRH agonists prior to myomectomy or hysterectomy can decrease blood loss, operating time, and postoperative pain (American College of Obstetricians and Gynecologists, 2008a, reaffirmed 2010; Parker, 2007).

Uterine Artery Embolization Uterine artery embolization (UAE) is performed by an interventional radiologist and involves injecting polyvinyl alcohol particles into the uterine arteries. The resulting embolization causes fibroid devascularization and infarction. UAE is used for women who do not desire future childbearing as loss of fertility may occur; moreover, there are only limited data about pregnancy outcomes after this procedure (American College of Obstetricians and Gynecologists, 2008a, reaffirmed 2010; Bradley, 2009).

When to Refer Acute torsion of a uterine fibroid is a surgical emergency requiring immediate referral. Most uterine fibroids present as a chronic condition, but acute hemorrhage can occur and is usually unresponsive to medical therapy. Collaborative management is often warranted in determining a plan for medical therapy, and referral is indicated when surgical options are being considered.

Emerging Evidence That May Change Management

Medical therapy with other progesterone modulators (Nieman et al., 2011) and aromatase inhibitors is being investigated (Parsanezhad et al., 2010; Varelas, Papanicolaou, Vavatsi-Christaki, Makedos, & Vlassis, 2007).

Special Considerations

Pregnant Women Based on ultrasound measurements, most fibroids appear to remain stable in size during pregnancy, and growth during this period is rare (Neiger, Sonek, Croom, & Ventolini, 2006). Potential complications of fibroids during pregnancy include failed implantation, spontaneous abortion, preterm labor, placental abruption, malpresentation, cesarean birth, peripartum hysterectomy, and postpartum hemorrhage (Klatsky, Tran, Caughey, & Fujimoto, 2008). Rapid fibroid growth during pregnancy can lead to infarction with bleeding into the fibroid itself rather than vaginally (red infarction or red fibroids), necrosis, and hemorrhage. In the postpartum period, rapid estrogen loss and vasculature reduction can lead to fibroid degeneration with attendant bleeding and pain.

Older Women The spontaneous decrease in hormone production at menopause often leads to a reduction in uterine fibroid size. Exogenous hormone therapy (HT; see Chapter 13) after menopause can cause modest fibroid growth and abnormal bleeding, but withholding hormone therapy is not warranted on this basis (American College of Obstetricians and Gynecologists, 2008a, reaffirmed 2010). Uterine sarcoma should be considered in postmenopausal women who present with an enlarging pelvic mass or vaginal bleeding.

Influences of Culture Abnormal bleeding can cause significant sexual difficulties for women from cultures in which sex during bleeding is taboo. The lack of proven alternative therapies for treatment of uterine fibroids and the potential need for surgery may cause cultural difficulty for those who prefer to avoid allopathic medicine. The effects of surgeries that cause loss of reproductive capability in women from cultures where fertility is equated with value should be considered when developing the treatment plan, and medical therapies may be more appropriate. Aspects of these cultural influences also apply to the conditions discussed in the remainder of this chapter: adenomyosis, endometriosis, and ovarian cysts.

Adenomyosis

Adenomyosis is the presence of endometrial tissue in the myometrium. It can be divided into two types of lesions: diffuse and local. The diffuse lesions are distributed within the myometrium. The local form involves nodular adenomyosis lesions within the myometrium that are called adenomyomas (Meredith, Sanchez-Ramos, & Kaunitz, 2009) (**Color Plate 37**).

Incidence

The estimated incidence of adenomyosis varies because the final diagnosis can be made only from histologic examination. Reported prevalence ranges from 5% to 70%, with a mean frequency of 20% to 30% at hysterectomy (Garcia & Isaacson, 2011). Adenomyosis is frequently underdiagnosed, likely because it has similar symptoms to other pelvic pain conditions and is somewhat more difficult to identify on ultrasound (Basak & Saha, 2009). Adenomyosis occurs more frequently in multiparous women (Garcia & Isaacson).

Etiology and Pathophysiology

The exact etiology of adenomyosis is unknown. The prevailing theory is that the endometrium invaginates the myometrium. The mechanism that causes the endometrium to grow into the myometrium has not been determined (Garcia & Isaacson, 2011).

Clinical Presentation

The most commonly noted symptoms of adenomyosis are menorrhagia and dysmenorrhea. Women may also report dyspareunia and pelvic pain. As with uterine fibroids, many women who have adenomyosis are asymptomatic or experience only mild changes that are usually attributed to aging or perimenopause. Therefore, to make a timely diagnosis and institute management, it is important to maintain a high index of suspicion for adenomyosis.

Assessment

History Obtain a detailed menstrual history and information about pain, including onset, location, frequency, quality, intensity, and aggravating and alleviating factors. If alterations in the menstrual pattern have occurred, identify when they began and what the specific changes have been. Ask the patient if she has experienced dyspareunia and if so, note the onset and location (e.g., at the introitus, deep in the pelvis). Inquire about previous evaluation or treatment for the symptoms she is experiencing. Complete general health and gynecologic histories should also be obtained (see Chapter 6).

Physical Examination Inspect and palpate the abdomen, then perform a complete pelvic examination. Bimanual examination with adenomyosis typically reveals a diffusely larger-than-average uterus that is somewhat boggy and tender to palpation. If the adenomyosis is of the nodular type, the uterus may be asymmetrical. Unlike with fibroids, distinct, firm, raised lesions are not palpable.

Diagnostic Testing Laboratory testing cannot be used to diagnose adenomyosis, but measurement of hemoglobin or hematocrit should be performed to assess the severity of any irregular bleeding. Assessment for adenomyosis is generally performed as part of the process of ruling out the differential diagnoses, and additional testing may be warranted if another condition is suspected and has not been excluded. In particular, endometrial biopsy should be strongly considered in the evaluation of women 35 years and older who present with menorrhagia.

Transvaginal ultrasound, the most commonly used diagnostic tool, has an estimated sensitivity of 83% and specificity of 85% (Meredith et al., 2009). Accuracy of ultrasound decreases when other uterine abnormalities, such as fibroids, are present. MRI can be a useful adjunct to ultrasound in women with more than one uterine abnormality (Garcia & Isaacson, 2011).

Differential Diagnosis

Uterine fibroids, endometrial hyperplasia and malignancy (see Chapter 28), abnormal uterine bleeding (see Chapter 25), and other causes of chronic pelvic pain (see Chapter 29) should be considered in the differential diagnosis. It is important to differentiate adenomyosis from uterine fibroids because the treatments for fibroids can make the symptoms of adenomyosis worse, or at least delay their proper management. The presence of pain on examination helps distinguish fibroids and adenomyosis. Fibroids are generally painful only at times of rapid growth or if degenerating, whereas tenderness to uterine palpation is usually present with adenomyosis. In addition, women with adenomyosis are more likely to report pelvic pain, dyspareunia, and dysmenorrhea than women with fibroids (Taran, Weaver, Coddington, & Stewart, 2010).

Management

Medical Management The LNG-IUS (see Chapter 12) improves dysmenorrhea and menorrhagia in women with adenomyosis and is associated with high patient satisfaction (Sheng, Zhang, Zhang, & Lu, 2009). It is likely to be the most effective medical therapy option for this condition. Combined estrogen and progestin contraceptives (i.e., pill, ring, and patch) may also be useful in adenomyosis management. Consider extended or continuous regimens for menstrual suppression (see Chapter 12). NSAIDs can be used for dysmenorrhea.

Surgical Management Hysterectomy provides definitive diagnosis and treatment for adenomyosis. Endometrial ablation or resection is most likely to be effective if adenomyosis is superficial. Other surgical therapies that have been used include myometrium or adeno-myoma excision and myometrial reduction (Garcia & Isaacson, 2011).

Uterine Artery Embolization Based on the success of UAE in treating fibroids, this proce-dure has also been used in women with adenomyosis. The embolization is thought to cause thrombosis and platelet aggregation in the adenomyosis lesions. While a sufficient body of evidence has not yet been published to recommend UAE as a first-line treatment for adeno-myosis, it is a potential option for women who wish to avoid surgery (Popovic, Puchner, Berzaczy, Lammer, & Bucek, 2011).

Emerging Evidence That May Change Management

Medical therapy with valproic acid is under investigation (Liu, Yuan, & Guo, 2010).

Endometriosis

Endometriosis is the presence of endometrial glands and stroma outside of the uterus (**Color Plate 38**). The most common sites for endometrial implants are—in decreasing order of frequency—the ovaries, anterior and posterior cul-de-sac, posterior broad ligaments, ute-rosacral ligaments, fallopian tubes, sigmoid colon, appendix, and round ligaments (Jenkins, Olive, & Haney, 1986). Endometrial implants have also been found in the vagina, vulva, cervix, perineum, inguinal canal, bladder, gastrointestinal tract locations other than those noted previously, peritoneum, and umbilicus (Douglas & Rotimi, 2004; Honoré, 1999). The appearance and size of implants vary widely. Endometriomas are cystlike structures that contain endometrial tissue and are often found on the ovaries (see the section on ovarian masses later in this chapter for further information).

Incidence

The true prevalence of endometriosis is unknown. Prevalence estimates for endometriosis are 71% to 87% in women with chronic pelvic pain, 9% to 50% in women with infertility, 50% in adolescents with chronic pelvic pain or dysmenorrhea, and 3% to 10% in the general popu-lation of reproductive-aged women (American College of Obstetricians and Gynecologists, 2010; Fritz & Speroff, 2011). The condition is 6 to 7 times more prevalent among women who have a first-degree relative with endometriosis as compared to the general population. Early menarche and short menstrual cycles have also been associated with increased risk of endometriosis. Endometriosis is rare in premenarcheal girls and postmenopausal women (Fritz & Speroff).

Etiology and Pathophysiology

Several theories have been proposed to explain the pathogenesis of endometriosis, but no single theory explains all cases of the condition. The retrograde menstruation theory sug-gests that reverse flow of menses out of the fallopian tubes allows endometrial cells to enter the pelvis and become implanted on the pelvic organs or peritoneal surface. The coelomic metaplasia theory proposes that endometriosis develops from spontaneous metaplasia of cells derived from the coelomic epithelium. The induction theory, which is related to the coelomic metaplasia theory, indicates that endogenous biochemical or immunologic factors stimulate cells to differentiate into endometrial tissue. The theory that endometrial cells can be directly implanted during surgery or episiotomy repair best explains the presence of endo-metriosis in surgical scars and the perineum. Endometriosis outside the pelvis is explained by the theory that cells are carried to distant sites in the lymphatic system or blood vessels. The most widely accepted theory for the origin of endometriosis is retrograde menstrua-tion, which occurs in 75% to 90% of women. Nevertheless, other factors must be involved in the development of endometriosis because the actual prevalence of endometriosis is much lower than the prevalence of retrograde menstruation. Potential contributing factors include immunologic and hormonal abnormalities, heredity, and environmental toxins (Fritz & Speroff, 2011; Seli, Berkkanoglu, & Arici, 2003).

Clinical Presentation

Endometriosis is often asymptomatic, but it can also be a severe and debilitating condition. The most common symptoms of endometriosis involve pelvic pain—specifically, secondary dysmenorrhea with symptoms frequently occurring before menses begins, deep dyspareunia that becomes worse during menses, and sacral backache during menses. Other symptoms include diarrhea, constipation, dyschezia, dysuria, hematuria, and infertility (American College of Obstetricians and Gynecologists, 2010). Unfortunately, these same symptoms occur with many other conditions, which can lead to a delay in the diagnosis of endometriosis (Husby, Haugen, & Moen, 2003). The extent of disease and severity of pain are not necessarily cor-related. Women with mild disease can have significant pain, whereas women with advanced disease can have minimal or no pain. However, there does appear to be a correlation between the severity of disease and the incidence of decreased fertility (Fritz & Speroff, 2011).

Assessment

History When endometriosis is suspected, the clinician should obtain a detailed history of any pelvic pain, including information on its onset, location, frequency, quality, intensity, and aggravating and alleviating factors. If dyspareunia is present, identify the location. Ask about menstrual cycle patterns, symptoms with menses (e.g., dysmenorrhea, nausea and vomiting, and diarrhea), and infertility. Note specifically if there have been any time periods when the woman was having intercourse without using contraception and did not become pregnant to assess for undiagnosed infertility. Document any family history of endometriosis. Complete general health and gynecologic histories should also be obtained (see Chapter 6).

Physical Examination Perform abdominal and pelvic examinations, paying particular atten-tion to the bimanual examination. Findings on physical examination may be limited, if present at all. The most common finding is pain during palpation of the posterior fornix.

Tenderness or induration of the uterosacral ligaments, palpation of nodules in the cul-de-sac or on the rectovaginal septum, tenderness with uterine motion, and a tender enlarged adnexal mass may also be identified during palpation. If the disease is extensive, the uterus may be fixed, and is most often in a retroflexed position.

Diagnostic Testing There are no specific laboratory tests for endometriosis. Transvaginal ultrasound can identify only endometriomas and, in some cases, deeply infiltrating endometriosis in the bladder, uterosacral ligaments, rectum, or rectovaginal septum. MRI can also identify endometriomas and may detect some endometrial implants, but it is not sufficiently sensitive to make a diagnosis (American College of Obstetricians and Gynecologists, 2010; Fritz & Speroff, 2011).

Laparoscopy with biopsy is the gold standard for the diagnosis of endometriosis. Laparoscopic findings can be used to stage the disease according to the classification system developed by the ASRM (1997). In this system, disease stages I to IV are based on the sites and severity of endometrial implants and adhesions. The ASRM classification system can be helpful for reporting operative findings and interpreting study results, but it does not correlate well with a woman's symptoms or prognosis for fertility (American College of Obstetricians and Gynecologists, 2010).

Differential Diagnosis

Differential diagnoses include other gynecologic and nongynecologic causes of chronic pelvic pain (see Chapter 29). The woman may also be experiencing menstrual pelvic pain and discomfort (see Chapter 24), infertility caused by another etiology (see Chapter 19), or abnormal uterine bleeding related to other causes (see Chapter 25).

Management

Treatment options for endometriosis include expectant management, medical therapy, and surgery. The woman's level of pain, desire for pregnancy, and desire for future fertility must be considered in developing the management plan (American College of Obstetricians and Gynecologists, 2010). Additional considerations used in the management of endometriosis-associated infertility are discussed later in the Special Considerations section.

Medical Management Options for medical therapy include combined estrogen and progestin contraceptives, progestins, GnRH agonists, and danazol. The rationale for their use is to eliminate or reduce menses, thereby minimizing the potential for retrograde menstruation. There is no evidence that any of these medications improve fertility, and they are all equally effective for pain relief (American College of Obstetricians and Gynecologists, 2010; Fritz & Speroff, 2011; Practice Committee of the ASRM, 2008). Recurrence of symptoms may occur after discontinuation of medical therapy. Medical therapy may be used as the primary treatment, or it may be administered after surgery to prevent recurrence of endometriosis. In addition to the options described in this section, NSAIDs can be used for pain relief.

Combined estrogen and progestin contraceptives (i.e., the pill, ring, and patch—see Chapter 12) provide effective pain relief and may prevent disease progression. They can be used indefinitely, unlike some of the other medical therapies (Fritz & Speroff, 2011). Continuous regimens (omitting the pill-, ring-, or patch-free week) may be more effective in the control of pain than cyclic regimens (Vercellini et al., 2003).

Progestins inhibit endometrial growth, and multiple progestin formulations can be used to treat endometriosis (American College of Obstetricians and Gynecologists, 2010; Fritz & Speroff, 2011). Oral options include medroxyprogesterone acetate (20–100 mg daily), norethindrone acetate (5–15 mg daily), and megestrol acetate (40 mg daily). Medroxyprogesterone acetate can also be given via intramuscular (150 mg) injection every 3 months. The LNG-IUS offers an alternative route of progestin delivery that provides effective pain relief and reliable contraception (Rodriguez et al., 2010). Side effects of progestins include irregular menstrual bleeding, breast tenderness, fluid retention, weight gain, and depression or mood instability.

GnRH agonists (Table 27-2) induce a hypogonadal state and amenorrhea, such that there is no estrogen to support existing disease and development of new disease is prevented. GnRH agonists can also decrease the size of endometriomas but do not eliminate them. These agents have significant side effects, including vasomotor symptoms and bone loss; add-back therapy is given to attenuate these effects. Estrogen-only add-back therapy is not recommended for women with endometriosis, as it may increase their pain. A combination of estrogen and progestin can be used to protect bone and prevent symptoms of estrogen deficiency (e.g., hot flashes and atrophic vaginitis). Other medications that can be used in add-back therapy include progestins alone, tibolone, bisphosphonates, and selective estrogen receptor modulators (SERMs). Recurrence of symptoms is common after discontinuation of GnRH agonists, which are typically used for limited periods due to their side effects (American College of Obstetricians and Gynecologists, 2010; Fritz & Speroff, 2011; Practice Committee of the ASRM, 2008) These agents are not superior to combined oral contraceptives (Davis, Kennedy, Moore, & Prentice, 2007).

Danazol (given orally at 400–800 mg per day) creates a hyperandrogenic hypoestrogenic hormonal milieu that inhibits endometrial growth. These hormonal changes are associated with significant side effects, including weight gain, muscle cramps, decreased breast size, acne, hirsutism, oily skin, hot flashes, mood changes, and depression. Danazol must be used in conjunction with highly effective contraception due to the potential for virilization of a female fetus (American College of Obstetricians and Gynecologists, 2010; Fritz & Speroff, 2011; Practice Committee of the ASRM, 2008).

Surgical Management Surgery for endometriosis is indicated for severe or debilitating symptoms that have not been controlled by medical therapy, anatomic distortion, urinary or bowel obstruction, and otherwise advanced disease. Surgery may also be indicated during infertility treatment (Practice Committee of the ASRM, 2006). The procedures performed can be conservative or definitive.

The goal of conservative surgery, which is usually performed laparoscopically, is to treat the endometriosis while preserving the uterus and as much ovarian tissue as possible. Most women experience improvement in pain after conservative surgery, but symptoms may recur (American College of Obstetricians and Gynecologists, 2010). In one study with a median of 7 years of follow-up, more than half of women (54%) who had initial conservative surgery for endometriosis went on to have further surgical treatment for pelvic pain (Shakiba, Bena, McGill, Minger, & Falcone, 2008).

The definitive surgery for endometriosis is a hysterectomy with salpingo-oophorectomy. Hysterectomy is indicated when significant disease is present and future fertility is not desired, when incapacitating symptoms persist despite medical therapy or conservative surgery, and/or if coexisting pelvic pathology requires hysterectomy. Conservation of the ovaries can be attempted, especially if endometriotic implants are removed. Symptoms may persist if the ovaries are left intact, however, such that an oophorectomy will be required later.

Emerging Evidence That May Change Management

Aromatase inhibitors are being investigated as a potential therapy for endometriosis (Ferrero, Gillott, Venturini, & Remorgida, 2011).

Special Considerations

Adolescents   Combined contraceptives are the first-line treatments for adolescents (Laufer, 2008). Some families object to adolescent use of contraception, fearing that their use will encourage sexual activity or that their daughter's ability to have children will be harmed; however, lack of treatment can pose a more severe risk to future fertility. It is important to include the family (with the patient's permission) when planning management, and to find balance in explaining the necessity of long-term treatment without promoting unnecessary fear. Diagrams to demonstrate anatomy and physiology and handouts that can be reviewed at home may be particularly helpful when caring for adolescents. Regardless of age, patients who do not respond to medical therapy should be referred for diagnostic laparoscopy (Laufer).

Infertility   Despite the clear association between endometriosis and infertility, the mechanisms of this relationship remain unclear. In addition, there is not universal agreement on the indications for surgical evaluation and therapy during infertility treatment. Age, duration of infertility, family history, pelvic pain, and stage of endometriosis should be taken into account when developing the management plan. For women with infertility and stage I/II endometriosis, treatment may include expectant management after laparoscopy, superovulation (with gonadotropins) and intrauterine insemination, or in vitro fertilization (see Chapter 19). Conservative surgical treatment is indicated for women with stage III/

IV endometriosis. In vitro fertilization may be necessary if pregnancy does not occur after surgery (Practice Committee of the ASRM, 2006).

Ovarian Masses

Ovarian masses can arise from all of the differentiated tissues of the ovary. There are many benign causes of ovarian masses, and most ovarian masses are benign. However, clinicians must always be vigilant for cancer when an ovarian mass is encountered. This section focuses on ovarian masses that are most likely benign; ovarian malignancies are discussed further in Chapter 28. Ovarian masses can cause women to have significant anxiety that may remain unspoken. When such statements are accurate, reassuring a woman of the nonmalignant nature of her condition or the unlikely loss of her fertility can be helpful.

Incidence

The actual incidence of ovarian masses is difficult to estimate because many are asymptomatic and never diagnosed.

Etiology and Pathophysiology

Common benign ovarian masses include functional ovarian cysts, mature cystic teratomas, serous or mucinous cystadenomas, and endometriomas (**Color Plate 39**). Functional ovarian cysts, also called physiologic cysts, can be classified by whether they occur in the follicular or luteal phase of the menstrual cycle. Follicular cysts, which develop from an unruptured follicle, are more common. These masses are usually asymptomatic and go undiagnosed unless they spontaneously rupture or cause pain with ovulation (mittelschmerz). If ovulation does not occur, the follicular cyst may continue to grow, with the risk of torsion or rupture increasing with size of the cyst. A corpus luteum cyst develops from the corpus luteum that is normally formed with each menstrual cycle after ovulation occurs. Functional hemorrhagic cysts can also occur (Liu & Zanotti, 2011; Stany & Hamilton, 2008).

Mature cystic teratomas arise from the ovarian germ cell and are the most common ovarian tumors. They are filled with sebaceous material and often also contain hair, bone, teeth, or other tissues from the germ layers. Ovarian torsion occurs in as many as 10% of teratomas (Liu & Zanotti, 2011; Stany & Hamilton, 2008).

Serous or mucinous cystadenomas arise from the ovarian epithelium. One-fourth of benign ovarian tumors are serous cystadenomas, which tend to persist but can be managed expectantly if they are small and have no concerning features. Mucinous cystadenomas can become very large and are prone to torsion because of their size (Liu & Zanotti, 2011; Stany & Hamilton, 2008).

Endometriomas, also known as chocolate cysts, are caused by endometriosis. These masses are a very common cause of ovarian enlargement and are found more frequently on the left ovary. They may be associated with dyspareunia and dysmenorrhea (Liu & Zanotti, 2011; Stany & Hamilton, 2008).

Clinical Presentation

The presentation of ovarian masses varies greatly because there are diverse etiologies with different clinical courses, and masses can range in size from those spanning a few centimeters to those weighing several pounds. All ovarian masses can be asymptomatic, though this is more likely with functional cysts and masses that are small in size. Functional cysts may cause pain but are often an incidental finding on examination or ultrasound. Other benign masses may present as a unilateral or bilateral pelvic mass or with abdominal pain or pressure. Pain may be either intermittent or persistent and have either a gradual or an abrupt onset. Usually pain with abrupt onset represents bleeding or spilling of cystic fluid into the abdomen with resultant peritoneal irritation. Pain can also occur with ovarian torsion. When masses become large, abdominal girth can increase from the tumor or ascites and may be mistaken for pregnancy. Urinary frequency without dysuria can occur if a large mass presses on the bladder.

Assessment

History Obtain a detailed history of any symptoms the woman is experiencing, including information about their onset, location, frequency, quality, intensity, and aggravating and alleviating factors. Note the last menstrual period and determine whether the menstrual cycles are regular. The menstrual history can help differentiate follicular and luteal cysts and identify irregular menstrual patterns that may result from functional cysts. Complete general health and gynecologic histories should also be obtained (see Chapter 6).

Physical Examination Measure vital signs and weight. Infection and thus fever are unlikely with ovarian masses, but heart rate and blood pressure changes may occur with significant pain. A disproportionate change in abdominal girth without a concomitant weight gain may indicate large tumor growth. Inspect, auscultate, and palpate the abdomen. Large masses may cause visible changes in the abdomen or may be palpable abdominally. Guarding or rebound tenderness can indicate irritation of the peritoneum. Perform a complete pelvic examination. Assess the location, size, shape, texture, mobility, and tenderness of any palpable mass.

Diagnostic Testing Perform pregnancy testing in all women of reproductive age to rule out ectopic pregnancy. Gonorrhea and chlamydia testing and complete blood count are warranted if a tubo-ovarian abscess is suspected. Additional laboratory testing can be deferred until after an ultrasound is completed. Measurement of tumor markers, such as the CA 125, alpha fetoprotein (AFP), lactate dehydrogenase (LDH), and human chorionic gonadotropin (hCG), should be considered if there is a strong suspicion of a malignant mass. The CA 125 test has higher specificity in postmenopausal women than in premenopausal women (American College of Obstetricians and Gynecologists, 2007, reaffirmed 2009). A new multivariate index assay (OV1), which assists in determining the risk that a mass is malignant, is available for women who are undergoing surgery for an ovarian mass (Liu & Zanotti, 2011; Ueland et al., 2011). Use of biomarker tests must be judicious and based on clear indications from patient characteristics and clinical findings. These tests are not appropriate for screening purposes and can lead to unnecessary evaluation, intervention, and cost if used inappropriately.

Transvaginal ultrasound is the first-line imaging modality for evaluation of ovarian masses. Ultrasound will classify a mass as cystic, solid, or complex. Color Doppler ultrasound is sometimes used as an adjunct to transvaginal ultrasound to measure blood flow in and around a mass. MRI and CT imaging are not appropriate for initial evaluation, however; rather, they should be reserved for specific indications such as determining the origin of nonovarian pelvic masses (MRI) and evaluating for metastases when cancer is suspected (CT) (American College of Obstetricians and Gynecologists, 2007, reaffirmed 2009).

Differential Diagnosis

Ectopic pregnancy, tubo-ovarian abscess, and ovarian cancer are the most likely other causes of an ovarian mass. Polycystic ovary syndrome should be considered if ultrasound identifies multiple follicular cysts (see Chapter 26). Numerous other gynecologic and nongynecologic causes of acute and chronic pelvic pain exist. If the pain is acute, pelvic inflammatory disease and appendicitis particularly warrant consideration as potential causes. Differential diagnoses for chronic pelvic pain can be found in Chapter 29.

Management

Asymptomatic simple ovarian cysts less than 10 cm in diameter, including functional cysts and benign neoplasms, have a low probability of malignancy and can be followed without intervention. There is no evidence-based guidance for timing of repeat ultrasound. One or two ultrasounds at 3- or 6-month intervals are frequently reported in the literature and appear reasonable (Liu & Zanotti, 2011). Most functional cysts will resolve within 3 months. The woman should be cautioned to consult a clinician for any significant increase in pain that might represent rupture or torsion. Repeated episodes of functional cysts can be reduced by using contraceptives to suppress ovulation. Contraceptives do not promote resolution of cysts that are already formed.

Complex and solid ovarian masses warrant further assessment to ascertain the likelihood of malignancy and need for surgery. A gynecologist should be consulted in such cases. The woman with a mass that is suspicious for ovarian cancer needs referral to a gynecologic oncologist because survival rates are higher when the initial surgery is performed by a gynecologic oncologist compared to a general gynecologist (Engelen et al., 2006).

Special Considerations

Adolescents Functional cysts, both follicular and luteal, are common in adolescents. Their immature pituitary–hypothalamic–ovarian axis allows for more anovulatory cycles, leading to more persistent simple cysts. Early evidence of polycystic ovarian syndrome may also manifest in members of this age group (see Chapter 26).

Pregnant Women More ovarian masses are being diagnosed during early pregnancy owing to the increasing use of first-trimester ultrasound. Corpus luteum cysts and mature cystic teratomas are the most commonly reported adnexal masses during pregnancy. The risk of malignancy and acute complications from an ovarian mass during pregnancy is low, and expectant management is appropriate (American College of Obstetricians and Gynecologists, 2007, reaffirmed 2009).

Older Women Postmenopausal women have an increased incidence of ovarian cancer, and benign functional cysts are rare in this age group. Therefore, an ovarian mass in a postmenopausal woman should be considered highly suspicious for malignancy and thoroughly evaluated.

References

American College of Obstetricians and Gynecologists. (2007, reaffirmed 2009). Management of adnexal masses. Practice Bulletin No. 83. *Obstetrics & Gynecology, 110*, 201–214.

American College of Obstetricians and Gynecologists. (2008a, reaffirmed 2010). Alternatives to hysterectomy in the management of leiomyomas. Practice Bulletin No. 96. *Obstetrics & Gynecology, 112*, 387–400.

American College of Obstetricians and Gynecologists. (2008b, reaffirmed 2010). Diagnosis and management of vulvar skin disorders. Practice Bulletin No. 93. *Obstetrics & Gynecology, 111*, 1243–1253.

American College of Obstetricians and Gynecologists. (2010). Management of endometriosis. Practice Bulletin No. 114. *Obstetrics & Gynecology, 116*, 223–236.

American Society for Reproductive Medicine (ASRM). (1997). Revised American Society for Reproductive Medicine classification of endometriosis: 1996. *Fertility and Sterility, 67*(5), 817–821.

Assman, T., Becker-Wegerich, P., Grewe, M., Megahed, M., & Ruzicka, T. (2003). Tacrolimus ointment for the treatment of vulvar lichen sclerosus. *Journal of the American Academy of Dermatology, 48*(6), 935–937.

Basak, S., & Saha, A. (2009). Adenomyosis: Still largely under-diagnosed. *Journal of Obstetrics and Gynaecology, 29*, 533–535.

Beecker, J. (2010). Therapeutic principles in vulvovaginal dermatology. *Dermatologic Clinics, 28*, 639–648.

Bradley, L. D. (2009). Uterine fibroid embolization: A viable alternative to hysterectomy. *American Journal of Obstetrics and Gynecology, 201*, 127–135.

Burrows, L. J., Shaw, H. A., & Goldstein, A. T. (2008). The vulvar dermatoses. *Journal of Sexual Medicine, 5*, 276–283.

Casey, P. M., Long, M. E., & Marnach, M. L. (2011). Abnormal cervical appearance: What to do, when to worry? *Mayo Clinic Proceedings, 86*, 147–151.

Clayton, R., Chaudhry, S., Ali, I., Cooper, S., Hodgson, T., & Wojnarowska, F. (2010). Mucosal (oral and vulva) lichen planus in women: Are angiotensin-converting enzyme inhibitors protective, and beta-blockers and non-steroidal anti-inflammatory drugs associated with the condition? *Clinical and Experimental Dermatology, 35*, 384–387.

Cooper, S. M., & Wojnarowska, F. (2006). Influence of treatment of erosive lichen planus of the vulva on its prognosis. *Archives of Dermatology, 142*, 289–294.

Cramer, S. F., & Patel, A. (1990). The frequency of uterine leiomyomas. *American Journal of Clinical Pathology, 94*(4), 435–438.

Davis, L., Kennedy, S. S., Moore, J., & Prentice, A. (2007). Modern combined oral contraceptives for pain associated with endometriosis. *Cochrane Database of Systematic Reviews, 18*(3), CD001019.

Douglas, C., & Rotimi, O. (2004). Extragenital endometriosis: A clinicopathological review of a Glasgow hospital experience with case illustrations. *Journal of Obstetrics and Gynaecology, 24*, 804–808.

Duhan, N., & Sirohiwal, D. (2010). Uterine myomas revisited. *European Journal of Obstetrics & Gynecology and Reproductive Biology, 152*, 119–125.

Engelen, M. J., Kos, H. E., Willemse, P. H., Aalders, J. G., de Vries, E. G., Schaapveld, M., et al. (2006). Surgery by consultant gynecologic oncologists improves survival in patients with ovarian carcinoma. *Cancer, 106*, 589–598.

Ferrero, S., Gillott, D. J., Venturini, P. L., & Remorgida, V. (2011). Use of aromatase inhibitors to treat endometriosis-related pain symptoms: A systematic review. *Reproductive Biology and Endocrinology, 21*, 89.

Fritz, M. A., & Speroff, L. (2011). *Clinical gynecologic endocrinology and infertility* (8th ed.). Baltimore: Lippincott Williams & Wilkins.

Funaro, D. (2004). Lichen sclerosus: A review and practical approach. *Dermatologic Therapy, 17*(1), 28–37.

Garcia, L., & Isaacson, K. (2011). Adenomyosis: Review of the literature. *Journal of Minimally Invasive Gynecology, 18*, 428–437.

Goldstein, A. T., Creasey, A., Pfau, R., Phillips, D., & Burrows, L. J. (2011). A double-blind, randomized controlled trial of clobetasol versus pimecrolimus in patients with vulvar lichen sclerosus. *Journal of the American Academy of Dermatology, 64*, e99–e104.

Goldstein, A. T., Thaci, D., & Luger, T. (2009). Topical calcineurin inhibitors for the treatment of vulvar dermatoses. *European Journal of Obstetrics & Gynecology and Reproductive Biology, 146*, 22–29.

Gupta, S., Jose, J., & Manyonda, I. (2008). Clinical presentation of fibroids. *Best Practice & Research Clinical Obstetrics & Gynaecology, 22*, 615–626.

Helgesen, A. L., Gjersvik, P., Jebsen, P., Kirschner, R., & Tanbo, T. (2010). Vaginal involvement in lichen planus. *Acta Obstetricia et Gynecologica Scandinavica, 98*, 966–970.

Honoré, G. M. (1999). Extrapelvic endometriosis. *Clinical Obstetrics and Gynecology, 42*(3), 699–711.

Husby, G. K., Haugen, R. S., & Moen, M. H. (2003). Diagnostic delay in women with pain and endometriosis. *Acta Obstetricia et Gynecologica Scandinavica, 82*(7), 649–653.

Jacoby, V. L., Fujimoto, V. Y., Giudice, L. C., Kuppermann, M., & Washington, A. E. (2010). Racial and ethnic disparities in benign gynecologic conditions and associated surgeries. *American Journal of Obstetrics and Gynecology, 202*, 514–521.

Jenkins, S., Olive, D. L., & Haney, A. F. (1986). Endometriosis: Pathogenetic implications of the anatomic distribution. *Obstetrics and Gynecology, 67*(3), 335–338.

Klatsky, P. C., Tran, N. D., Caughey, A. B., & Fujimoto, V. Y. (2008). Fibroids and reproductive outcomes: A systematic literature review from conception to delivery. *American Journal of Obstetrics and Gynecology, 198*, 357–366.

Kunstfeld, R., Kirnbauer, R., Stingl, G., & Karlhofer, F. M. (2003). Successful treatment of vulvar lichen sclerosus with topical tacrolimus. *Archives of Dermatology, 139*(7), 850–852.

Laufer, M. R. (2008). Current approaches to optimizing the treatment of endometriosis in adolescents. *Gynecologic and Obstetric Investigation, 66*(suppl 1), 19–27.

Lethaby, A., Vollenhoven, B., & Sowter, M. (2002). Efficacy of pre-operative gonadotrophin hormone releasing analogues for women with uterine fibroids undergoing hysterectomy or myomectomy: A systematic review. *British Journal of Obstetrics and Gynecology, 109*(10), 1097–1108.

Liu, X., Yuan, L., & Guo, S.-W. (2010). Valproic acid as a therapy for adenomyosis: A comparative case series. *Reproductive Sciences, 17*, 904–912.

Liu, J. H., & Zanotti, K. M. (2011). Management of the adnexal mass. *Obstetrics & Gynecology, 117*, 1413–1428.

Lonsdale-Eccles, A. A., & Velangi, S. (2005). Topical pimecrolimus in the treatment of genital lichen planus: A prospective case series. *British Journal of Dermatology, 153*, 390–394.

McPherson, T., & Cooper, S. (2010). Vulval lichen sclerosus and lichen planus. *Dermatologic Therapy, 23*, 523–532.

Meredith, S. M., Sanchez-Ramos, L., & Kaunitz, A. M. (2009). Diagnostic accuracy of transvaginal sonography for the diagnosis of adenomyosis: Systematic review and metaanalysis. *American Journal of Obstetrics and Gynecology, 107*, e1–e6.

Murphy, R. (2010). Lichen sclerosus. *Dermatologic Clinics, 28,* 707–715.

Neiger, R., Sonek, J. D., Croom, C. S., & Ventolini, G. (2006). Pregnancy-related changes in the size of uterine leiomyomas. *Journal of Reproductive Medicine, 51,* 671–674.

Nieman, L. K., Blocker, W., Nansel, T., Mahoney, S., Reynolds, J., Blithe, D., et al. (2011). Efficacy and tolerability of CDB-2914 treatment for symptomatic uterine fibroids: A randomized, double-blind, placebo-controlled, phase IIb study. *Fertility and Sterility, 95,* 767–772.

Okolo, S. (2008). Incidence, aetiology and epidemiology of uterine fibroids. *Best Practice & Research Clinical Obstetrics & Gynaecology, 4,* 571–588.

Panagiotopoulou, N., Wong, C. S. M., & Winter-Roach, B. (2010). Vulvovaginal–gingival syndrome. *Journal of Obstetrics & Gynaecology, 30,* 226–230.

Parker, W. H. (2007). Uterine myomas: Management. *Fertility and Sterility, 88,* 255–271.

Parker, W. H., Fu, Y. S., & Berek, J. S. (1994). Uterine sarcoma in patients operated on for presumed leiomyoma and rapidly growing leiomyoma. *Obstetrics and Gynecology, 83*(3), 414–418.

Parsanezhad, M. E., Azmoon, M., Alborzi, S., Rajaeefard, A., Zarei, A., Kazerooni, T., et al. (2010). A randomized, controlled clinical trial comparing the effects of aromatase inhibitor (letrozole) and gonadotropin-releasing hormone agonist (triptorelin) on uterine leiomyoma volume and hormonal status. *Fertility and Sterility, 93,* 192–198.

Popovic, M., Puchner, S., Berzaczy, D., Lammer, J., & Bucek, R. A. (2011). Uterine artery embolization for the treatment of adenomyosis: A review. *Journal of Vascular and Interventional Radiology, 22,* 901–909.

Practice Committee of the American Society for Reproductive Medicine (ASRM). (2006). Endometriosis and infertility. *Fertility and Sterility, 86,* S156–S160.

Practice Committee of the American Society for Reproductive Medicine (ASRM). (2008). Treatment of pelvic pain associated with endometriosis. *Fertility and Sterility, 90,* S260–S269.

Practice Committee of the American Society for Reproductive Medicine (ASRM) in collaboration with Society of Reproductive Surgeons. (2008). Myomas and reproductive function. *Fertility and Sterility, 90,* S125–S130.

Rodriguez, M. I., Warden, M., & Darney, P. D. (2010). Intrauterine progestins, progesterone antagonists, and receptor modulators: A review of gynecologic applications. *American Journal of Obstetrics and Gynecology, 202,* 420–428.

Schlosser, B. J. (2010). Contact dermatitis of the vulva. *Dermatologic Clinics, 28,* 697–706.

Seli, E., Berkkanoglu, M., & Arici, A. (2003). Pathogenesis of endometriosis. *Obstetrics and Gynecology Clinics of North America, 30*(1), 41–61.

Shakiba, K., Bena, J. F., McGill, K. M., Minger, J., & Falcone, T. (2008). Surgical treatment of endometriosis: A 7-year follow-up on the requirement for further surgery. *Obstetrics & Gynecology, 111,* 1285–1292.

Sheng, J., Zhang, W. Y., Zhang, J. P., & Lu, D. (2009). The LNG-IUS study on adenomyosis: A 3-year follow-up study on the efficacy and side effects of the use of levonorgestrel intrauterine system for the treatment of dysmenorrhea associated with adenomyosis. *Contraception, 79,* 189–193.

Spiewankiewicz, B., Stelmachow, J., Sawicki, W., Cendrowski, K., & Kuzlik, R. (2003). Hysteroscopy in cases of cervical polyps. *European Journal of Gynaecological Oncology, 24*(1), 67–69.

Stamatellos, I., Stamatopoulos, P., & Bontis, J. (2007). The role of hysteroscopy in the current management of the cervical polyps. *Archives of Gynecology and Obstetrics, 276,* 299–303.

Stany, M. P., & Hamilton, C. A. (2008). Benign disorders of the ovary. *Obstetrics and Gynecology Clinics of North America, 35,* 271–284.

Steinauer, J., Pritts, E. A., Jackson, R., & Jacoby, A. F. (2004). Systematic review of mifepristone for the treatment of uterine leiomyomata. *Obstetrics & Gynecology, 103,* 1331–1336.

Stewart, K. M. A. (2010). Clinical care of vulvar pruritus, with emphasis on one common cause, lichen simplex chronicus. *Dermatologic Clinics, 28,* 669–680.

Taran, F. A., Weaver, A. L., Coddington, C. C., & Stewart, E. A. (2010). Understanding adenomyosis: A case control study. *Fertility and Sterility, 94,* 1223–1228.

Ueland, F. R., Desimone, C. P., Seamon, L. G., Miller, R. A., Goodrich, S., Podzielinksi, I., et al. (2011). Effectiveness of a multivariate index assay in the preoperative assessment of ovarian tumors. *Obstetrics & Gynecology, 117,* 1289–1297.

Varelas, F. K., Papanicolaou, A. N., Vavatsi-Christaki, N., Makedos, G. A., & Vlassis, G. D. (2007). The effect of anastrazole on symptomatic uterine leiomyomata. *Obstetrics & Gynecology, 110,* 643–649.

Vercellini, P., Frontino, G., De Giorgi, O., Pietropaolo, G., Pasin, R., & Crosignani, P. G. (2003). Continuous use of an oral contraceptive for endometriosis-associated recurrent dysmenorrhea that does not respond to a cyclic pill regimen. *Fertility and Sterility, 80*(3), 560–563.

Vulvar Dermatology Resources

American Society for Colposcopy and Cervical Pathology. (2004). *Practice management: Vulva*. Retrieved from http://www.asccp.org/PracticeManagement/Vulva/tabid/7430/Default.aspx

Black, M. M., Ambros-Rudolph, D., Edwards, L., & Lynch, P. J. (2008). *Obstetric and gynecologic dermatology* (3rd ed.). Philadelphia, PA: Mosby.

Habif, T. P., Campbell, J. L., Chapman, M. S., Dinulos, J. G. H., & Zug, K. A. (2011). *Skin disease: Diagnosis and treatment* (3rd ed.). Philadelphia, PA: Saunders.

International Society for the Study of Vulvovaginal Disease. (2009). Retrieved from http:// www.issvd.org

Kaufman, R. H., Faro, S., & Brown, D. (2004). *Benign diseases of the vulva and vagina* (5th ed.). St. Louis, MO: Mosby.

National Lichen Sclerosus Support Group. (2011). Retrieved from http://www.lichensclerosus.org

National Psoriasis Foundation. (2011). Retrieved from http://www.psoriasis.org

Neill, S., & Lewis, F. (Eds.). (2009). *Ridley's the vulva*. West Sussex, UK: Wiley-Blackwell.

Stewart, E. G. (2002). *The V book: A doctor's guide to complete vulvovaginal health*. New York: Bantam Books.

Wilkinson, E. J., & Stone, I. K. (2008). *Atlas of vulvar disease* (2nd ed.). Philadelphia, PA: Lippincott Williams & Wilkins.

Wolverton, S. W. (2007). *Comprehensive dermatologic drug therapy* (2nd ed.). Philadelphia, PA: W. B. Saunders.

28

Gynecologic Cancers

Mary Wallace
Alison Boehm Barlow

G ynecologic cancers are serious, life-threatening diseases. Many symptoms of these diseases are vague and subtle, making early diagnosis, treatment, and successful recovery difficult.

A humanistic approach that integrates medical and sociopsychological perspectives and is patient centered serves to equalize the power imbalance between a woman and her clinician. Clinicians using this approach actively listen to their patients and assess them in the context of their lived experiences, ethnicity, culture, and socioeconomic class. These clinicians are less likely to miss hearing a woman as she describes vague symptoms that may be warnings of underlying disease, and instead encourage her to provide more information that may be helpful in making an accurate diagnosis. Clinicians using a humanistic approach are cautious, thoughtful, and think critically, using the most recent evidence in assessing and formulating treatment for the disease. They arm their patients with information that is critical to informed consent and decision making. Sensitive clinicians who use good listening skills are the ones who have helped decrease the number of cancer deaths in women who were misdiagnosed when their voices were ignored.

The focus of this chapter is gynecologic cancers. Such cancers account for approximately 78,490 new cases of cancer each year and are responsible for 28,490 deaths of women annually (American Cancer Society [ACS], 2008a). Preventive health is the primary goal of clinicians who provide health care for women. Genetic, behavioral, and environmental factors influence the risk of developing a gynecologic malignancy.

Vulvar Cancers

Scope of the Problem

Vulvar cancer accounts for approximately 5% of all reproductive-organ cancers in women (Centers for Disease Control and Prevention [CDC], 2010) and has an age-adjusted rate of 1.7 cases per 100,000 women in the United States (Joura, 2002). If detected, vulvar cancer is usually curable (ACS, 2008a). The overall 5-year survival rate for a woman with vulvar cancer is 90% if there is no lymph node involvement (ACS). Lymph node involvement and primary lesion size are the two most important prognostic factors. When the regional lymph nodes are involved, the presence of one or two involved lymph nodes confers a better prognosis than if three or more lymph nodes are malignant, or if there is bilateral node involvement. Patients who have multiple positive lymph nodes in the groin have a very poor prognosis. The overall 5-year survival rate for patients with lymph node involvement ranges from 50% to 60% (ACS).

Approximately 85% of vulvar cancers occur in women older than the age of 50; half of these cases occur in women older than age 70. However, 15% of new cases of vulvar cancer are diagnosed in women who are younger than the age of 40 (Chambers, 2001; Holschneider & Berek, 2002; National Cancer Institute [NCI], 2003b).

Etiology and Pathophysiology

DNA mutations resulting in vulvar cancer are acquired over the course of an individual's life; therefore, the risk for vulvar cancer is not inheritable. Research suggests that vulvar cancer evolves as two separate types of cancer. The first type is related to human papillomavirus (HPV) infection; this type of infection frequently leads to vulvar intraepithelial neoplasia (VIN) in younger women. The second type of vulvar cancer is usually diagnosed in women 65 to 75 years of age and is related to vulvar non-neoplastic epithelial disorders such as lichen sclerosus, squamous cell hyperplasia, and Paget's disease of the vulva (Chambers, 2001; Guarnieri & Klemm, 2000; Holschneider & Berek, 2002; Lee, 2000a).

HPV types 16, 18, 31, and others confer a high risk of vulvar cancer and appear to play a role in 30% to 50% of diagnosed cases (Chambers, 2001). Women who have HPV as a risk factor tend to be younger and frequently have multiple areas of VIN over their vulvas. Early sexual contact and infection with HPV provides more time for malignant transformation. Women who smoke cigarettes and have HPV also have a higher risk of vulvar cancer. The aforementioned 15% of newly affected women younger than the age of 40 often smoke and are infected with HPV (Chambers, 2001; Guarnieri & Klemm, 2000; Holschneider & Berek, 2002; Lee, 2000a).

VIN (formerly known as Bowen's disease) is a premalignant finding associated with HPV that confers an increased risk of vulvar cancer even though most cases do not progress to squamous cell cancer. An estimated 80% of women with untreated warty VIN develop invasive disease (Holschneider & Berek, 2002). The combination of HPV and smoking is known to increase the risk for vulvar and cervical cancer (Chambers, 2001; Guarnieri & Klemm, 2000; Lee, 2000a, 2000b). Vulvar intraepithelial neoplasia is classified according to degree of severity (**Table 28-1**).

Lichen sclerosus (see Chapter 27) slightly increases the risk for vulvar cancer in affected women. Approximately 4% of women with lichen sclerosus will develop vulvar cancer (Tucker Edwards & Saunders-Goldson, 2003). Lichen sclerosus, which causes a severe itch–scratch cycle, is thought to cause squamous hyperplasia, which then progresses to cellular atypia and finally to invasive squamous cell carcinoma. Aggressive evaluation and treatment have the potential to decrease the incidence of vulvar cancer in this subgroup of patients (Chambers, 2001; Guarnieri & Klemm, 2000; Lee, 2000b). Older women with lichen sclerosus who are not infected with HPV rarely have VIN, but often will have mutations of the p53 tumor suppressor gene, which may be identified through DNA testing (Guarnieri & Klemm). The p53 protein stops cell growth and division in DNA-damaged cells; when the damage cannot be repaired, the p53 protein triggers cell suicide, thereby preventing unregulated cell growth by damaged cells (NCI, 2003b).

Additional risk factors for vulvar cancer include human immunodeficiency virus (HIV), previous gynecologic malignancy, and a history of smoking (CDC, 2010; Lee, 2000a). HIV infection causes immunosuppression, thereby making tissues susceptible to persistent HPV infections, which in turn increases the risk of vulvar cancer (Lee).

Clinical Presentation

The most common presentation of vulvar cancer is a woman's report of a vulvar lump or mass with a prolonged history of vulvar pruritus; however, as many as 50% of women with vulvar cancer are asymptomatic (Chambers, 2001). Symptoms include vulvar bleeding, discharge, dysuria, and pain. On rare occasions, a woman will present with a large, fungating mass or lesion. On physical examination, the lesion is usually raised, and may be ulcerated, warty, or fleshy in appearance, or it may appear to be an area of squamous cell hyperplasia (see Chapter 27). Most lesions are solitary, and approximately 50% of the lesions are found on the labia majora. The labia minora, clitoris, and perineum are other possible primary sites (Chambers, 2001; Guarnieri & Klemm, 2000; Holschneider & Berek, 2002; Lee, 2000b; Tyring, 2003).

More than 90% of vulvar carcinomas are squamous cell carcinomas and are usually preceded by dysplasia or VIN (Chambers, 2001; Holschneider & Berek, 2002). Malignant melanoma of the vulva accounts for 2% to 4% of all vulvar cancers and usually occurs on the labia minora and clitoris (Chambers). Adenocarcinomas can develop in Bartholin's glands or

TABLE 28-1 Cellular Classification of Vulvar Intraepithelial Neoplasia (VIN)	
I.	Mild dysplasia (formerly mild atypia)
II.	Moderate dysplasia (formerly moderate atypia)
III.	Severe dysplasia (formerly severe atypia)
IV.	Carcinoma in situ
Source: National Cancer Institute, 2003b.	

with vulvar Paget's disease. A tumor of the Bartholin's gland is easily mistaken for a cyst, so delay in accurate diagnosis is common. Fewer than 2% of vulvar carcinomas are sarcomas; these tumors tend to grow rapidly and can occur at any age (Holschneider & Berek, 2001).

Assessment

Early identification of women at risk for developing vulvar cancer is important. Thorough patient education about when and how to perform a vulvar self-examination, and visual inspection of the external genitalia during the clinical pelvic examination are essential to early identification. Although annual Papanicolaou (Pap) tests are no longer recommended for all women (see Chapter 8), the American College of Obstetricians and Gynecologists (2009) recommends an annual pelvic examination for all women age 21 and older, as the incidence of vulvar cancer increases with age. Genital neoplasia in women is often multifocal. Thus careful examination of the entire vulva, vagina, cervix, perineum, and perianal area, including the anus, should be performed on women as part of the routine pelvic examination. The femoral and inguinal lymph nodes should be palpated routinely with pelvic examination.

All women reporting or found to have a vulvar lesion must be thoroughly evaluated to rule out malignancy. Colposcopy may assist in defining the extent of disease. A biopsy, which can be done in the outpatient setting, is required for definitive diagnosis (see Chapter 27).

Both patients and clinicians may contribute to the delay in diagnosis of vulvar cancers. Common causes of late-stage diagnosis of vulvar cancer include women not seeking treatment when initial symptoms occur, and clinicians providing symptomatic treatment for months prior to obtaining a biopsy. Experts recommend that any condyloma that does not respond to therapy or any lesion that increases in size or has an unusual appearance be biopsied (Chambers, 2001; Guarnieri & Klemm, 2000; Holschneider & Berek, 2002; Lee, 2000b; Tyring, 2003).

Staging, using the tumor–node–metastasis (TNM) classification system, identifies vulvar cancer growth with direct extension first, and then focuses on local lymph node involvement (American Joint Committee on Cancer [AJCC], 2002; NCI, 2003b). The TNM classification is a widely used carcinoma classification system that provides a way of describing the size, location, and spread of a tumor:

- The "T" describes the primary tumor according to its size and location.
- The "N" refers to the lymph nodes that drain fluid from the area of the tumor and indicates whether the cancer has spread to the lymph nodes.
- The "M" identifies whether the cancer has spread to distant areas in the body (e.g., from the vulva to the lungs).

The American Joint Committee on Cancer's TNM categories correspond to the stages accepted by the International Federation of Gynecology and Obstetrics (FIGO). Vulvar cancer staging according to the FIGO guidelines is outlined in **Table 28-2**.

TABLE 28-2 International Federation of Gynecology and Obstetrics (FIGO) Staging for Cancer of the Vulva

Stage	Characteristics
Stage 0	In situ disease, no lymph node metastases, no distant metastases
Stage I, IA, & IB	Primary tumor confined to vulva, < 2 cm, no lymph node metastases, no distant metastases
Stage II	Primary tumor > 2 cm, no lymph node metastases, no distant metastases
Stage III	Primary tumor of any size with adjacent spread to lower urethra, vagina, perineum, or anus, or unilateral lymph node metastases
Stage IVa	Primary tumor of any size with adjacent spread to the upper urethra, bladder mucosa, rectal mucosa, or pelvic bone, and/or bilateral regional lymph node metastases
Stage IVb	Primary tumor of any size, any lymph node metastases, and any distant metastases

Source: American Joint Committee on Cancer, 2002.

Vulvar cancer lesions tend to be minimally invasive and poorly differentiated, whereas anaplastic lesions tend to be deeply invasive. Local spread may extend to the urethra, vagina, perineum, and anus. Lymphatic spread usually occurs first in the inguinal lymph nodes, then involves the femoral lymph nodes, and finally spreads to the external iliac chain of the pelvic lymph nodes. The incidence of lymph node involvement is approximately 30% (ACS, 2008a). The risk of metastasis to the regional lymph nodes increases with increasing size and depth of the primary lesion. Hematogenous spread to distant sites is uncommon but may involve the lungs, liver, and bone (AJCC, 2002; NCI, 2003b).

Management

Prevention Preventive measures for vulvar cancer include the following:

- Avoiding exposure to HPV by limiting the number of sexual partners
- Seeking treatment for vulvar itching caused by chronic vulvar diseases such as lichen sclerosus
- Not smoking
- Routine vulvar self-examination (Guarnieri & Klemm, 2000)

Culturally sensitive interventions are still needed to address the educational needs of diverse communities of women to provide them with accurate prevention and screening information (Cohen & Frank-Stromborg, 2000; Guarnieri & Klemm, 2000).

Definitive Treatment Surgical resection is the standard treatment for patients with vulvar cancer. Patients presenting with symptoms or questionable lesions need to be referred to a gynecologist or gynecologic oncologist who has expertise in cancer surgery (Chambers, 2001). The preoperative work-up may include a chest x-ray, complete blood count (CBC), and imaging studies such as computed tomography (CT) and magnetic resonance imaging (MRI). The surgery involves removing the tumor and at least a 1-cm margin of normal tissue surrounding the tumor. Wide local excision and radical vulvectomy are the most commonly performed surgical procedures, with radical local excision being performed most often today. The inguinal and femoral lymph nodes are surgically evaluated as part of staging the disease because microscopic metastases may be present in clinically nonsuspicious nodes. Local recurrences are treated with local excision when possible and are followed by postoperative radiation therapy. Chemotherapy is reserved for metastatic disease (Chambers, 2001; NCI, 2003b).

Follow-Up Care of the Woman Who Has Been Treated for Vulvar Cancer

The primary early postoperative complications experienced by women who undergo radical local excision with groin dissection or radical vulvectomy are groin wound infection and tissue breakdown (Holschneider & Berek, 2002). One-third of patients will develop a recurrence within 2 years of primary treatment (Coulter & Gleeson, 2003). Some recurrences are seen at 5 or more years after treatment; consequently, lifelong follow-up on a regular schedule is important (Fischer, 1996). Many patients may return to their primary care clinicians for follow-up after surgical recovery and resolution of any postoperative wound healing complications. Typically a woman who has been treated for vulvar cancer is seen for follow-up every 3 months for the first 2 years, every 6 months for the next 3 years, and annually thereafter (Fischer).

A comprehensive annual history and physical examination are standard components of follow-up care. Post-treatment monthly self-examination of the vulva should be taught and emphasized, because recurrent disease is always a possibility. Early identification of a recurrence offers the best chance for effective treatment (Chambers, 2001; Guarnieri & Klemm, 2000; Holschneider & Berek, 2002; Lee, 2000b). New or persistent symptoms need to be reported promptly and carefully evaluated. Every follow-up visit should focus on the history of any new vulvar lesion, bladder function, bowel function, bone pain, and lower extremity lymphedema. The physical examination should include assessment of the breasts, abdomen, and lymph nodes, as well as a thorough pelvic and rectal examination (Fischer, 1996).

Chronic lymphedema of the lower extremities occurs in 20% to 50% of patients who have undergone lymph node dissection and may develop either early or late after treatment (Chambers, 2001; Ryan et al. 2003). Lymphedema may cause the urinary stream to change direction, causing urine to "spray" rather than "stream." If this occurs, a cone-shaped urinal (sometimes used by women when camping outdoors) may be helpful. Urinary stress incontinence, introital stenosis, altered body image issues, depression, and sexual dysfunction are other late complications associated with the extent of the surgery.

Regular (three times a week) use of vaginal dilators or regular sexual intercourse can help to stretch vaginal tissues and should be initiated before the vaginal introitus becomes stenotic. If introital stenosis occurs, the clinician may need to use a pediatric speculum for vaginal visualization, and only a single digit when palpating the vagina. Some degree of sexual dysfunction is almost always present with definitive treatment of vulvar cancer. In particular, problems with arousal, orgasm, vaginal dryness, and sexual relationship issues are commonplace. Vaginal dryness may be helped by the use of vaginal lubricants such as Astroglide or vaginal moisturizers such as Replens. Changing positions for sexual intercourse may reduce discomfort (Holschneider & Berek, 2002).

Counseling that explores relationship issues and discusses possible alternatives to vaginal intercourse allows for the expression of grief over the loss of normal sexual function. It is also important to address the ever-present fear of recurrence or metastasis. Choice of a personal caregiver for these women should be carefully considered; her sexual partner may not always be the best choice. Some women have attributed significant negative change in their sexual relationship to the participation of a sexual partner in postoperative wound care.

Cervical Cancer

Scope of the Problem

Cervical cancer is the third most common genital malignancy in women in the United States, after cancers of the endometrium and the ovary. An estimated 11,070 new cervical cancer cases and 3,070 cervical cancer deaths were estimated to occur in the United States in 2008 (ACS, 2008a). Although regular screening with Pap testing has dramatically decreased the incidence and mortality of cervical cancer, an additional 1,250,000 women are diagnosed with precancers annually (NCI, 2008a). Unfortunately, evaluation of these lesions is associated with a large number of diagnostic procedures (NCI). Women with precursor lesions have a 5-year survival rate of nearly 100%; when cervical cancers are detected at an early stage, the 5-year survival rate is approximately 92%. The overall (all stages combined) 5-year survival rate is approximately 72% (ACS).

In the United States, cervical cancer remains a disease of socioeconomic disparity, with Hispanic and African American women being both more likely to be diagnosed with the disease and more likely to die of it than white women. The high mortality rates are indicative of barriers to health care among the poor and minority women (ACS, 2008a; Garcia, 2007).

Etiology and Pathophysiology

HPV is now recognized as the most important causative agent in cervical carcinogenesis, and it is generally accepted that women must be infected by HPV before they develop cervical cancer (ACS, 2009; Saksouk, 2008). HPV is the most common sexually transmitted infection (STI) worldwide. It is estimated that more than 6.2 million people in the United States become infected with HPV each year, and more than 20 million Americans are believed to be already infected with the virus (CDC, 2007; Gearhart, 2007). Although HPV is considered an STI, it can be spread by skin-to-skin genital contact without intercourse. Most women are infected shortly after beginning their first sexual relationship, with the highest prevalence seen in women younger than 25 years of age. Thereafter, prevalence decreases rapidly. Condoms reduce but do not eliminate the risk of transmission (ACS, 2009; CDC, 2006; Garcia, 2007; Saksouk, 2008).

HPV is found in 95% of cervical malignancies (NCI, 2008b; Saksouk, 2008). Despite the significant correlation between HPV infection and cervical cancer, 80% to 90% of infections are transient, sometimes causing only mild cytologic abnormalities, and they usually become undetectable within 1 to 2 years. A successful immune response results in viral control or clearance. Nevertheless, 10% to 20% of women are at risk for HPV persistence; of these women, approximately 2% will develop cervical carcinoma. A persistent infection with high-risk HPV is the most significant risk factor for the development of invasive cervical cancer (Fey & Beal, 2004; Vachani, 2008).

More than 100 different HPV strains have been identified, approximately 40 of which infect the genital area. Genital HPV types can be divided into two broad categories based on their risk of oncogenesis. The low-risk HPV types include 6, 11, 42, 43, 44, 54, 61, 70, 72, and 81. Types 6 and 11 are responsible for 90% of genital warts (condylomata acuminata) and low-grade cervical changes such as mild dysplasia. Lesions due to low-risk HPV infections have a higher likelihood of regression and rarely progress to cancer (ACS, 2008b, 2009; Gearhart, 2007). The high-risk HPV types include 16, 18, 31, 33, 35, 39, 45, 51, 52, 56, 58, 59, 68, 73, and 82. These types are known to cause persistent infection, leading to high-grade cervical changes such as moderate or severe dysplasia and neoplasia. At the same time, these strains are frequently found to be the etiologic factor in minor lesions and mild dysplasia. Types 16 and 18 are found in 70% of cervical cancer cases and are also found in other types of anogenital cancers (ACS, 2008b, 2009; Gearhart, 2007; Mayeux & Spitzer, 2005) (see **Table 28-3**).

The major difference between the two types of HPV is that after infection, the low-risk HPV types are maintained as extrachromosomal DNA episomes, while the high-risk HPV genome becomes integrated into the host cells' DNA in malignant lesions. Integration of the viral genome into the host cell genome is considered a hallmark of malignant transformation (Garcia, 2007). High-risk HPV produces viral protein products (E6, E7) that bind and

TABLE 28-3 Common HPV Types Associated with Benign and Malignant Disease

	HPV Types	**Manifestations**
High Risk	Types 16 and 18	Low-grade cervical changes
		High-grade cervical changes
		Cervical cancer
		Cancers of the vagina, vulva, anus, and penis
Low Risk	Types 6 and 11	Benign low-grade cervical changes
		Genital warts

inactivate the host's tumor suppressor genes p53 and Rb. The inactivation of p53 and Rb tumor suppressor genes blocks apoptosis (programmed cell death) and induces chromosomal abnormalities (CDC, 2007; Garcia; Gearhart, 2007).

Cervical cancer is characterized by a well-defined premalignant phase that can be identified through cytological examination of exfoliated cells (Pap test) and confirmed on histological examination. These premalignant changes can represent a spectrum of cervical abnormalities referred to as squamous intraepithelial lesions (SIL) or cervical intraepithelial neoplasia (CIN). Such early lesions form a continuum that is divided into low-grade or high-grade SIL or CIN 1, 2, 3 and reflects the increasingly abnormal changes of the cervical epithelium. Over time, the premalignant lesions can persist, regress, or progress to invasive malignancy. CIN 1 often regresses spontaneously; whereas CIN 2 and 3 are more likely to persist or progress. The premalignant changes almost always occur in metaplastic epithelium at the squamocolumnar junction. Unfortunately, cytological and histological examinations cannot reliably distinguish the few women with abnormal cytology who will progress to invasive cancer from the vast majority of those whose abnormalities will spontaneously regress (ACS, 2008b; Garcia, 2007; Godfrey, 2007; Saksouk, 2008).

The latency period between HPV exposure and the development of cervical cancer is usually measured in years or decades. Longitudinal studies have shown that in untreated patients with carcinoma in situ (CIS) lesions, 30% to 70% will develop invasive carcinoma over a period of 10 to 12 years. In approximately 10% of patients, however, lesions progress from in situ to invasive in a period of less than 1 year (NCI, 2008c). The long natural history provides the opportunity to screen women for premalignant lesions, thereby preventing the lesions from evolving into cervical cancer.

Two main types of cervical cancer are distinguished. The most common type of cervical cancer is squamous cell carcinoma (SCC), which accounts for 80% to 90% of all cervical cancers. SCC arises from the squamous cells that cover the ectocervix. Adenocarcinoma, the second most common cancer type, accounts for 10% to 12% of cervical cancer cases. It most often arises from the columnar epithelium—a group of mucus-producing glandular cells—located in the endocervix. An increase in the incidence of adenocarcinomas has been observed during the past 20 to 30 years: Among women younger than 35 years, the incidence more than doubled between 1970 and the mid-1980s. On rare occasions, cervical cancers have features of both SCC and adenocarcinoma; these cases are called adenosquamous carcinomas or mixed carcinomas (ACS, 2008b; Saksouk, 2008).

Multiple risk factors are associated with acquiring HPV.

Age Early age at first intercourse (age 18 or younger) is a risk factor for HPV, because it is believed the younger-developing cervix is more likely to be infected due to the normal physiologic process called squamous metaplasia. The process of squamous metaplasia occurs at the squamocolumnar junction, or transformation zone, in which the more fragile columnar epithelial cells are replaced with hardier squamous epithelial cells. Squamous metaplasia is initiated by the eversion of the columnar epithelium onto the ectocervix under the influence of estrogen and its ensuing exposure to the acidic vaginal pH. Although metaplasia occurs throughout the reproductive years, it is most active during adolescence and first pregnancy. Cells undergoing metaplasia are more vulnerable to carcinogenic agents such as HPV (American Society for Colposcopy and Cervical Pathology[ASCCP], 2009).

Sexual Behavior Having multiple sexual partners or having a partner with multiple sex partners increases the risk of multiple exposures to HPV (Shumann, McFadden, & Shumann, 2001). However, only a small proportion of those women infected with HPV go on to develop cervical cancer (CDC, 2011). The cofactors discussed next are thought to play a contributing role in this evolution.

Smoking Among women infected with HPV, current and former smokers have approximately two to three times the incidence of high-grade cervical intraepithelial lesions or invasive cancer. Passive smoking is also associated with increased risk, albeit to a lesser extent (NCI, 2008a). Women who smoke cigarettes are twice as likely as nonsmokers to develop cervical cancer. Smoking exposes the body to many carcinogens that affect more than just the lungs, as carcinogens are absorbed by the lungs and carried in the bloodstream throughout the body. Tobacco by-products have been found in the cervical mucus of women who smoke, and it is believed these by-products damage DNA in cervical cells. Smoking may also impair the immune response, thereby interfering with the body's ability to clear the HPV infection (ACS, 2008b, 2009; Schumann et al., 2001).

Immunosuppression Patients who are immunocompromised from HIV, AIDS, or other causes (e.g., medications) have an increased prevalence and persistence of HPV infection. The immune system plays an important role in destroying cancer cells and slowing their growth and spread (ACS, 2008b, 2009; Garcia & Bi, 2007).

Oral Contraceptives Moreno et al. (2002) examined the impact of oral contraceptive (OC) use in women with HPV. Data were pooled from eight case-control studies of patients with histologically confirmed invasive cervical carcinoma (ICC) and from two studies of patients with CIS. Information about OC use was obtained from personal interviews. The findings suggest that women with HPV who have taken the pill for 5 to 9 years have approximately three times the incidence of invasive cancer, and those who have used them for 10 years or longer have approximately four times the risk. In the same study, cervical cancer risk was also more closely linked to duration of OC use than to age at first use (Moreno et al.).

While the connection between OCs and cervical cancer is not yet fully understood, it appears that the estrogenic effect of OCs may prevent the ectopy of the cervix from receding into the cervical canal, leaving the vulnerable area exposed (Schumann et al., 2001). Moreover, OC users are less likely to use barrier protection, thereby increasing their risk of contracting HPV. Findings to date do not warrant discontinuing OC use in the case of an abnormal Pap test (ACS, 2008b, 2009; Bertram, 2004; Schumann et al., 2001; Moreno et al., 2002; NCI, 2008a).

High Parity Munoz et al. (2002) also examined the effects of parity on the progression of HPV infection to cancer. As noted previously, data were pooled from eight case-controlled studies of patients with histologically confirmed ICC and from two studies of patients with CIS. The study found that women with HPV who had one or two full-term pregnancies had a 2.3 times greater risk of developing SCC, whereas those with a history of seven or more full-term pregnancies had a 4 times greater risk of developing SCC. Cervical cancer risk was also closely linked to age at first birth. Women who gave birth at age 16 or younger had a 4.4 times greater risk of developing cervical cancer, whereas women who gave birth at age 20 or older had a 2.2 times greater risk (Munoz et al.).

While the association between parity and ICC is unclear, hormonal factors related to pregnancy may influence the progression of HPV infection. However, women who reported cesarean births in the Moreno et al. (2002) study showed a reduced risk compared with those who had vaginal births. Although the number of cesarean births in this study was small, the purported influence of cervical trauma during vaginal birth on cancer risk remains uncertain. High parity did not seem to increase the probability of HPV infection in women in the study (ACS, 2008b, 2009; Munoz et al., 2002; NCI, 2008a).

Genetic Predisposition Studies suggest that women whose mother or sisters have had cervical cancer are more likely to develop the disease. Twin studies also suggest a familial susceptibility to cervical cancer is possible. Some researchers suspect this familial tendency is caused by an inherited condition that makes some women more susceptible to HPV infection than others (ACS, 2009; Gibson & Hainer, 2003).

Nutritional Status Diets low in fruits and vegetables have been identified as potential contributing factors in the development of cervical cancer. Low levels of vitamins C and E, folate, and carotenoids have been linked to cervical cancer (ACS, 2009; Gibson & Hainer, 2003; Snyder, 2003).

Diethylstilbestrol Daughters of women who took diethylstilbestrol (DES) are 40 times more likely to develop clear cell adenocarcinoma (CCA) of the vagina and cervix than women who were not exposed to DES in utero. Clear cell adenocarcinoma is a rare form of vaginal and cervical cancer (ACS, 2009).

Infectious Agents The specific role of herpes simplex virus 2 (HSV-2) or other infectious agents in the pathogenesis of cervical cancer remains unclear. Nevertheless, HSV-2 and *Chlamydia trachomatis* infections are known to be associated with a chronic inflammatory response and micro-ulceration of the cervical epithelium. Such an inflammatory response is associated with the generation of free radicals, which are thought to play important roles in the initiation and progression of cancers. Free radicals directly damage DNA and DNA repair proteins and inhibit apoptosis, allowing the development of genetic instability (ACS, 2009; Hawes & Kiviat, 2002). The postulated steps in the pathogenesis of cervical cancer are depicted in **Figure 28-1**.

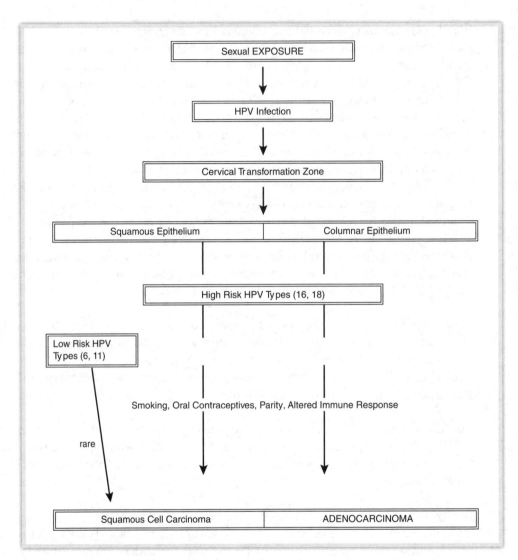

FIGURE 28-1 Postulated steps in the pathogenesis of cervical cancer.

Source: Adapted from Cotran et al., 1999.

Clinical Presentation

Early cervical cancer is usually asymptomatic, and as many as 20% of patients who have invasive cervical cancer are asymptomatic when the disease is diagnosed. Approximately 80% to 90% of patients with cervical cancer experience a form of abnormal vaginal bleeding, such as postmenopausal bleeding, irregular menses, heavy menstrual flow, painless metrorrhagia, or postcoital bleeding. Abnormal vaginal discharge is present in approximately 10% of patients. This discharge may be watery, purulent, or mucoid. Late symptoms that herald metastatic spread include bladder outlet obstruction, constipation, back pain, and leg swelling (ACS, 2008b; Garcia, 2007; Saksouk, 2008).

Assessment

History Key areas of inquiry that assist clinicians in identifying women at high risk for cervical cancer include the following:

- Abnormal vaginal bleeding (intermenstrual or postcoital bleeding), unusual vaginal discharge, or dyspareunia
- Sexual history—age at first intercourse, number of sexual partners in the past 6 months, number of lifetime partners, and presence of lesions in sexual partners
- Contraceptive history, including use of barrier methods
- HPV and other STIs in the patient and her partners
- Immunosuppression, including HIV infection
- Prior history of cancer or cancer therapy (e.g., radiation, chemotherapy, surgery)
- In utero DES exposure
- Date and result of the most recent Pap test
- Prior abnormal cervical cytology
- Menstrual history, including the date of the last menstrual period
- Pregnancy history
- History of tobacco, drug, or alcohol use
- Family history of cervical cancer

Physical Examination Physical examination should include a thorough pelvic, abdominal, inguinal lymph node, and rectal examination. Cervical cancer usually begins around the cervical os. In its earliest stages, a cancerous cervix cannot be distinguished from a normal cervix. As the disease progresses, the cervix may appear abnormal with gross erosion, ulcer, or a mass that bleeds easily on contact. In the late stages, an extensive, irregular, cauliflower-like growth may develop. The cervix may be hard and indurated, and its mobility may be restricted or lost. As the tumor enlarges, it grows by extending upward into the endometrial cavity, downward into the vagina, and laterally to the pelvic wall. It can invade the bladder and rectum directly. Common sites for distant metastasis include the pelvic lymph nodes, liver, lungs, and bones (Garcia, 2007; Saksouk, 2008).

Diagnostic Testing

See Chapter 6 for information on obtaining a Pap test and Chapter 8 for cervical cancer screening recommendations. The traditional Pap test has been used to screen women for cervical cancer since 1940 and has been credited with reducing the cervical cancer death rate by 70% since its introduction. However, a number of problems with the Pap test have been described: (1) poor quality of the cervical sample (e.g., incomplete sampling of the transformation zone, poorly prepared slide with drying artifact, clumping of cells, and obscuring elements); (2) the subjective nature of the reading of the slide, and (3) the repetitive nature of the reading, which can lead to greater number of interpretive errors. The low sensitivity of cytology has major medical, economic and legal implications (Cox & Cuzick, 2006; Jones, 2003; Stein, 2003; Yeoh, Chan, Lauder, & Lam, 1999).

Liquid-based cytology (ThinPrep, SurePath) was developed to improve the sensitivity of screening. However, recent studies suggest that this technique is not any more sensitive than standard Pap tests in detecting cervical cancers and precancerous lesions (Ronco et al., 2007; Siebers et al., 2009). Ronco et al. (2007) conducted a randomized control trial and compared the accuracy of conventional cytology with liquid-based cytology for primary screening of cervical cancer. The study included women aged 26 to 60 who attended 9 screening programs in Italy, with 22,466 women randomized to the traditional cytology and 22,708 women randomized to the liquid-based cytology. The median age was 41 in both arms of the study. The results showed no statistically significant differences in sensitivity between the liquid-based cytology and the traditional cytology for detection of CIN 2 or later-stage lesions. However, a significant reduction in the overall proportion of women with unsatisfactory cytology due to obscuring inflammation was observed. Other established advantages of liquid-based cytology include a shorter time needed for the cytologist to interpret the slide and the ability to use the same sample for testing HPV. A disadvantage of the liquid-based test is its higher cost compared to the traditional Pap test (Ronco et al.).

A more recent study by Siebers et al. (2009) assessed the performance of liquid-based cytology compared with conventional cytology in detecting CIN using a randomized controlled trial (RCT). In this study, 122 practices screened 49,222 women using liquid-based cytology and 124 practices screened 40,562 women using the conventional Pap test. The RCT spanned 2 years and patients were followed for 18 months. At the conclusion of the study, the researchers found no difference between liquid-based cytology and conventional Pap testing in terms of their sensitivity for and detection of cervical cancer.

Most laboratories use the Bethesda System for reporting the results of cervical cytology. The Bethesda System consists of a uniform system of terminology that provides guidance for the clinical management of Pap test results (see **Table 28-4**). **Table 28-5** provides a description of the 2001 Bethesda System for reporting cervical cytology results (Solomon et al., 2002).

HPV DNA The Hybrid Capture 2 (HC2) was once the only test approved by the U.S. Food and Drug Administration (FDA) for diagnosing HPV DNA. The HC2 detects 13 of the high-risk HPV types associated with cervical cancer (types 16, 18, 31, 33, 35, 39, 45, 51, 52, 56, 58, 59, and 62). In March 2009, the FDA approved two new HPV DNA diagnostic tests: Cervista HPV HR, which detects 14 high-risk types of HPV (16, 18, 31, 33, 35, 39, 45, 51, 52, 56, 58, 59, 66, and 68), and Cervista HPV, which detects types 16 and 18. Both tests are approved for use with ThinPrep cervical specimens ("Get Ready for Changes," 2009). In women who are age 30 and older and have borderline cytology, the Cervista HPV 16/18 can be used with cytology and the Cervista HPV HR can be used to assess the risk of cervical disease. Such

TABLE 28-4 The 2001 Bethesda Categories of Epithelial Cell Abnormalities

ASC-US	Atypical squamous cells of undetermined significance
	This term is used when the squamous cells do not appear completely normal but it is not possible to determine the cause of the abnormal cells.
ASC-H	Atypical squamous cells—cannot exclude HSIL
LSIL	Low-grade squamous intraepithelial neoplasia
	Encompasses:
	HPV
	CIN 1 (mild dysplasia): lesion involves the initial 1/3 of the epithelial layer
HSIL	High-grade squamous intraepithelial neoplasia
	Encompasses:
	CIN 2 (moderate dysplasia): Lesion involves 1/3 to < 2/3 of the epithelial layer
	CIN 3 (severe dysplasia, carcinoma in situ): Lesion involves 2/3 to full thickness
Squamous carcinoma	Malignant cells penetrate basement membrane of cervical epithelium and infiltrate stromal tissue (supporting tissue)
	In advanced cases, cancer may spread to adjacent organs such as bladder or rectum, or to distant sites in the body via the blood stream and lymphatic channels.

Note: CIN = cervical intraepithelial neoplasia.

testing can identify which women need a colposcopy as soon as possible and which ones can be followed by repeat cytology and high-risk HPV testing in 12 months (see Figure 28-12 later in this chapter) (ASCCP, 2009).

High-risk HPV DNA testing and genotyping is not recommended in the following circumstances:

- Adolescents (women age 20 years and younger), regardless of their cytology results
- Routine screening
- Women considering vaccination against HPV
- Routine STI screening
- Women with atypical squamous cells of undetermined significance (ASC-US)
- Initial screening of women 30 years and older
- Women 21 years and older with atypical squamous cells cannot rule out high-grade lesion (ASC-H) ("Get Ready for Changes," 2009)

The American Society for Colposcopy provides guidelines for the appropriate use of the tests on its website (http://www.asccp.org/pdfs/consensus/clinical_update_20090408.pdf).

TABLE 28-5 The 2001 Bethesda System for Reporting Cervical Cytologic Diagnoses (Abridged)

Adequacy of Specimen

Satisfactory for evaluation (note presence or absence of endocervical or transformation zone components)

Unsatisfactory for evaluation (specify reason)

General Categorization (optional)

Negative for intraepithelial lesion or malignancy

Epithelial cell abnormality

Other

Interpretation/Result

Negative for intraepithelial lesion or malignancy

Include findings of the following:

- Trichomonas, bacterial, viral, and fungus infection
- Nonneoplastic findings including reactive cellular changes associated with inflammation, radiation, and IUD; glandular cells (posthysterectomy); and atrophy

Epithelial Cell Abnormalities

Squamous cell

- Atypical squamous cells (ASC) are divided into two categories:
  - ASC-US: Atypical squamous cells of undetermined significance
  - ASC-H: Cannot exclude high-grade squamous intraepithelial lesion
- Low-grade squamous intraepithelial lesion (LSIL)
  - Refers to cervical cancer precursors encompassing the following: human papillomavirus, mild dysplasia, and cervical intraepithelial neoplasia 1 (CIN 1)
- High-grade squamous intraepithelial lesion (HSIL)
  - Refers to cervical cancer precursors encompassing: moderate and severe dysplasia, carcinoma in situ, and cervical intraepithelial neoplasias 2 and 3 (CIN 2 and CIN 3)
- Squamous cell carcinoma

Glandular cell

- Atypical glandular cell (AGC)
  - Specify: Endocervical, Endometrial, or Not otherwise specified (NOS)
- Atypical glandular cells, favor neoplastic
  - Specify: Endocervical or Not otherwise specified
- Endocervical adenocarcinoma in situ (AIS)
- Adenocarcinoma

Other (List Is Not Comprehensive)

Endometrial cells in a woman 40 years or older

Sources: Adapted from Bethesda System, 2002; Solomon et al., 2002; Wilbur, Wright, & Young, 2002.

Further Testing Additional laboratory testing that might be indicated to rule out other causes of vaginal discharge or bleeding includes the following:

- *STI testing.* Chlamydia and gonorrhea are commonly encountered STIs that may produce symptoms similar to those of cervical cancer—namely, dysuria, urinary frequency, vaginal discharge, and postcoital bleeding. However, most women are asymptomatic with these STIs. Both infections can be tested using a single vaginal or cervical swab (Jarvis, 2008) (see Chapter 6).
- *Wet mount preparation.* Women who have vulvovaginal candidiasis, bacterial vaginosis, or trichomoniasis can present with a variety of symptoms, including vaginal discharge, malodor, irritation, burning or itching, dysuria, and dyspareunia. Accurate identification of the pathogen requires microscopic examination of vaginal secretions. The microscopic examinations include a saline wet mount and a potassium hydroxide (KOH) preparation (see Chapter 6).

Differential Diagnoses

Differential diagnoses for cervical cancer include the following conditions, which must be ruled out prior to diagnosing cancer: cervicitis or STI, vaginitis, and cervical polyps.

Management

Prevention The identification and treatment of early precancerous lesions is critical to the prevention of cervical cancer. Scheduling and keeping appointments for regular gynecologic examinations and Pap tests decreases the incidence and mortality of cervical cancer (NCI, 2008a). Abnormal changes in the cervix are readily detected by the Pap test and are easily cured before cancer develops. Preventive measures should include educating women that the risk of infection can be decreased by delaying the onset of sexual activity, decreasing the number of sexual partners, using condoms consistently, and eliminating tobacco use.

Definitive Treatment The choice of treatment depends primarily on the stage of disease at the time of diagnosis, but other factors, such as a woman's general health and preferences, should also be considered. Treatment of precancerous lesions and CIS may include removal of the lesion by cryosurgery, laser ablation, loop electrosurgical excision procedure (LEEP), or conization (NCI, 2008c). After treatment, patients require lifelong surveillance at regular intervals. The clinician determines the timing and frequency of follow-up based on Pap test results and colposcopy examinations (NCI).

Treatment of advanced cervical cancer includes surgery, radiation therapy, and chemotherapy. Usually two or more approaches are used. Surgery can include simple or radical hysterectomy with pelvic lymph node dissection, or pelvic exenteration (removal of all pelvic organs including the bladder, rectum, vulva, and vagina). Radiation therapy can involve external beam or intracavitary irradiation. Radiation is often combined with chemotherapy. Recent clinical trial results suggest a combination of radiation therapy and chemotherapy with cisplatin is more effective than radiation alone (Garcia, 2007; NCI, 2008c). The treatment of disseminated cervical cancer is primarily palliative, because cure is not possible. Palliative radiation may be used to control bleeding, pelvic pain, or urinary or bowel obstruction from pelvic disease (Garcia).

Referral Abnormal Pap test results may require a referral for colposcopic examination. The American Society for Colposcopy and Cervical Pathology (ASCCP, 2006) provides algorithms for the management of women with cervical cytologic abnormalities. Algorithms are shown in **Figures 28-2 through 28-12**.

New and Emerging Evidence for Practice

HPV Vaccines In June 2006, the FDA approved the quadrivalent HPV vaccine, Gardasil (manufactured by Merck), which protects against the four types of HPV (6, 11, 16, and 18) that cause the majority of genital warts and cervical cancers. Gardasil is not a live vaccine, so it does not pose risks to individuals who are immunocompromised (Widener, 2008). The vaccine, which was originally licensed for use in females aged 9 to 26, was approved by the FDA in 2009 for use in males aged 9 to 26. The vaccine has proved to be effective for as long as 5 years, but it is unknown whether a booster after 5 years is necessary to extend the protective effect (Widener).

The HPV vaccine is delivered through a series of three intramuscular injections over a 6-month period (0 months, 2 months, and 6 months). If a dose is missed, the series should be continued, not started over (Widener, 2008). It is critical to impress upon patients and their caregivers the importance of receiving all doses. As with all vaccines delivered intramuscularly, mild to moderate swelling may occur at the injection site. Because of the risk of anaphylaxis, the patient should be observed for at least 15 minutes after receiving the vaccination.

Clinical trials in females (age 16 to 26) have demonstrated that Gardasil has 100% efficacy in preventing cervical precancers caused by HPV types 16 and 18. The vaccine has also been found to be almost 100% effective in preventing genital warts. Ideally, the vaccine would be administered before the onset of sexual activity, but females who are sexually active may also benefit from vaccination. Those who have not been infected with any HPV type prevented by the vaccine would receive the full benefit of vaccination. Those who have already been infected with one or more HPV types would still get protection from the vaccine types they have not yet acquired. Women who receive the vaccine will still need regular cervical cancer screening, because the vaccine does not provide protection against all HPV types that cause cervical cancer (CDC, 2006, 2007).

The cost for the three-dose Gardasil series is approximately $360. Although many insurers cover the cost, some do not; also, many women do not have health insurance. Thus this vaccine is inaccessible to many women; a patient rebate program is available.

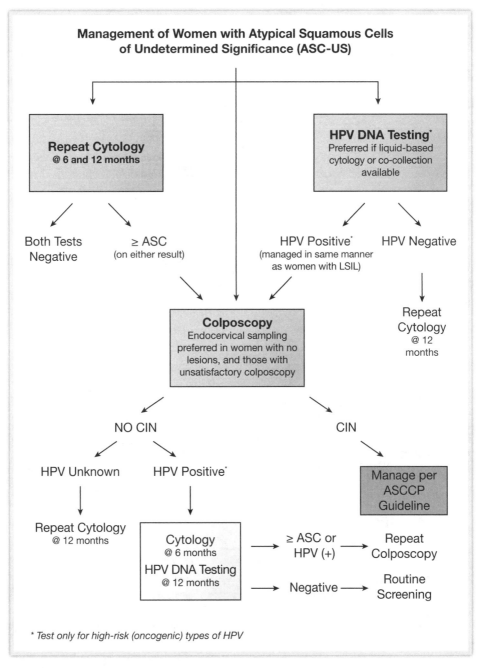

FIGURE 28-2 Management of women with atypical squamous cells of undetermined significance (ASC-US).

Source: American Society for Colposcopy and Cervical Pathology. (2007). The Consensus Guidelines algorithms are reprinted from *The Journal of Lower Genital Tract Disease*, Vol. 11, Issue 4, with permission of ASCCP. Copyright © American Society for Colposcopy and Cervical Pathology.

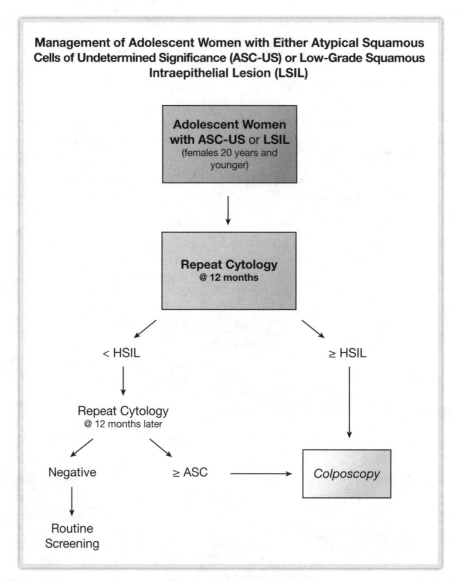

FIGURE 28-3 Management of adolescent women with either atypical squamous cells of undetermined significance (ASC-US) or low-grade squamous intraepithelial lesion (LSIL).

Source: American Society for Colposcopy and Cervical Pathology. (2007). The Consensus Guidelines algorithms are reprinted from *The Journal of Lower Genital Tract Disease*, Vol. 11, Issue 4, with permission of ASCCP. Copyright © American Society for Colposcopy and Cervical Pathology.

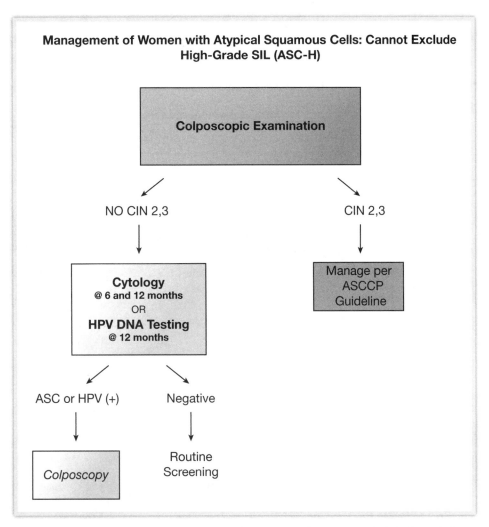

FIGURE 28-4 Management of women with atypical squamous cells: Cannot exclude high-grade SIL (ASC-H).

Source: American Society for Colposcopy and Cervical Pathology. (2007). The Consensus Guidelines algorithms are reprinted from *The Journal of Lower Genital Tract Disease*, Vol. 11, Issue 4, with permission of ASCCP. Copyright © American Society for Colposcopy and Cervical Pathology.

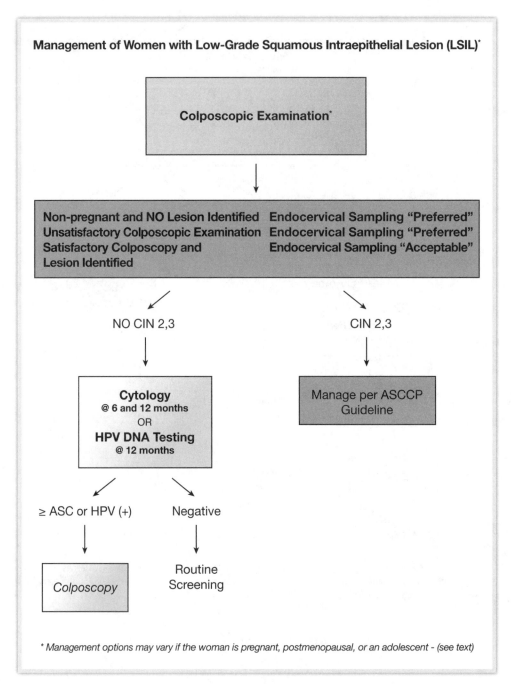

FIGURE 28-5 Management of women with low-grade squamous intraepithelial lesion (LSIL).

Source: American Society for Colposcopy and Cervical Pathology. (2007). The Consensus Guidelines algorithms are reprinted from *The Journal of Lower Genital Tract Disease*, Vol. 11, Issue 4, with permission of ASCCP. Copyright © American Society for Colposcopy and Cervical Pathology.

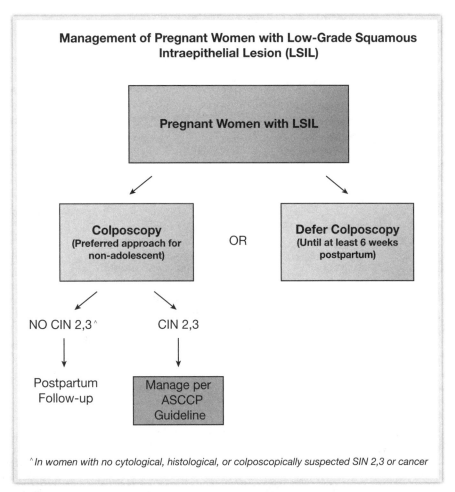

FIGURE 28-6 Management of pregnant women with low-grade squamous intraepithelial lesion (LSIL).

Source: American Society for Colposcopy and Cervical Pathology. (2007). The Consensus Guidelines algorithms are reprinted from *The Journal of Lower Genital Tract Disease*, Vol. 11, Issue 4, with permission of ASCCP. Copyright © American Society for Colposcopy and Cervical Pathology.

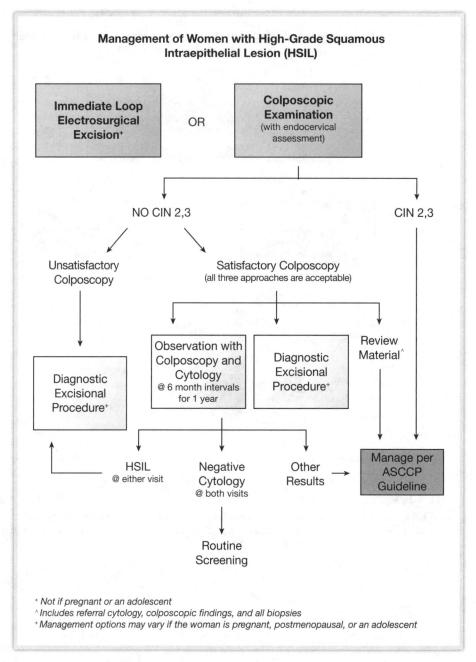

Management of Women with High-Grade Squamous Intraepithelial Lesion (HSIL)

Immediate Loop Electrosurgical Excision⁺ OR **Colposcopic Examination** (with endocervical assessment)

NO CIN 2,3 — CIN 2,3

Unsatisfactory Colposcopy

Satisfactory Colposcopy (all three approaches are acceptable)

Diagnostic Excisional Procedure⁺

Observation with Colposcopy and Cytology @ 6 month intervals for 1 year

Diagnostic Excisional Procedure⁺

Review Material^

HSIL @ either visit

Negative Cytology @ both visits

Other Results

Manage per ASCCP Guideline

Routine Screening

⁺ Not if pregnant or an adolescent
^ Includes referral cytology, colposcopic findings, and all biopsies
⁺ Management options may vary if the woman is pregnant, postmenopausal, or an adolescent

FIGURE 28-7 Management of women with high-grade squamous intraepithelial lesion (HSIL).

Source: American Society for Colposcopy and Cervical Pathology. (2007). The Consensus Guidelines algorithms are reprinted from *The Journal of Lower Genital Tract Disease*, Vol. 11, Issue 4, with permission of ASCCP. Copyright © American Society for Colposcopy and Cervical Pathology.

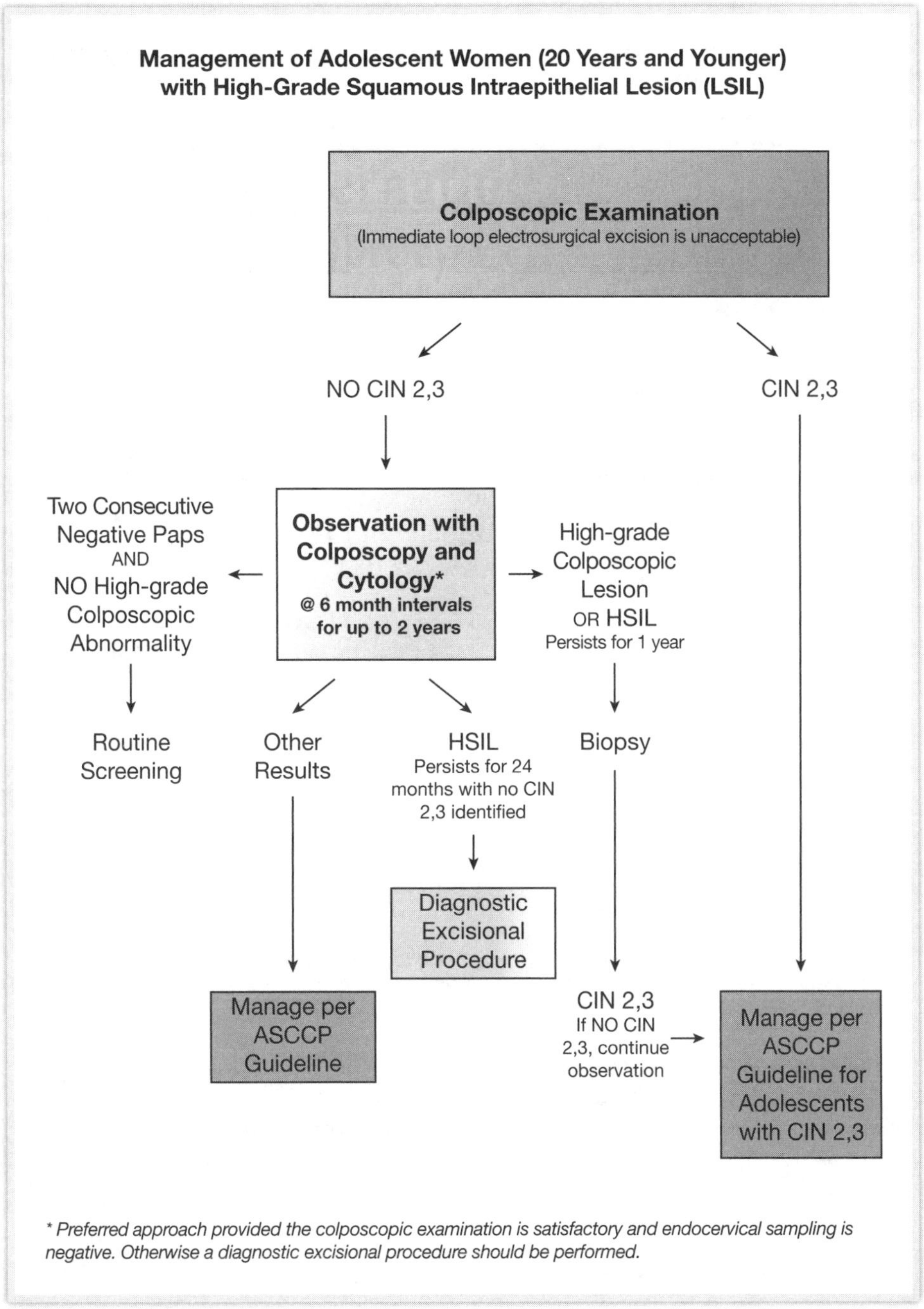

Management of Adolescent Women (20 Years and Younger) with High-Grade Squamous Intraepithelial Lesion (LSIL)

Colposcopic Examination
(Immediate loop electrosurgical excision is unacceptable)

NO CIN 2,3   CIN 2,3

Two Consecutive Negative Paps AND NO High-grade Colposcopic Abnormality

Observation with Colposcopy and Cytology* @ 6 month intervals for up to 2 years

High-grade Colposcopic Lesion OR HSIL Persists for 1 year

Routine Screening

Other Results

HSIL Persists for 24 months with no CIN 2,3 identified

Biopsy

Diagnostic Excisional Procedure

Manage per ASCCP Guideline

CIN 2,3 If NO CIN 2,3, continue observation

Manage per ASCCP Guideline for Adolescents with CIN 2,3

* Preferred approach provided the colposcopic examination is satisfactory and endocervical sampling is negative. Otherwise a diagnostic excisional procedure should be performed.

FIGURE 28-8 Management of adolescent women (20 years and younger) with high-grade squamous intraepithelial lesion (HSIL).

Source: American Society for Colposcopy and Cervical Pathology. (2007). The Consensus Guidelines algorithms are reprinted from *The Journal of Lower Genital Tract Disease*, Vol. 11, Issue 4, with permission of ASCCP. Copyright © American Society for Colposcopy and Cervical Pathology.

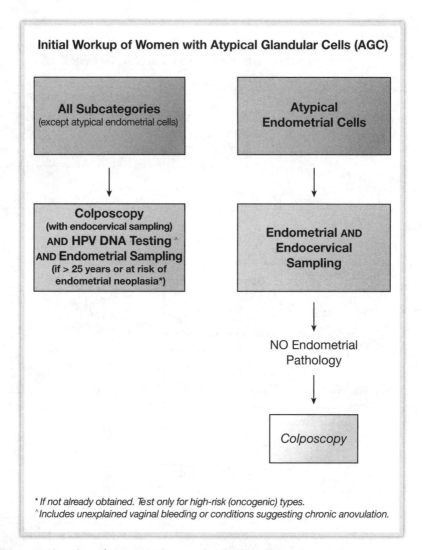

Initial Workup of Women with Atypical Glandular Cells (AGC)

All Subcategories
(except atypical endometrial cells)

Atypical Endometrial Cells

Colposcopy
(with endocervical sampling)
AND **HPV DNA Testing** ^
AND **Endometrial Sampling**
(if > 25 years or at risk of
endometrial neoplasia*)

Endometrial AND Endocervical Sampling

NO Endometrial Pathology

Colposcopy

* If not already obtained. Test only for high-risk (oncogenic) types.
^ Includes unexplained vaginal bleeding or conditions suggesting chronic anovulation.

FIGURE 28-9 Initial workup of women with atypical glandular cells (AGC).

Source: American Society for Colposcopy and Cervical Pathology. (2007). The Consensus Guidelines algorithms are reprinted from *The Journal of Lower Genital Tract Disease*, Vol. 11, Issue 4, with permission of ASCCP. Copyright © American Society for Colposcopy and Cervical Pathology.

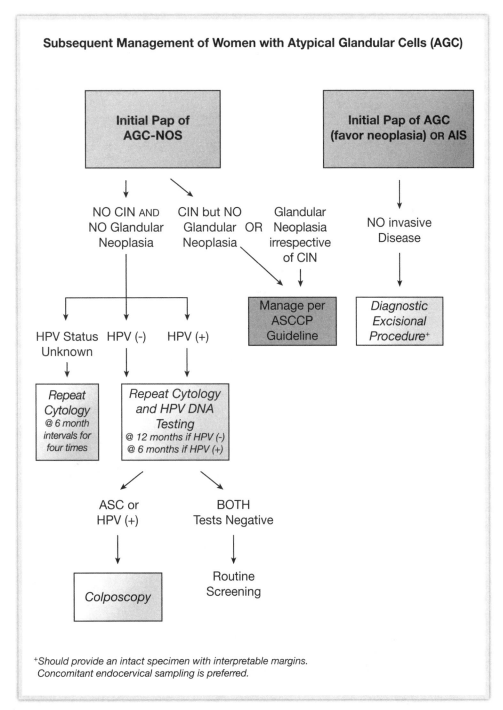

FIGURE 28-10 Subsequent management of women with atypical glandular cells (AGC).

Source: American Society for Colposcopy and Cervical Pathology. (2007). The Consensus Guidelines algorithms are reprinted from *The Journal of Lower Genital Tract Disease*, Vol. 11, Issue 4, with permission of ASCCP. Copyright © American Society for Colposcopy and Cervical Pathology.

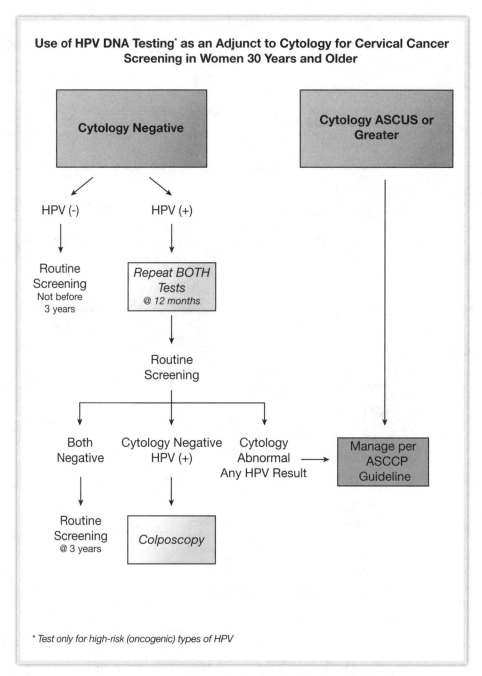

FIGURE 28-11 Use of HPV DNA testing* as an adjunct to cytology for cervical cancer screening in women 30 years and older.

Source: American Society for Colposcopy and Cervical Pathology. (2007). The Consensus Guidelines algorithms are reprinted from *The Journal of Lower Genital Tract Disease*, Vol. 11, Issue 4, with permission of ASCCP. Copyright © American Society for Colposcopy and Cervical Pathology.

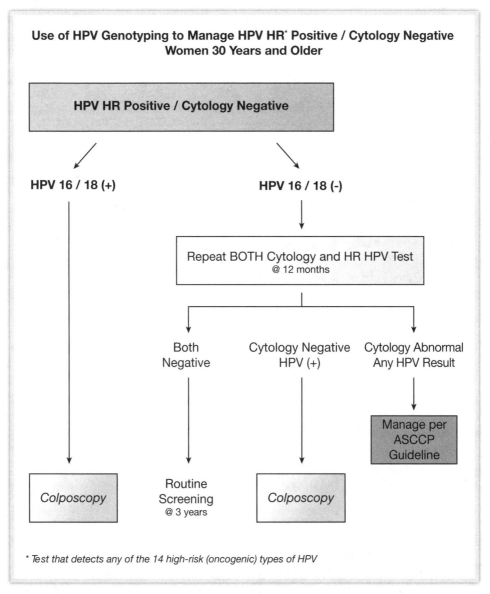

FIGURE 28-12 Use of HPV genotyping to manage HPV HR positive/cytology negative women 30 years and older.

Source: Copyright © 2004, 2009 American Society for Colposcopy and Cervical Pathology. All rights reserved.

A new HPV vaccine, Cervarix (manufactured by GlaxoSmithKline), was approved by the FDA in October 2009 for use in females. Initial studies of this vaccine, which also targets HPV types 16 and 18, have shown that Cervarix protects against persistent infection with these two HPV types and may also confer some protection against very closely related HPV types (31, 45, and 52). Together with HPV types 16 and 18, these types are collectively responsible for more than 80% of cervical cancer cases (NCI, n.d.). Cervarix is also administered by intramuscular injection in a three-dose series at 0, 1, and 6 months (Keam & Harper, 2008).

As a result of the approval of Gardasil and Cervarix, new guidelines for prophylactic vaccination for HPV and cervical cancer have been developed (see Chapter 21).

Other Vaccines   Researchers are also working to develop a vaccine targeted against a minor surface protein of HPV, known as L2, which contains regions that induce neutralizing antibodies against a broad range of HPV types. This property means that a single vaccine targeting the L2 protein may have the potential to provide broad protection against many HPV types. Other vaccine studies are targeting two HPV oncogenic proteins, E6 and E7, which play important roles in inducing and maintaining cellular transformation (NCI, n.d.).

Special Considerations

Adolescent Women   Adolescent women (aged 19 and younger) have a high prevalence of HPV infections with more minor-grade cytologic abnormalities (ASC-US and low-grade squamous intraepithelial lesion [LSIL]) but are at very low risk for invasive cervical cancer compared with older women. The vast majority of HPV infections clear spontaneously within 2 years and have little long-term significance. Thus performing colposcopy is discouraged because it can potentially result in harm through unnecessary treatment. However, colposcopy is recommended for adolescents with high-grade squamous intraepithelial lesion (HSIL) (Wright et al., 2005).

Pregnant Women   No treatment is warranted for preinvasive lesions of the cervix during pregnancy, although expert colposcopy is recommended to exclude invasive cervical cancer. Treatment of invasive cervical cancer depends on the stage of the cancer and gestational age at diagnosis. When the cancer is diagnosed before fetal maturity, the traditional approach is to recommend immediate therapy appropriate for the stage of disease. Other reports suggest that if the cancer is in the early stages, delaying therapy may be a reasonable option to allow for improved fetal viability (NCI, 2008c). Most experts advocate a cesarean birth because of the risk of disease recurrence with vaginal birth (NCI; Sood et al., 2000).

Talking with the Patient   Many women associate precancerous lesions detected by a Pap test with a diagnosis of cancer. Clinicians should clarify any misperceptions and emphasize the importance of treating these early lesions to prevent the development of cancer. Treatment protocols should be reviewed with the patient. The clinician should address

STI-prevention strategies and provide guidelines for safer sexual practices. Counseling should include information about the association between HPV infection and cervical cancer. Women should be encouraged to reduce their risk of HPV exposure by delaying the onset of sexual activity, decreasing their number of sexual partners, and eliminating tobacco products. Condom use should be encouraged, especially with new, multiple, and nonmonogamous partners.

Endometrial Cancer

Scope of the Problem

Carcinoma of the endometrium is the most prevalent gynecologic malignancy and is the fourth most common malignant neoplasm in women, after breast, lung, and colon cancers (ACS, 2008a). Approximately 40,100 new cases of endometrial cancer and 7,470 endometrial cancer deaths were estimated to occur in 2008 in the United States (ACS). The incidence of endometrial cancer is higher in white women than in black women, but the mortality rate in black women is nearly twice as high as that in white women. A major factor explaining the increased mortality rate in black women is the significant occurrence of higher-grade and more aggressive histologies in this population (NCI, 2008d). Five-year survival rates for localized, regional, and metastatic disease are 95%, 67%, and 23%, respectively (ACS).

Etiology and Pathophysiology

Endometrial cancer is classified into three types. Type I, or estrogen-dependent endometrial cancer, is the most common type (80% of cases). It is caused by an excess of endogenous or exogenous estrogen, unopposed by progesterone. Long-term unopposed estrogen exposure allows for continued endometrial growth, and the development of hyperplasia with or without atypia. The resulting tumors are usually low grade and have a favorable prognosis. Type I cancers commonly occur in women who are younger, obese, and perimenopausal (American College of Obstetricians and Gynecologists, 2005, reaffirmed 2011; Sorosky, 2008).

Type II endometrial cancer accounts for approximately 10% of cases and is unrelated to estrogen or endometrial hyperplasia. The endometrium is generally atrophic or has polyps. These neoplasms occur spontaneously and tend to present with higher-grade tumors or poor prognostic cell types, such as papillary serous or clear cell tumors. These patients are often multiparous and normal weight. Type II cancers tend to occur in women who are older and postmenopausal, and are more common in African American women (American College of Obstetricians and Gynecologists, 2005, reaffirmed 2011; Sorosky, 2008).

Finally, familial endometrial carcinoma is a hereditary form of the disorder that accounts for as many as 10% of cases, of which 5% are associated with Lynch II syndrome, also known as hereditary nonpolyposis colorectal cancer (HNPCC). While endometrial cancer is the most common cancer seen in association with HNPCC (40% to 60% lifetime risk), other malignancies may also occur (e.g., ovarian cancer). HNPCC is an autosomal dominant condition characterized by germline mutations in any one of six genes located on chromosomes 2, 3, and 7. Although it may produce a neoplasm of any grade or histology, as many as 35% of endometrial cancers in this syndrome are associated with high-grade tumors (American College of Obstetricians and Gynecologists, 2005, reaffirmed 2011; Sorosky, 2008).

While the exact cause of endometrial cancer is not known, the current understanding of risk factors helps to identify women at risk for type I endometrial cancer due to estrogen excess. Risk factors associated with exogenous sources of estrogen include the following:

- *Estrogen therapy (ET).* For women with a uterus, the risk of endometrial cancer associated with unopposed estrogen use for 5 or more years is more than 10-fold higher compared with women not taking ET. However, adding progestogen therapy to estrogen eliminates the risk of endometrial cancer (NCI, 2008d; Sorosky, 2008).
- *Tamoxifen (Nolvadex).* Tamoxifen, when used for chemoprevention of breast cancer, increases the risk of endometrial cancer nearly threefold (Sorosky, 2008). A selective estrogen receptor modulator (SERM), Tamoxifen has site-specific activity in different tissues. It suppresses growth in breast tissue, but stimulates the growth of the endometrial lining (NCI, 2008d; Sorosky, 2008).

Risk factors associated with endogenous sources of estrogen include the following:

- *Early menarche.* Starting menstruation before the age of 12 years increases the number of years the endometrium is exposed to estrogen (ACS, 2008c; Winter & Gosewehr, 2006).
- *Late menopause.* Menopause occurring after the age of 52 increases the duration of estrogen exposure (ACS, 2008c; Winter & Gosewehr, 2006).
- *History of infertility or nulliparity.* During pregnancy, the hormonal balance shifts toward more progesterone, which protects the uterus. As a consequence, women who have had many pregnancies have a reduced risk of developing endometrial cancer, and women who are infertile or who have never been pregnant have an increased risk (ACS, 2008c).
- *Obesity.* The majority of women who develop endometrial cancer tend to be obese. Women who are 30 pounds over ideal weight have a 3-fold increased risk of developing endometrial cancer, whereas those who are 50 pounds or more over ideal weight have a 10-fold increased risk (Porth, 2007; Winter & Gosewehr, 2006). Women who are obese have higher levels of endogenous estrogen as a result of the conversion of androstenedione to estrone and the aromatization of androgens to estradiol, both of which occur in peripheral adipose tissue (ACS, 2008c; Sorosky, 2008; Winter & Gosewehr, 2006).
- *Chronic anovulation.* Anovulation is a common cause of infertility and may be caused by several factors. However, one of the leading causes of chronic anovulation is polycystic ovary syndrome (PCOS; see Chapter 26). Women with PCOS have excess androgens and elevated luteinizing hormone (LH) and normal or low follicle-stimulating hormone (FSH) levels. Patients may also have elevated levels of free estrogen, owing to the peripheral conversion of androgens to estrogens and the decreased production of sex hormone-binding globulin (SHBG) in the liver, which serves to increase the unopposed effects of estrogen over time (ACS, 2008c; Marrinan, 2007).

- *Diabetes.* Diabetes is associated with twofold to threefold increased incidence of endo-metrial cancer that appears to be related to obesity (ACS, 2008c; Sorosky, 2008).
- *High-fat diet.* Consumption of a high-fat diet may lead to obesity, and obesity is a well-documented risk factor for endometrial cancer. Some researchers believe that fatty foods may also have a direct effect on estrogen metabolism, thereby increasing the risk for endometrial cancer (ACS, 2008c; Winter & Gosewehr, 2006).
- *Ovarian cancer.* Certain ovarian tumors, such as granulosa theca cell tumors, produce estrogen, thereby increasing a woman's risk of developing endometrial cancer (ACS, 2008c).

The most common endometrial cancer cell type is endometrioid adenocarcinoma, which constitutes 75% to 80% of endometrial carcinoma cases (NCI, 2008f). Adenocarci-nomas arise from glandular epithelial cells of the endometrium. Less common types include the following: papillary serous carcinoma (less than 10%), mixed (10%), clear cell carcinoma (4% to 5%), mucinous (1%), and squamous cell (less than 1%) (NCI). Both papillary serous and clear cell carcinomas tend to be more aggressive than endometrial adenocarcinoma and tend to be detected at advanced stages (NCI; Sorosky, 2008).

Clinical Presentation

Endometrial cancer occurs most frequently in postmenopausal women. The average age at diagnosis is approximately 61 years, with most patients being diagnosed between the ages of 50 and 60. Women diagnosed with endometrial cancer at an age younger than 40 account for only 5% of the total number of cases. These women usually have specific risk factors such as morbid obesity, chronic anovulation, and hereditary syndromes. The most common symptom, present in 90% of women, is abnormal uterine bleeding. In women who are menstruating, this symptom can take the form of bleeding between periods or excessive, prolonged menstrual flow. In postmenopausal women, any bleeding is abnormal and should be evaluated (Porth, 2007; Sorosky, 2008; Winter & Gosewehr, 2006).

Assessment

History Key pieces of information that assist the clinician in identifying women at high risk for endometrial cancer include the character of the bleeding, the pattern of the flow, and the number of pads used when bleeding occurs. Inquire about accompanying problems (e.g., dyspareunia, pain, bladder or bowel problems); ask the woman if she is experiencing any unusual vaginal discharge or if she has ever been diagnosed with an STI. Obtain a menstrual history (see Chapter 6) and inquire if the woman is taking any hormones. Ask about the possibility of pregnancy and whether she has experienced any symptoms of pregnancy (e.g., missed period, breast tenderness, or nausea and vomiting). If she has previously been preg-nant, obtain a pregnancy history in addition to medical and family histories (see Chapter 6). Be sure to ask the woman if she has a personal or family history of breast, ovarian, or colon cancer. Ask her if she has experienced infertility problems or if she has a history of PCOS (Dains, Baumann, & Scheibel, 2003; Jarvis, 2008).

Physical Examination The physical examination should include a thorough abdominal, inguinal lymph node, pelvic, vaginal, and rectal examination. Abnormal bleeding from the genital tract can occur from the vagina, cervix, uterus, or fallopian tubes. Inspect the external genitalia for lesions or atrophic vaginitis, which may be the cause of the bleeding. Perform a vaginal examination to determine whether the bleeding is caused by vaginal or cervical infection. Note the amount, color, consistency, and odor of the vaginal discharge; determine whether the cervix is friable or has an unusual discharge; and examine the patient for cervical polyps.

Perform a bimanual examination. Palpate the cervix, which normally feels smooth, firm, evenly rounded, and mobile. Note any cervical motion tenderness. Next palpate the uterus, ovaries, and inguinal lymph nodes. Note uterine size and contour. Endometrial cancer seldom causes much uterine enlargement, and any increase in size usually occurs slowly. Uterine fibroids usually feel firm and may make the uterus asymmetrical. Note any enlargement of the ovaries and lymph nodes. Lastly, perform a rectal examination to identify lesions or other abnormalities.

Metastatic spread of endometrial cancer occurs in a characteristic pattern, which is commonly to the pelvic and para-aortic nodes. Common sites for distant metastasis include the lungs, inguinal and supraclavicular lymph nodes, liver, bones, brain, and vagina (Dains et al., 2003; Jarvis, 2008).

Screening Tests There is no screening test currently available to detect endometrial cancer. In particular, a Pap test is not effective in detecting endometrial cancer. Nevertheless, the finding of atypical glandular cells in a postmenopausal woman is strongly suggestive of uterine malignancy. If endometrial cancer is suspected or if a woman is at high risk for its development, a gynecologist or gynecologic oncologist should be consulted immediately (ACS, 2008c; Winter & Gosewehr, 2006).

Endometrial Biopsy Endometrial biopsy is an office procedure that is generally accepted as the first step in the diagnosis of endometrial cancer in the patient with postmenopausal bleeding. The biopsy is obtained through the use of an endometrial suction catheter that is inserted through the cervix into the uterine cavity. Endometrial biopsy detects 80% to 90% of endometrial cancers if an adequate tissue sample is obtained. However, if the biopsy result fails to provide sufficient diagnostic information or if abnormal bleeding persists, a dilation and curettage (D & C) with or without a hysteroscopy is recommended (NCI, 2008e; Winter & Gosewehr, 2006).

Transvaginal Ultrasound Transvaginal ultrasound is used as an adjunctive means of evaluation for endometrial hyperplasia as well as polyps, myomas, and structural abnormalities of the uterus. An endometrial thickness of greater than 5 mm in a menopausal women is considered an indication for further evaluation (NCI, 2008e; Sorosky, 2008; Winter & Gosewehr, 2006).

Dilatation and Curettage Dilatation and curettage is the gold standard for assessing uterine bleeding and diagnosing endometrial cancer. If endometrial biopsy findings are negative or inadequate, if the endometrial thickness by transvaginal ultrasound is greater than 5 mm, or if a high degree of suspicion exists, the patient needs a D & C under anesthesia to exclude malignancy (NCI, 2008e; Sorosky, 2008; Winter & Gosewehr, 2006).

Hysteroscopy Hysteroscopy is used in the office setting to directly visualize the uterine cavity. In conjunction with the D & C, hysteroscopy is a helpful tool in providing a diagnosis for abnormal bleeding and guiding directed biopsies of suspicious area. However, concern exists regarding transtubal intraperitoneal expulsion of cancer cells (NCI, 2008e; Winter & Gosewehr, 2006).

Differential Diagnosis

Differential diagnosis of genital bleeding depends on the clinical picture. Bleeding from the lower genital tract can occur from the vagina (carcinoma, lacerations, trauma, or infections) or the cervix (cervicitis, STIs, polyps, or cervical carcinoma). It may also occur from the uterus (carcinoma, fibroids, polyps, pregnancy, or dysfunctional uterine bleeding) or the fallopian tubes (pelvic inflammatory disease [PID], ectopic pregnancy) (Beckman et al., 2006; Collins, 2003).

Management

Prevention Although most cases of endometrial cancer cannot be prevented, several factors are associated with a decreased incidence of endometrial cancer:

- *Combined oral contraceptives (COCs).* The risk of endometrial hyperplasia is increased by the presence of unopposed estrogen. Thus using a COC instead of an estrogen-only contraceptive prevents the proliferative effect of estrogen, thereby decreasing the risk of developing abnormal endometrial hyperplasia resulting in endometrial cancer (Marsden & Sturdee, 2009). The chance of developing endometrial cancer due to unopposed estrogen is both risk and duration related, and it remains increased for years after stopping unopposed estrogen (Paganini-Hill, Ross, & Henderson, 1989). These effects are ameliorated by adding progestogens in the correct dose and duration (Marsden & Sturdee, 2009).
- *Physical activity.* Studies investigating the relationship between physical activity and the risk of endometrial cancer have shown a weak to moderate inverse relationship between the two (Linkov et al., 2008; NCI, 2008d). It is believed that physical activity modifies the risk of endometrial cancer by reducing obesity, a known risk factor for endometrial cancer (NCI).
- *Low-fat diet.* A number of observational studies have demonstrated that consumption of a diet low in saturated fats and high in fruits and vegetables intake is associated with reduced risk of developing endometrial cancer (NCI, 2008d). However, a prospective study of a cohort of postmenopausal women with a case-cohort analysis reported that energy intake was not strongly related to risk (Zheng et al., 1995).

- *Controlling other risk factors.* Women with PCOS need appropriate treatment to avoid the effect of unopposed estrogen on the uterus. Menopausal women with an intact uterus should avoid using unopposed estrogen to relieve menopausal symptoms. Women with a history of breast or ovarian cancer or HNPCC need to be closely monitored for endometrial cancer. The American Cancer Society recommends that women with or at increased risk for HNPCC should be offered annual testing for endometrial cancer with endometrial biopsy beginning at the age of 35 years. These women should also be counseled about preventive measures such as the option of prophylactic hysterectomy with bilateral salpingo-oophorectomy at the completion of childbearing (ACS, 2008c; Sorosky, 2008).

Definitive Treatment   The choice of treatment for endometrial cancer depends primarily on the type and stage of the disease, the level of differentiation, the woman's overall health, and her personal preferences. Treatment options for endometrial cancer include hysterectomy, radiation therapy, and hormonal therapy. Chemotherapy may be used in recurrent or advanced cases of endometrial cancer, although there are no standard chemotherapy programs for patients with metastatic disease. Treatment options with single-agent and combination drugs are currently under clinical investigation (NCI, 2008f; Winter & Gosewehr, 2006).

Surgery   The recommended surgery is a total abdominal hysterectomy with bilateral salpingo-oophorectomy. Patients with localized disease are usually cured with surgery alone. In contrast, patients with myometrial invasion are usually treated with a combination of surgery and adjuvant radiation therapy. Lymph node sampling may be done at the same time as surgery. Recovery usually takes 4 to 6 weeks (ACS, 2008c; NCI, 2008f; Winter & Gosewehr, 2006).

Radiation Therapy   Radiation treatments may be given externally (external beam radiation), via an intracavitary method (brachytherapy), or both. Diarrhea and fatigue are common side effects of radiation therapy. Pelvic radiation may also cause vaginal stenosis (narrowing of the vagina from scar tissue), which may make vaginal intercourse painful. The use of a vaginal dilator or having vaginal intercourse several times per week helps prevent scar tissue formation. Use of vaginal lubricants may also be helpful (ACS, 2008c; NCI, 2008f; Sorosky, 2008; Winter & Gosewehr, 2006).

Hormone Therapy   Patients who are not candidates for surgery or radiation, or who have advanced disease, are treated with hormonal therapy. The hormonal agents most commonly used for this purpose are progestational drugs such as hydroxyprogesterone (Delalutin), medroxyprogesterone (Provera), and megestrol (Megace). Response to hormones reflects the presence and level of hormone receptors and the degree of tumor differentiation (NCI, 2008f).

Follow-Up   An important part of the treatment plan is a specific schedule of follow-up visits after surgery, chemotherapy, or radiation therapy. Follow-up visits are scheduled every 3 to 4 months during the first 3 years and then usually twice yearly. Approximately 75% to 85%

of recurrences are found within the first 3 years (ACS, 2008c; American College of Obstetricians and Gynecologists, 2005; reaffirmed 2011, Winter & Gosewehr, 2006). An examination of the abdomen and inguinal lymph nodes, along with speculum and rectovaginal examinations, should be done at each visit. History questions should focus on symptoms that might indicate cancer recurrence, because most recurrences are discovered during evaluation of symptomatic patients. If the patient's symptoms or physical examination results suggest recurrent cancer, imaging tests such as a CT scan, ultrasound, CA-125 blood test, or biopsies should be ordered. Conversely, if no symptoms or physical examination abnormalities are identified, routine blood tests and imaging tests are not recommended (ACS, 2008c; Sorosky, 2008; Winter & Gosewehr, 2006).

Ovarian Cancer

Scope of the Problem

Ovarian cancer has the highest mortality rate of all gynecologic cancers and is the fifth leading cause of all cancer deaths among women. Approximately 21,650 new cases of ovarian cancer were diagnosed in the United States in 2008 (Jemal et al., 2008). Advancing age is a significant risk factor in the development of ovarian cancer, with the risk increasing at menopause. The average age of women in the United States who are diagnosed with ovarian cancer is 63 years (NCI, 2004d), although primary diagnoses of ovarian cancer occur most commonly in women who are 40 to 70 years of age. African American women have a lower lifetime risk of ovarian cancer than Caucasian women, but the 5-year survival rates are similar in both groups (ACS, 2008a).

The prognosis for most women with ovarian cancer remains poor, primarily because early diagnosis of the disease is infrequent (Berek, 2002; NCI, 2004d). The 5-year survival rates have improved only slightly with advances in surgery and chemotherapy. If the disease is confined to the ovary (Stage I) at the time of diagnosis, 5-year survival rates approach 95%; however, only 25% of women have localized disease at the time of their diagnosis. The overall 5-year survival rate for ovarian cancers is less than 50% (NCI). Clinical and technological advances in early detection are urgently needed to decrease the morbidity and mortality associated with this disease.

Etiology and Pathophysiology

Epithelial ovarian carcinomas are the most common type of ovarian cancer and account for approximately 90% of diagnoses. The majority of these cases occur in postmenopausal women (Ozols, Schwartz, & Eifel, 2001).

Epithelial ovarian cancers arise from the epithelial lining of the ovary. As the ovary enlarges with tumor growth, cells from the surface of the ovary are shed into the peritoneal cavity, where they are implanted on the peritoneal surface and omentum and become small tumor sites (Ozols et al., 2001). Invasive spread to the regional para-aortic and pelvic lymph nodes, bowel, and bladder, accompanied by ascites with peritoneal seeding of the liver surface, diaphragm, bladder, and intestines, is common (Ozols et al.).

Epithelial ovarian cancer can be further subdivided into the following histologic subtypes: serous or mucinous (the two most common cell types), endometrioid, clear cell, transitional, or undifferentiated carcinomas (NCI, 2004a). Epithelial tumors of low-malignancy potential (borderline ovarian carcinoma) are usually found in younger women and are often confined to the ovary at diagnosis (Ozols et al., 2001). Germ cell and sex cord-stromal tumors account for 5% of all ovarian cancers (NCI, 2003a; Ozols et al., 2001).

Risk Factors

The most important risk factor for ovarian cancer is a family history in a first-degree relative. Women who have a first- or second-degree relative with ovarian cancer are approximately three times more likely to develop ovarian cancer than those who do not (Ozols et al., 2001). When a woman carries the BRCA1 or BRCA2 genetic mutation, her hereditary ovarian cancer risk is increased to as high as 50%. She is also at significantly increased risk for developing breast cancer (Berek, 2002; NCI, 2004a; Ozols et al.). Nevertheless, it is estimated that only 5% to 10% of all ovarian cancers are hereditary (NCI, 2004b; Ozols et al.).

Age is also a significant risk factor in the development of ovarian cancer (Luce, Hassey Dow, & Holcomb, 2003; O'Rourke & Mahon, 2003). The risk of ovarian cancer increases with age, and half of all ovarian cancers are diagnosed in women older than the age of 63 (ACS, 2008a).

Women who have never been pregnant have a slightly higher risk of developing ovarian cancer than women who have gone through at least one full-term pregnancy. This risk continues to decline with each additional pregnancy and breastfeeding. In contrast, the age at menarche and menopause, and the woman's age at the time of her first live birth, appear to be unrelated to the risk of developing ovarian cancer (NCI, 2004d).

Three often suggested, but as yet unproven, risk factors for the development of ovarian cancer are body weight, use of talcum powder, and hormone therapy. The relationship between body weight and the development of ovarian cancer remains unclear. Presently there is no clearly identified relationship between increasing body weight and risk of ovarian cancer (O'Rourke & Mahon, 2003). The use of talcum powder has been suggested as a possible risk factor in the development of ovarian cancer because of its similarity to asbestos; however, studies demonstrate talcum powder use for more than 20 years confers no increased risk (Huncharek, Geschwind, & Kupelnick, 2003; O'Rourke & Mahon). Studies evaluating the relationship between hormone therapy and the risk for ovarian cancer also have yielded inconsistent results (O'Rourke & Mahon). Prolonged hormonal estrogen therapy in postmenopausal women may be associated with an increased risk of developing ovarian cancer (NCI, 2008c).

Women who have used fertility drugs have also been suggested to be at an increased risk for ovarian cancer; however, an NCI study of 12,000 women found no association between the use of medications that stimulate ovulation and ovarian cancer (Brinton et al., 2004).

Clomiphene citrate (Clomid) users actually had slightly fewer ovarian cancers than would be expected in the general population, and gonadotropin users had slightly more cancers. Women who use fertility drugs and then conceive and give birth are not believed to be at increased risk for developing ovarian cancer (Brinton et al.; O'Rourke & Mahon, 2003).

Clinical Presentation

The majority of cases of ovarian cancer are diagnosed when the disease has already reached an advanced stage. Symptoms of the disease are vague and offer only subtle signs of its presence, such as abdominal bloating and discomfort, dyspepsia, and fatigue or weakness—all of which can be caused by many factors (Goff, Mandel, Melancon, & Muntz, 2004; Ozols et al., 2001). Additional symptoms that may or may not accompany ovarian cancer include back pain, changes in bowel or bladder function (e.g., constipation or diarrhea, and a sensation of urinary fullness or urge), urinary incontinence, and unexplained weight gain or loss (Goff et al.; Ozols et al.). Signs of advanced disease include anorexia, nausea or vomiting, ascites, abdominal or back pain, an abdominal mass, or pleural effusion (Goff et al.; Ozols et al.). Effective screening is difficult because of the lack of specific symptoms in the premalignant or very early stages of the disease (Berek, 2002). **Table 28-6** identifies the early and late symptoms that may occur with ovarian cancer.

Assessment

Screening Routine population-based screening for ovarian cancer is not recommended (NCI, 2004c; U.S. Preventive Services Task Force [USPSTF], 2004). Neither pelvic examination, nor tumor-associated antigen CA-125, nor transvaginal ultrasound is considered sufficiently sensitive or specific enough to be recommended for screening asymptomatic women for this disease (NCI). Ovarian cancer is occasionally detected during the pelvic examination and, when detected, it almost always indicates advanced disease. Palpation of the ovaries during pelvic examination has not proved to be useful in identifying ovarian

TABLE 28-6 Clinical Presentation of Ovarian Cancer

Early Symptoms	Later Symptoms
Abdominal bloating/discomfort	Ascites
Early satiety	Anorexia
Indigestion	Nausea or vomiting
Fatigue/weakness	Palpable abdominal or pelvic mass
Vague abdominal pain/painful areas in abdomen on palpation	Distinct abdominal pain
Urinary fullness and/or urge urinary incontinence	Back pain
Diarrhea or constipation	Pleural effusion
Unexplained weight gain or loss	

740 CHAPTER 28   Gynecologic Cancers

cancer in women who are premenopausal. A palpable pelvic mass in a woman who is post-menopausal is always considered abnormal and should be evaluated further.

CA-125 is a tumor-associated antigen (glycoprotein) that has been used to monitor the clinical status of patients with ovarian cancer (Ozols et al., 2001). This marker is most useful when the CA-125 level is elevated at the time of diagnosis and then drops after definitive primary therapy such as surgical debulking of the primary tumor followed by chemotherapy (Ozols et al.). CA-125 is shed from the surface of the fallopian tubes, endometrium, endo-cervix, peritoneum, pleura, pericardium, and bronchus. Elevation of CA-125 levels is not specific for ovarian cancer; indeed, this level may be elevated in women with endometriosis, other nongynecologic malignancies, PID, fibroids, and menstruation, and during the first tri-mester of pregnancy (Ozols et al.). Therefore, CA-125 is not a recommended screening test. It can be useful as part of the follow-up of treated patients if the CA-125 level was obtained and found to be elevated at the time of diagnosis and then observed to drop significantly after definitive treatment of the ovarian cancer (Berek, 2002; Ozols et al.).

Ultrasound has demonstrated value in the detection of advanced ovarian cancer, but its ability to provide accurate detection in the early stage of the disease is poor (O'Rourke & Mahon, 2003). The finding of a palpable pelvic mass combined with a positive transvaginal ultrasound and elevated CA-125 level decreases the number of false positives and improves the rate of accurate detection (Berek, 2002; NCI, 2004d; USPSTF, 2004).

New developments in the screening for ovarian cancer include a search for biomark-ers that can be detected by a simple blood or urine test and evaluation of the laparoscopic ovarian Pap test, transvaginal sonography, and multimodal screening (Anderson, 2009). Proteomics—an area of genetics that examines the proteins encoded by a genome—is a new approach to screening for ovarian cancer that may have potential for identifying stage I ovarian cancer, although much more research is needed before its use becomes widespread (Anderson).

Management

Prevention Factors that inhibit ovulation appear to reduce the risk of developing ovarian cancer. For example, COC use for 5 or more years reduces the risk of ovarian cancer by 40% to 50%, and the protective effect continues for 10 to 15 years following discontinuation of their use (Barnes, Grizzle, Grubbs, & Partridge, 2002; NCI, 2009). Pregnancy resulting in at least one full-term birth and breastfeeding also reduce ovarian cancer risk (NCI). The more times a woman has been pregnant, the lower her risk of ovarian cancer (NCI). Tubal ligation and hysterectomy without oophorectomy also appear to reduce the risk of ovarian cancer.

Bilateral salpingo-oophorectomy is often recommended to women who have docu-mented mutations in the BRCA1 or BRCA2 gene. This procedure appears to reduce the risk of both breast cancer and ovarian cancer in carriers of these mutated genes (Berek, 2002; Hogg & Friedlander, 2004; Martin, 2000). It is important to note that patients who choose a risk-reducing bilateral salpingo-oophorectomy continue to have a 5% lifetime chance of developing a primary peritoneal cancer and need to continue to be followed. Women considering this option need genetic counseling and testing as well as education regarding the clinical effects of premature menopause so they may make an informed decision.

Staging Persistent ovarian masses in premenopausal women and any palpable pelvic mass in postmenopausal women should be evaluated by obtaining a transvaginal ultrasound and CA-125 level (Berek, 2002; Martin, 2000; NCI, 2009; Ozols et al., 2001). Color-flow Doppler ultrasound may also be used to further evaluate a suspicious mass (Berek). Malignancy is suspected if the mass has irregular borders, solid areas with papillary projections, or multiple, dense, irregular septae (Martin). Ascites is present in one-third of women at the time of diagnosis (Martin). Referral to a gynecologic oncologist is appropriate at this point. Not only are appropriate staging and debulking of tumor much more likely to be achieved when done by a gynecologic oncologist, but this approach has also been noted to produce a 5- to 8-month median survival benefit for patients with advanced disease (Vernooij, Heintz, Witteveen, & van der Graaf, 2007).

The initial work-up prior to surgery may include a CT of the abdomen and pelvis with contrast, chest x-ray, and mammogram (Berek, 2002; Ozols et al., 2001). Surgical exploration is required to make a definitive diagnosis of cancer, stage the extent of the disease, and debulk (remove) all of the visible tumor in the abdomen and pelvis. The goal is to leave tumor bulk less than 1 cm in diameter. A total abdominal hysterectomy, bilateral salpingo-oophorectomy, peritoneal cytology, omentectomy, pelvic and para-aortic lymph node sampling, scraping of the undersurface of the diaphragm, multiple peritoneal biopsies, and random biopsies are all part of the standard surgical procedure (Berek; NCI, 2004d; National Institutes of Health [NIH] Consensus Conference, 1995; Ozols et al.).

Ovarian cancer is surgically staged, and the FIGO staging system is used to provide important prognostic information (**Table 28-7**). The volume of postoperative residual tumor is also of prognostic significance, with greater volumes conferring a poorer prognosis.

Postoperative Treatment All women diagnosed with ovarian cancer are potential candidates for clinical trials and should be offered participation in them if they meet the selection criteria.

TABLE 28-7 FIGO Ovarian Cancer Staging System

Stage	Characteristics
Stage I	Tumor limited to the ovaries
Stage II	Tumor involves one or both ovaries and extends into pelvis
Stage III	Tumor involves one or both ovaries and pelvis; has extended to bowel, peritoneum, or lymph nodes
Stage IV	Tumor involves one or both ovaries with distant metastases to areas such as liver and chest

Source: International Federation of Gynecology and Obstetrics, 2002.

Women with early Stage I disease with well-differentiated or moderately well-differentiated histologies require no further treatment and have a 5-year survival rate of greater than 90%, provided they have undergone total abdominal hysterectomy and bilateral salpingo-oophorectomy with omentectomy, visualization and biopsy of the undersurface of the diaphragm, pelvic and peritoneal biopsies, and peritoneal washings (NCI, 2004d). Standard treatment for women who fall into the unfavorable or high-risk categories includes postoperative chemotherapy with a platinum-based regimen (NCI).

Surgery for Stage II disease should include total abdominal hysterectomy, bilateral salpingo-oophorectomy, and omentectomy with tumor debulking (to remove as much tumor bulk as possible), followed by combination chemotherapy (NCI, 2004d). The role of total abdominal and pelvic radiation therapy remains controversial as adjuvant treatment and is not included in the 2008 Guidelines for Ovarian Cancer (National Comprehensive Cancer Network [NCCN], 2008).

Advanced disease (Stages III and IV) is treated with a combination of debulking surgery and postoperative chemotherapy. Standard combination chemotherapy includes the use of platinum-based compounds and the taxanes (NCI, 2004d; Ozols et al., 2001), administered either intravenously or intraperitoneally. In 2006, NCI recommended a combination of intravenous and intraperitoneal chemotherapy for women with optimally debulked Stage IIIc ovarian cancer. After several cycles of chemotherapy have been completed, interval debulking surgery is performed in women who did not have a primary debulking procedure (NCI; Ozols et al.). Secondary debulking surgery is sometimes performed if there is a relapse. Second-look surgery or exploratory surgery at the completion of chemotherapy is an option for women with Stages III and IV disease who have a normal CA-125 level and a negative CT scan. Second-look surgery is controversial because it does not improve survival, and if the patient is found to have residual cancer, available treatment is not curative (Berek, 2002; Ozols et al.).

Follow-Up Care of the Woman Who Has Been Treated for Ovarian Cancer

Factors that positively influence the prognosis of ovarian cancer include diagnosis at a younger age, a lower stage of disease at diagnosis, a well-differentiated tumor, no ascites present, a tumor that has a smaller volume prior to debulking surgery such that there is smaller residual volume following debulking surgery, and a cell type other than mucinous or clear cell (NCI, 2004d).

The annual mortality rate from ovarian cancer is approximately equal to the incidence rate, because most patients have widespread disease at the time of diagnosis (Ries et al., 2004). As more effective treatments have become available, increasing numbers of women with advanced disease at diagnosis are surviving, and they are having remissions of 2 years or longer.

The majority of recurrences of ovarian cancer happen within the first year after initial treatment. The majority of patients with advanced-stage ovarian cancer who develop recurrent disease do so within 2 years after treatment (Berek, 2002). Major metastatic sites include the abdomen and pelvis, pelvic and para-aortic lymph nodes, diaphragm, lungs, liver, serosa, pleura, peritoneum overlying the kidneys, adrenal glands, bladder, and spleen. Ascites is present in two-thirds of women at the time of their death (Martin, 2000). Intestinal obstruction with tumor or adhesions causing extrinsic compression of the bowel occurs in approximately 25% to 50% of women with ovarian cancer (Martin). Obstruction can be either partial or complete, and either acute or chronic. The most common presenting symptom is cramping abdominal pain (Martin). Pleural effusion and lymphedema are other possible complications of recurrent disease.

The primary goal of follow-up care is the early identification of recurrence, in the hope that additional treatment will offer the possibility of disease control. A therapeutic alliance and partnership between clinician and patient improves the likelihood that early, subtle signs of recurrence will be promptly reported and evaluated. Lifelong follow-up will be required at regularly scheduled intervals. Follow-up needs to be coordinated with the primary care provider and the gynecologic oncologist, or medical and radiation oncologists. Patients are usually seen for follow-up every 3 months during the first year, with follow-up thereafter determined by the initial stage of their disease and the potential for delayed effects of definitive treatment (Fischer, 1996). History taking should include questions about changes in appetite, increase in abdominal size or mass, weight gain or loss, changes in bowel or bladder function, pelvic pain, and leg edema. Physical examination should focus on the breasts, lungs, abdomen, pelvis, and extremities (Ozols et al., 2001). A rising CA-125 level is highly suggestive of recurrent disease. Nevertheless, it is important to keep in mind that not all ovarian carcinomas are revealed by CA-125; ovarian cancer may recur without a corresponding rise in the CA-125. Options for treatment of recurrent disease include surgical debulking of gross tumor, additional chemotherapy, and radiation therapy (Ozols et al.).

The fear of recurrence is always present for a woman who has been treated for ovarian cancer. Periods of remission followed by recurrence and the need for retreatment keep women in an ongoing state of uncertainty and anxiety (Ferrell, Smith, Ervin, Itano, & Melancon, 2003; Steginga & Dunn, 1997). Even in women with a good prognosis, the fear of recurrence commonly persists for years after completion of definitive treatment and may surface at some follow-up appointments and not others. All symptoms should be taken seriously by the woman and her clinician, because the initial symptoms of ovarian cancer are subtle, vague, and ill defined. The woman who reports symptoms should be seen promptly even though the symptoms may be a result of sometimes minor, transient problems such as indigestion or a muscle strain. Each follow-up assessment must always include the consideration of the possibility of recurrent disease as well as the delayed effects of surgery, chemotherapy, and radiation therapy.

Quality of life and the meaning of life itself are important issues for ovarian cancer survivors. When the diagnosis of ovarian cancer is first received, women commonly feel isolated and wish to avoid others who have the disease, particularly those women whose disease is at an advanced stage. Later, women recently diagnosed with ovarian cancer often will seek relationships with other women who have the disease so that they can share the lived experience and find emotional support. Many women have difficulty coping with the wish that the cancer had been diagnosed sooner. Women with ovarian cancer often will take control of their treatment by seeking out alternative and complementary therapies that they will combine with conventional treatment. Some women worry about passing a genetic predisposition for ovarian cancer on to their daughters (Ferrell et al., 2003; Zebrack, 2000). Relationships are reevaluated and personal beliefs about life and death are examined, as well as the woman's spirituality (Zebrack). Loss of fertility and the permanent physical changes that accompany total abdominal hysterectomy and bilateral salpingo-oophorectomy, followed by chemotherapy, add to the stress that the cancer diagnosis places on women's personal relationships. Menopausal symptoms such as hot flashes and vaginal dryness, and the side effects of chemotherapy such as peripheral neuropathy and temporary hair loss, often leave women feeling as though they have lost their femininity and sexuality (Ferrell et al.).

In spite of these negative aspects of the disease and the treatment process, quality of life is moderately high for most women with ovarian cancer (Ersek, Ferrell, Dow, & Melancon, 1997). These women derive great benefit and support from the presence of consistent, sensitive clinicians who take their symptoms and concerns seriously and provide prompt, thorough follow-up that does not offer any false sense of reassurance or undue sense of alarm.

References

American Cancer Society (ACS). (2008a). *Cancer facts and figures.* Retrieved from http://www.cancer.org/downloads/STT/2008CAFFfinalsecured.pdf

American Cancer Society (ACS). (2008b). *Detailed guide: Cervical cancer.* Retrieved from http://www.cancer.org/docroot/CRI/CRI_2_3x.asp?dt=8

American Cancer Society (ACS). (2008c). *Detailed guide: Endometrial (uterine) cancer.* Retrieved from http://documents.cancer.org/140.00/140.00.pdf

American Cancer Society (ACS). (2009). *Detailed guide: What are the risk factors for cervical cancer?* Retrieved from http://www.cancer.org/docroot/CRI/content/CRI_2_4_2X_What_are_the_risk_factors_for_cervical_cancer_8.asp?rnav=cri

American College of Obstetricians and Gynecologists (2005, reaffirmed 2011). Management of endometrial cancer (ACOG Practice Bulletin No. 65). *Obstetrics & Gynecology, 106,* 413–425.

American College of Obstetricians & Gynecologists. (2009). Routine pelvic examination and cervical cytology screening (ACOG Committee Opinion No. 431). *Obstetrics & Gynecology, 113*(5), 1190–1193.

American Joint Committee on Cancer (AJCC). (2002). *AJCC cancer staging manual and handbook* (6th ed.). New York: Springer.

American Society for Colposcopy and Cervical Pathology (ASCCP). (2006). *2006 consensus guidelines for the management of women with cervical intraepithelial neoplasia or adenocarcinoma in situ.* Retrieved from http://www.asccp.org/pdfs/consensus/algorithms_cyto_07.pdf

American Society for Colposcopy and Cervical Pathology (ASCCP). (2009). *HPV genotyping update.* Retrieved from http://www.asccp.org/consensus.shtml

Anderson, L. (2009). Ovarian cancer: The search for an accurate screening technique. *Journal of American Association of Physician Assistants, 22*(2), 22–25.

Barnes, M. N., Grizzle, W. E., Grubbs, C. J., & Partridge, E. E. (2002). Paradigms for the primary prevention of ovarian carcinoma. *CA: Cancer Journal for Clinicians, 52*(4), 216–225.

Beckmann, C. R. B., Ling, F. W., Smith, R. P., Barzansky, B. M., Herbert, W. N., & Laube, D. W. (2006). *Obstetrics and gynecology.* Philadelphia: Lippincott Williams & Wilkins.

Berek, J. S. (2002). Ovarian cancer. In J. S. Berek (Ed.), *Novak's gynecology* (13th ed., pp. 1245–1319). Philadelphia: Lippincott Williams & Wilkins.

Bertram, C. C. (2004). Evidence for practice: Oral contraception and risk of cervical cancer. *American Academy of Nurse Practitioners, 16,* 455–461.

Bethesda System: Terminology for reporting results of cervical cytology. (2002). *Journal of the American Medical Association, 287*(16), 2114–2119.

Brinton, L. A., Lamb, E. J., Moghissi, K. S., Scoccia, B., Althuis, M. D., Mabie, J. E., et al. (2004). Ovarian cancer risk after the use of ovulation-stimulating drugs. *Obstetrics and Gynecology, 103*(6), 1194–1203.

Centers for Disease Control and Prevention (CDC). (2006). *HPV and HPV vaccine: Information for healthcare providers.* Retrieved from http://www.cdc.gov/STD/hpv/STDFact-HPV-vaccine-hcp.htm

Centers for Disease Control and Prevention (CDC). (2007). *Quadrivalent human papillomavirus vaccine.* Retrieved from http://www.cdc.gov/mmwr/preview/mmwrhtml/rr56e312a1.htm

Centers for Disease Control and Prevention (CDC). (2010). *Vaginal and vulvar cancers.* Retrieved from http://www.cdc.gov/cancer/vagvulv/pdf/vagvulv_facts.pdf

Centers for Disease Control and Prevention (CDC). (2011). *Cervical cancer.* Retrieved from http://www.cdc.gov/cancer/cervical.

Chambers, S. K. (2001). Gynecologic cancers. In V. T. DeVita, S. Hellman, & S. A. Rosenberg (Eds.), *Cancer: Principles and practice of oncology* (Vol. 2, pp. 1519–1525). Philadelphia: Lippincott Williams & Wilkins.

Cohen, R. F., & Frank-Stromborg, M. (2000). Assessment and interventions for cancer detection. In S. L. Groenwald, M. H. Frogge, M. Goodman, & C. H. Yarbro (Eds.), *Cancer nursing: Principles and practice* (5th ed., pp. 150–188). Sudbury, MA: Jones and Bartlett.

Collins, R. D. (2003). *Differential diagnosis in primary care.* Philadelphia: Lippincott Williams & Wilkins.

Cotran, R. S., Kumar, V., & Collins, T. (1999). *Pathologic basis of disease.* Philadelphia: W.B. Saunders.

Coulter, J., & Gleeson, N. (2003). Local and regional recurrence of vulval cancer: Management dilemmas. Best practice and research. *Clinical Obstetrics & Gynecology, 17,* 663–681.

Cox, T., & Cuzick, J. (2006). HPV DNA testing in cervical cancer screening: From evidence to policies. *Gynecologic Oncology, 1003,* 8–11.

Dains, J. E., Baumann, L. C., & Scheibel, P. (2003). *Advanced health assessment and clinical diagnosis in primary care.* St. Louis, MO: Mosby.

Ersek, M., Ferrell, B., Dow, K., & Melaneon, C. (1997). Quality of life in women with ovarian cancer. *Western Journal of Nursing Research, 19*(3), 334–350.

Ferrell, B. R., Smith, S. L., Ervin, K. S., Itano, J., & Melancon, C. (2003). A qualitative analysis of social concerns of women with ovarian cancer. *Psycho-oncology, 12,* 647–663.

Fey, M. C., & Beal, M. W. (2004). The role of human papilloma virus testing in cervical cancer prevention. *Journal of Midwifery and Women's Health, 49*(1), 4–13.

Fischer, D. S. (1996). *Follow-up of cancer: A handbook for physicians.* Philadelphia: Lippincott-Raven.

Garcia, A. A. (2007). *Cervical cancer.* Retrieved from http://www.emedicine.com/MED/topic324.htm

Garcia, A. A., & Bi, J. (2007). *Cervical cancer.* Retrieved from http://www.emedicine.com/med/topic324.htm.

Gearhart, P. A. (2007). *Human papillomavirus.* Retrieved from http://www.emedicine.com/med/TOPIC1037.HTM

Get ready for changes in HPV DNA testing. (2009). *Contraceptive Technology Update, 30*(6), 67–69.

Gibson, M., & Hainer, B., (2003). Women's health: Managing abnormal Pap smears. *Patient Care, 37*(5), 56–58.

Godfrey, J. R. (2007). Conversation with experts: Toward optimal health. *Journal of Women's Health, 16,* 1397–1401.

Goff, B. A., Mandel, L. S., Melancon, C. H., & Muntz, H. G. (2004). Frequency of symptoms of ovarian cancer in women presenting to primary care clinics. *Journal of the American Medical Association, 291,* 2705–2712.

Guarnieri, C., & Klemm, P. R. (2000). Vulvar and vaginal cancer. In C. H. Yarbro, M. Hansen Frogge, M. Goodman, & S. L. Groenwald (Eds.), *Cancer nursing: Principles and practice* (5th ed., pp. 1511–1525). Sudbury, MA: Jones and Bartlett.

Hawes, S. E., & Kiviat, N. B. (2002). Are genital infections and inflammation cofactors in the pathogenesis of invasive cervical cancer? *Journal of the National Cancer Institute, 94,* 1592–1593.

Hogg, R., & Friedlander, M. (2004). Biology of epithelial ovarian cancer: Implications for screening women at high genetic risk. *Journal of Clinical Oncology, 22*(7), 1315–1327.

Holschneider, C. H., & Berek, J. S. (2002). Vulvar cancer. In J. S. Berek (Ed.), *Novak's gynecology* (13th ed., pp. 1321–1351). Philadelphia: Lippincott Williams & Wilkins.

Huncharek, M., Geschwind, J. F., & Kupelnick, B. (2003). Perineal application of cosmetic talc and the risk of invasive epithelial ovarian cancer: A meta-analysis of

11,933 subjects from sixteen observational studies. *Anticancer Research, 23*(2C), 1995–1960.

International Federation of Gynecology and Obstetrics. (2002). Ovarian cancer staging system. In F. L. Green, D. L. Page, I. D. Fleming, A. Fritz, C. M. Balch, D. G. Haller, et al. (Eds.), *American Joint Committee on Cancer Staging manual and handbook* (6th ed.). New York: Springer.

Jarvis, C. (2008). *Physical examination and health assessment*. Philadelphia: W. B. Saunders.

Jemal, A., Siegal, R., Ward, E., et al. (2008). Cancer statistics 2008. *A Cancer Journal for Clinicians, 58*(2), 71–96

Jones, G. (2003). *Standard of care for Pap screening*. Retrieved from http://www.medscape.com/view article/450617

Joura, E. (2002). Epidemiology and precursors of vulvar cancer: Review article. *Journal of Women's Imaging, 4*(3), 126–129, 148–149.

Keam, S., & Harper, D. (2008). Human papillomavirus types 16 and 18 vaccine (recombinant, AS04 adjuvanted, adsorbed) [Cervarix]. *Drugs 2008, 68*(3), 359–372.

Lee, C. O. (2000a). Gynecologic cancers: Part I—risk factors. *Clinical Journal of Oncology Nursing, 4*(2), 67–71.

Lee, C. O. (2000b). Gynecologic cancers: Part II—risk assessment and screening. *Clinical Journal of Oncology Nursing, 4*(2), 73–77.

Linkov, F., Edwards, R., Balk, J., Yurkovetsky, Z., Stadterman, B., … Taioli, E. (2008). Endometrial hyperplasia, endometrial cancer and prevention: Gaps in existing research of modifiable factors. *European Journal of Cancer, 44*, 1632–1644.

Luce, T. L., Hassey Dow, K., & Holcomb, L. (2003). Early diagnosis for epithelial ovarian cancer. *The Nurse Clinician: The American Journal of Primary Health Care, 28*(12), 41–49.

Marrinan, G. (2007). *Polycystic ovarian disease (Stein-Leventhal syndrome)*. Retrieved from http://www.emedicine.com/radio/topic565.htm

Marsden, J., & Sturdee, D. (2009). Cancer issues. *Best Practice & Research Clinical Obstetrics & Gynecology, 23l*, 87–107. doi: 10.1016/j.bpobgyn.2008.10.005

Martin, V. R. (2000). Ovarian cancer. In C. H. Yarbro, M. Hansen Frogge, M. Goodman, & S. L. Groenwald (Eds.), *Cancer nursing: Principles and practice* (5th ed., pp. 1371–1399). Sudbury, MA: Jones and Bartlett.

Mayeux, E. J., & Spitzer, M. (2005). *Preventing cervical cancer and other HPV related diseases*. Retrieved from http://www.medscape.com/viewprogram/4331_pnt

Moreno, V., Bosch, F. X., Munoz, N., Meijer, C. J., Shah, K. V., Walboomers, J. M., et al. (2002). Effect of oral contraceptives on risk of cervical cancer in women with human papillomavirus infection: The IARC multicentric case-control study. *Lancet, 259*, 1085–1092.

Munoz, N., Franceschi, S., Bosetti, C., Moreno, V., Herrero, R., Smith, J. S., et al. (2002). The role of parity and human papilloma virus in cervical cancer: The International Agency for Research on Cancer (IARC) multicentric case-control study. *Lancet, 359*, 1093–1101.

National Cancer Institute (NCI). (n.d.). *Cancer advances in focus: Cervical cancer*. Retrieved from http://www.cancer.gov/cancertopics/cancer-advances-in-focus/cervical

National Cancer Institute (NCI). (2003a). *Ovarian low malignant potential tumors (PDQ): Treatment: Health professional version*. Retrieved from http://www.nci.nih.gov/cancertopics/pdq/screening/ovarian/healthprofessional

National Cancer Institute (NCI). (2003b). *Vulvar cancer (PDQ): Treatment: Health professional version*. Retrieved from http://www.nci.nih.gov/cancertopics/pdq/treatment/vulvar/HealthProfessional/page2

National Cancer Institute (NCI). (2004a). *Genetics of breast and ovarian cancer (PDQ): Health professional version*. Retrieved from http://www.cancer.gov/cancerinfo/pdq/genetics/breast-and-ovarian/HealthProfessional

National Cancer Institute (NCI). (2004b). *Hormone replacement therapy and breast cancer relapse*. Retrieved from http://www.cancer.gov/clinicaltrials/results/hrt-and-breast-cancer0204

National Cancer Institute (NCI). (2004c). *Ovarian cancer (PDQ): Prevention: Health professional version*. Retrieved from http://www.nci.nih.gov/cancertopics/pdq/screening/ovarian/healthprofessional

National Cancer Institute (NCI). (2004d). *Ovarian epithelial cancer (PDQ): Treatment: Health professional version*. Retrieved from http://www.nci.nih.gov/cancerinfo/pdq/treatment/ovarianepithelial/healthprofessional/

National Cancer Institute (NCI). (2008a). *Cervical cancer prevention (PDQ): Health professional version*. Retrieved from http://www.cancer.gov/cancertopics/pdq/prevention/cervical/healthprofessional/allpages/print

National Cancer Institute (NCI). (2008b). *Cervical cancer screening (PDQ): Health professional version*.

Retrieved from http://www.cancer.gov/cancertopics /pdq/screening/cervical/healthprofessional

National Cancer Institute (NCI). (2008c). *Cervical cancer treatment (PDQ): Health professional version.* Retrieved from http://www.cancer.gov/cancertopics /pdq/treatment/cervical/HealthProfessional

National Cancer Institute (NCI). (2008d). *Endometrial cancer prevention (PDQ).* Retrieved from http://www.cancer.org/docroot/CRI/CRI_2x.asp? sitearea=&dt=11

National Cancer Institute (NCI). (2008e). *Endometrial cancer screening (PDQ).* Retrieved from http://www .cancer.gov/cancertopics/pdq/screening/endometrial /healthprofessional/allpages/print

National Cancer Institute (NCI). (2008f). *Endometrial cancer treatment (PDQ).* Retrieved from http://www .cancer.gov/cancertopics/pdq/treatment/endometrial /healthprofessional/allpages/print

National Cancer Institute (NCI). (2009). *Ovarian cancer (PDQ): Screening: Health professional version.* Retrieved from http://www.nci.nih.gov/cancertopics /pdq/prevention/ovarian/HealthProfessional/page2# Section_62

National Comprehensive Cancer Network (NCCN). (2008). Ovarian cancer: Clinical practice guidelines in oncology. *Journal of the National Comprehensive Cancer Network, 6*(8), 766–794.

National Institutes of Health (NIH) Consensus Conference. (1995). Ovarian cancer: Screening, treatment, and follow-up. NIH Consensus Development Panel on Ovarian Cancer. *Journal of the American Medical Association, 273*(8), 491–497.

O'Rourke, J., & Mahon, S. (2003). A comprehensive look at the early detection of ovarian cancer. *Clinical Journal of Oncology Nursing, 7*(1), 41–47.

Ozols, R. F., Schwartz, P. E., & Eifel, P. J. (2001). Ovarian cancer, fallopian tube carcinoma, and peritoneal carcinoma. In V. T. DeVita, S. Hellman, & S. A. Rosenberg (Eds.), *Cancer: Principles and practice of oncology* (6th ed., pp. 1594–1632). Philadelphia: Lippincott Williams & Wilkins.

Paganini-Hill, A., Ross, R., & Henderson, B. (1989). Endometrial cancer and patterns of use of estrogen replacement therapy: A cohort study. *British Journal of Cancer, 59,* 445–447.

Porth, C. M. (2007). *Essentials of pathophysiology: Concepts of altered health states.* Philadelphia: Lippincott, Williams & Wilkins.

Ries, L. A. G., Eisner, M. P., Kosary, C. L., Hankey, B. F., Miller, B. A., Clegg, L., et al. (Eds.). (2004). *SEER cancer statistics review, 1975–2002.* Bethesda, MD: National Cancer Institute. Retrieved from http://seer .cancer.gov/csr/1975_2002/

Ronco, G., Cuzick, J., Pierotti, P., Cariaggi, M. P., Palma, P. D., Naldoni, C., et al. (2007). Accuracy of liquid based versus conventional cytology: Overall results of new technologies for cervical cancer screening randomized controlled trial. *British Medical Journal, 335*(1), 1–7.

Ryan, M., Stainton, M. C., Jaconelli, C., Watts, S., MacKenzie, P., & Mansberg, T. (2003). The experience of lower limb lymphedema for women after treatment for gynecologic cancer. *Oncology Nursing Forum, 30*(3), 417–423.

Saksouk, F. A. (2008). *Cervix, cancer.* Retrieved from http://www.emedicine.com/radio/topic140.htm

Schumann, L., McFadden, S. E., & Schumann, L. (2001). The role of human papillomavirus in screening for cervical cancer. *Journal of American Academy of Nurse Practitioners, 13,* 116–128.

Siebers, A., Klinkhamer, P., Grefte, J., Massuger, L., Vedder, J., Beijers-Broos, A., et al. (2009). Comparison of liquid-based cytology with conventional cytology for detection of cervical cancer precursors: A randomized controlled trial. *Journal of the American Medical Association, 302,* 1757–2322. doi: 10.1001 /jama.2009.1569

Snyder, U. (2003). *A look at cervical cancer.* Retrieved from www.medscape.com/viewarticle/452727

Solomon, D., Davey, D., Kurman, R., Moriarty, A., O'Connor, D., Prey, M., et al. (2002). The 2001 Bethesda System: Terminology for reporting results of cervical cytology. *Journal of the American Medical Association, 287*(16), 2114–2119.

Sood, A. K., Sorosky, J. L., Mayr, N., Anderson, B., Buller, R. E., & Niebyl, J. (2000). Cervical cancer diagnosed shortly after pregnancy: Prognostic variables and delivery routes. *Obstetrics & Gynecology, 95,* 832–838.

Sorosky, J. I. (2008). Clinical expert series: Endometrial cancer. *American College of Obstetricians and Gynecologists, 111,* 436–447.

Steginga, S. K., & Dunn, J. (1997). Women's experiences following treatment for gynecologic cancer. *Oncology Nursing Forum, 24*(8), 1403–1408.

Stein, S. R. (2003). ThinPrep versus the conventional Papanicolaou test: A review of specimen adequacy, sensitivity and cost-effectiveness. *Primary Care Update for Ob/Gyns, 10,* 310–314.

Tucker Edwards, Q., & Saunders-Goldson, S. (2003). Lichen sclerosus of the vulva in women: Assessment, diagnosis, and management for the nurse clinician. *Journal of the American Academy of Nurse Clinicians, 15*(3), 115–119.

Tyring, S. K. (2003). Vulvar squamous cell carcinoma: Guidelines for early diagnosis and treatment. *American Journal of Obstetrics and Gynecology, 189*(suppl 3), S17–S23.

U. S. Preventive Services Task Force (USPSTF). (2004, May). *Recommendation statement: Screening for ovarian cancer.* Retrieved from http://www.ahrq .gov/clinic/uspstf/uspsovar.htm

Vachani, C. (2008). *A new direction in cancer prevention: An interview with Christine Chu, MD.* Retrieved from http://www.oncolink.com/custom_tags /print_article.cfm?Page=2&id

Vernooij, F., Heintz, P., Witteveen, E., & van der Graaf, Y. (2007). The outcomes of ovarian cancer treatment are better when provided by a gynecologic oncologist and in specialized hospitals: A systematic review. *Gynecology and Oncology, 105*, 801–812.

Widener, M. (2008, August). Drug criteria and outcomes: Test your vaccine knowledge: Gardasil. *Drug Formulary Review* (suppl), 1–3.

Wilbur, D., Wright, T., & Young, N. (2002). The 2001 Bethesda System: Terminology for reporting results of cervical cytology. *Journal of the American Medical Association, 287*(16), 2114–2119.

Winter, W. E., & Gosewehr, J. A. (2006). *Uterine cancer.* Retrieved June 8, 2008, from http://www.emedicine. com/med/topic2832.htm

Wright, J. D., Davila, R. M., Pinto, K. R., Merritt, D. F., Gibb, R. K., Radar, J. S., et al. (2005). Cervical dysplasia in adolescents. *American College of Obstetricians and Gynecologists, 106*, 115–120.

Yeoh, G. P., Chan, K. W., Lauder, I., & Lam, M. M. (1999). Evaluation of the ThinPrep Papanicolaou test in clinical practice: 6-month study of 16,541 cases with histological correlation in 220 cases. *Hong Kong Medical Journal, 5*, 233–239.

Zebrack, B. J. (2000). Cancer survivor identity and quality of life. *Cancer Practice, 8*, 238–242.

Zheng, W., Kushi, L., Potter, J., Sellers, T., Doyle, T., Bostick, R., & Folsom, A. (1995). Dietary intake of energy and animal foods and endometrial cancer incidence: The Iowa Women's Health Study. *American Journal of Epidemiology, 142*(4), 388–394.

Pelvic Pain

Kerri Durnell Schuiling
Nanci Gasiewicz

H istorically, when a woman presented with pelvic or lower abdominal pain, the clinician automatically focused solely on the gynecologic organs, assuming they were the cause of the problem. This clinical "gynevision" promoted treatment modalities that encouraged the use of a surgical approach in which organ pathology was viewed as a priority (Ling, 1995; Martin & Ling, 1999). Such a narrow clinical view assumes pathology and risks categorizing normal female physiologic processes as abnormal. A number of the causes of pelvic pain in women are unrelated to the gynecologic organs. Often pelvic pain is caused by multiple factors, requiring clinicians to take a multidisciplinary, holistic approach to its assessment and management. An appreciation for the intertwining influence of the mind and the body during assessment and in planning interventions is important. This approach places the woman at the center of her management plan, and respects her credibility as the authoritative "knower."

Pain in the pelvic region concerns many women because of its significance to both sexuality and reproduction (Fogel, 1995). Some of the pelvic pain experienced by women is associated with normal physiologic functions such as menstruation and childbearing. Other common causes include pathologic processes such as endometriosis and infection (Fogel). In addition, a number of nongynecologic causes of pelvic pain must be considered. This chapter addresses pelvic pain that is primarily chronic and gynecologic in origin. Acute pelvic pain that is gynecologically related is discussed in greater detail elsewhere in this book. Nongynecologic acute and chronic pelvic pain is addressed in the context of providing differential diagnoses for the clinician to consider during assessment and evaluation.

Description and Definition

Pelvic pain is a broad term encompassing a number of etiologies, within or across body systems. The pain can be acute, chronic, cyclic, or noncyclic and gynecologically related or not. It may be symptomatic of an underlying cause or it can be a syndrome unto itself. Pelvic pain can be so severe it adversely affects a woman's normal functioning, prohibiting her from participating in her normal lifestyle. Although seeking treatment for pelvic pain is one of the most common reasons women come to a clinician for care, diagnosing its cause and prescribing the appropriate treatment is often difficult because of the complexity of the pathophysiology and the myriad contributing factors.

There is no universally accepted definition of chronic pelvic pain. For the purposes of this chapter, chronic pelvic pain is defined as "noncyclic pain of six or more months duration that localizes to the anatomic pelvis, anterior abdominal wall at or below the umbilicus, the lumbosacral back, or the buttocks, and is of sufficient severity to cause functional disability or lead to medical care" (American College of Obstetricians and Gynecologists, 2004, reaffirmed 2010). Other widely accepted definitions of chronic pelvic pain exist, however, and a consistent definition has not used in research (Williams, Hartmann, & Steege, 2004). For example, the "six months' duration of pain" guideline has been reduced by some clinicians to three months because so many women wait a long period of time before seeking treatment.

Acute pelvic pain is generally defined as pain that is in the pelvis or lower abdomen and is less than three months' duration (Kruszka & Kruszka, 2010). Acute pain is generally sudden in onset, is sharp yet intense, and runs a short course (Rapkin & Howe, 2007). Given that it is more often associated with an identifiable cause such as pelvic inflammatory disease or ectopic pregnancy, a wrong diagnosis can result in morbidity and even mortality (Karnath & Breitkopf, 2007; Rapkin & Howe).

Scope and Incidence of Chronic Pelvic Pain

Chronic pelvic pain is probably far more common than data from incidence reports suggest because of the variety of definitions and because many women do not seek care until the pain is unrelenting and debilitating, thus causing underreporting (Jarrell et al., 2005; Williams, Hartmann, & Steege, 2004; Zondervan et al., 1999). Estimates of women of reproductive age who live in the United States or the United Kingdom experiencing either acute or chronic pelvic pain range from 12% to 39% (Gunter, 2003; Vincent, 2009; Williams, Hartmann, Sandler, Miller, & Steege, 2004). This range represents more than 9 million women living in developed countries who suffer from pelvic pain (Gunter). Of women aged 18 to 50 years, 15% to 20% have chronic pelvic pain that lasts longer than 1 year (American College of Obstetricians and Gynecologists, 2004, reaffirmed 2010). Women experiencing chronic pelvic pain are reported to use significantly more medications, have nongynecologic operations much more often, and are more likely to have a hysterectomy and reduced quality of life than women who do not have pelvic pain (Williams, Hartmann, Sandler, et al.). In the

United States, 10% of gynecologic visits are for treatment of chronic pelvic pain, 40% of all laparoscopies performed are attributable to this condition, and 10% to 15% of hysterectomies performed because of chronic pain have no pathologic findings (Altman & Lee, 2009).

Clearly, chronic pelvic pain is a serious health problem for women and contributes significantly to healthcare costs. Estimates suggest that millions of healthcare dollars are spent each year in the United States by women who have pelvic pain (Beckman et al., 2002). Many women with chronic pelvic pain are unable to work and, therefore, unable to contribute to their family's household income. The loss of daily functioning because of pelvic pain creates increased psychosocial stressors including hopelessness, loss of interest in sexual intimacy, and despair compounded by financial stress, all of which can lead to depression (Rapkin & Howe, 2007).

Pain and Gender

Pain is an intimate experience that only the person experiencing it can comprehend. Because pain is a subjective phenomenon, it should be able to be reliably assessed from the woman's personal perspective. The emphasis on equality during the 1980s, however, downplayed gender differences; as a consequence, few studies assessed differences between men and women, including studies about pain. Pain research was based on the male response to pain and it was assumed the findings would generalize to women (Vallerand, 1995). Interestingly, as pain and gender studies became more prevalent, researchers observed that women were better able to verbalize the emotions they experienced with pain. Unfortunately, this finding caused women's responses to pain to be viewed as a psychologic issue and treated accordingly (Vallerand). Women's responses to pain were often viewed with suspicion and the treatment for their pain was less aggressive (Vallerand).

In the late 1990s, the National Institutes of Health (NIH) Pain Research Consortium hosted a conference that focused on gender and pain. Also during this time, the International Association of the Study of Pain (IASP) formed a special-interest group—Sex, Gender, and Pain—which held its first meeting in 1999 in Vienna (Fillingim, King, Ribeiro-Dasilva, Rahim-Williams, & Riley, 2009). These two meetings served as springboards for the dramatic increase in research focusing on sex, gender, and pain.

In 2005, Mogil and Chanda repeated the call to include women in research about pain. According to these authors, from 1997 to 2007 the majority (79%) of the animal studies published in the journal *Pain* used only male subjects. Mogil and Chanda conjectured that the reason for this dominance was because the estrous cyclicity adds variability to the data and scientists do not have a solid understanding of the size and direction of the mean effects. Even so, it is imperative to include females in studies about pain because of the significant number of women who experience chronic pain and the widespread acknowledgment that women suffer more pain than men (Collett & Berkley, 2007). Women have more pain than men for myriad reasons, including female-specific conditions that occur across the life span (e.g., gynecologic conditions). In addition, women tend to live longer than men and, therefore, may be more exposed to degenerative conditions due to aging (Collett & Berkley). It is also suspected that genetics and hormones play important roles in women's experience of pain.

In 2007, the IASP launched the Global Year Against Pain in Women, in recognition of the fact that a significant number of women worldwide have chronic pain conditions that negatively affect their lives, their families, and their communities. The call to include more women in studies about pain also reflects the imperative that sex and gender differences be addressed by clinicians. Moreover, studying pain in women is important for driving attitudinal changes among clinicians who provide health care for women. Attitude can influence healthcare treatment, as can culture. When women are held in low esteem, they often do not receive adequate treatment for their pain (Collett & Berkley, 2007).

Also in 2007, a consensus report was published that was to serve as a guide to researchers studying sex and gender differences in pain and analgesia (Greenspan et al., 2007). This report underscored the point that there is no longer any debate about whether there are sex and gender differences in pain. The evidence reveals that they do, indeed, exist. What is needed now is (1) to develop a better understanding of which conditions lead to these differences, (2) to determine which mechanisms underlie the differences, (3) to learn how these differences inform pain management, and (4) to explore differences in outcomes when similar treatments are used (Greenspan et al.).

Research suggests that women have a lower threshold for pain, have less tolerance for pain, are better able to discriminate painful sensations, and will rate the same type of pain higher than men (Berkley, 1997). It appears that gender is a mediating variable in response and perception of pain (Vallerand & Polomano, 2000). Interestingly, women with chronic pain seem to be more concerned with the effect the pain will have on their lives (Vallerand & Polomano). In fact, women who have multiple responsibilities as part of caring for their family view chronic pain as more of a threat because of its potential to affect their daily lives. For all these reasons, it is very important that the clinician carefully interview the woman who presents with chronic pelvic pain to assess the level of interference the pain may be having with her life and activities of daily living. Part of effective treatment may be working with her to identify how some of the activities can be accomplished.

Etiology and Pathophysiology

The model for chronic pain is entirely different from the model for acute pain (Butrick, 2007). Understanding the differences between the models is important so that the clinician can provide effective care. Also important is the knowledge that it is rare for the pain to stem from only one etiology (Butrick). In fact, many women with pelvic pain have more than one diagnosis as the possible cause of their pain, and women who have multiple diagnoses related to pelvic pain have been shown to suffer greater pain than their counterparts who have one diagnostic cause (American College of Obstetricians and Gynecologists, 2004, reaffirmed 2010).

Pelvic pain generally arises from either a visceral source, such as the gynecologic, genitourinary, or gastrointestinal tracts, or from a somatic source, such as the pelvic bones, ligaments, muscles, and fascia (American College of Obstetricians and Gynecologists, 2004, reaffirmed 2010). Somatic pain may be superficial or deep. Superficial pain occurs when the body surface is stimulated, whereas deep pain originates in muscles, joints, bones, or connective tissue. Somatic pain is often described as being either sharp or dull, is usually localized, and is found on either the right or the left within dermatomes that correspond to the innervations of the involved tissues (Hoffman, 2008). Chronic pelvic pain is often sensed as deep pain.

Visceral pain arises from internal organs and is often associated with strong contractions of visceral muscles. Stretching, distention, ischemia, or spasm of abdominal organs can stimulate visceral pain (Hoffman, 2008). This type of pain is transmitted through the sympathetic tracts of the autonomic nervous system, and is usually described as being dull or poorly localized. It frequently localizes to the midline of the body because of the innervations of the abdominal organs. Nausea, vomiting, and diaphoresis are typical visceral pain phenomena (Gunter, 2003).

Inflammatory pain results from tissue injury and is experienced as acute pain. When tissues are injured, inflammation often follows. When the noxious stimulus is removed, the activity of the sensory pain receptors (also known as nociceptors) quickly ceases (Hoffman, 2008).

Neuropathic pain occurs when noxious stimuli have sustained action, producing continuous central sensitization and loss of neuronal inhibition that becomes permanent (Hoffman, 2008). The result is a decreased pain threshold. This type of pain is often seen in chronic pelvic pain and explains why it is common for the person to experience pain that is disproportionate to the amount of coexisting disease (Hoffman).

The etiologies of pelvic pain include gynecologic, urologic, gastrointestinal, musculoskeletal, and psychoneurologic conditions and abnormalities—a vast range of possibilities that makes diagnosis and management challenging (Olson & Schnatz, 2007). In turn, the approach to health care for the woman with pelvic pain must be multifaceted. The process of determining the cause of pelvic pain and developing a successful treatment plan is often difficult, time consuming, and costly for the woman, and difficult and confusing, at best, for even the most experienced clinician. Many of the diseases believed to cause pelvic pain do not meet epidemiologic criteria for causality; that is, the evidence may strongly suggest such criteria as the cause, but research results do not yet provide definitive support for such a relationship. This ambiguity increases the difficulty in assessment, diagnosis, and treatment of pelvic pain (American College of Obstetricians and Gynecologists, 2004, reaffirmed 2010). Because the causes of many disorders that are associated with pelvic pain are not well established, the majority of clinicians treat the condition empirically.

Clinical Presentation

Acute pelvic pain is generally accepted to comprise pain in the lower abdomen or pelvic region that has occurred within the last seven days and has been ongoing for less than three months (Hoffman, 2008); it may or may not be recurrent or related to the menstrual cycle. The woman usually describes pain that is rapid in onset and sharp in intensity. The discomfort may consist of colicky pain, or it may come and go like menstrual cramps. Vital signs may be unstable because of the sharpness of the pain. The cause of acute pelvic pain must be quickly diagnosed because delay can result in increased morbidity and mortality (Rapkin & Howe, 2007). If the woman is of reproductive age, pregnancy must first be ruled out.

Chronic pelvic pain is often classified as either gynecologic or nongynecologic. Categorizing the pain further into cyclic or noncyclic categories assists the clinician in determining whether the pain may be related to the woman's menstrual cycle. Sometimes, however, cyclic pain has no relationship to the menstrual cycle and is totally unrelated to the pelvic organs. Pelvic pain that is gynecologic in origin and cyclic is addressed in various chapters within this book, such as those dealing with dysmenorrhea and endometriosis; the reader is referred to Chapters 24 and 27 for further information on conditions that cause this type of pain.

Women presenting with chronic pelvic pain often have had the pain for some time and do not come for treatment until they are so negatively affected by the pain that they can no longer perform activities of daily living. They do not always appear to be experiencing the amount of distress that individuals with severe pain often display. This affect may reflect the fact that these patients have lived with the pain for so long that they have normalized it and, therefore, do not present as the typical patient suffering from significant pain. Frequently they will describe an inability to work or function at home and describe a pain that is unrelenting. It is also not unusual to observe that a woman has seen a variety of clinicians over several years with a variety of concerns, all of which center on her pelvic pain.

Assessment

A detailed history and physical examination are essential to make an accurate diagnosis. Using a formatted, widely accepted questionnaire can be helpful in ensuring that all critical points are covered. The International Pelvic Pain Society provides a pelvic pain assessment form that can be downloaded at no cost from www.pelvicpain.org/pdf/FRM_Pain_Questionnaire.pdf. This form is also available in Appendix 29-A.

History

The approach to assessment and diagnosis of pelvic pain needs to be systematic and detailed for the cause to be identified and an appropriate treatment plan developed. Care must be taken during the first visit to validate the woman's symptoms and acknowledge her agency in the healthcare process. It is important to allow enough time during the visit so that she can tell her story in entirety. She needs to feel that she has been listened to and heard. Establishing a good rapport increases the likelihood that she will be comfortable sharing relevant sensitive topics (Olson & Schnatz, 2007).

Focused questioning is important for obtaining an accurate history, and active listening is essential. Valuing the woman's description of her pain and validating her feelings are paramount in developing trust and rapport. A holistic approach considers how the pain a woman describes is affecting every facet of her life. The multiple roles most women play are all altered by pain, and obtaining information about how the pain affects her physically and emotionally, how it impacts her activities of daily living, and how it changes her relationships is important.

The importance of a meticulous health history cannot be overemphasized. It is critical that a pain history be taken during the first visit, including "the nature of each pain symptom: location, radiation, severity, aggravating and alleviating factors; effect of menstrual cycle, stress, work, exercise, intercourse, orgasm; the context in which pain arose; and the social and occupational toll of the pain" (Rapkin & Howe, 2007, pp. 521–522).

Rapkin and Howe (2007, p. 522) offer the mnemonic "OLD CAARTS" as an aid for performing a pain history:

O = Onset: When and how did the pain start?

L = Location: Specific location of the pain. Can you put a finger on it?

D = Duration: How long does it last?

C = Characteristics: What is the pain like—cramping, aching, stabbing, burning, tingling, itching, and so on?

A = Alleviating or aggravating factors: What makes the pain better (e.g., medication, position change, heat) and what makes it worse (e.g., specific activity, stress, menstrual cycle)?

A = Associated symptoms: Gynecologic (dyspareunia, dysmenorrhea, abnormal bleeding, discharge, infertility), gastrointestinal (constipation, diarrhea), genitourinary (dysuria, urgency, incontinence), and neurologic (specific nerve involvement).

R = Radiation: Does the pain move to other areas on your body?

T = Temporal: What time of day is it worse and better?

S = Severity (on a scale of 1 to 10).

The use of a pain-rating scale may assist clinicians to comprehend the intensity of the woman's pain. Pain-rating scales, such as the numeric-ranking scale, visual-analog scales, and verbal-descriptive scales, allow the patient to identify the severity of the pain. If there is a language barrier related to culture or mental ability, the Wong-Baker FACES pain-rating scale (smile to frown) may be helpful (Ignatavicius & Workman, 2002).

An accurate and nonjudgmental sexual history is very important. Clinicians should not allow heterosexism to blind their objectivity; a woman's partner may be female. Keep in mind that although a woman may believe she is monogamous with one partner, her partner may have other partners. Additionally, a woman may report a monogamous relationship, but fail to mention that it is her third monogamous relationship in the past year. Given these possibilities, it is important to ask about her number of sexual partners and the possibility of her partner having multiple partners.

Obtain a detailed obstetric history because pregnancy and vaginal birth can be traumatic to neuromuscular structures and have been linked to pelvic floor, symphyseal, and sacroiliac joint pain (Hoffman, 2008). Cesarean birth has been linked to lower abdominal wall pain and adhesions.

Include a surgical history. It provides information about the patient's risk for adhesions, peritoneal injuries, infections, and related diagnoses that may be responsible for the pain (e.g., endometriosis).

Many studies have documented an association between chronic pelvic pain and abuse (Karnath & Breithopf, 2007). The reason for the association is unknown, and research on this topic is ongoing. If the abuse is currently occurring, it is important that the woman be counseled appropriately (see Chapters 14 and 15). Therefore, obtaining a careful psychosocial history is important.

The evidence also suggests that women with pelvic pain should be screened for depression (Kassab & Rollins, 2011). In Kassab and Rollins's study, patients who had chronic pelvic pain were found to have depression more often than their counterparts and experienced significantly more issues with social impairment and decreased quality of life.

Substance abuse, as a pain mitigator, is unfortunately higher in women with chronic pelvic pain (Gunter, 2003). Always inquire about the use of narcotics, alcohol, and recreational drugs when assessing clients who have chronic pelvic pain.

Physical Examination

Always obtain baseline vital signs, including blood pressure, temperature, pulse, and respirations, prior to performing the physical examination. If the woman has not had a complete physical examination in the last year, one should be performed during the first visit (see Chapter 6). Because the examination may be painful for the woman, especially if she has chronic pelvic pain, be sure to let her know that she has the ability to halt the examination at any time (Hoffman, 2008).

Proceed with the examination in a slow, deliberate step-by-step fashion to allow for the woman to relax between steps (Hoffman, 2008). Observe the woman's gait and stance—women with intraperiotoneal pathology may compensate for it with changes in posture (Hoffman). Also, musculoskeletal structures may be the site of referred pain from these organs; thus an orthopedic evaluation is important in women with pelvic pain.

Examine the head, neck, cardiac, and respiratory systems to rule out abnormalities. A brief, but succinct neurologic examination, including inspection, palpation, and percussion of the spinal column, can be helpful in ruling out radiculopathy. When the woman is in a supine position, inspect the abdomen, noting any scars, auscultating for bowel sounds, percussing, and palpating for organomegaly. While she is in the supine position, have her raise her head off of the table or have her straight-raise her legs to differentiate abdominal wall and visceral sources of pain (Rapkin & Howe, 2007); this technique is known as the Carnett test.

Palpating over the area the woman identifies as the origin of the pain and pain mapping may also aid diagnosis and can be accomplished during this part of the physical examination. Pain mapping enables clients who feel as if they "hurt all over" to identify the location of their pain. It is done by asking the client to point or specify the exact location of the pain or painful areas. Sometimes it is useful to have the client use a diagram of the body to identify the locations. It may be necessary to focus on one area at a time and move methodically to ensure that all areas that hurt are identified or mapped. Clients who feel as if they hurt all over are often relieved to realize their pain is actually localized and that other areas are not painful. Conscious pain mapping is a newer technique that is performed under local anesthesia during laparoscopy. During this procedure, the patient remains awake and can be questioned about her pain (Hoffman, 2008).

During the pelvic examination, pay particular attention to the woman's reaction when the vagina is palpated to observe if she experiences discomfort from pressure along the pelvic floor; this finding may be indicative of myofascial pain syndrome. Tenderness of the urethra or bladder may indicate involvement of the genitourinary system. Pain with deep palpation may indicate endometriosis, whereas cervical motion tenderness is suggestive of PID, adhesions, and other conditions. A rectal examination should always be included in the pelvic examination of a woman with pelvic pain. Guidelines for the pelvic examination are provided in Chapter 6.

General Screening and Diagnostic Testing

Laboratory testing for women with chronic pelvic pain should include the following elements:

- Complete blood count (CBC)
- Erythrocyte sedimentation rate (ESR)
- Serologic testing for syphilis
- Urinalysis and urine culture (where appropriate)
- Pregnancy testing (if appropriate)
- Vaginal smears or cultures to rule out infection
- Stool guaiac to evaluate gastrointestinal pathology
- Thyroid-stimulating hormone (TSH)

The last test is performed because thyroid disease affects body functions and may be found in women with bowel or bladder symptoms (Hoffman, 2008).

Diagnostic Imaging

Historically, the evaluation of pelvic pain in women who were of reproductive and post-menopausal ages was conducted by ultrasound (US). Today, advances in computed tomography (CT) and magnetic resonance imaging (MRI) have made use of these technologies in diagnosing causes of pelvic pain commonplace (Kalish, Patel, Gunn, & Dubinsky, 2007). The modality of choice for initial imaging remains US, although it is often followed by CT scan. Whereas diffuse and focal adenomyosis and pelvic varices can be identified readily with high-resolution sonography and color Doppler, endometriosis, endometriomas, adhesions, and neoplastic processes are better identified by CT because of its sensitivity (Olson & Schnatz, 2007; Potter & Chandrasekhar, 2008).

Other imaging studies may be used if the patient's symptoms indicate the need. For example, a barium enema study may be performed in women with bowel symptoms; in contrast, if pelvic congestion is suspected, pelvic venography is the tool of choice (Hoffman, 2008). If urinary symptoms are primary with the pelvic pain, then a cystoscopy is typically advised (Hoffman). Laparoscopy is used when pelvic pathology is unable to be detected by physical examination or other testing; it allows direct visualization and may enable direct treatment of intra-abdominal pathology (Hoffman).

Differential Diagnoses

Pathology within systems (nongynecologic and gynecologic) needs to be considered when developing a list of differential diagnoses for pelvic pain. It is important to remember that there may be more than one cause of pelvic pain, and involvement of more than one body system. **Table 29-1** lists differential diagnoses of pelvic pain organized by system.

Evaluation of the pain must differentiate between acute and chronic etiologies as well as gynecologic and nongynecologic causes (Forrest, 2004). **Table 29-2** lists common differential diagnoses related to acute pelvic pain of gynecologic origin and **Table 29-3** lists common differential diagnoses of acute pelvic pain that are not related to a gynecologic problem.

TABLE 29-1 Differential Diagnoses of Pelvic Pain

Diagnoses of Gynecologic Origin	Nongynecologic Diagnoses
Endometriosis	**Gastrointestinal**
Chronic pelvic inflammatory disease (PID)	Irritable bowel syndrome (IBS)
Dysmenorrhea	Diverticulitis
Pelvic adhesions	Constipation
Pelvic congestion	Bowel obstruction
Mittelschmerz	Appendicitis
Vulvodynia	Colon cancer
Uterine prolapse	**Genitourinary**
Ovarian cyst	Interstitial cystitis
Adenomyosis	Urinary tract infection
Fibroids	Urinary retention
Ovarian cancer	Renal calculi
Cervical cancer	**Musculoskeletal**
	Scoliosis
	Radiculopathy
	Arthritis
	Herniated disk

TABLE 29-2 Acute Pelvic Pain of Gynecologic Origin (Noncyclic): Common Differential Diagnoses and Signs, Symptoms, and Location of Pain

Condition	Symptoms	Signs
Abortion: threatened, inevitable, or incomplete (see also Chapter 7)	Crampy, intermittent pain that is in the midline or bilateral lower abdomen	Pregnancy test usually + Vaginal bleeding usually present If infection: elevated WBC and ESR
Ectopic pregnancy (see also Chapter 7)	Unilateral crampy pain that is often continuous	Usually vaginal bleeding is present May have very slight elevation of temperature ESR and WBC may be slightly elevated Serum β-hCG is + US may help with diagnosis PE may reveal an adnexal mass
Pelvic inflammatory disease (see also Chapter 21)	Lower abdominal, uterine adnexal, and cervical motion tenderness Pain is often described as dull or achy and may radiate to back or upper thighs May have nausea and vomiting due to pain	Low-grade fever Purulent discharge Elevated WBC Elevated ESR
Ovarian cysts (see also Chapter 27)	Pain is mild to moderate and self-limiting unless it is due to a hemorrhagic corpus luteum cyst, which can result in significant blood loss and hemoperitoneum Onset of pain is usually sudden and midcycle Note: a corpus luteum cyst is the most prone to rupture and mimics ectopic pregnancy	Hypovolemia only if there is hemoperitoneum Most critical sign is significant abdominal tenderness, often associated with rebound tenderness due to peritoneal irritation May be able to palpate a mass during the pelvic examination if the cyst is still leaking and not entirely ruptured
Adnexal torsion	Results in ischemia and rapid onset of acute pelvic pain Pain is usually severe and constant unless torsion is intermittent, in which case then pain will come and go Pain may worsen with lifting, exercise, and intercourse	Tender abdomen with PE and localized rebound tenderness in lower abdominal quadrants Most important sign: large pelvic mass on PE Mild temperature elevation Mild elevated WBC

(continues)

TABLE 29-2 Acute Pelvic Pain of Gynecologic Origin (Noncyclic): Common Differential Diagnoses and Signs, Symptoms, and Location of Pain *(Continued)*

Condition	Symptoms	Signs
Uterine fibroids (see also Chapters 25 and 27)	Often asymptomatic, can have increased uterine bleeding, pelvic pressure or pain, and dyspareunia (pain with intercourse) Acute pain with torsion or rupture Note: may be confused with subacute salpingo-oophoritis	Palpation of abdomen reveals mass(es) arising from uterus May note tenderness with palpation May have elevated temperature and WBC
Endometriosis (see also Chapters 24 and 27)	Often asymptomatic Most common symptoms are dysmenorrhea, deep dyspareunia, and sacral backache during menses	Physical examination findings may be absent or limited Laparoscopy with biopsy is the gold standard for diagnosis

Note: ESR = erythrocyte sedimentation rate; hCG = human chorionic gonadotropin; PE = physical examination; US = ultrasound; WBC = white blood cell.

Sources: Adapted from Berek, 2007; Karnath & Breitkopf, 2007; Katz, Lentz, Lobo, & Gershenson, 2007; Schorge, Schaffer, Halvorson, Hoffman, Bradshaw, & Cunningham, 2008.

After all other causes of pelvic pain are ruled out, psychogenic pain needs to be considered as a possibility. Psychiatric and psychosocial disorders include substance abuse, depression, physical and emotional abuse, somatization, and hypochondriasis (Shulman & Winer, 2004).

Common Noncyclic Gynecologic Causes of Chronic Pelvic Pain

The most common gynecologic-related causes of chronic pelvic pain identified by laparoscopy are endometriosis (see Chapter 27) and adhesions (Rapkin & Howe, 2007). Other common causes include ovarian remnant, retained ovary syndrome, pelvic congestion syndrome, pelvic relaxation causing prolapse of gynecologic organs (e.g., uterine prolapse; see Chapter 26), subacute salpingo-oophoritis (see Chapter 21), cancer of gynecologic origin (see Chapter 28), and ovarian hyperstimulation syndrome (OHSS).

Pelvic Adhesions

Pelvic adhesions are coarse bands of tissue that connect organs to other organs or to the abdominal wall in places where there should be no connection. Adhesions can be caused by previous surgeries, infection, or endometriosis (Hoffman, 2008; Karnath & Breitkopf, 2007; Rapkin & Howe, 2007). They may be the etiology for infertility, dyspareunia, and bowel obstruction (Hoffman; Karnath & Breitkopf). Adhesions are the most common cause of recurrent or acute bowel obstruction (Karnath & Breitkopf). Currently, the causal role of adhesions in pelvic pain is unknown. Lysis of adhesions is often the treatment of choice,

TABLE 29-3 Acute Pelvic Pain of Nongynecologic Origin: Common Differential Diagnoses, Signs, Symptoms, and Location of Pain

Condition (System)	Symptoms	Signs	Comment
Appendicitis (GI)	Diffuse abdominal pain, generally periumbilical Anorexia, nausea, vomiting Pain usually in RLQ (McBurney's point) Chills	May have low-grade fever High fever if ruptured Chills Rebound tenderness + Psoas sign* + Obturator sign† Rovsing's sign‡ elicited May observe leukocyte shift to left	Most common source of acute pelvic pain in women May be confused with gastroenteritis, pelvic inflammatory disease, urinary tract infection, or ruptured ovarian cyst
Diverticulitis (GI)	Often asymptomatic May experience abdominal bloating, constipation and diarrhea Severe LLQ pain	Distended abdomen with LLQ tenderness with palpation Localized rebound tenderness May palpate a doughy, mobile mass in the LLQ Hypoactive bowel sounds May see elevated WBC	Mimics IBS Fistulas can occur Note: diverticulitis can present with perforations or abscess that produce peritonitis
Intestinal obstruction (GI)	Colicky abdominal pain Abdominal distention Vomiting Constipation and obstipation Higher and acute obstruction presents with early vomiting Colonic obstruction presents with greater degree of abdominal distention and obstipation	Significant abdominal distention Bowel sounds are abnormal: at onset they are high pitched during pain and later will decrease and may be absent due to ischemia Elevated WBC and fever are noted as the condition progresses	
Irritable bowel syndrome (GI)	Acute abdominal pain (may also cause chronic pelvic pain) Bloating Urgency of defecation Diarrhea Constipation	Abdominal pain with palpation May note blood with stool and/or rectal bleeding	IBS is the most commonly identified functional bowel disorder It is diagnosed more often in women than men

(continues)

TABLE 29-3 Acute Pelvic Pain of Nongynecologic Origin: Common Differential Diagnoses, Signs, Symptoms, and Location of Pain *(Continued)*

Condition (System)	Symptoms	Signs	Comment
Gastroenteritis (GI)	Vomiting Diarrhea Abdominal cramping and pain	May have systemic toxicity such as fever and tachycardia Marked abdominal tenderness with palpation	Causes generally are viral or bacterial Usually self-limited
Ureteral lithiasis (GU)	Severe, colicky pain in suprapubic area and in pelvis Urinary frequency Dysuria Nausea, vomiting	Hematuria Flank and costovertebral angle pain	Can mimic ectopic pregnancy
Cystitis (GU)	Lower abdominal or pelvic pain usually midline Dysuria, urinary urgency and frequency	Urine dipstick positive for leukocyte esterase or nitrite	See Chapter 22
Abdominal wall hernia (MU)	Sharp pain sometimes radiates to lower back	Pain intensity is related to position Abdominal tenderness increases when abdominal wall is tensed	

*Psoas sign: Passively lift the patient's thigh against the examiner's hand above the knee. A positive sign is pain in the RLQ.
†Obturator sign: Patient passively flexes the right hip and knee and internally rotates the right leg at the hip. A positive sign is when the acute pain travels from the periumbilical region to the RLQ.
‡Rovsing's sign: Pressing the LLQ produces pain in the RLQ when pressure is released.
GI = gastrointestinal; GU = genitourinary; IBS = irritable bowel syndrome; LLQ = left lower quadrant; MU = musculoskeletal; RLQ = right lower quadrant; WBC = white blood cells.

Sources: Adapted from Berek, 2007; Karnath & Breitkopf, 2007; Katz et al., 2007; Merlin, Shah, & Shiroff, 2010; Schorge et al., 2008.

although it should be attempted only after a thorough evaluation because it can cause the development of more adhesions (Hoffman; Rapkin & Howe). To prevent adhesiogenesis following laparoscopy, the clinician is encouraged to handle the tissues gently, assure hemostasis during the procedure, and consider the use of adhesion barriers, which have been shown to be helpful in preventing formation of adhesions (Hoffman). **Table 29-4** summarizes diagnosis and treatment recommendations related to pelvic adhesions.

Ovarian Remnant Syndrome and Ovarian Retention Syndrome

Although ovarian remnant syndrome and ovarian retention syndrome are two separate etiologies for chronic pelvic pain, they produce almost the same symptoms, and are diagnosed

TABLE 29-4 Common Noncyclic Gynecologic Causes of Chronic Pelvic Pain: Signs, Symptoms, Diagnosis, and Management

Condition	Symptoms	Signs	Diagnosis	Management
Adhesions	Lower abdominal or pelvic pain that occurs or increases when the peritoneum or organ serosa are stretched Dyspareunia	May elicit abdominal pain with light palpation Decreased motility of pelvic organs Adnexal enlargement	Laparoscopy is the diagnostic tool of choice if somatic causes are ruled out and the psychosocial evaluation is negative	Surgical lysis of adhesions only after a thorough evaluation
Ovarian remnant syndrome	Lateral pelvic pain described as sharp and stabbing or dull and not radiating May have dyspareunia, constipation, or flank pain May have genitourinary and/or gastrointestinal symptoms that accompany the pelvic pain	Pelvic mass identified during bimanual examination May observe that the vulva and vagina remain in a persistent estrogenized state	Ultrasound (US) Note: US may be improved by treating the woman with *clomiphene citrate* (Clomid) 100 mg for 5–10 days prior to the US to stimulate follicular development	Initial treatment with *danazol* or high-dose progestins may be helpful in some cases Gonadotropic-releasing hormone (GnRH) agonist may help but cannot be used for long-term therapy Surgical excision is often required
Pelvic congestion syndrome	Bilateral lower abdominal and back pain The following symptoms may accompany pelvic congestion syndrome: • Dysmenorrhea • Dyspareunia Abnormal uterine bleeding Chronic fatigue Irritable bowel syndrome	Bulky feeling to uterus when palpated during the bimanual examination Ovaries may be enlarged and there may be many functional cysts on the ovaries Uterus, parametria, and uterosacral ligaments are tender to touch	Transuterine venography is the primary method used for diagnosis Other methods include the following: • Ultrasound • Magnetic resonance imaging • Laparoscopy	Begin with the least invasive measures Hormonal measures include progestin or GnRH agonist administration Ovarian vein embolization or ligation Hysterectomy with bilateral salpingo-oophorectomy should be the last resort

Sources: Adapted from Berek, 2007; Karnath & Breitkopf, 2007; Katz et al., 2007; Schorge et al., 2008; Tu, Hahn, & Steege, 2010.

and managed similarly. Ovarian remnant syndrome occurs when some of the ovarian tissue is left behind after an oophorectomy; ovarian retention syndrome occurs when an ovary is purposely left behind after hysterectomy (Hoffman, 2008; Rapkin & Howe, 2007). Table 29-4 summarizes diagnosis and treatment recommendations related to these conditions.

Ovarian Hyperstimulation Syndrome

Ovarian hyperstimulation syndrome (OHSS) can result from treatment for infertility. OHSS refers to a combination of ovarian enlargement caused by multiple ovarian cysts that may rupture creating a shift of fluids from the intravascular spaces. This can potentially become a life-threatening complication of ovulation induction.

Mild OHSS is a self-limiting disease, and treatment should be conservative and aimed at symptoms. Medical therapy suffices for most women (Horwitz, Pundi, & Blankstein, 2011).

Mild OHSS can evolve into moderate or severe disease, particularly if conception occurs (Horwitz et al., 2011). Symptoms of increasing severity include enlarging abdominal girth, acute weight gain, and abdominal discomfort. Treatment of moderate to severe disease includes careful fluid management particularly directed at maintenance of intravascular blood volume.

After a few days, third-spaced fluid is absorbed into intravascular spaces, hemoconcentration reverses, and natural dieresis occurs (Horwitz et al., 2011). Intravenous fluids can be discontinued as oral intake of fluids becomes adequate. Complete resolution usually takes 10–14 days after initial onset of symptoms (Horwitz et al.).

Surgery is required in extreme cases, such as in the case of a ruptured cyst, ovarian torsion, or internal hemorrhage. Aggressive palpation of the abdomen can precipitate follicular rupture and should be avoided if OHSS is suspected.

Pelvic Congestion Syndrome

Pelvic congestion syndrome is typically seen in a woman of reproductive age. It occurs when uterine arteries and veins remain chronically dilated and cause pelvic vascular congestion. The pathophysiology involved is unclear, but the syndrome is believed to result from mechanical dilation, ovarian hormone dysfunction, or both (Hoffman, 2008). Table 29-4 summarizes diagnosis and treatment recommendations related to pelvic congestion syndrome.

General Treatment Modalities

The treatment options discussed in this section focus on gynecologic causes of chronic pelvic pain. Enlisting the woman's input in developing her treatment plan, and encouraging her to take an active role in and feel ownership of the plan, is encouraged and often critical to the success of the management plan. Treatment needs to be comprehensive and may include both pharmacologic and complementary approaches. Treatment is most often dictated by the diagnosis. If no pathology is identified, however, treatment is aimed at alleviating symptoms (Hoffman, 2008).

Exercise and physical therapy have been shown to be helpful but require a specialized physiotherapist for initial evaluation to determine an appropriate plan (Bruckenthal, 2011). Aerobic exercises as well as nonaerobic exercises, such as weight lifting, have shown positive results. Determining which type of exercise a woman is likely to do and encouraging that activity may be helpful in reducing the severity of the pain, especially in cases where no known cause can be found.

Pharmacologic treatment for chronic pelvic pain frequently begins with an oral analgesic such as acetaminophen (Tylenol) or nonsteroidal anti-inflammatory drugs (NSAIDs), both nonselective and the cyclo-oxygenase 2 (COX-2) inhibitors (American College of Obstetricians and Gynecologists, 2004, reaffirmed 2010; Hoffman, 2008). If pain relief is not satisfactory with these options, the next pharmacologic agent to consider is a mild opioid such as codeine or hydrocodone. Risk of addiction with these drugs has been shown to be low in patients with chronic pain (American College of Obstetricians and Gynecologists). If the pain persists, stronger opioids such as morphine or fentanyl can be considered, although close and regular surveillance is important with these agents (Gunter, 2003).

Hormonal treatment offers another alternative, and several options are available. Combined oral contraceptives (COCs) are useful in providing relief from primary dysmenorrhea and endometriosis (American College of Obstetricians and Gynecologists, 2004, reaffirmed 2010). The gonadotropin-releasing hormone (GnRH) agonist goserelin may be helpful in reducing pelvic pain from endometriosis and dyspareunia (American College of Obstetricians and Gynecologists). Progestogen therapy can be useful in treating chronic pelvic pain that results from endometriosis and pelvic congestion syndrome (American College of Obstetricians and Gynecologists).

If the chronic pelvic pain is neuropathic in origin, then tricyclic antidepressants may be helpful. These agents are also useful in treating the depression that often accompanies chronic pain. Amitriptyline (Elavil) and its metabolite nortriptyline (Pamelor) have well-documented efficacy in the treatment of both neuropathic and non-neuropathic pain (Hoffman, 2008).

The clinician may also have to consider combining drugs that work via differing mechanisms of action to increase pain relief. For example, an NSAID and an opioid may be prescribed as dual therapy, particularly if inflammation is present (Hoffman, 2008). Transcutaneous electrical nerve stimulation (TENS) can be useful for treatment of localized or regional chronic pelvic pain. TENS therapy involves placement of electrodes near nerve pathways. The electrodes deliver electrical impulses that may help to control or alleviate some types of pain.

Surgical intervention may be necessary and has been shown to be helpful in reducing chronic pelvic pain that is unrelieved by any other measure. When endometriosis is present, excision or laser ablation of the endometrial tissue may be performed, though these procedures have varying success rates (American College of Obstetricians and Gynecologists,

2004, reaffirmed 2010). Presacral neurectomy has been useful in treating chronic pelvic pain associated with dysmenorrhea after other treatment methods have failed. Hysterectomy is, of course, a last resort, and should be considered only after other methods have failed. If the woman is of reproductive age, every attempt should be made to treat her pain with nonsurgical methods before considering hysterectomy.

Psychotherapy should always be considered for a woman with chronic pelvic pain. Physical and sexual abuse is a significant cause of pelvic pain, and as many as 50% of women with chronic pelvic pain have experienced either physical or sexual abuse, or both (American College of Obstetricians and Gynecologists, 2004, reaffirmed 2010). Psychotherapies found to be useful include cognitive therapy, operant conditioning, and behavioral modification (American College of Obstetricians and Gynecologists). If an infection has been confirmed as the source of chronic pelvic pain, antibiotics should be prescribed. The type and length of antibiotic treatment is often dependent on culture and sensitivity results from the infectious source(s).

Alternative and Complementary Treatment

Alternative and complementary therapies are now much more widely accepted and available within developed countries. It is not unusual for even small towns to hold yoga and Tai Chi classes. Additionally, women have increased access to massage, therapeutic touch, acupressure, acupuncture, and reikki therapies (Blonna, 2000). Techniques such as biofeedback, hypnosis, relaxation, and desensitization have all been used to treat pelvic pain, albeit with varying degrees of success (Proctor & Farquhar, 2003). Pain causes muscular contraction; therefore, techniques that relax muscles may help to reduce some types of chronic pelvic pain. Often these relaxation techniques can be used adjunctively with a combination of pharmaceutical agents and alternative therapies (Blonna). Hypnosis has been shown to be helpful for women who are experiencing chronic pelvic pain, particularly that caused by vaginismus and endometriosis (Hornyak & Green, 2000). Knowing what is available in the community and talking with the patient to gain an understanding of what she would favor are important parts of the multifaceted approach needed to resolve symptomatology. The patient needs to be receptive to trying these measures to obtain any degree of effectiveness.

Some clinicians have used herbal, nutritional, and other forms of complementary therapy for the treatment of pelvic pain; however, the evidence base for these treatments is lacking (American College of Obstetricians and Gynecologists, 2004, reaffirmed 2010). Although these alternatives to allopathic procedures may hold promise in the future, there are no current evidence-based recommendations for their use.

Common Nongynecologic Causes of Chronic Pelvic Pain

In a number of instances, the cause of chronic pelvic pain is not gynecologic in origin. The more common nongynecologic causes are addressed here because they should be considered when the clinician is developing a list of differential diagnoses during the work-up for chronic pelvic pain (see Table 29-1). An in-depth discussion is beyond the scope of this book; instead, the reader is referred to the appropriate references at the end of this chapter.

Gastrointestinal Causes: Irritable Bowel Syndrome

Irritable bowel syndrome (IBS) is the most common functional gastrointestinal disorder (Shen & Nahas, 2009). A functional disorder means that the affected organ or system is not working correctly. IBS is characterized by a chronic, relapsing pattern of abdominal and pelvic pain, and is usually accompanied by constipation or diarrhea (American College of Obstetricians and Gynecologists, 2004, reaffirmed 2010; Hammer & Talley, 2008).

Women are diagnosed with IBS at about twice the rate of men (Hammer & Talley, 2008; Heitkemper & Jarrett, 2008). This higher incidence in women may, however, be attributed to the fact that women are overrepresented in clinical and epidemiologic studies of IBS and the potential effect of the menstrual cycle and its hormones may have on IBS (Heitkemper & Jarret). The gender-based difference in the rates of diagnosis may also be related to culture, psychosocial, or healthcare access issues (Heitkemper & Jarrett). A prospective study of 325 women with IBS and 104 men revealed that gender distribution of IBS was proportional to the severity of the constipation related to the diarrhea (Herman, Pokkunuri, Braham, & Pimentel, 2010). Constipation was significantly more prevalent in the women in the study than in the men, whereas the incidence of diarrhea was about the same in the two genders.

Clinical features of IBS include shifting abdominal pain accompanied by constipation or diarrhea, or both. Bloating, nausea, and vomiting are also common symptoms. The pain may be identified in one quadrant of the abdomen but then relocate during the next attack. Typically, defecation provides relief from the pain. Although the exact etiology of IBS is unknown, its cause is believed to involve dysregulation in interactions between the central nervous system and the enteric nervous system (Hoffman, 2008).

The patient's history is critical to the diagnosis of IBS because the diagnosis is based on the symptoms. The Rome criteria are used to categorize the symptoms and make the diagnosis. These criteria constitute a system developed to classify functional gastrointestinal disorders (FGIDs), disorders of the digestive system in which symptoms cannot be explained by the presence of structural or tissue abnormality, based on clinical symptoms (Rome Foundation, 2011). The Rome III Diagnostic Criteria for IBS include the following findings: recurrent abdominal pain or discomfort that has occurred for at least 3 days each month for the past 3 months and has been accompanied by at least two of the following: (1) improvement with defecation, (2) onset associated with a change in frequency of stool, and (3) onset associated with a change in form (appearance) of stool.

During physical examination of the abdomen, areas of hard feces may be felt in the transverse and descending colon, and the rectal examination may reveal the presence of a hard, lumpy stool if constipation is one of the symptoms. Women with IBS often experience bloating and general intestinal irritability. Passage of mucus rectally is common. Less frequently, women with IBS may experience blood in their stools, so guaiac testing is important. Additional gastrointestinal causes of pelvic pain to keep in mind (although not as common as IBS) include chronic appendicitis, adhesions from previous bowel surgery, and abdominal wall hernia, including umbilical hernias.

Management of IBS depends on the symptoms and the presence of any comorbidities. Often psychologic support is helpful. Many clinicians recommend an increase in fiber consumed as part of the diet, although there is no evidence to support this recommendation. Medications to decrease anxiety have been used with some success. Other medications are prescribed to treat the symptoms of diarrhea and constipation. Antispasmodics such as dicyclomine (Bentyl) and hyoscyamine (Levsin) have been used to decrease abdominal pain due to spasm (Hoffman, 2008). Current research is directed at probiotics, and preliminary findings are encouraging regarding their action, particularly in symptom improvement (Longstreth et al., 2006).

Musculoskeletal Causes

Although musculoskeletal disorders have not been routinely considered as causes of pelvic pain, their importance is increasingly becoming recognized. For example, myofascial pain originating from trigger points in skeletal muscle has been identified as the cause in some cases of pelvic pain. The incidence of myofascial disease is unknown. Testing for Carnett's sign assists in making the diagnosis and identifying the trigger points. Once these sites have been identified, they can be injected with local anesthetic—a technique that has been shown to bring relief of the symptoms.

Abdominal wall hernias may be another musculoskeletal source of pelvic pain. While a detailed discussion of hernias is beyond the scope of this book, the clinician should suspect an abdominal wall hernia if the pelvic pain intensity is related to the patient's position and if she has increased pain when she tenses her abdominal wall (Karnath & Breitkopf, 2007).

Urologic Causes

Interstitial cystitis (see Chapter 22) occurs more often in women than in men, and most patients diagnosed with this condition are between 40 and 60 years of age (Rapkin & Howe, 2007). Cystoscopy findings of petechiae or decreased bladder capacity (less than 350 mL) are considered diagnostic (American College of Obstetricians and Gynecologists, 2004, reaffirmed 2010). Symptoms of interstitial cystitis include severe urinary frequency and pain, nocturia, and dysuria. Hematuria may also be present. Anterior pain that occurs when palpating the vaginal wall over the border of the bladder is suggestive of interstitial cystitis. Diagnosis of this disorder is made based on symptoms and findings on cystoscopy. The etiology of interstitial cystitis is unknown; thus its management is empirical. Diet changes, stress reduction, and behavior changes are often suggested, and the woman is encouraged to do pelvic floor exercises, which sometimes bring relief of urge frequency.

Urethral syndrome, defined as a symptom complex including dysuria, frequency, and urgency of urination, should also be considered in the work-up of the woman with pelvic pain. Typically the woman with urethral syndrome presents with the aforementioned symptoms plus suprapubic tenderness, urinary incontinence, and dyspareunia. Diagnosis is made by exclusion; for this reason, a clean catch or catheterized urine specimen should be ordered to rule out urinary tract infection. Sometimes sterile pyuria is present; if it is, a course of doxycycline or erythromycin is helpful. A trial of local estrogen therapy is suggested, though if there is no improvement after 2 months, urethral dilation is a consideration (Rapkin & Howe, 2007).

Current and Emergent Evidence for Practice

Recommendations based on limited or inconsistent scientific evidence (Level B) include using GnRH agonists to treat chronic pelvic pain that is not caused by endometriosis or IBS. These agents are often tried only because they have been shown to be effective in treating pelvic pain associated with endometriosis; there is no scientific evidence to support their use for long-standing chronic pelvic pain. Other Level B treatments that the American College of Obstetricians and Gynecologists (2004, reaffirmed 2010, p. 11) suggests for consideration include the following:

- Surgical adhesiolysis for adhesions other than bowel adhesions
- Hysterectomy to treat chronic pelvic pain associated with gynecologic tract symptoms
- Sacral nerve stimulation
- Various physical therapies
- Nutritional supplementation with vitamin B_1 or magnesium for pain associated with dysmenorrhea
- Injection of trigger points of the abdominal wall, vagina, and sacrum with local anesthetic
- Treatment of abdominal trigger points by application of magnets to the trigger points
- Acupuncture, acupressure, and transcutaneous nerve stimulation for treatment of pain related to primary dysmenorrhea

Recommendations identified by the American College of Obstetricians and Gynecologists (2004, reaffirmed 2010, p. 11) that are based primarily on consensus and expert opinion (Level C) include the following:

- A detailed history and physical examination as the basis for differential diagnoses
- Antidepressants
- Opioid analgesics

Special Considerations

Adolescents

Pelvic pain in adolescents is almost always gynecologic in origin, cyclic, and not as uncommon as one would think (Hewitt & Brown, 2000). Common causes of pelvic pain in adolescents, listed in order of frequency, include gynecologic, urologic, gastrointestinal, musculoskeletal, and psychosocial sources (Hewitt & Brown). Interestingly, pelvic pain is more likely to be of gynecologic origin than of gastrointestinal origin (specifically IBS) within this age group. PID is important to rule out as a cause of pelvic pain in adolescents because it is so commonly diagnosed in this age group. Rarely do adolescents present with pelvic pain that is chronic. Estimates of the percentage of adolescent women presenting with chronic pelvic pain have not been published in the literature.

Adolescents, because of their emotional and physical development, pose challenges to clinicians that are different from those associated with women in their 20s and beyond. Developing a rapport with any teenager may be the biggest challenge facing the clinician working with this age group. Suggestions for developing rapport include maintaining eye contact, demonstrating a nonjudgmental attitude, treating the patient with respect, and giving her undivided attention. It is important to validate her symptoms and the feelings she associates with them.

It is important to be familiar with state and local statutes regarding health care for minors. Many states have parental consent laws. Each practice needs to have its own policy that must follow the legal parameters already in place.

Culture

Knowing and appreciating the cultural background of a patient is a significant component of culturally competent health care. Cultural and social stratification influences decision making for both patient and clinician, as well as the treatment options that are offered and accepted. Should the clinician be shaking hands, making eye contact, or addressing the patient directly? If her husband is present, does the couple's culture dictate that the clinician include him in the conversation as well? How close should the clinician stand or sit when taking a history? These are all culturally significant questions to consider. In addition, women of different cultures express pain differently. The expression of pain may vary from stoicism to wailing (Luckmann, 1999). Validating a patient's feelings and recognizing and appreciating her cultural and ethnic background are important not only in gaining her trust and establishing rapport, but also in helping the clinician understand the scope of the problem the woman presents.

Culture can also affect symptom reporting and diagnosis. A retrospective review of charts of Mexican American patients with IBS was performed to determine whether the symptoms reported met the Rome II criteria (Barakzai & Gregory, 2007). Only 63% of the patients in the study reported symptoms that met any of the Rome II criteria. These findings emphasize that the clinician must have a clear understanding of what the illness means to the patient to make accurate diagnoses and create appropriate treatment plans (Barakzai & Gregory).

References

Altman, G., & Lee, C. (2009). Chronic pelvic pain and associated disorders. *Kansas Nurse, 84*, 12–15.

American College of Obstetricians and Gynecologists. (2004, reaffirmed 2010). *Chronic pelvic pain: Clinical management guidelines for obstetrician-gynecologists.* Practice Bulletin No. 51. Washington, DC: Author.

Barakzai, M. D., & Gregory, J. (2007). The effect of culture on symptom reporting: Hispanics and irritable bowel syndrome. *American Academy of Nurse Practitioners, 19*, 261–267.

Beckman, C. R., Ling, F. W., Laube, D. W., Smith, R. P., Barzansky, B. M., & Herbert, W. N. (2002). *Obstetrics and gynecology* (4th ed.). Philadelphia, PA: Lippincott, Williams & Wilkins.

Berek, J. (2007). *Berek and Novak's gynecology* (14th ed.). Philadelphia, PA: Lippincott, Williams & Wilkins.

Berkley, K. J. (1997). Sex differences in pain. *Behavioral Brain Science, 20*, 371–380, 435–513.

Blonna, R. (2000). *Coping with stress in a changing world* (2nd ed.). New York: McGraw-Hill.

Bruckenthal, P. (2011). Chronic pelvic pain: Approaches to diagnosis. *Pain Management in Nursing, 12*(1), S4–S10.

Butrick, C. (2007). Chronic pelvic pain: How many surgeries are enough? *Clinical Obstetrics and Gynecology, 50*, 412–424.

Collett, B. J., & Berkley, K. (2007). Editorial: The IASP Global Year Against Pain in Women. *Pain, 132*, S1–S2.

Fillingim, R. B., King, C. D., Ribeiro-Dasilva, M. C., Rahim-Williams, B., & Riley, J. L. (2009). Sex, gender, and pain: A review of recent clinical and experimental findings. *Journal of Pain, 10*(5), 447–485.

Fogel, C. I. (1995). Common symptoms. In C. I. Fogel & N. F. Woods (Eds.), *Women's health care: A comprehensive handbook* (pp. 517–570). Thousand Oaks, CA: Sage.

Forrest, D. E. (2004). Common gynecologic pelvic disorders. In E. Youngkin & M. Davis (Eds.), *Women's health* (3rd ed., pp. 303–350). Upper Saddle River, NJ: Pearson Prentice Hall.

Greenspan, J. D., Craft, R. M., LeResche, L., Arendt-Nielsen, L., Berkley, K., Fillingim, R. B., & Pain SIG of the IASP. (2007). Studying sex and gender differences in pain and analgesia: A consensus report. *Pain, 132*, S26–S45.

Gunter, J. (2003). Chronic pelvic pain: An integrated approach to diagnosis and treatment. *Obstetrical & Gynecological Survey, 58*, 615–623.

Hammer, J., & Talley, N. J. (2008). Value of different diagnostic criteria for the irritable bowel syndrome among men and women. *Clinical Gastroenterology, 42*(2), 160–166.

Heitkemper, M. M., & Jarrett, M. E. (2008). Update on irritable bowel syndrome and gender differences. *Nutrition in Clinical Practice, 23*(3), 275–283.

Herman, J., Pokkunuri, V., Braham, L., & Pimentel, M. (2010). Gender distribution in irritable bowel syndrome is proportional to the severity of constipation relative to diarrhea. *Gender Medicine, 7*(3), 240–246.

Hewitt, G. D., & Brown, R. T. (2000). Chronic pelvic pain in the adolescent. *Female Patient, 84*(4), 1009–1025.

Hoffman, B. (2008). Pelvic pain. In J. Schorge, J. Schaffer, L. Halvorson, K. Bradshaw, and F. G. Cunningham (Eds.), *Williams gynecology* (pp. 244–268). New York: McGraw-Hill Medical.

Hornyak, L. M., & Green, J. P. (Eds.). (2000). *Healing from within: The use of hypnosis in women's health care*. Washington, DC: American Psychological Association.

Horwitz, J., Pundi, R. S., & Blankstein, J. (2011). Ovarian hyperstimulation syndrome treatment & management. *Medscape Reference*. Retrieved from http://emedicine.medscape.com/article/1343572 -treatment

Ignatavicius, D., & Workman, M. (2002). *Medical–surgical nursing: Critical thinking for collaborative care*. Philadelphia, PA: W. B. Saunders.

Jarrell, J., Vilos, G., Allaire, C., Burgess, S., Fortin, C., Gerwin, R.,... Abu-Rafea, B. (2005). Consensus guidelines for the management of chronic pain. *Journal of Obstetrics Gynecology Canada, 164*, 781–801.

Kalish, G. M., Patel, M. D., Gunn, M. L. D., & Dubinsky, T. J. (2007). Computed tomographic and magnetic resonance features of gynecologic abnormalities in women presenting with acute or chronic abdominal pain. *Ultrasound Quarterly, 23*(5), 167–175.

Karnath, B., & Breitkopf, D. (2007). Acute and chronic pelvic pain in women. *Hospital Physician, 43*(7), 41–48.

Kassab, D., & Rollins, V. (2011). Should we screen patients with chronic pelvic pain for depression? *Evidence-Based Practice: Patient-Oriented Evidence That Matters, 14*(1), 13.

Katz, V., Lentz, G., Lobo, R., & Gershenson, D. M. (2007). *Comprehensive gynecology* (5th ed.). Philadelphia, PA: Mosby Elsevier.

Kruszka, P., & Kruszka, S. (2010). Evaluation of acute pelvic pain in women. *American Family Physician, 82*, 141–147.

Ling, F. (1995). Pelvic pain. In D. Nichols & P. Sweeney (Eds.), *Ambulatory gynecology* (pp. 200–212). Philadelphia, PA: JB Lippincott.

Longstreth, G. F., Thompson, W. G., Chey, W. D., Houghton, L. A., Mearin, F., & Spiller, R. C. (2006). Functional bowel disorders. *Gastroenterology, 130*, 1480–1491.

Luckmann, J. (1999). *Transcultural communication in nursing.* New York: Delmar.

Martin, D., & Ling, F. (1999). Endometriosis and pain. *Clinical Obstetrics and Gynecology, 42*(3), 664–686.

Merlin, M. A., Shah, C. N., & Shiroff, A. M. (2010). Evidence-based appendicitis: The initial work-up. *Postgraduate Medicine, 122*(3), 189–195.

Mogil, J. S., & Chanda, M. L. (2005). The case for the inclusion of female subjects in basic science studies of pain. *Pain, 117*, 1–5.

Olson, C., & Schnatz, P. F. (2007). Evaluation and management of chronic pelvic pain in women. *Journal of Clinical Outcomes Management, 14*(10), 563–573.

Potter, A.W., & Chandrasekhar, C. A. (2008). US and CT evaluation of acute pelvic pain of gynecologic origin in nonpregnant premenopausal patients. *Radiographics, 28*, 1645–1659.

Proctor, M. L., & Farquhar, C. M. (2003, June). Dysmenorrhea. *Clinical Evidence, 9*, 1994–2013.

Rapkin, A., & Howe, C. (2007). Pelvic pain and dysmenorrhea. In J. Berek (Ed.), *Berek and Novak's gynecology* (14th ed., pp. 505–540). Philadelphia, PA: Lippincott Williams & Wilkins.

Rome Foundation. (2011). *About the Rome Foundation.* Retrieved from www.romecriteria.org

Schorge, J. O., Schaffer, J. I., Halvorson, L. M., Hoffman, B. L., Bradshaw, K. D., & Cunningham, F. G. (2008). *Williams gynecology.* New York: McGraw-Hill.

Shen, Y., & Nahas, R. (2009). Complementary and alternative medicine for treatment of irritable bowel syndrome. *Canadian Family Physician, 55*, 143–148.

Shulman, L. P., & Winer, S. (2004). Chronic pelvic pain. *The Forum, 1*, 12–17.

Tu, F. F., Hahn, D., & Steege, J. F. (2010). Pelvic congestion syndrome–associated pelvic pain: A systematic review of diagnosis and management. *Obstetrical and Gynecological Survey, 65*(5), 332–340.

Vallerand, A. (1995). Gender differences in pain. *Image: Journal of Nursing Scholarship, 27*, 235–237.

Vallerand, A. H., & Polomano, R. C. (2000). The relationship of gender to pain. *Pain Management Nursing, 1*(3 suppl 1), 8–15.

Vincent, K. (2009). Chronic pelvic pain in women. *Postgraduate Medicine, 85*, 24–29.

Williams, R., Hartmann, K., Sandler, R., Miller, W., & Steege, J. (2004). Prevalence and characteristics of irritable bowel syndrome among women with chronic pelvic pain. *American College of Obstetrics & Gynecology, 104*, 452–458.

Williams, R., Hartmann, K., & Steege, J. (2004). Documenting the current definitions of chronic pelvic pain: Implications for research. *American College of Obstetrics and Gynecology, 103*, 686–691.

Zondervan, K., Yudkin, P., Vessey, M., Dawes, M., Barlow, D., & Kennedy, S. (1999). Prevalence and incidence of chronic pelvic pain in primary care: Evidence from a national general practice database. *British Journal of Obstetrics & Gynecology, 106*(11), 1149–1155.

29-A

The International Pelvic Pain Society Pelvic Pain Asssessment Form

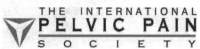

Pelvic Pain Assessment Form

Physician: _____

Initial History and Physical Examination   *Date:* _____

This assessment form is intended to assist the clinician with the initial patient assessment and is not meant to be a diagnostic tool.

Contact Information

Name: _____   Birth Date: _____   Chart Number: _____

Phone: Work: _____   Home: _____   Cell: _____

Referring Provider's Name and Address: _____

Information About Your Pain

Please describe your pain problem (use a separate sheet of paper if needed) : _____
_____
_____
_____
_____
_____

What do you think is causing your pain? _____

Is there an event that you associate with the onset of your pain? ☐ Yes   ☐ No   If so, what? _____

How long have you had this pain? ____ years ____ months

For each of the symptoms listed below, please "bubble in" your level of pain over the last month using a 10-point scale:
0 - no pain   10 – the worst pain imaginable

	0	1	2	3	4	5	6	7	8	9	10
How would you rate your pain?											
Pain at ovulation (mid-cycle)	O	O	O	O	O	O	O	O	O	O	O
Pain just before period	O	O	O	O	O	O	O	O	O	O	O
Pain (not cramps) before period	O	O	O	O	O	O	O	O	O	O	O
Deep pain with intercourse	O	O	O	O	O	O	O	O	O	O	O
Pain in groin when lifting	O	O	O	O	O	O	O	O	O	O	O
Pelvic pain lasting hours or days after intercourse	O	O	O	O	O	O	O	O	O	O	O
Pain when bladder is full	O	O	O	O	O	O	O	O	O	O	O
Muscle / joint pain	O	O	O	O	O	O	O	O	O	O	O
Level of cramps with period	O	O	O	O	O	O	O	O	O	O	O
Pain after period is over	O	O	O	O	O	O	O	O	O	O	O
Burning vaginal pain after sex	O	O	O	O	O	O	O	O	O	O	O
Pain with urination	O	O	O	O	O	O	O	O	O	O	O
Backache	O	O	O	O	O	O	O	O	O	O	O
Migraine headache	O	O	O	O	O	O	O	O	O	O	O
Pain with sitting	O	O	O	O	O	O	O	O	O	O	O

Provider Comments

_____
_____
_____
_____

Information About Your Pain
What types of treatments / providers have you tried in the past for your pain?   **Please check all that apply.**

☐ Acupuncture
☐ Anesthesiologist
☐ Anti-seizure medications
☐ Antidepressants
☐ Biofeedback
☐ Botox injection
☐ Contraceptive pills / patch / ring
☐ Danazol (Danocrine)
☐ Depo-provera
☐ Gastroenterologist
☐ Gynecologist

☐ Family Practitioner
☐ Herbal Medicine
☐ Homeopathic medicine
☐ Lupron, Synarel, Zoladex
☐ Massage
☐ Meditation
☐ Narcotics
☐ Naturopathic mediciation
☐ Nerve blocks
☐ Neurosurgeon
☐ Nonprescription medicine

☐ Nutrition / diet
☐ Physical Therapy
☐ Psychotherapy
☐ Psychiatrist
☐ Rheumatologist
☐ Skin magnets
☐ Surgery
☐ TENS unit
☐ Trigger point injections
☐ Urologist
☐ Other _____

Pain Maps
Please shade areas of pain and write a number from 1 to 10 at the site(s) of pain. (10 = most severe pain imaginable)

Vulvar / Perineal Pain
(pain outside and around the vagina and anus)

If you have vulvar pain, shade the painful areas and write a number from 1 to 10 at the painful sites. (10 = most severe pain imaginable)

Is your pain relieved by sitting on a commode seat?   ☐ Yes   ☐ No

Right   Left

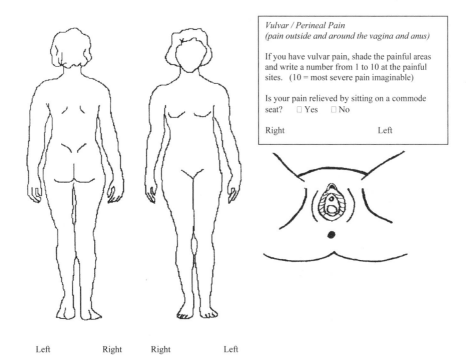

Left   Right   Right   Left

What physicians or health care providers have evaluated or treated you for **chronic pelvic pain**?

Physician / Provider	Specialty	City, State, Phone

Demographic Information
Are you (check all that apply):
      ☐ Married   ☐ Widowed   ☐ Separated   ☐ Committed Relationship
      ☐ Single   ☐ Remarried   ☐ Divorced
Who do you live with? _____

Education: ☐ Less than 12 years   ☐ High School graduate
            ☐ College degree   ☐ Postgraduate degree
What type of work are you trained for? _____
What type of work are you doing? _____

Surgical History
Please list all surgical procedures you have had **related to this pain**:

Year	Procedure	Surgeon	Findings

Please list all **other** surgical procedures:

Year	Procedure	Year	Procedure

Provider Comments
_____
_____
_____
_____

Medications

Please list **pain medication** you have taken for your pain condition in the past 6 months, and the providers who prescribed them (use a separate page if needed):

Medication / dose	Provider	Did it help?		
		☐ Yes	☐ No	☐ Currently taking
		☐ Yes	☐ No	☐ Currently taking
		☐ Yes	☐ No	☐ Currently taking
		☐ Yes	☐ No	☐ Currently taking
		☐ Yes	☐ No	☐ Currently taking
		☐ Yes	☐ No	☐ Currently taking
		☐ Yes	☐ No	☐ Currently taking
		☐ Yes	☐ No	☐ Currently taking

Please list all **other medications** you are presently taking, the condition, and the provider who prescribed them (use a separate page if needed):

Medication / dose	Provider	Medical Condition

Obstetrical History

How many pregnancies have you had? _____

Resulting in (#): _____ Full 9 months _____ Premature _____ Miscarriage / Abortion _____ Living children

Where there any complications during pregnancy, labor, delivery, or post partum?

☐ 4° Episiotomy   ☐ C-Section   ☐ Vacuum   ☐ Post-partum hemorrhaging

☐ Vaginal laceration   ☐ Forceps   ☐ Medication for bleeding   ☐ Other _____

Family History

Has anyone in your family had: ☐ Fibromyalgia ☐ Chronic pelvic pain   ☐ Irritable bowel syndrome

☐ Depression   ☐ Interstitial Cystitis   ☐ Other Chronic Condition _____

☐ Endometriosis ☐ Cancer, Type(s) _____

Medical History

Please list any medical problems / diagnoses _____

_____

_____

Allergies (including latex allergy) _____

Who is your primary care provider? _____

Have you ever been hospitalized for anything besides childbirth?   ☐ Yes   ☐ No   If yes, please explain_____

_____

Have you had major accidents such as falls or a back injury?   ☐ Yes   ☐ No

Have you ever been treated for depression? ☐ Yes ☐ No   Treatments: ☐ Medication ☐ Hospitalization ☐ Psychotherapy

Birth control method: ☐ Nothing   ☐ Pill   ☐ Vasectomy   ☐ Vaginal ring   ☐ Depo provera

☐ Condom   ☐ IUD   ☐ Hysterectomy   ☐ Diaphragm   ☐ Tubal Sterilization

☐ Other _____

Menstrual History

How old were you when your menses started? _____

Are you still having menstrual periods? ☐ Yes ☐ No

Answer the following only if you are still having menstrual periods.

Periods are: ☐ Light   ☐ Moderate   ☐ Heavy   ☐ Bleed through protection

How many days between your periods? _____

How many days of menstrual flow? _____

Date of first day of last menstrual period _____

Do you have any pain with your periods? ☐ Yes   ☐ No

    Does pain start the day flow starts? ☐ Yes   ☐ No   Pain starts _____ days before flow

    Are periods regular? ☐ Yes   ☐ No

Do you pass clots in menstrual flow? ☐ Yes   ☐ No

Gastrointestinal / Eating

Do you have nausea?   ☐ No   ☐ With pain   ☐ Taking medications   ☐ With eating   ☐ Other

Do you have vomiting?   ☐ No   ☐ With pain   ☐ Taking medications   ☐ With eating   ☐ Other

Have you ever had an eating disorder such as anorexia or bulimia?   ☐ Yes   ☐ No

Are you experiencing rectal bleeding or blood in your stool?   ☐ Yes   ☐ No

Do you have increased pain with bowel movements?   ☐ Yes   ☐ No

The following questions help to diagnose irritable bowel syndrome, a gastrointestinal condition, which may be a cause of pelvic pain.

Do you have pain or discomfort that is associated with the following:

    Change in frequency of bowel movement   ☐ Yes   ☐ No

    Change in appearance of stool or bowel movement?   ☐ Yes   ☐ No

    Does your pain improve after completing a bowel movement?   ☐ Yes   ☐ No

---

Health Habits

How often do you exercise?   ☐ Rarely   ☐ 1-2 times weekly   ☐ 3-5 times weekly   ☐ Daily

What is your caffeine intake (number cups per day, include coffee, tea, soft drinks, etc)?   ☐ 0   ☐ 1-3   ☐ 4-6   ☐ >6

How many cigarettes do you smoke per day? _____   For how many years? _____

Do you drink alcohol?   ☐ Yes   ☐ No

    Number of drinks per week _____

Have you ever received treatment for substance abuse? ☐ Yes   ☐ No

What is your use of recreational drugs? ☐ Never used   ☐ Used in the past, but not now   ☐ Presently using   ☐ No answer

    ☐ Heroin   ☐ Amphetamines   ☐ Marijuana   ☐ Barbiturates   ☐ Cocaine   ☐ Other _____

How would you describe your diet? (check all that apply)   ☐ Well balanced   ☐ Vegan   ☐ Vegetarian   ☐ Fried food

    ☐ Special diet _____   ☐ Other _____

Urinary Symptoms

Do you experience any of the following?

Loss of urine when coughing, sneezing, or laughing? ☐ Yes   ☐ No
Difficulty passing urine? ☐ Yes   ☐ No
Frequent bladder infections? ☐ Yes   ☐ No
Blood in the urine? ☐ Yes   ☐ No
Still feeling full after urination? ☐ Yes   ☐ No
Having to void again within minutes of voiding? ☐ Yes   ☐ No

The following questions help to diagnose painful bladder syndrome, which may cause pelvic pain

Please circle the answer that best describes your bladder function and symptoms.

	0	1	2	3	4
1. How many times do you go to the bathroom **DURING THE DAY** (to void or empty your bladder)?	3-6	7-10	11-14	15-19	20 or more
2. How many times do you go to the bathroom **AT NIGHT** (to void or empty your bladder)?	0	1	2	3	4 or more
3. If you get up at night to void or empty your bladder does it bother you?	Never	Mildly	Moderately	Severely	
4. Are you sexually active? ☐ Yes ☐ No					
5. If you are sexually active, do you now or have you ever had pain or symptoms during or after sexual intercourse?	Never	Occasionally	Usually	Always	
6. If you have pain with intercourse, does it make you avoid sexual intercourse?	Never	Occasionally	Usually	Always	
7. Do you have pain associated with your bladder or in your pelvis (lower abdomen, labia, vagina, urethra, perineum)?	Never	Occasionally	Usually	Always	
8. Do you have urgency after voiding?	Never	Occasionally	Usually	Always	
9. If you have pain, is it usually	Never	Mild	Moderate	Severe	
10. Does your pain bother you?	Never	Occasionally	Usually	Always	
11. If you have urgency, is it usually		Mild	Moderate	Severe	
12. Does your urgency bother you?	Never	Occasionally	Usually	Always	

© 2000 C. Lowell Parsons, MD Reprinted with permission.

KCl ____ *Not Indicated* ____ *Positive* ____ *Negative*

Coping Mechanisms

Who are the people you talk to concerning your pain, or during stressful times?

☐ Spouse / Partner   ☐ Relative   ☐ Support group   ☐ Clergy

☐ Doctor / Nurse   ☐ Friend   ☐ Mental Health provider   ☐ I take care of myself

How does your partner deal with your pain?

☐ Doesn't notice when I'm in pain   ☐ Takes care of me   ☐ Not applicable

☐ Withdraws   ☐ Feels helpless

☐ Distracts me with activities   ☐ Gets angry

What helps your pain?

☐ Meditation   ☐ Relaxation   ☐ Lying down   ☐ Music

☐ Massage   ☐ Ice   ☐ Heating pad   ☐ Hot bath

☐ Pain medication   ☐ Laxatives / Enema   ☐ Injection   ☐ TENS unit

☐ Bowel movement   ☐ Emptying bladder   ☐ Nothing

☐ Other _____

What makes your pain worse?

☐ Intercourse   ☐ Orgasm   ☐ Stress   ☐ Full meal

☐ Bowel movement   ☐ Full bladder   ☐ Urination   ☐ Standing

☐ Walking   ☐ Exercise   ☐ Time of day   ☐ Weather

☐ Contact with clothing   ☐ Coughing / sneezing   ☐ Not related to anything

☐ Other _____

Of all the problems or stresses or your life, how does your pain compare in importance?

☐ The most important problem   ☐ Just one of many problems

Sexual and Physical Abuse History

Have you ever been the victim of emotional abuse? This can include being humiliated or insulted ☐ Yes ☐ No ☐ No answer

	As a child (13 and younger)	As an adult (14 and over)
Check an answer for <u>both</u> as a child and as an adult.		
1a. Has anyone ever exposed the sex organs of their body to you when you did not want it?	☐ Yes ☐ No	☐ Yes ☐ No
1b. Has anyone ever threatened to have sex with you when you did not want it?	☐ Yes ☐ No	☐ Yes ☐ No
1c. Has anyone ever touched the sex organs of your body when you did not want this?	☐ Yes ☐ No	☐ Yes ☐ No
1d. Has anyone ever made you touch the sex organs of their body when you did not want this?	☐ Yes ☐ No	☐ Yes ☐ No
1e. Has anyone forced you to have sex when you did not want this?	☐ Yes ☐ No	☐ Yes ☐ No
1f. Have you had any other unwanted sexual experiences not mentioned above?	☐ Yes ☐ No	☐ Yes ☐ No

If yes, please specify _____

2. When you were a child (13 or younger), did an older person do the following?

a. Hit, kick, or beat you?   ☐ Never   ☐ Seldom   ☐ Occasionally   ☐ Often

b. Seriously threaten your life?   ☐ Never   ☐ Seldom   ☐ Occasionally   ☐ Often

3. Now that you are an adult (14 or older), has any other adult done the following?

a. Hit, kick, or beat you?   ☐ Never   ☐ Seldom   ☐ Occasionally   ☐ Often

b. Seriously threaten your life?   ☐ Never   ☐ Seldom   ☐ Occasionally   ☐ Often

Leserman, J, Drossman D, Li Z. The reliability and validity of a sexual and physical abuse history questionnaire in female patients with gastrointestinal disorders. Behavioral Medicine 1995;21:141-148.

Short-Form McGill
The words below describe average pain. Place a check mark (√) in the column which represents the degree to which you feel that type of pain. Please limit yourself to a description of the pain in your pelvic area <u>only</u>.

What does your pain feel like?

Type	None (0)	Mild (1)	Moderate (2)	Severe (3)
Throbbing	_____	_____	_____	_____
Shooting	_____	_____	_____	_____
Stabbing	_____	_____	_____	_____
Sharp	_____	_____	_____	_____
Cramping	_____	_____	_____	_____
Gnawing	_____	_____	_____	_____
Hot-Burning	_____	_____	_____	_____
Aching	_____	_____	_____	_____
Heavy	_____	_____	_____	_____
Tender	_____	_____	_____	_____
Splitting	_____	_____	_____	_____
Tiring-Exhausting	_____	_____	_____	_____
Sickening	_____	_____	_____	_____
Fearful	_____	_____	_____	_____
Punishing-Cruel	_____	_____	_____	_____

Melzak R. The Short-form McGill Pain Questionnaire. Pain 1987;30:191-197.

Pelvic Varicosity Pain Syndrome Questions

Is your pelvic pain aggravated by prolonged physical activity?	☐ Yes	☐ No
Does your pelvic pain improve when you lie down?	☐ Yes	☐ No
Do you have pain that is deep in the vagina or pelvis *during* sex?	☐ Yes	☐ No
Do you have pelvic throbbing or aching *after* sex?	☐ Yes	☐ No
Do you have pelvic pain that moves from side to side?	☐ Yes	☐ No
Do you have sudden episodes of severe pelvic pain that come and go?	☐ Yes	☐ No

Physical Examination – For Physician Use Only

Name:_____ Chart Number:_____

Date of Exam:_____ Height:_____ Weight:_____ BMI:_____

BP:_____ HR: _____ Temp:_____ Resp:_____ LMP:_____

ROS, PFSH Reviewed: ☐ Yes ☐ No Physician Signature:_____

General Appearance: ☐ Well-appearing ☐ Ill-appearing ☐ Tearful ☐ Depressed
☐ Normal weight ☐ Underweight ☐ Overweight ☐ Abnormal Gait

_____

<u>*NOTE: Mark "Not Examined" as N/E*</u>

HEENT ☐ WNL *Lungs* ☐ WNL *Heart* ☐ WNL *Breasts* ☐ WNL
☐ Other _____ ☐ Other _____ ☐ Other _____ ☐ Other _____

Right   Left

Abdomen
☐ Non-tender ☐ Tender ☐ Incisions ☐ Trigger Points
☐ Inguinal Tenderness ☐ Inguinal Bulge ☐ Suprapubic Tenderness ☐ Ovarian Point Tenderness
☐ Mass ☐ Guarding ☐ Rebound ☐ Distention
☐ Other _____

Right   Left   Right   Left   Right   Left
Trigger Points   **Surgical Scars**   **Other Findings**

Back
☐ Non-tender ☐ Tender ☐ Alteration in posture ☐ SI joint rotation _____

Lower Extremities
☐ WNL ☐ Edema ☐ Varicosities ☐ Neuropathy ☐ Length Discrepancy _____

Neuropathy
☐ Iliohypogastric ☐ Ilioinguinal ☐ Genitofemoral ☐ Pudendal ☐ Altered sensation

9

Fibromyalgia / Back / Buttock

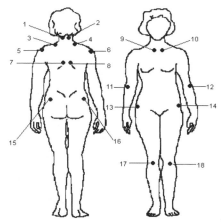

Left   Right   Right   Left

External Genitalia

☐ WNL   ☐ Erythema   ☐ Discharge   ☐ Q-tip test (show on diagram)   ☐ Tenderness (show on diagram)

Right   Left   Right   Left

Q-tip Test (score each circle 0-4) **Total Score** _____   **Other Findings**_____

Vagina

☐ WNL   ☐ Wet prep:_____

☐ Local tenderness_____   ☐ Vaginal mucosa_____   ☐ Discharge_____

Cultures: ☐ GC   ☐ Chlamydia   ☐ Fungal   ☐ Herpes

☐Vaginal Apex Tenderness (post hysterectomy – show on diagram)

Right   Left

Transverse apex closure   **Vertical apex closure**

Unimanual Exam
- ☐ WNL
- ☐ Introitus
- ☐ Uterine-cervical unction
- ☐ Urethra
- ☐ Bladder
- ☐ R ureter
- ☐ R inguinal
- ☐ Muscle awareness

- ☐ Cervix
- ☐ Cervical motion
- ☐ Parametrium
- ☐ Vaginal cuff
- ☐ Cul-de-sac
- ☐ L ureter
- ☐ L inguinal
- ☐ Clitoral tenderness

Rank muscle tenderness on 0-4 scale
- ☐ R obturator_____
- ☐ R piriformis_____
- ☐ R pubococcygeus_____
- ☐Total pelvic floor score_____

- ☐ L obturator_____
- ☐ L piriformis_____
- ☐ L pubococcygeus_____
- ☐ Anal Sphincter _____

Bimanual Exam

Uterus:			
	☐ Tender	☐ Non-tender	☐ Absent
Position:	☐ Anterior	☐ Posterior	☐ Midplane
Size:	☐ Normal	☐ Other_____	
Contour:	☐ Regular	☐ Irregular	☐ Other
Consistency:	☐ Firm	☐ Soft	☐ Hard
Mobility:	☐ Mobile	☐ Hypermobile	☐ Fixed
Support:	☐ Well supported	☐ Prolapse	

Adnexal Exam

Right:

- ☐ Absent
- ☐ WNL
- ☐ Tender
- ☐ Fixed
- ☐ Enlarged _____ cm

Left:

- ☐ Absent
- ☐ WNL
- ☐ Tender
- ☐ Fixed
- ☐ Enlarged _____ cm

Rectovaginal Exam
- ☐ WNL
- ☐ Tenderness
- ☐ Nodules
- ☐ Mucosal pathology
- ☐ Guaiac positive
- ☐ Not examined

Assessment:_____

_____

_____

_____

_____

_____

Diagnostic Plan:_____

_____

_____

Therapeutic Plan:_____

_____

_____

Index

Figures and tables are indicated with f and t following the page numbers.

About the Editors

Kerri Durnell Schuiling, PhD, NP-BC, CNM, FACNM, FAAN earned her master's degree in advanced maternity nursing from Wayne State University and a PhD in nursing and graduate certificate in women's studies from the University of Michigan. She received her nurse practitioner education from Planned Parenthood Association of Milwaukee, Wisconsin, and her nurse–midwifery education from Frontier Nursing University. She is dually certified as a women's health care nurse practitioner and nurse–midwife, and has been an advanced practice nurse and educator for more than 30 years. She has presented numerous times to national and international audiences on topics that focus on women's health, and twice was invited to provide formal presentations to maternal–child health committees of the Institute of Medicine. As a member of the American College of Nurse-Midwives (ACNM) Clinical Practice Committee, Kerri assisted in the development of clinical bulletins related to abnormal uterine bleeding. She has been an item writer for the national certification examination for women's health care nurse practitioners and currently is the Co-Editor-in-Chief of the *International Journal of Childbirth*, the official journal of the International Confederation of Midwives. Kerri has authored several articles and book chapters that focus on women's health. She has received numerous awards for her work including a Clinical Merit Award from the University of Michigan for outstanding clinical practice, and the Kitty Ernst award from the ACNM in recognition of innovative, creative endeavors in midwifery and women's health care. She is a Fellow of the ACNM and the American Academy of Nursing. Currently she is Professor and Dean of the School of Nursing at Oakland University and works with the ACNM as a senior researcher.

Frances E. Likis, DrPH, NP-BC, CNM, FACNM earned her bachelor's and master's degrees from Vanderbilt University and her doctorate in public health from the University of North Carolina at Chapel Hill. She received her nurse–midwifery and women's health care nurse practitioner education from Frontier Nursing University, and she earned a certificate in medical writing and editing from the University of Chicago. Francie is a women's health care nurse practitioner, family nurse practitioner, and certified nurse–midwife. Her clinical experience includes family practice in community health and urgent care centers, performing sexual assault examinations, and midwifery practice in a freestanding birth center and a large obstetrics and gynecology group practice. Francie has authored several journal articles, systematic reviews, and book chapters related to women's health, and she has given numerous presentations at national meetings and invited lectures. Her awards and honors include the Student Choice Award for Teaching Excellence at Frontier Nursing University; selection as a Vanderbilt University School of Nursing Top 100 Leader, one of 100 distinguished alumni and faculty honored in commemoration of the School's Centennial; the Kitty Ernst Award from the American College of Nurse-Midwives (ACNM); and induction as a Fellow of the ACNM. Currently she is an Investigator for the Vanderbilt Evidence-Based Practice Center at Vanderbilt University Medical Center, and the Editor-in-Chief of the *Journal of Midwifery & Women's Health*, the official journal of the ACNM.